# Against the Spirit of System

# Against the Spirit
of System

## THE FRENCH IMPULSE

## IN NINETEENTH-CENTURY

## AMERICAN MEDICINE

• *JOHN HARLEY WARNER* •

PRINCETON UNIVERSITY PRESS

PRINCETON, NEW JERSEY

Library of Congress Cataloging-in-Publication Data

Warner, John Harley, 1953–
Against the spirit of system : the French impulse in nineteenth-century
American medicine / John Harley Warner
p.   cm.
Includes bibliographical references and index.
ISBN 0-691-01203-2 (cl : alk. paper)
1. Medicine—United States—French influences.
2. Medicine—United States—History—19th century.
3. Medical education—France—Paris—History—19th century.
I. Title.
R152.W37   1998
610'.973'09034—dc21      97-15996

This book has been composed in Berkeley Medium

Princeton University Press books are printed on acid-free paper, and meet the guidelines
for permanence and durability of the Committee on Production Guidelines for Book
Longevity of the Council on Library Resources

http://pup.princeton.edu

Printed in the United States of America

1   3   5   7   9   10   8   6   4   2

FOR NAOMI
AND
FOR OUR *LIKHTIKN* NATHANIEL

# · C O N T E N T S ·

THIS PROJECT had its inception when I was a postdoctoral fellow at the Wellcome Institute for the History of Medicine in London, where I first noticed the difference between English and American depictions of the Paris Clinical School and began to sort out the meanings of that difference. I am grateful for the support I received there between 1984 and 1986 from a NATO Postdoctoral Fellowship in Science from the National Science Foundation and a Research Fellowship from the Wellcome Trust. My research in American archives was supported in 1989–1992 by National Institutes of Health Publication Grant LM 05013 from the National Library of Medicine and by Research Grants in the History of Medicine from Yale University in 1992 and 1994.

Ever since I joined the Program in History of Medicine and Science at Yale in 1986, Larry Holmes has fostered an environment that has encouraged this work while giving me the freedom to pursue other projects. I would have published sooner, and have been less satisfied with the product, without such nurturing of intellectual exploration. My work and my spirits have also benefited immensely from the workaday support of Selda Lippa, Joanne Gorman, and especially Pat Johnson.

I have been extremely fortunate in the groups that have listened to my work in process, raised questions I had not thought to ask, and both challenged and encouraged my interpretations. In addition to lectures and colloquia delivered to historical and medical communities at Yale, I am grateful for the opportunities to present various aspects of this project at other universities—Alabama at Birmingham, Connecticut College, Florida State, Harvard, Indiana, Johns Hopkins, McGill, Manchester, Melbourne, New South Wales, Pennsylvania, Pittsburgh, Sydney, Toronto, UCLA, University College London, and Wisconsin at Madison. Trained principally as an Americanist, I particularly benefited from invitations to contribute to historical conferences on British medicine at the Wellcome Institute and at the Royal Institution Centre for the History of Science and Technology in London, and on French medicine at the Virginia Polytechnic and State University in Blacksburg and at the Wood Institute of the College of Physicians of Philadelphia. I have also presented parts of this work at meetings of the Organization of American Historians, the History of Science Society, the British Society for the History of Science, and the Canadian Society for the History of Medicine. Criticisms and suggestions at these occasions have fundamentally helped shape this book.

In this work I draw on archival materials from nearly a hundred manuscript repositories, and I am greatly indebted for the generous guidance and help I have enjoyed from archivists across the United States and United Kingdom. I am particularly pleased to acknowledge the kind permission John Blackwell granted me to quote from the Blackwell Family Papers at Schlesinger Library. Of the many librarians who have been indispensable to my research, I owe special debts to Richard Wolfe at Harvard and to Ferenc Gyorgyey and Toby Appel at Yale. When I turned to a research assistant in my effort to identify Americans who officially registered for courses at the Faculté de Médecine in Paris, Donna Evleth approached a tedious task at the Archives Nationales with efficiency and humor. For their insight, encouragement, and patience, I am grateful to my editor Emily Wilkinson and to Lauren Lepow and Kevin Downing at Princeton University Press.

Of the community of scholars who have contributed to this project, helpful in diverse ways but at particularly critical junctures have been Gert Brieger, Tom Broman, Bill Bynum, Ann Carmichael, June Factor, Gina Feldberg, Gerry Geison, Faye Getz, Caroline Hannaway, Gwen Kay, Harry Marks, Russ Maulitz, Ron Numbers, Terrie Romano, Carolyn Shapiro, Molly Sutphen, Godelieve van Heteren, George Weisz, and most especially Nancy Tomes. Jackie Duffin, Ann La Berge, Sue Lederer, and Janet Tighe read the entire manuscript, and I am deeply indebted to each of them for making this book better than it would have been without their criticisms, suggestions, and sustaining friendship.

My parents have nurtured me during this project as they have all my life, and have helped me balance the tensions among teaching, writing, and family. My partner, Naomi Rogers, has been my most ruthless and caring critic. I have leaned on her fine historical sensibility, while I lean each day on her light-giving companionship. Our son Nathaniel was born two days after I submitted the first complete draft of my manuscript to the press, bringing a satisfying sense of closure and beginnings.

I HAVE retained the original spelling and grammar in all quotations, even though manuscripts left by nineteenth-century American physicians are often written in unconventional English or very poor French. (Typically, for example, the Parisian dissecting establishment Clamart often appears written phonetically as Clamar or Clamard.) I have used [*sic*] only when omitting it would make a passage confusing to the reader. I have modernized a few terms in my own prose: for example, I use *enfants* rather than the earlier *enfans*, a French spelling convention that changed during the nineteenth century, and Le Havre rather than Havre.

Against the Spirit of System

# Storytelling and Professional Culture:
# American Constructions of the Paris Clinical School

OUT OF the reorganization of medicine in the wake of the French Revolution, the Paris hospitals emerged as the most vibrant center of Western medicine. What has come to be called the Paris Clinical School is broadly identified with a distinctive complex of institutional arrangements, clinical techniques and teaching practices, modes of organizing knowledge, and structures of medical perception that characterized Paris medicine between 1794 and the mid–nineteenth century. After Waterloo and peace, Paris became a Mecca for foreign medical students and practitioners. Between 1815 and the 1850s, some one thousand crossed the Atlantic from the United States to study in the hospitals and dissecting rooms of the French capital, and many times that number made shorter journeys across the Rhine from German states and across the Channel from Britain.

Americans who joined this migration were characteristically enthusiastic about the vigor of medical activity in Paris contrasted with the lethargy of their own country, and reveled in both the spectacle of Parisian life and the exhilarating sense of being at the center of things. An example was the medical student and recent Harvard College graduate Oliver Wendell Holmes: "Merely to have breathed a concentrated scientific atmosphere like that of Paris," he wrote from Paris to his parents in 1833, "must have an effect on anyone who has lived where stupidity is tolerated, where mediocrity is applauded, and where excellence is defied."[1] The knowledge, techniques, and ideals these travelers brought back were leading ingredients in the transformation of American medicine in the decades before the Civil War, so much so that historians have called the antebellum era the "French period" in American medicine.[2]

This episode in the transmission of European culture to America was framed by wider changes in Western medicine that had profound and lasting scientific and human consequences. While the Paris School has come under intensive revisionist scrutiny, historical consensus persists in finding in it the origins of modern scientific medicine. Two divergent and not necessarily incompatible master narratives have governed accounts of Paris medicine, and together they trace how changes forged during this era fundamentally altered both clinical approaches to understanding disease and attitudes toward the human body as an object of scientific knowledge. The first narrative tracks the ways Parisian clinicians created new models of medical science by using the free access they were granted to the bodies of patients and the new tools they developed for investigating disease. The Paris School, this story recounts, boasted such technical and conceptual innovations as the stethoscope and physical examination, tissue pathology, systematic clinical instruction, clinical statistics, and an anatomo-clinical paradigm rooted in systematic correlation of signs and symptoms observed at the bedside with lesions found in the organs at autopsy— contributions of enduring importance that formed much of the foundation for modern clinical practice and investigation. This account, embodied in Erwin H. Ackerknecht's *Medicine at the Paris Hospital, 1794–1848* (1967), which remains the standard treatment of the Paris School, has been told and retold from the nineteenth century through the present, often as a story of progress.[3]

The second narrative tells a darker tale. Although it too locates the creation of modern medicine in the Paris School, it passes a very different judgment on Paris medicine and its legacy. According to this account, it was in the Paris Clinic that the human body was converted into an object of knowledge like any other, setting scientific medicine on a trajectory it continues to follow today. Michel Foucault's *The Birth of the Clinic* (1963), and his identification of the Paris School with an epistemic rift that for the first time made possible "a scientifically structured discourse about an individual," has come to emblemize this perspective.[4] But it is rooted in a larger critique of the dehumanizing tendencies of modern medicine that first grew strident in the 1960s and 1970s. Historians, sociologists, and medical ethicists have widely participated in depicting the Paris School as the decisive moment in the shift of clinical attention from individual sick people as the focus of healing to disease entities as the object of research, instigating what one sociologist has described as "the disappearance of the sick-man from medical cosmology."[5] Both narratives suggest that by tracing the French impulse in the United States, we can discover a formative stage in the emergence of modern American medicine, including enduring sources of both extraordinary clinical power and shortfalls in humane patient care.

What Paris medicine meant in nineteenth-century America, however, cannot be understood merely through the mapping of particular ideas, practices, and attitudes of French provenance onto a history of American science and medicine. It is an overarching argument of this book that the representations of French medicine deployed in the United States were highly selective constructions that made the Paris School stand for a celebration of empiricism and animus against rationalistic systems. Exploring these constructions, I will argue, tells us at least as much about American society and culture as it does about European realities. At the same time, this particular French impulse was intellectually the most powerful source of change in antebellum American medicine, and allegiances to its epistemological ideals persisted as a crucial ingredient in the reshaping of American conceptions of scientific medicine during the final third of the nineteenth century.

The Paris clinician Pierre-Charles-Alexandre Louis, a radical empiricist and enemy of rationalist medical system building who is most often remembered today as father of clinical statistics, wrote in 1840 to his Boston disciple Henry Ingersoll Bowditch, reminding him of the duty they both had embraced to stand stalwart, as Louis put it, at "la Barrière contre l'esprit du système."[6] If there is one dominant and recurrent image in nineteenth-century American representations of the Paris Clinical School, one trope that most fully expresses and embodies the French impulse in American medicine, it is this of a campaign *against the spirit of system*. This campaign was firmly rooted in the French medical tradition of sensual empiricism, yet it took on distinctive resonances in the United States that Louis would not fully have understood and acquired new meaning from the values and needs of American culture. It was under the banner of the empiricist crusade against the spirit of system that the American disciples of the Paris School mounted their program for the intellectual and social transformation of American medicine.

The Parisian medical world was diverse and ever changing: "the picture which offered itself," Ackerknecht noted, "was bound to be a rather chaotic one."[7] Yet the American physicians who described Paris, like other travelers who try to capture the essence of a foreign place, were inclined to impose unity and order upon otherwise bewildering complexity. As selective witnesses and selective reporters, they paid keen attention to some aspects of medical Paris while seeming just barely to notice others. Over time, their depictions increasingly were streamlined—simplified and distilled into symbols that stood for the whole, encompassing both their own experience abroad and the larger lessons of Paris. The texts they produced telling of French medicine (which they virtually equated with the Paris Clinic) were not just vehicles through which it was disseminated but also creative stories, and the ways the authors perceived medical Paris and composed their narratives are as revealing as the descriptions they provided. To a significant extent, the Paris Clinical School was something Americans made up for themselves.

This assertion neither diminishes Parisian intellectual, social, and institutional realities in informing and constraining American accounts nor devalues influence as an indispensable category of historical analysis. But even if essential resources for American representations of French medicine came from Paris, equally important resources came from American culture. The migration of American doctors to Paris for study, their transportation of French medical ways back to the United States, and their contested efforts to use French models to reform medicine in their own country: all these were *American* cultural practices. And while understanding these practices tells us much about the cardinal role French medicine played in changing American medicine, it reveals at least as much about the values, assumptions, expectations, and apprehensions of American culture itself.[8]

In medicine and science, as in other realms of culture, transmission is an active and selective process, not one of passive diffusion—irrespective of whether knowledge, techniques, and ideals are being transmitted across national boundaries, between disciplines, or among social classes. Sound knowledge does not simply travel to where it is in short supply: its dissemination or stasis depends upon cultural appraisals made by its potential couriers, whose agency is critical. The transferral of Parisian medicine to America was not an inevitable consequence of American physicians' studies in Paris, but rather the expression of choices and purposeful actions that must be accounted for. The truth value and utility of French knowledge and technique in such fields as pathological anatomy, clinical diagnosis, and surgery offer important but insufficient explanations for central issues: why Americans were attracted to Paris in the first place, why knowledge in these areas did or did not make the westward passage across the Atlantic, and how elements of French medicine were interpreted and assigned meaning in America. Studying the relationship between American physicians and French medicine therefore provides a platform for exploring the processes by which one realm of European culture was selectively transmitted to the New World, and for observing the machinery of nineteenth-century American culture at work in shaping professional knowledge, behavior, identities, and ideals.

This book is not a full study of the influence of the Paris School on nineteenth-century American medicine. The French impulse was a crucial ingredient in transforming American ideas about disease, the organization and function of hospitals, the education of physicians, the production of new medical knowledge, perceptions of the patient as an object of research, and the practices of diagnosis, surgery, and medical therapeutics. Yet in each of these instances, much of the complex nature of influence would best be revealed by more focused and intensive studies that explore French medicine as only one among myriad other factors in promoting change. Further—and partly because it has not been my aim to produce an exhaustive influence study—I have focused chiefly on internal medicine and surgery and have given little attention to certain other important medical fields, such as psychiatry, forensic medicine, pediatrics, or public health.

At the same time, this book is a good deal more than a study of influence. It uses the French impulse as a wedge to broaden understanding of how the social realities and cultural needs of the young United States shaped the ways that European cultural possibilities were perceived, reconstructed, and enlisted by one group of American professionals. American representations of Paris medicine, to be understood, must be rooted, on the one hand, in the intellectual, institutional, and marketplace realities of the American medical profession, and, on the other, in the lives of the individual physicians who deployed these images as part of their intertwined endeavors to build lucrative careers and to create satisfying identities. This, then, is a study of the relationships between Old World and New and of the cross-cultural transmission of science and medicine. But it is above all a study of American culture and the culture of American medicine.

Chronologically, my study begins with the small number of American physicians who crossed wartime borders to reach Napoleonic Paris during the first two decades of the nineteenth century, then moves through the influx after the close of hostilities to the height of American engagement with French medicine between Waterloo and the 1850s. But while the "French period" in American medicine that historians have conventionally identified with the 1820s through the 1850s is my central focus, I go on to pursue the French impulse through the late nineteenth century. I follow the migration of American medical men and women that persisted through the 1860s, and trace into the 1870s and 1880s both the perceived disintegration of the Franco-American medical relationship and the role that enduring commitments to French ideals played in shaping the American reception of German medicine and its hallmarks, experimental laboratory science and clinical specialism. By 1897, when William Osler wrote his well-known essay, "The Influence of Louis on American Medicine," he was partly paying historical homage to his teachers—and his teachers' teachers—and partly affirming a tradition of clinical science imparted by the Paris School that he believed had ongoing significance.[9]

The role of individual and collective memory is one theme that an expansive time frame encourages. Being in Paris could make a powerful and lasting impression, and many American physicians believed that study there conferred a duty to remember and to tell about what they had witnessed. Selective perceptions in France—recorded on the spot in diaries and letters—were one basis for selective memory. After their return, the American migrants tailored recollections of Paris to the needs and possibilities of their own country. What they publicly remembered and recounted changed in the shifting social, intellectual, and professional climate of the United States, where certain memories acquired special meaning. At the same time, memories of Paris became tools in professional reform and emblems of individual and collective identity. Over the ensuing decades, while some images of medical Paris were remarkably durable, other memories, and especially the meanings attached to them, were further transformed. With the decline of the Paris School and ascendancy of German medicine, remembering Paris yet again took on a different complexion. The meanings attached to private and public memories changed as older, French-experienced American physicians nearing the end of their lives recalled the medical Paris of their youth and reaffirmed their allegiance to what they saw as its enduring legacy.

An expansive time frame also makes it possible to explore and reassess large-scale shifts in American medical travel abroad. Historians have long treated it as self-evident that the migration to Paris should be attributed to that city's scientific supremacy, just as they have tended to assume more generally that the movement of foreign students to a scientific or medical center affirms its intellectual vibrancy. But if we look closely at the appraisals of Edinburgh, London, Paris, Vienna, and Berlin that Americans made during their sojourns abroad rather than at how they later remembered and reconstructed the story of their European experiences, we find little indication that putative superiority in medical science was the key factor in their decision making. Between the 1810s and 1850s, what led Americans to chose Paris over, say, London was unparalleled access to practical experience at the bedside and dissecting table, especially in small paid private courses, not so much instruction by the great professors or medical science at its cutting edge. So too while the shift begun in the late 1850s from Paris to German centers has been taken as evidence of the intellectual stagnancy of the Paris School—its "dead end," as Ackerknecht put it[10]—what most Americans chiefly sought in German-speaking lands was the same kind of ready access to experiential knowledge that for so long had drawn them to the Paris hospitals. The ascendancy of laboratory medicine in Germany was not what first turned the tide, which had more to do with shifting patterns of clinical access on both sides of the Rhine. The reasons Americans journeyed to Paris cannot be equated with the stories they later told about its significance or with the meanings they later came to attach to their experience. This warrants some rethinking of the historical meaning of cultural migration, for the influx of foreign students to a particular center is a highly problematic index of its intellectual vitality.

My analysis also leans heavily on comparison of the relationship between American doctors and French medicine with the relationship between English medical practitioners and French medicine.[11] I follow here the lead Marc Bloch suggested long ago, namely, that a comparative method can help the historian identify what it is that needs to be explained.[12] While I sketch the English case only lightly in this book, I have drawn on it heavily as a heuristic device.

When one looks comparatively at reports on the Paris School that the English and the Americans produced, it becomes apparent that they told rather different stories about French medicine—represented different images of what medical Paris was like and what it meant. The elements that went into their narratives were substantially the same, but the differences in selection and emphasis were pervasive, unmistakable, and remarkably durable. The Americans and the English constructed two nationally distinct models of the Paris Clinical School and of its significance.

In American portraits, the Paris School was made to stand above all else for *empiricism*—a strident, skeptical empiricism explicitly set against what was depicted as the legacies of Enlightenment rationalism. To Americans in Paris, what was most notable about French medicine was an attitude toward gaining and assessing medical knowledge that transcended the institutions of the Paris School and the experiences they afforded. After their return, they fixed upon empiricism with redoubled ardor. The most significant feature of Parisian medicine, according to their portrayal of it, was its allegiance to empirical fact, to knowledge gained and verified by direct observation and analysis of nature, coupled with opposition to rationalism, hypothesis, and speculative systems of pathology and therapeutics. In particular, Americans pointed to the sensual empiricism of the French medical idéologues—the tradition of Étienne Bonnot de Condillac and Pierre-J.-G. Cabanis—a radical reaction against the rationalism of the old medical regime. Yet in depicting the Paris School, they conferred upon empiricism a unifying power out of scale with the significance most French observers would have accorded it.

There was nothing inevitable about the American preoccupation with empiricism, and this fact is clearly displayed by the comparison between American and English accounts of Paris medicine. Whereas the Americans tended to stress French *epistemology*—its empiricism and antirationalism—the English instead tended to stress French medical *polity*, that is, the social and legal organization of the Paris School, its institutional arrangements and relationship with the state, and the value system that underpinned its mode of managing professional affairs. The English noted French empiricism but did not dwell on it; conversely, the Americans included elements of French polity in their reports on Paris but did not give them pride of place. A comparative perspective thus begins to disclose patterns that a focus on the American context alone would leave undetected.

Why did the English and the Americans construct different versions of the French medical model? Or, more precisely, why did they build and celebrate the particular model each of them did construct, rather than some other model? In both countries it was as a vehicle for urging professional change that the French model was most vigorously deployed. Those returning travelers who most stridently drew attention to French medicine were by and large the regular physicians—that is, practitioners who identified with an orthodox rather than irregular tradition—who were among the most eager of their cohort to promote professional reform. Together with reform-minded compatriots who had not made the journey in person but seized upon the reports of those who had, they boldly depicted the French model in the literature of their native lands and forced it into the consciousness of the wider medical profession. Representations of Paris medicine often were blueprints for reforming the profession and its place in society.

Between the 1810s and the 1850s, reformers in both countries were preoccupied with the degradation of the medical profession and saw in the French example a professional leaven. But they looked to different aspects of French medicine to effect professional uplift, and these were the aspects they made prominent in their depictions of it. The models they constructed therefore offer sensitive gauges both of the professional meanings assigned to Paris medicine and of the profession's perceived needs and problems in each country. A comparative perspective reveals what in some ways were singularly American approaches to professional reform and understandings of professional identity.

Comparison simultaneously presses us to explore and explain the special power an ideal of empirical truth commanded in antebellum America, and the expectations American doctors held about the social functions of epistemological change. The empiricist crusade was launched principally in the name of the Paris School, but its force must be sought in American culture. A proclaimed allegiance to empiricism—direct observation of fact open for all to see, an egalitarian foundation for knowledge not shrouded as a professional mystery—was singularly well-suited to the political tenor of antebellum American society. It gave regular physicians a defense against radical democratic assaults on the orthodox profession and its putative trickery of the public through the mystification of medical knowledge. It also promised to expose the falsehood of rationalistic medical systems, orthodox and antiorthodox alike. And in a society preoccupied with calculated deception and its social consequences, an ideal of empirical truth represented a touchstone of authenticity, something simple, honest, and certain in a world beset by imposture, artificial embellishment, and humbug. The program for empiricism and against rationalism thus provided a vehicle for expressing, comprehending, and beginning to address anxieties central both to the culture of medicine and to the broader culture of antebellum America.

Recognizing how stories about the Paris Clinical School were fitted to the audiences they were intended to reach and the purposes they were intended to serve offers yet another guide to discovering the contingency of their construction. Depictions of medical Paris varied according to the context in which they were cast: in diaries kept in Paris; in private letters sent home to family members or public reports sent back to a medical journal; in lectures to students at American medical schools recounting the advantages and dangers of Parisian experience; and in orations at ritual occasions, such as a medical school commencement, which often were civic events. Underscoring the malleability of American representations of French medicine in no sense trivializes them but rather invites the historian to take storytelling seriously as a medical practice that has important cognitive and social consequences.[13]

These were not *merely* stories, in the colloquial and dismissive sense of fabricated falsehoods. The stories Americans themselves told were the principal medium for infusing French ways into the fabric of American medicine. The writings of French physicians and surgeons—or, more often, translations and abstracts of them published in America—were another important conduit for transmission, as was the medical behavior of Paris-returned Americans. But even physical artifacts transported home from France—stethoscopes, pathological specimens, obstetric speculums, surgical instruments—acquired much of their meaning from the stories that accompanied them: a French-made stethoscope was just a wooden tube but became immeasurably more in the context of stories that explained its use and where it fit within a broader program for anatomizing the living body, advancing knowledge about disease, and defining a new tradition.

I have also paid attention to those elements of the Paris School that Americans glossed over or actively eschewed. This means listening for the silences in their stories, as well as attending to those aspects of Paris medicine they dismissed as irrelevant to American society and others they decried as dangerous, doubtfully moral, and potentially corrupting. Most American physicians were scornful of the patient care they witnessed in the Paris hospitals, which embodied what they interpreted as a perverse French valuation of knowledge above healing. Americans admired the French clinicians as the best medical scientists in the world but deplored them as healers—a paradox that raised disturbing questions about the relationship between science and healing. Even the most devout American disciples of the Paris School denounced the French clinicians' brutality, lack of interest in actively curing disease, objectification of the sick, and tendency to convert medical and surgical encounters into theatrical displays governed more by a passion for spectacle than by the aim of healing the sick. This was a French model not to emulate but to shun.

While they remained in France, American physicians tended to reassure themselves that American values—including practicality and sturdy morality—would shield them from taint: they would not succumb to the darker seductions of French science and French values precisely because they were Americans. To this extent, their demonization of French patient care was part of a larger process through which Americans abroad clarified their own culture and its virtues by contrasting themselves with Europeans. Once they returned home, however, and sought to define the place of science in American professional culture, matters became more difficult. This was especially the case for those eager to pursue practice and investigation along French lines at the American bedside while preserving untarnished their integrity and reputation as healers. The often uneasy compromises they made to reconcile their ideals as disciples of the Paris School with their obligations as American professionals offer an exceptionally revealing context for exploring the moral order of nineteenth-century American medicine. This was the moment when the tension between the physician's identity as healer and identity as scientist first became an intensely freighted issue in America. As the implications of French medical models were sorted out, the image of the hardened and heartless medical scientist became firmly established in American culture and concerns over transforming patients from subjects of healing into objects of scientific scrutiny emerged as a prominent theme in anxieties over the conduct of the American medical enterprise.

French medicine did not mean the same thing to all American physicians or occupy the same place in their lives and careers. The voices I have listened to include those of American physicians who never left their native shores as well as others who journeyed to France; those who assailed the Paris School and others who prided themselves as its disciples; and antiorthodox physicians intent on subverting established medicine as well as orthodox practitioners who saw French medicine as a tool for combating unorthodox competitors and reforming orthodoxy from within. Some American physicians who did not study in France, including some who longed to make the journey but never did, embraced French ideas and practices, eager to make them part of American medicine. Others were skeptical or openly hostile to French ways, resentful of the foreign pretensions of Paris-returned practitioners and fearful that Frenchification would not uplift but further degrade medical practice and the profession's standing in American society. Such hostility encouraged the disciples of the Paris School to reaffirm their fealty with redoubled fervor and to draw together as a professional network with a shared past and a common mission.

My central focus, however, is on those American men and women who *did* travel to the Paris School for medical study, especially those who came to see themselves as its disciples, and I have placed them and their lives at the heart of this book. They were not merely passive vehicles by which French influence was transported; to a significant extent they created what they purported to convey, deploying a representation of French medicine in America that had special meaning not only to their profession but to their own lives. By getting to know some of them rather well—and by trying to understand the place French medicine occupied within their wider aspirations, passions, apprehensions, disappointments, and identities as professionals and as Americans—I have tried to bring human texture to this study of professional culture and the cross-cultural transmission of science and medicine.

Among those who studied in Paris were many of the best-known figures from more than two generations of American physicians. Indeed, their prominence both in the medical world of their age and in medical historiography is out of all proportion to their numbers. That they could afford the time and expense of traveling to Europe often meant they enjoyed socioeconomic and familial privilege in the first place. On their return, these social advantages, enhanced by the technical and ornamental value of having studied abroad, eased their way into positions of eminence and influence. Collectively, they were the men and women most likely to teach at medical schools, to serve as medical officers at hospitals, to lead medical societies, and to edit and write for medical journals. Such positions, in turn, gave them powerful forums for promulgating the lessons of the Paris School, for applying French ideals to American practice in programs of research and professional reform, and for teaching French ways to the upcoming generation—ultimately the most effective means by which elements of French medicine became American medicine. Paris study correlated well with elite status, just as promoting the intellectual program of French medicine and building a lucrative career were reciprocally reinforcing activities.

Yet looking beyond these great doctors we see remarkable diversity among the Americans who found their way to Paris for medical study. It would be a grave mistake to accept a monolithic portrait of privilege and prominence as a fair depiction of these Americans as a group, for such an image is belied by the sheer variety in their backgrounds, in their motivations for studying in Paris and means of realizing the journey, and in the environments in which they led their lives after returning home. Some enjoyed the assurance of affluent families that expense was nothing when it came to their education, while others managed to reach Paris only after hard years of saving, or working their passage across the Atlantic, or—regarding the trip partly as a calculated investment in the financial future of their family—going into debt. Some were young medical graduates who hoped that time spent in Paris would bring both the experience of a seasoned practitioner and adventure, while others were older, established physicians who yearned for travel as a professionally respectable sabbatical from the unrelenting workaday routine of decades tied down to practice. Some returned from France to spend the remainder of their lives treating fevers, setting fractures, and attending childbirths in rural communities in the South or West, while others returned to Philadelphia, New Orleans, New York, Cincinnati, or Charleston, where they enjoyed control of wards at hospitals that, though dwarfed in scale by those of Paris, were the largest in their nation.

United by their shared experience in the Paris Clinic, the Americans who studied in France were divided by other social, political, and economic forces. Their ranks included both slave owners and ardent abolitionists. They included women who had become physicians out of feminist commitments and men who blocked educational opportunities and professional recognition for women physicians. Nearly all of them were European-American, but a few were African-American; most claimed English as their mother tongue and went for experience, not formal credentials, but some were Francophone Creoles from Louisiana who sought their M.D. degree abroad; and while the majority saw themselves as medically orthodox, some unorthodox practitioners gained Parisian experience as well. Most practiced medicine after their return—making calls by carriage to the houses of Boston Brahmins, or arduous rounds on horseback among the families of rural Kentucky—but some gave up practice to run a plantation, to pursue a career in natural history, or, in the instance of one American doctor who had studied in Paris, to lead a private invasion of Central America and establish a slave-holding republic with himself declared its president. From such individual experiences, and by trying to capture some measure of their diversity, I have constructed a collective portrait of the relationship with French medicine of the doctors who studied abroad, its place in their lives and careers, and the meaning they saw in it for American medicine.

For the diverse group of Americans who counted themselves as disciples of the Paris School, empiricism and antirationalism more than anything else represented the message and significance of the Paris School, and it was under the banner of empirical truth that they launched their crusade for reform. By the end of the antebellum period the campaign had been remarkably successful in transforming American medical ideas, practices, and, above all, epistemology; but the profession's social and economic problems, which many crusaders believed it would also resolve, proved more intractable. Nevertheless, the American disciples of the Paris School succeeded in establishing the crusade against the spirit of system as a central theme in nineteenth-century American medical discourse, shaping fundamentally a formative period in the creation of the modern scientific medicine we live with today.

In his review of Thomas Neville Bonner's 1963 book on the migration of American doctors to German universities between 1870 and 1914, Richard H. Shryock lamented that there was no comparable account of "the still-neglected French period in our medical past (1820–1850)."[14] Although helpful essays have appeared in subsequent decades, particularly several important articles on American doctors and the Paris School by Russell M. Jones published in the early 1970s, over a quarter of a century later there still has been no book-length study of the French impulse in American medicine.[15] Expressions of Parisian influence have been explored, however, as part of works on particular aspects of nineteenth-century American medicine, among them studies by Charles Rosenberg on the hospital, James Mohr on medical jurisprudence, Barbara

Gutmann Rosenkrantz on public health, Dale Smith on clinical education, and James Cassedy on statistics, as well as my own earlier studies on medical therapeutics.[16] Similarly, the relationship of English practitioners to the Paris School has been investigated by Russell Maulitz and Adrian Desmond, among others.[17] I have leaned on these studies and on a rich recent historical literature on Paris medicine.[18]

Published professional rhetoric—in medical journals, books, and prefaces to translations of French works—helped convey the technical content of Paris medicine to American practitioners and provide the historian with knowledge of public pronouncements that were broadly visible and widely circulated. These were also the forums in which accounts of Paris medicine were converted most openly into polemics designed to propel reform. Ceremonial addresses, such as inaugural speeches delivered to students at medical schools and presidential addresses to medical societies, were often published as well, and in them accounts of French medicine were frequently recounted not so much to convert the unenlightened as to reassure and inspire the faithful; to help create a sturdy past for an orthodox medical profession that appeared to be coming apart at the seams; and to display a plan for change that could be pursued with confidence. Other published sources, ranging from reports that physicians abroad sent to hometown newspapers to fictional depictions of medicine in novels and short stories, begin to give further clues to how French medicine and French experience were viewed by the wider society, including prospective patients.

Critical as published sources are, however, I could not have written this book without relying heavily on a remarkable manuscript record that offers accounts of French medicine composed for audiences and purposes sometimes different from those the authors of published sources had in mind, accounts that compel critical rethinking of public depictions. Particularly rich are journals, family letters, and other correspondence in which Americans contemplating a journey to Paris recounted their deliberations; diaries, student notebooks, and letters to relatives, colleagues, and former preceptors that Americans wrote while in France; and correspondence among these medical migrants after they returned home, as well as clinical casebooks, correspondence relating the travails of building a practice, and letters applying for hospital and teaching posts that reflect how they cast the meaning of Paris experience in their lives. Equally important are lecture notebooks, journals, M.D. theses, and letters home written by students at American medical schools, indicating some of the ways they perceived French medicine. Essential ingredients as well are the protean and often conflicting appraisals of Paris medicine made by other American physicians in, for example, editorial correspondence soliciting or evaluating articles and book reviews, letters of recommendation for professional posts, and medical school faculty minutes.

These unpublished sources do not offer somehow privileged access to *real* beliefs, a truer gauge of American perceptions. The letters an American physician in France wrote home to his wife or preceptor were sometimes no less polemical than addresses delivered before medical societies. And although some Americans kept diaries in Paris so intimate in recording their private lives and loves that clearly they were not intended for wider viewing—even (or especially) by other family members—nineteenth-century travel diaries were commonly written with the expectation that they would be passed around among friends and colleagues. Every text is written for an audience—even the most intimate of journals inscribed as part of the private construction of self. Rather, such sources offer us somewhat different access to how Americans perceived Paris medicine and why they represented it as they did. Private diaries and letters cannot be taken at face value, but reading them critically ensures that we cannot take other more public depictions of the French impulse at face value either, while it enriches our understanding of how Paris medicine took on meaning in the public careers and private lives of American medical men and women.

The first section of this study explores the reasons some American physicians and medical students elected to travel to Paris, their experiences abroad, and the ways they transmitted French medicine to the United States. Chapter 1 sketches the opportunities and rewards in antebellum America for acquiring advanced medical knowledge and experience, setting the stage for an understanding of why any American physician would undertake a program of professional improvement at home or abroad. Chapter 2 investigates the diverse motivations that led some American medical men and women to embark for Europe, rooting their deliberations and decisions in the realities of practice and career making in the United States, and clarifies the special attraction of Paris by showing why Americans so persistently chose it over London. Chapter 3 reconstructs the experience of a medical voyage to Paris—how newly arrived Americans spent their time (learning French, for example), how they planned their course of study, the communities they formed, their interactions with the Parisian medical world, their changing perceptions of self—and argues that access to sensual experience of the body, gained especially through paid private courses at the bedside and dissecting table, was what they most valued in their Parisian studies. Chapter 4 analyzes the vehicles Americans abroad employed in transmitting French ideas, ideals, and artifacts across the Atlantic, the platforms from which they proselytized for French medical ways after homecoming, and the personal and professional meaning of these endeavors. Chapter 5 examines the account of medical history that American disciples of French medicine told—both to promote the campaign against the spirit of system and to situate the Paris School, themselves, and the future they envisaged for their profession—and considers the counterhistory promoted by critics who saw the growing French impulse as corrupting.

   The middle section, the analytical core of the book, investigates how American physicians appraised Paris medicine, how this evaluation was shaped by the values and needs of their own culture, and how they selectively used French models in reforming medical knowledge, practice, institutions, and the place of the profession in American society. Chapter 6 shows that Americans found much to admire in French medical polity and patterned important institutional changes after this French model; yet because of their appreciation of American social, political, and cultural values they failed to see much promise in it for thoroughgoing professional changes that would be viable or desirable in the American context, and therefore did not make it central to programs for professional reform, as their English counterparts did. Chapter 7 establishes and explains the extraordinary American celebration of French medical epistemology (that is, radical empiricism and antirationalism), investigates the special social and cultural meaning this epistemological stance acquired in antebellum America, and shows how and why the Americans who looked to French medicine for models of professional reform—unlike the English—made it the central core of their program for professional salvation. Chapter 8 turns to an aspect of the Paris School that American and English observers alike openly deplored, the performance of the French clinicians as healers, appraising how this menaced the American physicians who sought to emulate them as scientists and exploring the searching self-reflection this promoted about relationships between science and healing and the wider moral order of American medicine.

The final section pursues the relationship between American physicians and French medicine through the decades after the Civil War, an age of German ascendancy in science and medicine. Chapter 9 scrutinizes both those postbellum Americans who traveled to Paris for medical study and the changing character of their experience there, and traces and reinterprets the animus and meaning of the growing shift in American medical migration from France to German centers. Chapter 10 concludes by tracking the deprecation of the French medical impulse in America expressed by physicians consecrated to new ideals of German medicine, especially experimental laboratory science, and assesses how, during the final decades of the nineteenth century, older physicians still firm in their allegiance to the Paris School tried to keep alive and convey to their descendants both the memory of the Paris of their youth and its enduring lessons for America.

# Professional Improvement and the Antebellum Medical Marketplace

WHY would an American physician go to Paris? If the rich resources and intellectual vitality of the Paris Clinical School seem to offer an obvious answer, in fact it is not self-evident why an antebellum American physician would invest time and money in what was termed "professional improvement" either at home or abroad. Antebellum society required little formal training of those recognized as professional physicians, and during the decades when the numbers of Americans traveling to Paris for medical study grew, the revocation of already minimal medical-licensing laws meant that all those who wished could call themselves physicians regardless of their training or lack of it. To frame the migration to Paris as postgraduate medical education, as some historians have done, not only glosses over the diversity in the backgrounds and experiences of those who went, but also anachronistically implies a system of formal structures for recognizing and certifying educational programs quite absent in antebellum America.

To understand why so many Americans made the journey to Paris, then, we must first explore briefly why *any* American physician would voluntarily labor for advanced education in a society notorious for neither recognizing nor rewarding superior professional knowledge. The decision to travel to France was fundamentally rooted in the peculiar limitations and possibilities of American culture, and was governed by broader American assumptions about how a professional career should be made and advanced. Accordingly, instead of isolating a journey to Paris from the other choices Americans made in piecing together a medical education, we should see it as only one part of a complex and largely voluntary system of medical education.

By and large, antebellum American physicians took their medical education far more seriously than later historians have done. While late-nineteenth- and early-twentieth-century medical education has recently received sophisticated historical scrutiny, the nature of antebellum education remains strongly shaped by a Flexnerian caricature of the past. To become a regular physician required very little, but the education that American physicians actually undertook varied enormously. At worst, even minimal formal requirements were circumvented. But at best, American doctors received rigorous albeit eclectic preparations for their profession that gave them a merited rank among the leading people of learning in their society. The plan of medical education that prevailed was remarkably flexible and largely voluntary, a system in which a whole host of options for professional improvement—among them, study abroad—were selectively pursued by physicians in accordance with their own ambitions, talents, and means.

There was, to be sure, a core program that most Americans aspiring to a regular medical practice more or less followed. Throughout this period the foundation of a typical medical training was apprenticeship for three years to an established practitioner, an experience that varied according to the knowledge and conscientiousness of the preceptor. Such training was sufficient to win acceptance (for men, at least) into the regular professional brotherhood, formally expressed early in the century by a license granted by a medical society. Some practitioners also elected to supplement their apprenticeship with didactic training in a medical school, a choice that by the second quarter of the century shifted from exception to norm. The M.D. degree was granted in return for the aspirant's attending a three- to four-month course of didactic lectures (usually taken twice), submitting a thesis (ordinarily twenty to thirty handwritten pages), undergoing a brief oral examination, and paying required fees. Sometimes anatomical dissection or clinical lessons were part of the curriculum, but with or without such experience the holder of an M.D. degree usually had automatic entitlement to a license, bypassing the requirement of approval by medical society members.[1]

By the 1830s and 1840s, the rapid proliferation of for-profit medical schools, often small operations with low standards, had led to vigorous competition for paying students. Existing schools began to trim their requirements to the demands of the market. As competition encouraged schools to keep standards low, and as training in schools came to supplant functions once assumed to be the responsibility of preceptors, the production of poorly trained medical practitioners increased. The revocation of virtually all medical-licensing laws by state legislatures between the 1830s and midcentury made even this training inessential to the aspiring medical practitioner, for any American who wished could set up practice as a physician. The growing number and popular appeal of irregular physicians—especially adherents of antiorthodox medical movements that possessed a formal structure and shared creed, often called *sects* by contemporary critics and later historians—redoubled competition for regular practitioners. During the 1820s and 1830s the number of professional Thomsonian practitioners grew markedly, and during the 1840s and 1850s Eclecticism began to flourish, as did hydropathy. At the same time homeopathy, first introduced into the United States in the mid-1820s, grew to become the country's most prominent nonorthodox medical system.[2]

Possession of a regular medical education nonetheless remained one mark of an orthodox physician, and throughout the antebellum period the majority of Americans who hoped to earn their living by practicing medicine continued to chose a program of apprenticeship and lectures that led to a regular M.D. degree. Even they, however, often circumvented the already minimal requirements of the system. As students sought M.D. degrees in schools located far from the communities where they and their backgrounds were known, it became easy to claim an apprenticeship without having served it in full or at all.

"Ma, you must tell Cousin Roth, that I took the liberty of claiming him as my *preceptor*, as I must need claim one," one young man of doubtful experience wrote home to Alabama from his school in New Orleans.[3] Equally, it was not in the financial interests of proprietary schools to be rigorous about requiring attendance. Sometimes, moreover, an M.D. was granted to a practitioner who had never set foot in the school. In 1859, the Board of Trustees of the Cincinnati College of Medicine approved the motion from the faculty "that the regular degree of Doctor of Medicine be conferred on Alexander Mc'Pheters upon a full compliance of the school as to fees, the faculty waving attendance upon Lectures in consideration of his having been in honorable practice for Twenty five years."[4] But similar arrangements were also made for other practitioners who lacked Mc'Pheters's experience. A regular medical education, in other words, was not necessarily a demanding undertaking. Indeed, a father who wrote in 1846 from Gosport, Alabama, informing his son of his decision that the young man should prepare for medical practice, reassured him that "it is an easy profession to acquire" and "it will not prevent you from being a farmer," adding that "you could attend to both."[5]

The ease of becoming a physician drew a growing number of Americans to compete for patients within what became an acutely overcrowded medical marketplace. Although building a practice had never been regarded as easy, through the first two decades of the century regularly educated physicians tended to speak with confidence of their prospects for winning public patronage. But with the growth of proprietary schools, the revocation of licensing laws, and the proliferation of irregular practitioners, many regular graduates found it difficult or impossible to earn a living practicing medicine. At first those educated in eastern schools could migrate to the South or West, but during the second quarter of the century the multiplication of medical schools in those regions led to vigorous and often divisive competition for patients in all parts of the United States. "There are so many physicians so little business & so much competition," a physician trying to build a practice in Utica, New York, complained in 1829.[6] "Should any young medical protegee of yours wish a position wherein to commence his professional labours, you may inform him that at present there is no vacancy"—thus Philadelphia physician George B. Wood, traveling in the lower South, wrote back to the Philadelphia chemist and physician Franklin Bache in 1844. "I have not come across a single spot, which is not full and overflowing with physicians. It is the universal cry. The practitioners ascribe it to the medical schools, which stimulate young men to become candidates for the doctorate, and afford them great facilities for its attainment. They say out here that a year and a half is quite sufficient to make a Doctor."[7]

Such overcrowding compelled physicians to take sometimes extreme measures to win a practice. As revealed by the letters they wrote home to their parents, young physicians searching for a place to settle often chose to live in disease-ridden districts, resigned to risk their own health in the hope that the call for medical services there would be greater. And they explicitly sized up the likely longevity of older physicians already established in the community. "There is not much chance of either of those physicians dying," one physician who considered settling in Williamsport, Maryland, wrote to his brother in 1828 about the entrenched competition. "The practice too is very laborious & some of the Physicians make use of every meaness to obtain practice by undercharging and some times slandering each other, so that the most experienced physicians is never sure of retaining his practice."[8] The depressing surplus of regular physicians, aggravated by the rising power of irregular practitioners, led to a widespread perception that the regular medical profession was degraded. The complaint that the lower ranks of the regular profession were inadequately educated became routine in demands for educational reform, yet their numbers continued to grow and the level of their training worsened. This concern was articulated by Philadelphia physician Alfred Stillé, who had recently returned from study in Paris: "This country is overrun with half educated physicians," he wrote in 1844 to a medical friend in Boston, "and the chance of earning one's meat & drink are just about in proportion to one's disregard of truth, honor, and modesty."[9]

The educational system that produced many poorly trained holders of M.D. degrees, the public complaints of reformers, and the private frustration of physicians established in practice—all would persist past the Civil War. Yet many medical students and physicians aspired to a more thorough education than the prevailing system demanded of them, and pursued what was usually termed *professional improvement* through a variety of channels. Professional improvement referred to the enhancement of knowledge and skills, the improvement of the physician's ability to allay patients' ills. Equally, it referred to the enhancement of the physician's professional standing, chances to win recognition and esteem from other physicians, and prospects for recruiting affluent patients. Antebellum physicians understood the double entendre of the expression but saw no conflict between its multiple meanings: improving one's knowledge and performance at the bedside and improving one's professional standing and income went comfortably hand in hand. The various motivations that would lead some Americans to Paris for professional improvement reflected the limitations of American medical institutions, but they also reflected many of the same incentives and expectations that led other physicians to pursue plans of professional improvement within the United States.

The voluntary system of medical education and its assorted options for professional improvement often baffled Americans trying to shape their own professional lives. For them, as for later historians, it was hard to reconcile formal requirements with informal expectations. Although such frustration was shared by nineteenth-century medical students and practitioners elsewhere, the American experience was in many respects singular. In England, for example, especially during the period between the passage of the Apothecaries Act in 1815 and the Medical Act in 1858, private correspondence between medical students and their preceptors displayed their uncertainties and misunderstandings about what was required to become a qualified medical practitioner. It was particularly difficult for provincial students and preceptors to keep up with the changing regulations of the Apothecaries Hall and Royal College of Surgeons, or to remain abreast of the many reform bills brought before Parliament.[10]

But in England, at least there were clear answers to questions about what kind of education a person needed in order to become medically qualified, even if the answers changed over time. In the United States, however, nowhere were the answers spelled out, making it difficult for aspiring medical practitioners to gauge what was expected of them or what they should reasonably expect of themselves. The *qualified* practitioner was not first of all a person educated, duly examined, and certified by a legally chartered body, as was the case in Britain and all of Europe. In America, physicians instead established themselves as *qualified* in an open market by winning the confidence of patients and fellow physicians in their practice. Thus a North Carolina physician concerned with his son's career wrote in 1819 to David Hosack that "it is my desire to endeavour to qualify him for a City Practitioner," confident that Hosack, a New York medical professor, would have a better grasp than he did of what that process might entail.[11] A young physician trained in Philadelphia wrote back from Mississippi to his former professor, "I do not think of locating myself for some time yet to come. It is probable I [will] spend this summer and next winter in New Orleans for the purpose of better qualifying myself to commence the practice of Medicine."[12] The kinds of education, experience, and credentials appropriate to becoming qualified in a system based not on formal certification so much as on informal claims to confidence depended very much on the professional aspirations of each individual.

In the absence of formal requirements, seeking advice was crucial to putting together a program of study; yet the advice would-be physicians received often compounded the ambiguities of the open educational system. When in 1845 a Mississippi man asked about the best plan for the medical education of his grandson, his friend in New Orleans had to reply, "I have consulted with several of our Physicians and they all give different advice so that I have been left without any thing positive to say."[13] He outlined the opportunities for medical instruction the city afforded, however, and suggested that if the young man would come to New Orleans, he would introduce him to physician-acquaintances who could give further direction. More frustrating still was the situation of a young man who thought he had completed his education and was ready to open an office, only to be persuaded by another physician that his preceptor's advice had been misleading. "Since you left me I have applied myself closely to the studies, that were before me at that time. It was my impression then, from what my preceptor had told me, that at this period I might with propriety began the practice of medicine," the young physician wrote in 1845. "It was natural, you know, for me to believe it—and had it not been through your instrumentality in enabling me to attend a course of lectures, I might have run heedlessly into that about which I know comparatively nothing."[14]

One of the most prominent themes in the advice aspiring physicians received from medical kinsfolk and friends was that they should regard the requirements of the formal system of training merely as the skeleton on which to flesh out a fuller education. "I do not wish to see you a mere *Blue Pill Pedlar*," a medical student attending lectures at Transylvania University in Lexington, Kentucky, wrote to his brother, still in apprenticeship. He sent a list of books for his brother to read, "for be assured that nothing but the knowledge of the great *principles* of medicine can keep the most sagaceous man from doing more harm than good by his prescriptions."[15] Success in the marketplace was cited as often as success at the bedside as the reason for aiming at more than a degree, but some emphasized as well the value of intellectual achievement for sustaining self-esteem in a degraded profession. Josiah Clark Nott, recently returned from study in Paris nearly a decade after receiving his M.D. from the University of Pennsylvania in 1827, replied to a young physician's request for advice about medical study in Philadelphia by noting, "As to professional improvement, there is no doubt you will reap incalculably benefit," and suggested in particular that he attend William Wood Gerhard's clinical course. "Pay particular attention to the diseases of the chest, for you will never enjoy such another opportunity, the advantage of the physical signs must be evident to you & as the science is comparatively, a new one, in the United States, and as yet but little studied by the profession it will be more likely to give an eclat to your practice than any other." Nott cautioned that if the young physician returned to Alabama to practice, "time & money will have been thrown away, if with regard to pecuniary advancement, for here, science and mental cultivation weigh not a feather in the scale of reputation. Nay they even act deleteriously than other wise." Yet, he urged, "on the other hand, there is the inward consolation . . . of feeling yourself superior to the common herd, ignorant pretenders, and unblushing quacks with which you are surrounded. A consolation which no time or circumstance can ever rob you of."[16]

Nott's advice might well be read as noble but irrelevant to the concerns of physicians confronting the harsh, mundane realities of earning a living. "'Tis noble to breathe from time to time the sublime aspiration of arriving at eminence," a Louisville practitioner wrote to a medical friend in 1825, "but, I fear, that to be great is not in the reach of [the] country town physician, who has only the ordinary interest of getting a livelihood actuating his mind."[17] Yet as they weighed the costs of professional improvement against the rewards, many physicians and medical students felt deeply the desire to rise above "the common herd." In 1860, during his second course at the University of Nashville, a medical student confided to his fiancée his growing anxiety at knowing that he was "soon to have the permission to take upon myself the awful responsibility of the care of human lives, which I do not feel that I will be prepared to do, though I make every possible exertion. Every moment that I waste I feel as though I had committed some terrible sin that it was one human life gone."[18] He felt both a heady sense of self-importance and a humbling sense of self-doubt. Distinction in a highly competitive marketplace was one leading incentive for seeking professional improvement, but its meaning for antebellum physicians cannot be reduced to that alone, for reputation, community respect, self-esteem, and above all confidence were not just means of attracting custom but ends to be sought for their intrinsic value in composing a physician's life.

Professional improvement could mean as little as obtaining an M.D. degree. This was a modest enough goal for most students, though for some, like a student at the University of Louisiana Medical Department fearful of his forthcoming examination, it could seem formidable. "All I want is a sheepskin even if I am a sheep in knowledge," he wrote to his father, pledging two months later, "I cannot but feel despondency in view of the approaching examination but whether I *graduate* or *not* I will commence the practice of medicine next April so surely as I like. This I am as determined to do as a man can be. If I fail to graduate I will go to some country locality and practice until I can make money enough to try again. I will graduate if I have to attend lectures for the next fifty years."[19]

Many of the students who filled the classrooms of antebellum medical schools were not fresh from apprenticeship, however, but seasoned practitioners seeking something more than they had received in apprenticeship, years or even decades earlier. The M.D. theses written by those who sought degrees often testify to the professional lives they had led before entering a medical school. In the 1850s, one student presented the faculty of the Medical College of the State of South Carolina with a thesis summarizing his experience treating over four hundred cases of typhoid fever in his practice; another, who had been in practice for eleven years before seeking a degree at the University of Nashville, offered a statistical summary of the diseases afflicting the twenty-four hundred patients he had cared for, including the eighty-three who had died; while yet another student gave his thesis the revealing title "Finale of Twenty Years Study and Practice of Medicine."[20] A student at the University of Pennsylvania reported in his thesis that after studying medicine in Ireland with his physician-father, spending two years under the instruction of a physician in Canada and five more with a preceptor in the United States, and then practicing for eight years on his own, he had concluded that "to graduate in college was not at all necessary for me, as I could get what instructions I required from my books." Yet he went on to flatter his professors by asserting, "In this, I must say, I was entirely mistaken. My conviction is now, that more sound fundamental medical knowledge can be acquired within the walls of that noble institution University of Pennsylvania, in the course of one winter, than would by any other means that may be adopted, in ten." "Being a man of family," he wrote, "it was making extraordinary exertion, for me to attend this winter," but, pointing to what had led him to seek a diploma in the first place, he noted that "I most abominably hated the character of Quack."[21]

However little importance historians have attached to an antebellum M.D. degree, to practitioners such as these the distinction of receiving a diploma and seeing that fact duly reported in the local newspaper clearly mattered. "The possession of a Diploma is no infallible testimony of merit, but . . . we are cast into a society whose good opinion & confidence is principally made up from the exterior of appearance of things," a Philadelphia medical student suggested.[22] With the repeal of licensing and proliferation of medical colleges, even though an M.D. was not required, it became increasingly important as one identifiable source of professional recognition for those practitioners trained by apprenticeship who wanted to be regarded as members of the regular profession.[23]

Many of the students who attended lectures at antebellum medical schools also took quite seriously the task of mastering the material presented to them. At some institutions students were tested throughout the term; the University of Virginia even issued report cards, printed forms that graded students on a "scale of preparation" in such subjects as physiology, medicine, and pathology.[24] And although the final examination for the degree was brief and oral, many students anguished for months over the coming trial of what was usually called the "green room," often forming "quizzing clubs" to strengthen their preparation.[25] Most students passed, in part because the income of the professors depended largely on the graduation fees and a reputation for flunking candidates would soon have driven potential students to competing schools and gentler examiners. Yet as important is the fact revealed by faculty minutes that many antebellum schools did fail some of the students they examined.[26] Despite the caricature of antebellum medical education historians have come to accept, the receipt of an M.D. degree was not the inevitable outcome of making an appearance at lectures and paying fees.

Students attending medical school often aimed at more than an M.D. alone. Some evidence of this can be seen in medical activities they pursued while at school that went beyond the curriculum, such as regularly reading medical journals, observing in hospital wards, and frequenting medical society meetings. But it is best illustrated by the fact that a remarkably large number of antebellum physicians returned to medical school long after they had received their own M.D. degree to listen to another season of lectures. A medical student in Philadelphia noted that a mistreated case he had just observed "shows plainly that unless a Physician reads continually or will occasionally attend a course of Lectures, he will certainly forget the simplest parts of his profession, especially the surgical department."[27] Many attended only for a course rather than for a degree, but multiple M.D. degrees were not uncommon. One Ohio physician who earned his M.D. degree in 1844 from the Cleveland Medical College received a second M.D. from Jefferson in Philadelphia seventeen years later; a Lexington student in 1820 decided at the outset of his studies to attend three rather than the usual two courses of medical lectures.[28] Such patterns were fully in accord with the fundamentally voluntary nature of medical education. Especially in the late antebellum period it grew common for students to attend their first course at a relatively easy school near home, then travel to a more rigorous school such as Pennsylvania to attend a second course and win their M.D. degree. Indeed, Philadelphia functioned as a center within the United States where ambitious medical Americans pursued professional improvement in much the same way that Paris functioned as a center on a larger stage.

More elusive than the didactic lessons was access to practical instruction, especially at the bedside and dissecting table. In principle, the medical student was supposed to learn the practical business of healing in apprenticeship by assisting and observing a preceptor in action. And some apprentices were able to try their hand at anatomical dissection as well. A medical apprentice in Columbia, South Carolina, reported in a letter to his mother in 1854, "I have a large *negroid disecting* which I have been wishing to get for a long-time. I have had him about a week and a-half—and expect to keep him about 2 weeks longer." Two weeks later he was again able to report that "I have been Dissecting all of this week. On last Saturday Night I had an opportunity of getting a Subject, as one of the *Crazy men* of the *Assilum* Dyed. So I have been over a fellow Dissecting Ever since. I like dissecting very much, only here of late, people do-not die fast enough to get many."[29]

For most apprentices and medical schools alike, however, access to an adequate supply of bodies for dissection was a serious problem that persisted throughout the antebellum period, even where provisions made legal access possible.[30] A Boston medical student wrote in 1819 with enthusiasm that a ship long thought lost had finally reached the harbor, and that "the pirates she brought home have received their trial and four of them are to be hanged." With evident anticipation of an unusually rich legal supply of dissection material, he added, "It will be a fine chance for Doctor Warren's lectures which I again attend."[31] Most were compelled to rely on the illegal and sometimes dangerous practice of grave robbing. "We have had a high times here this spring in the line of resurrectionising; which has kept the rabble, & the Police department in a compleat stew," a Rochester student wrote to a friend in 1841. "The subject, was supposed to be an old negro, who died in a fit of intoxication some six miles out of the city. He was buried in the clothing in which he died, & had not a friend on Earth, and probably not in Heaven, or any other place, whose feelings could [be] injured." After the partly dissected body was discovered on the third story of a building on Main Street, "by order of the Police justice, three students were commited to prison for contempt of court; in as much as they refused to answer certain questions, which they feared might criminate themselves." In this case, the letter-writer could go on to note that one of the students was the son of an ex-governor and another the son of a judge, and that "the justice is now under an arrest for false imprisonment." He concluded smugly, "Thus you see, we have water sufficiently hot to wash off the scurf."[32]

Some students relished their clandestine night labor in the graveyard, as an adventure and as a rite of initiation, but others resented the risk imposed upon them. "Shall we expose our lives our property and our reputations for nought?" wrote one student who objected to the "invariable rule" at a Boston school that the students "dig & shovel" to procure the bodies for anatomical lectures.[33] Dissection was a leading point of conflict between medical schools and their communities. "It is expedient to abolish as soon as practicable the present mode of obtaining anatomical subjects through the agency of the students," the faculty of the Medical College of Ohio in Cincinnati resolved in

1828, "& to arrange some mode of obtaining them at some fixed price through the agency of a resurrection man—& that ten dollars per subject be considered not an unreasonable price."[34] But the supply obtained this way remained sparse, and by 1843 the faculty was forced to decree "that any Student who shall be convicted before the Faculty of having, during the Collegiate Session, engaged without knowledge or approbation of the Professor of Anatomy or of Surgery in procuring an Anatomical subject, shall be debarred from all further admission to the Classes of this Institution."[35] Several years later they again insisted, "Pupils shall not divulge the secrets of the dissecting room, on pain of forfeiting their privileges to the same."[36] The problem remained, however, and in the late 1870s the faculty again had to sort out the legal problems that resulted from the discovery of an untoward body in their dissecting room.[37]

Anatomical dissection, if not by the student then at least by a demonstrator, was part of virtually every school's advertised curriculum. But the opportunity to gain extensive experience as part of a regular medical school education was rare. Those few schools that were well supplied with cadavers made a point of drawing attention to the opportunities they offered. The Medical College of Louisiana, for example, asserted (probably justly) in its annual announcement of the 1842–1843 term that "the advantages offered by the city of New Orleans for acquiring a practical knowledge of Medicine and Surgery are not surpassed by those of any other city in the United States," boasting that "subjects for dissection will be provided in any number free of charge."[38] Charleston too could claim "advantages of a peculiar character." As the dean explained in a petition to the state legislature for support, "No place in the United States offers so great opportunities for the acquisition of Anatomical knowledge, subjects being obtained from among the coloured population in sufficient number for every purpose, and proper dissection carried on without offending any individual in the community." He went on to note, "Those impediments which exist elsewhere in so many other places, to the prosecution of this study, are not here thrown in the path of the Student, public feeling being rather favourable than hostile to the advancement of the Science of Anatomy."[39] By defining both "the community" and "public feeling" in ways that referred only to the European-American population of Charleston, while at the same time drawing subjects for dissection exclusively from the African-American population, he neatly circumvented tensions between the school and the "community." Both class and race were key factors in determining susceptibility to dissection, and slaves were particularly vulnerable.[40] While this surely gave southern schools an edge, even in the South the supply of available bodies ordinarily fell far short of what anatomy professors and students would have liked.

The place of clinical education in medical schools was more checkered still, and the perceived inadequacies grew to provoke a leading complaint about American medical education. Early in the century it was assumed that experience at the preceptor's side would give the student all the practical training required, and apprenticeship continued to give many students a good deal of practical experience. "I have had a very good opportunity myself for observing the different stages [of disease], as I saw every one of his patients, and losed a great many hours of sleep on their account," one apprentice wrote in 1855 to his brother. "The Dr has me trotting around Town pritty constantly indeed I have a great deal of the Prescribing to do. I am glad he has had such a run of Pneumonia this spring, as it will be all the better for me. Night before last, I spent the whole night with a case."[41] As study at a medical school became the norm, however, and as the expectations of what apprenticeship would provide were diluted, students increasingly looked to schools for not just didactic but also practical training, often in vain. At the same time, as some Americans returned from Paris to proselytize for the French example of systematic clinical instruction, reformers insisted that clinical education should become an important part of the curriculum at American schools. The reform program (explored in chapter 6) did somewhat increase the practical clinical experience offered in American schools during the antebellum period and even more later in the century.

Clinical access became one of the chief devices that medical schools used in competing with one another for paying pupils, giving city schools a clear advantage. "I asked Dr. Watson if it were not equally well to study in the country, and attend lectures in the city," a young man trying to decide on the best course for learning medicine wrote to his uncle in 1840, having just spoken with a prospective preceptor in New York. "He said in that way I might get a theoretical knowledge from books, but that by studying in the city the practical knowledge obtained from having access to Hospitals was much more beneficial."[42] The faculties of schools located in small towns were routinely defensive, and more so as calls for clinical instruction became louder. Thus in 1825 a medical professor in Lexington refuted the charge that the absence of a hospital made his institution inferior, telling incoming students that the kind of patients who crowded into urban hospitals "are not such as will be met with in practice," and urged that "the insight into practice from living with a skillful practitioner in the country, seeing diseases at the bedside noting all changes, the effects of treatment—hearing the causes & history of the disease is of incomparably more utility to a Student."[43]

Medical schools that could offer access to a hospital, on the other hand, made the most of it. As a Philadelphia medical professor told his students, "For those who study in large towns, abundant clinical opportunities are usually afforded in hospitals, dispensaries, and other public institutions, which a student would be quite unpardonable in wholly neglecting, if he have any view ultimately of taking upon himself the care of the sick."[44] The Medical Department of the University of Louisiana in New Orleans, with access to one of the largest hospitals in the country, could confidently assert in its 1859 catalog that "the Student can visit patients in the Charity Hospital from morning until night, and . . . can question and examine for himself."[45] Yet throughout the antebellum period, institutions such as the New Orleans schools were exceptions, and the clinical education most medical schools offered remained meager.

What emerged was a widely shared understanding that young medical graduates would have to find ways on their own of gaining practical experience
before they could reasonably expect to build a practice of citizens able to pay
for a doctor's services. Professional improvement of this sort was regarded not
as an extravagance, even for physicians bound for country practice, but as a
necessary step to insure competent patient care and public recognition. It was
a truism that the public had little faith in young physicians, and young physicians not only recognized this but understood the reasons why.

Country practitioners tended to learn their art by practicing on the poor
gratis; their city counterparts who held higher professional aspirations did the
same in the wards of urban hospitals. "As to my professional prospects, they
are not very bright: my practice is *very* limited indeed & even to that extent
almost exclusively confined to paupers," a Richmond physician lamented in
1845. "Not one of my relations or *friends* have ever employed me (except our
own immediate family) or given me any encouragement to hope that they ever
would."[46] But more seasoned practitioners counseled that paying patients
would come only with experience. To an equally forlorn young physician in
Augusta, Georgia, his father stressed that "the main advantage of your locality
is that you get practice, *& that* practice gives you experience,"[47] while a friend
similarly told him that "it is always better for a Physician to practice for nothing, than not practice at all. There are many paupers in yr. City. My advice then
w$^d$ be to mingle freely among them & get from that source all the cases you can.
This kind of practice is a sort of rough & tumble business, but will only prepare you the better, for the roughness of a country practice."[48]

The acquisition of experience could be accelerated if, after graduation, the
young physician gained access to a hospital or dispensary. Some did this informally, as in the case of a student completing lectures in Philadelphia who
informed his preceptor in Savannah, "I have paved the way to combine the
speculations of authors with the experience of practitioners, by cultivating an
acquaintance with the officers of the two great medical institutions of this
city—viz—the Hospital and the Alms-House."[49] But in addition to such informal arrangements, private programs emerged explicitly designed to supplement the ordinary course of training in apprenticeship and medical school.
What these "private" or "preparatory" schools stressed was access to practical
experience, that is, anatomical dissection and clinical instruction.

One of the best-known of these schools for professional improvement was
the Tremont Street School in Boston, where the faculty members of Harvard's
medical school offered additional instruction during the summer for additional fees. Its 1830 advertisement in the *Boston Medical and Surgical Journal*
promised that "the pupils are admitted to the practice of the Mass. General
Hospital, and receive Clinical Lectures on the cases from Drs. Jackson, Channing and Ware," and that "Private Instruction will be given in Practical Anatomy, by means of demonstrations and dissections."[50] Similarly, an announcement in the *Charleston Medical Journal and Review* for 1859 noted that the
preparatory school in that city would offer clinical instruction "in the Marine

and Roper Hospitals by lectures, autopsies, etc., and the Professors will endeavor as often as practicable to exhibit obstetrical and surgical cases as well as medical cases to the class."[51] Such schools proliferated, so much so that in 1852, one physician telling another of his plan to found a new one felt constrained to insist that his would be a reputable venture. "We all of us despise any thing like the little, two-penny establishments, with which our country is being filled, and should we engage in a movement of this kind, we should aim to have a respectable board of teachers, and a class of stable-sturdy pupils."[52]

The multiplication of such programs testified to the growing demand for systematic means of gaining practical experience. Even if the experience was voluntary and not recognized by any formal degree, students expected it to be well rewarded. "My friends here seem to think I will do well in a reasonable time," Cornelius G. W. Comegys, a young physician who had just moved to Cincinnati, reported to a friend in 1848. "My long observations in the abundant practice of the Hospitals in Philad[a] as well as my time in the Dispensary there and in private, has given me much familiarity with a great variety of affections & the mode of treating them."[53]

Those who aspired to eminence in the profession might seek more extensive hospital experience than a course of clinical instruction could offer. The hospital remained marginal to the professional lives of most antebellum physicians; yet, as Charles Rosenberg has shown, even during this period it was one important platform on which the elite constructed their careers.[54] Securing a position for a year or more as resident physician to a hospital, or being attached to a dispensary, was recognized as a way for a young physician to both gain experience and draw the notice of those whom he might most welcome as patients. A young physician in Cincinnati sought the aid of his uncle in 1851 to get a post as resident physician to the hospital there, noting that "it is generally thought, that the position in the Hospital for one year, is equivalent to six or eight years practice; that is such as Young Physicians generally have at first."[55] Enterprising physicians sometimes established their own modest clinical institutions as a way of gaining experience and prominence. Nott reported in 1836 that along with another physician, he planned to build a hospital in Mobile, "which will give 1st money and 2[d] reputation."[56] So too a young physician in Baltimore wrote to his father in 1845, describing the dispensary that he and others had just opened. "To many it seems a most strange method of getting practice: constantly spending money to get patients, and receiving nothing from them," he admitted; but "knowing men in the profession, who are our seniors by many years, tell us that the experiment will pay for itself the first year by the good practice [it] will bring us."[57]

Older physicians followed avenues of professional improvement somewhat different from those pursued by young graduates, but by reading a medical journal, participating in a medical society, or returning to a medical school to attend a course of lectures, they too participated in an open-ended, voluntary system in which no clear sign marked the completion of professional education. Even the distinction between student and practitioner often was blurred:

sometimes experienced practitioners shared benches in the classroom with in-experienced apprentices, while medical students tried to attract patients while they were learning medicine. Changing aspirations could also prompt an older physician to search for ways of expanding knowledge and skill. Elisha Bartlett, who had received an M.D. from Brown University in 1826, was already well established in life when he began to be preoccupied with, as he described it to a friend in 1838, "dreams of distinction and aspirations for a broader and higher theatre of professional exertion." He had a highly lucrative medical practice, was mayor of Lowell, Massachusetts, and lectured at various New England medical schools during the winters. But the ambitions that had sent him to Paris to study a dozen years earlier reawakened in his middle age. "I am very far from feeling satisfied and contented with my present position," he confided to the Philadelphia physician Isaac Hays. "I have a practice, to be sure, pleasant and respectable enough, and by many of my brother doctors my situation would be regarded as an enviable and desirable one. But the opportunities here, for the study of medicine, as a great and progressive science, are almost nothing, and I feel, every day, with more and more earnestness, the want of these opportunities, and of kindred and co-operating associates in medical studies." Prompted by these feelings, he explained, "I have been, for some time past, brooding over the subject of a removal to some of our metropolitan cities. I long for the ward of a hospital, to which, in due time, I might attend a class for clinical instruction."[58] Bartlett left Lowell to study fevers in the hospitals of Baltimore, New York, and Philadelphia. In a typical letter from this transition period in his career, he wrote from Philadelphia saying he had made "arrange-ments to attend Dr. Gerhards Clinique the forenoon of three days in the week, & his consultations at the Dispensary on the afternoon of this alternate days:— so that in a professional point of view my time is very profitably disposed of."[59] Bartlett went on to become a prominent professor, medical author, and con-sultant physician.

Through a variety of channels, then, antebellum medical students and phy-sicians, working within the peculiar limitations and possibilities of American society, pieced together educations they believed would prepare them for prac-tice in a highly competitive medical world. Because medical education was largely a voluntary affair, it was up to the aspiring professional to make choices that often were not clear-cut—choices informed by the weighing of aspirations against means, by the institutional realities of American medical culture, and by the expectations of those sought as paying patients. Physicians often de-scribed their efforts at professional improvement as philanthropic acts, as an exercise of duty to patients motivated by the desire to do good; yet at the same time they clearly hoped to do well by doing good. Professional improvement unmistakably served the economic and social interests of career building.

It would be a mistake to reduce the motivations for professional improve-ment to socioeconomic self-interest alone, however, for often they had broader meaning as well in the lives of people whose sense of self-worth could not be disentangled from their sense of duty. Jonathan T. Updegraff decided to spend the final few minutes of 1847 reflecting on his medical practice and wrote his thoughts down in the private daybook he ordinarily used only to record the case histories of his patients. Son of a Quaker minister, trained by apprenticeship in the town where he later would practice, and holder of an M.D. degree from the University of Pennsylvania, Updegraff worked in the small hill town of Mount Pleasant on the eastern border of Ohio, managing the ills of families he had grown up with. "Nearly midnight," he began his entry on New Year's Eve of 1847. "It is now nearly the last moment of this year—I have just finished putting up my accounts—(no great task—) so as to begin the New Year square, if I shall live to enjoy it—I have been practicing here, nearly two years now, & I hope done some little good, & I think not much harm yet—I feel my responsibilities increasing as my practice increases—It is indeed a fearful thing to have the lives of our fellow creatures entrusted to our care—I pray that I may be helped rightly to discharge these high responsibilities—I feel encouraged to hope I may if I use exertion on my part, which I am determined to do."[60] Doing well in the world and doing good for one's fellows were, for Updegraff as for other Quakers, ends that went hand in hand. And within several years, Updegraff, like many other American physicians, would seek to advance both ends simultaneously by embarking on a journey of professional improvement to Paris.

# Why Paris?

BY THE mid-1820s, with the French capital readily accessible, the American of ambition and means who considered the options for professional improvement in medicine more than likely would have included a journey to Paris among them. This was a recent development, however, and had not been the case a decade earlier. The pattern of Americans' traveling to Europe for medical study had old roots, stretching back to those who studied in Leyden in the seventeenth century and the substantial number who visited Edinburgh and London in the eighteenth. Between 1769 and 1819, over 300 Americans attended medical lectures in Edinburgh, and 145 received medical degrees there.[1] Some Americans, including Philadelphia physician John Morgan as early as 1763, made their way to Paris as well, but before the end of the Napoleonic Wars this remained an unusual step.[2] How did it happen that some Americans came to seriously consider a journey to Paris for medical study as the most desirable option available to them?

The technical and cognitive innovations and scientific preeminence of medical Paris suggest a ready answer, but it is an inadequate and in some ways misleading one. What Americans depicted as being most important about the Paris School after their return—a new departure in medical science—was not what drew them across the Atlantic in such large numbers in the first place; and it is important not to equate later recollection and storytelling with earlier motivation and expectation. American physicians were attracted to Paris for a wide variety of reasons, reflecting the diversity of those who made the journey. But overwhelmingly it was experiential knowledge—the promise of gaining practical experience at the bedside and dissecting table—that drew most of them to Paris, not intellectual vigor or the chance to witness the vanguard of medical science. Later, once in Paris, many Americans were recruited to French ideals of medical science, on behalf of which, after their return, they proselytized other physicians as a way of propelling the campaign against the spirit of system—a campaign that they believed would bring an intellectual and social transformation in American medicine. No American was to become a more ardent disciple of French medical science than James Jackson, Jr.; yet shortly after his arrival in Paris in 1831 he could write to his father in Boston, "I have learned very little that is *new*—but it was not for novelty that I crossed the waters to visit foreign hospitals."[3]

Two interrelated processes combined during the first two decades of the nineteenth century to make medical Americans consider the possibility of visiting Paris. The first was a growing awareness of the vigor of Parisian medical activity in the wake of the French Revolution. Thoughtful physicians, like

Americans interested in other realms of natural science, were acquainted with French work in such areas as pathology and chemistry well before many had made the trip to Paris to study these sciences in person. Just as those who cultivated chemistry in the Early Republic knew the work of Antoine-Laurent Lavoisier and the French chemists who came after him, the larger community of physician-intellectuals knew the writings of the pathologist Xavier Bichat and his successors. Yet one could read Bichat without traveling to Paris.

Equally important were reports by those few medical Americans who did find their way to Paris in the years before Waterloo that the French capital offered opportunities vastly exceeding anything available in London or Edinburgh. Before the end of the Napoleonic Wars the number of these travelers remained small, for the political situation rendered travel to Paris difficult and risky. In 1805, Yale's recently appointed young professor of chemistry, Benjamin Silliman, traveled to Europe to learn something of the science he was expected to teach. He divided his time in Edinburgh between lectures in chemistry and in medicine and spent a profitable period in London, but wanted to visit France— to buy books and especially to visit the laboratories of leading French chemists in search of a model for the one he would establish in New Haven. He reached the Continent by sailing to Rotterdam, an illegal crossing during this time of war but one that ships made regularly nonetheless. He was disappointed, however, in being flatly refused entry from Holland into France, which left him no real alternative but to make the illicit passage back to Britain, his letter of introduction to the chemist Antoine-François de Fourcroy unused.[4]

The experiences and perceptions of one American who did make it to Paris to study medicine from 1806 to 1808 exemplify both the circumstances that made this undertaking difficult and the enthusiasm for access to experience in Paris that, broadcast back in America, encouraged a brisk influx of medical Americans once the political situation changed. In August 1805, the young George Watson, who had studied medicine at the University of Pennsylvania with Benjamin Rush but had not yet earned an M.D. degree, sailed from Hampton in his native Virginia for Liverpool. He proceeded directly to Edinburgh, where he found a community of two dozen American medical students and made arrangements to attend lectures. His first impressions of Scottish medicine were not favorable. "From what little conversation which I have heard here on medical subjects I am more and more impressed with the absurdity of young men's leaving a school in their own country to study Medicine in a foreign one," Watson wrote to his brother. He was appalled by the lives that would be sacrificed were American students to apply Scottish ideas about curing fever without bloodletting to the very different diseases of North America. Equally scornful of Scottish views on the nature and treatment of yellow fever, he noted that "here they teach the old and now exploded opinion in the United States, that it is contagious, and that it is a Putrid fever, forbidding the use of the lancet." Such opinions, he insisted, "are to be unlearned by the American students educated at this place."[5] Nevertheless, and despite the nationalist pique he felt at Scottish disparagements of American culture, Watson wrote with satisfaction of the "opportunities of improvement" that Edinburgh afforded, and planned to follow lectures and graduate there the following summer.[6]

Yet after only a few months in Edinburgh, Watson began to speak of his growing desire to study in Paris. He had met an American physician, James Morris, who was about to leave for the French capital in search of medical improvement, and the idea took hold.[7] Watson had planned to spend some time in London but wrote to his father, "It seems the unanimous opinion of every student, who has been at both places, that Paris would be much the best and cheapest place, for the prosecution of the studies I wish to pursue."[8] At first he thought that passage to France would be difficult, but then—encouraged by the knowledge that a Virginian acquaintance from Williamsburg, Charles Carter, had just completed the journey—concluded that "the war will not prevent me from going."[9] As Watson told his father in January 1806, "The late decisive victories of the French Army have nearly made peace on the Continent."[10] Two months later he was making plans to engage a French tutor in Edinburgh.[11]

What Watson hoped most to gain in Paris was extensive practical experience at anatomical dissection, difficult to come by in Edinburgh. He was satisfied with the lectures, especially James Gregory's clinical lectures at the Royal Infirmary. As he described them, "Dr. Gregory has sicks [sic] rooms in the Royal Infirmary, in which he puts all those cases of sick people, which he thinks will be most improving for his students to attend to. Dr Gregory has the treatment of these patients himself: the students see his practice and observe its effects and he gives lectures to them upon these particular cases."[12] The deficiency that remained was "such a minute knowledge of Anatomy, and expertness at dissection, as is only to be acquired, by much practice on the human subject. My opportunities here have been very bad," he explained to his brother. "Subjects are so dear, that a course of lectures, which would require twenty five, or thirty subjects, if they could have been easily obtained, has been delivered with only three. If I get to Paris next winter, I do not despair of making myself an accurate Anatomist, and a good dissector, in twelve months."[13]

Because of the unstable political situation, it was impossible to make firm plans. Watson still hoped to visit Paris, "but considering the turbulent times among the nations on the continent, you will not be surprised, that any views of mine, which are connected with its situation, are soon changed," he told his father in April 1806. "The only passage which has been open, for some time, from this country to France, has been through the dominions of the King of Prussia. He has lately declared war against this country; so that pass is obstructed; and it is thought impossible, that I can be able to get from this to France at all, in the present state of things. This being the case, I must put in practice my old plan, of going to London, if no change takes place."[14]

Watson did go to London, writing that during his month-long stay he had "visited such places and things, as usually attract the attention of strangers," but about a week after composing this letter he and three other Americans were sailing to Holland, headed for France.[15] They reached Rotterdam by mid-October, obtained passports in Antwerp, and hired a private coach to take them to Paris, where they arrived without difficulty toward the end of the month. Though sick for six weeks after his arrival, Watson began to explore what Paris had to offer. In a letter sent home with a returning Virginian, he reported that while the costs of lodging, food, and clothing were high, "those expenses however, which attend the study of Anatomy are next to nothing. For three Guineas a pupil, [has] as many subjects as we want, a fine nice room with every thing pertaining to dissection, and a teacher too, if we want one, are found us." And in contrast to Britain, "every other branch of science may be studied here, without any expense at all. Lectures upon each of them, by the greatest men in the country, are heard by any one who pleases for nothing: Museums, cabinets, picture-galleries, libraries &c are open to every one upon the same terms. These things are supported at the public expense."[16]

His hopes for anatomical experience were more than fulfilled. In April, several months after he started dissecting, he had another chance to send a letter by a Philadelphian returning home and reported that he was engaged in "the study of Anatomy, in the only way in which it can be learned; I mean by dissecting with my own hands." He told his brother with some amazement that "the place where I work is open to every one who choses to come and see, and almost every day we have curious visitants without ceremony. The yard in which the Pavilions stand is often the play place of the neighboring children who see through the doors and windows the business going on without interruption to their mirth." He noted particularly that "men, women, and children here, see each others bodies dissected with at least as little emotion, as you see Davy cut up a beef or a hog. More than once this winter, I have been shocked at seeing women, young, genteel in their appearance, and one very *handsome* standing by a dissecting table, and witnessing with idle curiosity the examine of the human intestines. If this is philosophy, it is such as I do not like." But contrasting this with sensibilities in his own country, Watson noted that "where this is the case superstition is out of the question; the practice is not only licensed but encouraged by the Government; and in such a place as Paris deaths are frequent enough." From anatomical dissection and from "investigating as far as it can be done the causes and seats of disease from opening dead bodies," he concluded that "with respect to my profession I feel myself prepared for what is a much rarer thing than every body knows it to be,—I mean *to learn from experience.*"[17]

Counterbalancing his enthusiasm was a growing sense of isolation. "Much more rigorous measure[s] have just been adopted, than have been hitherto employed, to prevent all communication between this country . . . and Britain," he had reported to his father a month after arriving. "This circumstance, as you may easily conceive, has produced much alarm in all those who expect their supplies of money from England; as it will not be possible for remittances to be made as long as the present state of affairs continues. I beg, therefore, that you will send me, as soon as it possibly can be done, a letter of credit upon some mercantile house in France."[18] Over the ensuing months, without money his debts mounted and his isolation intensified. "What could be more vexatious, than that I should have been here now going on seven months, and never have seen the scratch of a pen from any of my friends?" he told his brother in May 1807. Plaintively he wrote that "by the time I get money, I shall be what might be called *ragged*," adding, "For God's sake, try and get me out of this situation and keep me out in the future."[19]

What made Watson's isolation worse was that he still could not speak French. Ill when he arrived, he had moved into a house with Morris where nearly everyone was a native speaker of English, "so that I had as well be in London or any where else to learn French."[20] By the time he was well again, he was so much in debt to his landlord that he could not move.[21] When letters and money finally reached him, though, his spirits lifted and his resolve to master the language was renewed.

Although his family urged him to come home, at the end of spring Watson told his brother that he had determined to remain for another year. "After having been at all the trouble, and a great part of the expense in getting an opportunity of profit from the immense sources of information which are open here, it would be unpardonable to leave them at this period," he explained. "I shall redouble my diligence & increase my opportunities of learning French," he wrote, outlining the plan he envisioned. "I will attend one of the best Hospitals constantly. When the Lectures in the Medical Schools begin which will be in November, I shall dissect with the preparer for Anatomical lecture at the school of Medicine, who is without doubt I suppose the best in the world." With this grounding, "I shall be well prepared in the Spring and summer, to commence a course of Natural History and comparative Anatomy." Looking forward to the distinction this course of study would give him, he urged that in America, "I expect to proceed in the practice of my profession with a confidence in my opinions and a boldness in doing operations when they are necessary which nothing else would justify."[22]

During the ensuing year in Paris, Watson largely stayed the course he had sketched. He again ran out of money and heard with concern about the embargo of America; but he wrote that "I comfort myself with the reflection that I could not be in a better place without money than in Paris. Schools of every kind are open for nothing so that one is not obliged to be idle."[23] By April 1808, having resumed his natural history study at the Jardin des Plantes after the close of the winter lectures at the École de Médecine, he wrote that "in my own opinion I am spending my time to greater advantage than I ever was in my life."[24]

When Watson left Edinburgh, he had planned to return there to obtain its M.D. degree after visiting Paris, but instead he sailed directly for the United States and, early in 1809, received his degree from the University of Pennsylvania.[25] When his family opposed his plan of settling in Philadelphia, Watson pressed them to defend their choice of Richmond: "Is it a place which you think might be made to afford the means of becoming eminent, by a person who possessed the ambition and the abilities to become so?" he asked his brother. "Is there any science there?"[26] His education in Paris had given Watson the confidence to aspire to something higher than a lucrative practice alone. He would go on to serve as a surgeon in the War of 1812, as a founding member of the Medical Society of Virginia early in the 1820s, and as a member of the Richmond Board of Health during the 1832 cholera epidemic.[27] Yet even though Watson's reports on Parisian opportunities might have whetted the appetite of other Americans, while the political situation remained so uncertain, his difficult journey hardly served as an appealing exemplar for others to emulate.

The end of hostilities after Waterloo, however, brought a large influx of foreigners into the French capital, including many Americans. Physicians who visited Paris during the second half of the 1810s witnessed the same advantages that Watson had reported, and told others about them after their return home. But unlike Watson, they could go on to point out the free commerce with France that made medical study in Paris easily available to Americans. John W. Francis, a twenty-six-year-old New York professor of materia medica, traveled to Europe in 1815–1816 for ill health ("induced by too strict attention to his studies," as a medical friend put it)[28] and took advantage of the occasion to visit the medical institutions of the newly opened French capital; he then returned home urging the opportunities for study there on his own pupils.[29] Usher Parsons, who took leave from the United States Navy in the Mediterranean on account of ill health, traveled in 1819 to Paris, where he spent several months studying at the École de Médecine and in the hospitals. "These establishments are so numerous and employ so many lecturers and professors that a stranger at first sight would believe the attention of the whole city is directed toward them," he wrote to the New York physician Lyman Spalding. Reporting that he had seen more than sixty lecturers on medicine and natural science, Parsons boasted that "I have attended the lectures of some whose names are familiar to you particular Duboi's Boyer's Dupuytren's Richerand's Alibert's Larrey's on surgery—Vauquelin Chaptal, Guy Lussac, Thenard & Abby Hauy." He noted that "Béclard a young anatomist and Thénard the chemist are the most popular lecturers. I have seen 2500 persons at Béclard's lectures, and not more than three fourths of those who go to hear Thénard can gain admittance." He went on to catalog the physicians and surgeons famous in the United States through their publications whom he had met, and to brag of his acquaintance with Philippe Pinel and Georges Cuvier.[30]

At the same time that some Americans were reporting on the medical vitality of Paris, others were reporting on the shortcomings of Edinburgh. Antagonism against the British, growing since Watson's time and brought to crisis by the War of 1812, was one factor that made some Americans look more favorably on study in France. Other Americans confirmed Watson's perception that the practical anatomical experience to be had in Britain was meager, especially as contrasted with Paris. And as opportunities for study in the Paris hospitals increasingly became known, those offered by the Edinburgh Royal Infirmary, once impressive, appeared by comparison modest. David Gittings, a young physician from Baltimore, wrote in 1818 to his father from Edinburgh that even though he was entitled to examine patients at the Royal Infirmary, "it is really a sin in the winter season when there are four or five hundred medical students here to tease the poor devils to death, and on that account I do not expect to derive as much instruction from the hospital this winter as when they disperse throughout the country during the summer season."[31] His clinical activity chiefly consisted of "copying off cases from the journal of the institution about 1 or 2 hundred of the most interesting of which I intend transcribing into a book for the purpose of taking to America with me."[32] Compared with study under his preceptor in Baltimore, Edinburgh afforded Gittings welcome clinical exposure; but compared with the clinical access other Americans began to report in Paris, opportunities for gaining practical experience in Edinburgh were slim. Throughout the nineteenth century, Americans would continue to visit Edinburgh and especially London. But by the 1820s, for those who traveled to Europe for serious medical study, the tide unmistakably was turning.

It is not possible to know how many Americans traveled to Paris during the antebellum period. In the early 1970s historian Russell M. Jones said that 105 went in the 1820s, 222 in the 1830s, 128 in the 1840s, and 279 in the 1850s. His conclusions, however, were based upon a tacit assumption that the numbers of names he was able to find in published and manuscript sources closely approximated the numbers of Americans who actually did study medicine in Paris; whereas in fact his sample was eclectic, favored physicians who were or became prominent, and yielded tallies unmistakably low. The further limitation on our ability to know is built into the nature of American medical studies in Paris: nothing in the French system required the visiting foreign student to register even for the didactic and clinical courses that were part of the official curriculum, much less for the private courses that flourished outside of the official program of instruction.[33]

The Registres des Inscriptions for the Faculté de Médecine have survived from the years 1815 to 1839, and from them we learn that 108 Americans formally registered for the official course of medical instruction. Yet registration was unnecessary for the foreign student who did not seek to graduate in Paris, and nearly half of the Americans who did inscribe were from Louisiana, often students from Creole families who were considering taking a Parisian medical degree. Others, like John Dix Fisher in 1825 and James Jackson, Jr., in 1831, inscribed for one trimester shortly after arriving in Paris but then discontinued the practice, realizing that such formal registration was unnecessary for their purposes. The vast majority, however, never inscribed at all; the Philadelphian Thomas Hun, to cite only one example, who studied medicine in Paris from 1833 to 1839, appears nowhere in the official inscription lists.[34]

Contemporary accounts estimating as many as three to four hundred Americans studying medicine in Paris at a single time during the 1850s were no doubt inflated.[35] Yet it is surely conservative to say that over a thousand medical Americans studied in Paris during the antebellum decades. What is clear, in any event, is that contrasted with the handful of medical Americans who found their way to Paris before 1815, the growing number who made the journey after Waterloo testifies to the marked migration that came with peace and intensified through the remainder of the antebellum decades.

## THE ATTRACTIONS OF PARIS

Contemporary characterizations of American physicians' reasons for traveling to Paris employed catchwords that, like *professional improvement*, implied much but made little explicit. When Caspar Wistar Pennock set off for Paris in 1830, having received his M.D. from the University of Pennsylvania in 1828 and then spent a year at the Philadelphia Almshouse, he carried with him a large bundle of letters to prominent medical figures in London and Paris, written in language that typified the ways such a journey was ordinarily cast. "Pray give me leave to introduce to your acquaintance Dr. C. W. Pennock a gentleman whose devotion to medical science has induced him to visit Europe," one stated. "He visits Europe for the enlargement of his knowledge, more particularly in medical science, which he will seek at the schools on the Continent," said another. Pennock traveled to Europe, as others put it, "with a view of becoming acquainted with its medical and literary institutions"; "to enlarge the sphere of his information by foreign residence and study"; and "to complete his medical education." One Philadelphian wrote to John James Audubon in London that Pennock "visits Europe with the desire of perfecting his medical education," while another used almost identical language in writing to toxicologist Mathieu-J.-B. Orfila in Paris that Pennock "part pour l'Europe, avec le désir de se perfectionner dans l'étude de votre Profession." [36] Like the phrases of social convention urged by nineteenth-century guides to the etiquette of letter writing, such language masked the multiple incentives that converged in leading individual Americans to cross the Atlantic.

These travelers went to Paris for a variety of reasons, which included most of the motivations that led physicians to seek professional improvement at home. Yet no list can begin to capture the texture of deliberations in which the sizable costs of a journey abroad were weighed against the anticipated rewards. The decision to go to Paris must ultimately be understood in the context of individual lives and individual choices. However, certain broad patterns of motivation and decision making remained remarkably durable across the entire antebellum period, despite the marked changes between Waterloo and the American Civil War.

Many of the Americans who made the journey (and an increasing proportion over time) were still establishing the basic foundation for a career. These were people who had not yet begun to practice on their own, but who typically had served an apprenticeship and received an M.D. degree. Some had pursued additional clinical training, such as a year as resident physician in a hospital. It was not necessary even to have earned an M.D. before visiting Paris, however; Jackson, Jr., traveled to France in 1831 with a good medical education under his father, the Harvard medical professor James Jackson, Sr., but with no intention of earning a diploma until after his return to Boston. Most young medical travelers, though, had received an M.D. degree shortly before setting off, and it was for this reason that Parisian study was often framed as a process of *completing* their education. While such a trip bore some of the hallmarks of the gentleman's grand tour, it never served this function for young Americans in anything approaching the extent it did for their English counterparts. Nevertheless, cultural broadening (and, although seldom articulated, adventure) routinely figured among the incentives for Parisian study. The trip completed their education in more than medicine alone and had an ornamental value— what one physician later termed "Parisian polish"—that went beyond the knowledge and experience acquired in hospitals.[37]

Medical students became aware of the opportunities for study Paris afforded through descriptions that appeared in letters Americans abroad sent to medical journals, in introductory addresses and classroom lectures at medical schools, in papers read and discussions that followed at the meetings of medical societies, and in guidebooks to medical Paris written for Americans contemplating the journey. As important as such public rhetoric was informal communication between those who had been to Paris and others studying in America. When in 1833 Jackson, Jr., wrote from Paris to Charles Gideon Putnam, a young physician in Salem, Massachusetts, Putnam replied, "You can scarcely conceive the restlessness that tries one at hearing your tales of Louis, Andral[,] Bichat and other medical worthies—surely never was [a] Knight more devoted to his lady love than you to your chère amie La Medecine." When a letter from his preceptor, then visiting Paris, seconded Jackson's enthusiastic reports, Putnam continued, "I then all but vowed to cross the water."[38] So too Francis Peyre Porcher, who in 1847 had just received his M.D. degree in South Carolina and was pursuing clinical study in New York, could see the patina of authority that Paris experience conferred. Telling his brother of an evening spent at the house of Henry Daggett Bulkley, Porcher wrote that Bulkley "was for some years in Paris & is said to be more au fait in Diseases of the skin than any one in these cases, certainly he is final umpire in settling all doubtful diagnoses in reference to affections of that class." The reputation that accrued from Parisian study was apparent to Porcher, who, reporting on his own clinical studies, noted, "No place could suit me better than New York (barring Paris)."[39]

The most persistent refrain heard in America about medical study in Paris was that in the French capital the young physician found access to practical experience unrivaled anywhere in the New World or the Old. "I enjoy advantages here which I could never have elsewhere, for improvement in every branch of human knowledge," Charles Thomas Jackson wrote home from Paris in 1832, and Edward E. Jenkins reported in 1853 that "of the opportunities for studying diseases of every nature you will be able to form an opinion when

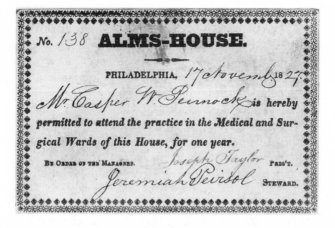

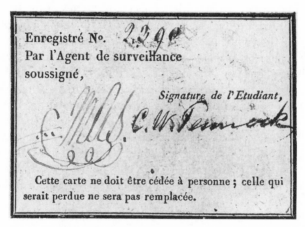

Fig. 2.1. Tickets admitting Caspar Wistar Pennock to study
at the Philadelphia Almshouse in 1827 and at the Hôtel Dieu
in Paris in 1831. Like many Americans, Pennock, who
received his M.D. degree from the University of Pennsylvania
in 1828, traveled to France largely for access to extensive
clinical experience that was difficult to obtain in his
own country. (Courtesy of Francis A. Countway Library
of Medicine, Boston.)

informed that during the course of a year eighty thousand persons are admitted
to the Hospitals."[40] Porcher, when he finally did make it to Paris, wrote back
to readers of the *Charleston Medical Journal and Review* in 1852 that "the facilities for seeing a great and endless variety of medical and surgical cases has far
surpassed our expectation."[41] And in an 1845 guide to the Paris hospitals, F.
Campbell Stewart, who had received his M.D. at the University of Pennsylvania, asserted flatly that "in no part of the world can the same practical experience be acquired by the attentive student as in the French capital."[42]

Such rhetoric spoke powerfully to the professional needs of physicians yet to start practice. The message was that just as young physicians could gain experience by treating the poor in dispensary or private practice, by taking a course of instruction at a private medical school, or by securing an appointment at an American hospital, they could acquire experience in Paris by what one physician called a "tour of professional improvement."[43] But what took time to gain in the best of American circumstances came quickly in France. Thus in 1848 Augustus Kinsley Gardner, in a book reporting his experiences in Paris, argued that while American students were soundly educated in the principles of medicine, "still, without practice, it is nothing. This is the reason, why the young physician is inferior to the old, though his head is stuffed with book information to the crown of his hat. The hospital is the place for supplying this deficiency." Gardner, who had worked for nearly three years in Massachusetts hospitals after receiving his M.D. from Harvard in 1844, went on to claim that in Paris, the student's access to bodies of the living and the dead was unrivaled, noting that "every patient who enters a hospital is, in a certain degree, Government property, and, not only through life, but even after death, is subject, in some sense, to the control of the physician." He urged on young physicians at home the example of some fifty American medical students he had encountered in Paris, "perfecting themselves in their science" in the French hospitals. "Those who imagine that the obtaining of a degree denotes the end of study, of course will say that it is useless," he concluded, "but those who consider that they have then but entered the threshold only, will look upon it in a far different light."[44] To young physicians reading Gardner's book, the point was unambiguous: study in the Paris hospitals offered one means of eroding distinctions between them and physicians of greater age and experience.

Study in Paris, then, represented a catalyst for transforming the inexperienced graduate into a seasoned practitioner, with all the material and emotional rewards anticipated from such a change. Experience at the bedside, moreover, gave the physician self-assurance and poise that generated confidence in patients, as a North Carolina physician reminded a young family friend studying in Paris in 1852. The older physician approved of his younger colleague's decision to extend his stay, counseling that "one of the chief sources of pleasure to you—resulting from this undertaking of yours—will arise from that confidence and self-reliance on your own resources which the knowledge you acquire and the practice you witness will certainly give." Experience, he continued, "gives the calm minded steady purpose to the Physician and, the cool deliberation—unwavering determination and quiet nerve to the surgeon."[45]

The decision to go to Paris did not begin with formal statements of the rewards that warranted it, which frequently had more to do with justification than motivation. As one among many options in the voluntary system of medical education that prevailed in antebellum America, it often captured the student's attention only gradually. The best way to begin to understand how and why some medical students reached that decision is to see how it took shape within the broader context of choices they made about their educations.

Levin Smith Joynes provides one unexceptional example of someone who drew from among various options for study in America and then, as part of the same ongoing process, sailed for France to continue his studies. Born in Accomack County, Virginia, Joynes, in 1835, at the age of sixteen, graduated with an A.B. degree from Washington and Jefferson College in Pennsylvania. "I was amused at a remark in your letter on the subject of choosing a profession," his father wrote to him early that year. "You think that the practice of medicine is too laborious, and you seem to think you will in the end select the ancient and honourable profession of a farmer, but if you do 'it will not be in a slave-holding state.'—Now I want to know if you do not think, that a farmer in a non-slaveholding state, has to work as hard as a doctor."[46] The matter remained unresolved for the time being, leading the father to write toward the end of the year, "With respect to your future pursuit in life, I will repeat for, perhaps, the hundredth time, that I intend to leave that matter entirely to your own choice." But he ventured that success in law was even more uncertain than success in medicine, and added "that *all* your friends here and in Washington think that the Medical profession would particularly suit your disposition and talents."[47]

Joynes began studying at the University of Virginia, still undecided about his profession, reading history and considering taking a master's degree. His father reassured him of financial support for whatever course he chose, even should he decide to study in Europe.[48] But within a year the son settled on medicine. "I think I should prefer your graduating at the university of V^a and then going to Phila^a and graduating there, too. All this can be accomplished before you are 21 years of age, which will be early enough to commence practice," the father advised.[49] Nearly nine months later he again wrote his son, "My object is not so much that you should be studying *in any particular place*, as that you should be *studying*—I cannot bear for you to be idle."[50]

Joynes received an M.D. degree from the University of Virginia and then proceeded to Philadelphia for further medical lectures, filling letters to his father with reassurances of his diligence. While still in Virginia, however, he had begun to think about studying in Paris, an ambition he described to his brother William. "I was informed by William sometime past that you wished to spend a year or two in Europe after completing your studies at the University of Va and in Philadelphia," Joynes's father wrote to him at the start of 1839. "It is my wish to afford you every opportunity for your improvement and for qualifying you to practice your profession with reputation,—and if it is thought by your professors, to whom I shall write on the subject, that the advantages will be equivalent to the time and expense I shall not hesitate to permit you to spend two or three years in the best schools of Europe."[51]

In Philadelphia, Joynes prepared for a trip to Paris by finding a boarding-house where only French was spoken. Picking and choosing from the city's medical offerings, at the opening of the 1839 winter term he attended intro-

ductory lectures both at Jefferson Medical College and at the University of
Pennsylvania before settling on lectures at the latter. He dispensed with materia medica and chemistry, as he felt he had a good grasp of both subjects, and
explained that instead "I have taken Dr Gerhard's ticket for his private course
of lectures on diseases of the chest, & practical instructions in the use of that
fashionable and useful instrument, the stethoscope. Dr. G's ticket will also
entitle me to the privilege of attending the clinical lectures at the Dispensary &
Almshouse, (for which students generally have to pay $10)."[52] It was an eclec-
tic course of professional improvement; and it was this eclecticism, not its
specific elements, that made it typical.

The arrangement with Gerhard was satisfying, especially the opportunity to
study specimens Gerhard preserved from autopsies at the Almshouse, but trying to gain anatomical experience in Philadelphia proved frustrating. In the
same letter in which he complained of finding "subjects so scarce in Philadelphia," even in the private dissecting room reported to be better supplied than
the university, Joynes spoke with renewed resolve of his plan to travel to Paris
for the experience that came so slowly in America.[53] A lecture by William
Gibson, his professor of surgery, especially piqued his enthusiasm. "He has
lately returned from Europe, and in one of his first lectures he gave an account
of the school & hospital, & other means of acquiring medical instruction in
Paris," Joynes told his father. "The interesting statement which he gave of the
decided superiority of Paris in this respect over every other city in the world
greatly increased my desire to enjoy its advantages."[54] It is likely that Gibson
told his class something along the lines of the account he later published of his
1839 trip to Paris, in which he depicted the French capital as a place "where the
science of medicine in all its branches is taught with an assiduity and accuracy,
enthusiasm and fidelity, unknown in most other parts of the world; where the
student . . . may go at almost any moment and witness important operations on
the living body, listen to a lecture on the case and reasons for performing it,
and with an unfavorable result, have an opportunity of seeing the injection and
dissection of the parts, and their mode of preservation; where he may perform
with his own hand operation after operation, guided by some able assistant,
until he acquires a perfect knowledge of the principles which govern him, the
instruments he employs, and the nature of the case in which he resorts to
which measures."[55] Half a year later Joynes was on shipboard sailing to Europe,
where he would remain until 1843.[56]

Similar only in the eclectic course of study that preceded travel to Paris was
the case of James Lawrence Cabell, whose choices display the voluntary system
of education in which requirements for an M.D. degree could play only a minor
role in charting the course of professional improvement. Cabell, born in 1813
in Virginia, entered the University of Virginia in 1829 and earned an A.M. there
in 1833. During this period he also took a course of lectures on medicine and
the following year attended a second course in Baltimore, where in spring 1834
he received his M.D. Earlier that year he had told his uncle and guardian that
not only had he been attending six lectures a day, but also "Dr. Dunglison has

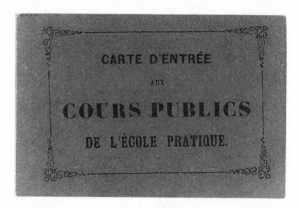

Fig. 2.2. Tickets admitting William J. Holt to a course on
practical anatomy at the University of Georgia in 1850 and to
L'École Pratique, one of the two largest dissecting establishments in Paris, in 1854. Like most of the medical Americans who
studied in France, Holt sought to supplement the meager opportunities for human dissection available in his own country with
the extraordinarily free access to the body in Paris. (William
Joseph Holt Papers, courtesy of Manuscripts Division, South
Caroliniana Library, University of South Carolina, Columbia.)

been kind enough to examine me twice a week on the subjects of all the lectures & this will be of great advantage to me," noting that "the professors
having but an hour a day for four months, do not examine the class publickly,
but many of them have private classes & examine them on the whole course."
He sent his uncle the bill for his professor's fees, anatomical instruments, dissecting ticket, subjects for dissection, and one book (the French surgeon Armand Velpeau's treatise on midwifery).[57]

As graduation approached, Cabell began to talk about summer plans. His uncle wanted him to return to Richmond, making it impossible for him to remain for the entire course of supplementary lectures that the professors gave during the summer for additional fees. So Cabell proposed instead a combination of dissecting and clinical study under Robley Dunglison at the infirmary. At the same time, Cabell raised the possibility of continuing his medical studies in Paris. A year earlier, his uncle had actually suggested study in Paris, but in chemistry and mathematics, not medicine, with the idea that the young man would then return to become a professor of one of these subjects. The younger Cabell had rejected the idea, explaining, "I knew that I had no certainty of obtaining a professorship on my return to this country & I would then either have the mortification of turning my attention to some other profession or quietly wait until some employment should present itself—on the contrary by obtaining a degree in medicine I but added another string to my bow." Proposing his plan to study medicine in Paris tentatively—"as a suggestion & not a request"—he wrote to his uncle, "You were willing then to borrow the money necessary to prosecute my studies in Paris & go my security for its payment; I now say that if you are still willing to bear that responsibility, I will at once decide to exert all my powers of body and mind." To underscore the advantages of the trip, Cabell added that "I am still more convinced by the reports of one or two young men whom I have just seen & who spent a year or more in Paris. The mere fact, generally known, that they studied in France has gained them more distinction than other young men would acquire in double the time, & this coupled with the information obtained there will give them a standing which it would require years of labour to obtain."[58]

The plan went unrealized, at least for the time being, and late in 1834 Cabell returned to Baltimore, this time as resident student at the Almshouse. "My present situation offers great advantages to the medical student, & I rejoice that I did not neglect the only opportunity which might be offered for many years," he told his uncle. "I shall probably see almost every variety of disease which the climate & season present," he wrote, noting that "the house is now crowded with the sick & every moment of my time will be engaged until I become more ready and expert in practice."[59] Within a few months Cabell was already lobbying his uncle to extend his studies.[60]

Despite possession of an M.D. degree a year old and supplemented by elective study, Cabell made it clear that he still saw himself as a student, continuing to gain the knowledge and experience that would prepare him for practice. "The medical student has a long & arduous apprenticeship to serve and I have just commenced," he wrote to his uncle in February 1835. "I am thus anxious to continue here at least a year longer than the term of six months for which I have paid." He proposed a modified and cheaper version of the now defunct plan of studying in France, that is, borrowing half the money a trip to Paris would have required and using it to prolong his studies in Baltimore. "I think $600 will not only support all my necessary expenses, but enable me to procure suitable books & instruments—& probably medicines—I wish to see diseases of all seasons and have another winter for dissection & the study of practical surgery."[61]

Behind this maneuver was Cabell's growing resolve not only to stay in medicine but to aim for professional eminence. In summer 1836 he returned to Richmond, where his uncle helped him find an office. But Cabell found the profession there "greatly overstocked" and complained that "superior attainments or a period of professional pupilage which would justify the supposition of superior attainments, have little to do with a physician's success in Richmond." His deeper dissatisfaction stemmed from his experience of the professional lethargy of Richmond in the wake of the vigor he had enjoyed in Baltimore. "I have no means of continuing the study of my profession," he explained. "No man can keep pace with its improvement who had not the means of testing the truth or fallacy of what he reads. These means are afforded in a large city by the hospitals & infirmaries always accessible to practitioners." In Richmond, he lamented, "we have no hospital—no professional intercourse between the physicians, each moving in his own separate sphere & knows nothing of the practice of a brother physician."[62]

Insisting that medicine in Richmond was "a mere trade," Cabell told his uncle, "If I have not the means of making myself eminent in the profession, I would rather not offer for practice at all. I do not wish to be a quack." He proposed returning to Baltimore to gain further experience, even if it was without remuneration: "The only chance I have of acquiring eminence, is to throw myself prominently before the profession in a large city where the facilities for study & of making oneself an author are greater than in Richmond."[63] His uncle finally relented, but instead of an indefinite residence in Baltimore, Cabell's course was to be a period of intensive study in Paris. At the start of December 1836, scarcely five weeks after proposing the move to Baltimore, Cabell was in New York about to embark for France.[64] And indeed, less than two months after arriving in Paris, he wrote to his uncle that "the opportunities for medical instruction are so very great & there is so much to be learned, so much to keep one constantly employed, that I should like to stay longer than I expected to do."[65] He remained in Paris until 1837, when he was offered the chair in anatomy, physiology, and surgery at the University of Virginia that he occupied for the next two decades.

Joynes and Cabell were led to Paris largely by the limited advantages American institutions afforded for extensive clinical experience. Yet as white men, they could expect vastly greater access to the facilities that did exist in the United States—meager as these were—than others among their medical compatriots. Mid-nineteenth-century women physicians and African-American physicians—even when they were enabled to earn the M.D. degree, increasingly at separatist medical schools founded in the third quarter of the century—were barred from study at most American hospitals, dispensaries, and medical schools, and had particular reason to explore the possibility that abroad they might find the experience that gender and race barriers denied them in the United States. In 1852 William P. Powell, an African American,

wrote to the faculty of the Liverpool Royal Infirmary School of Medicine asking that his son William P. Powell, Jr., be admitted as a "free student" to the
lectures necessary to qualify him as a physician. The elder Powell stated in his
petition that he, his wife, and seven children had emigrated from America to
Britain "for the purpose of having the eldest taught useful professions," explaining that "owing to the *prejudice, customs,* and *usages* of the American
people it is impossible for him to give his children, that Education and secure
to them those opportunities for a livelihood, and a respectable position in
society to which as human beings they are entitled." Powell, Sr., told the faculty that he was "unable to defray the necessary expenses to have his eldest
son taught the Science of *medical* and *surgical* practice"; lectures would complete his education, for the Medical Board of the Liverpool Infirmary had already granted his son admission as a "free student" to clinical study.[66] The
record of the faculty meeting summarized this memorial "from Mr. W. P.
Powell a coloured American," noting that "free admission" was requested "on
the grounds that he was prevented being educated at the Colleges in America
on account of his colour—and that he was unable to pay." After what the
minutes called "a long discussion," the faculty voted three to two to grant the
application.[67]

James McCune Smith, the first African American to receive a medical degree,
headed to Paris after graduating in Glasgow in 1837, though the nature of his
studies in France before he returned to practice medicine in New York is uncertain.[68] John Van Surly de Grasse, after receiving his M.D. degree from Bowdoin, not only set off in 1849 for two years' study in the Paris hospitals but
became an assistant there to the surgeon Velpeau. De Grasse had been admitted
to Bowdoin through the efforts of the American Colonization Society with the
expectation that he would emigrate to Liberia, but in 1852 he instead chose to
practice in Boston and, during the Civil War, served as an assistant surgeon in
the United States Army.[69] So too physician and abolitionist Martin Robison
Delany, writing in 1852, pointed to a compatriot studying medicine in Paris as
evidence of African-American advancement in the professions. "Daniel Laing,
Jr., Esq., a fine intellectual young gentleman of Boston, a student also of Dr.
Clarke of that city, of the Surgeons of the Massachusetts General Hospital, who
attended the course of Lectures at the session of 1850–51, at the Medical
School of Harvard University," Delany wrote with satisfaction, "is now in Paris,
to spend two years in the hospitals, and attend the Medical Lectures of that
great seat of learning."[70]

American women physicians were particularly drawn to Paris by the promise of clinical instruction and experience difficult if not impossible to acquire
in their own country. From midcentury, when women in the United States
first began to receive M.D. degrees from a few male-dominated schools and
especially from newly established women's medical colleges, there was a remarkably uniform consensus that the leading deficiency was inadequate access to practical hospital instruction. Even the kind of clinical lectures Joynes
attended at the Philadelphia Dispensary and Almshouse, and the practical

knowledge Cabell gained as resident student at the Baltimore Almshouse, were ordinarily inaccessible to women. The problem was alleviated as gradual inroads were made into male-dominated institutions and as separate hospitals and dispensaries were founded to give women clinical experience. Yet it was hardly resolved.[71] Frances Emily White, who had traveled to Paris for clinical study, was echoing a complaint that had been commonplace for nearly half a century when in 1895 she told the graduating class of the Woman's Medical College of Pennsylvania that "the chief disadvantages from which medical women in this country now suffer arise from the exclusion (during their professional career) from the work of the great public hospitals." Separate schools assured that women could earn an M.D. degree, but, as White told the graduates, "the hospital is no less important than the college in the training of doctors."[72]

Compounding the problem, the first generation of women physicians believed, was the tendency of the public to hold them to a different, higher standard than their male counterparts. "If we as *women* should fail in any one of the particulars, wherein our brothers, *do* sometimes fail," a student at the Female Medical College of Pennsylvania wrote in her 1861 M.D. thesis, "it would be readily seized upon and heralded to the discredit of ourselves."[73] Florence Nightingale stated the case even more pointedly in a private letter to Elizabeth Blackwell, who in 1849, by earning her medical degree from the Geneva Medical College in New York State, became the first American woman to receive an M.D. degree. A "pioneer" in the movement for women's medical education "must have both natural talent and experience and undoubted superiority," Nightingale told Blackwell in 1856. "A mistake, such as ignorance of her profession," Nightingale observed, "would wreck that cause for fifty years."[74]

Blackwell's decision to embark for Paris three months after receiving her M.D. degree, while motivated by the same quest for practical experience that drew many male physicians abroad, was also informed by her understanding of the singular difficulties women faced in obtaining clinical education in America. Indeed, in 1847, when she was still searching for an American medical school willing to admit a woman, Blackwell noted in her diary that the idea was repeatedly urged upon her "of giving up the attempt in America and going to France."[75] If no American school would admit a woman, her advisers reasoned, perhaps she could obtain medical instruction in Paris. "The free Government lectures, delivered by the faculty, are confined to men, and a diploma is strictly denied to a woman, even when (as in one instance, as it is said) she has gone through the course in male attire," Blackwell wrote in late spring 1847. "Yet every year thorough courses of lectures are delivered by able physicians on every branch of medical knowledge, to which I should be admitted without hesitation and treated with becoming respect. The true place for study, then, seems open to me."[76] Blackwell would later recall Joseph Warrington, a Philadelphia Quaker physician who had supported her efforts to enroll at an American medical college, advising her, "'Elizabeth, it is no use trying. Thee cannot gain admission to these schools. Thee must go to Paris and don masculine attire to gain the necessary knowledge.'"[77] Joseph Pancoast proposed that she try the same strategy of disguise in his medical classes in Philadelphia: as Blackwell put it, Pancoast "told me that although my public entrance into the class was out of the question, yet if I would assume masculine attire and enter the college he could entirely rely on two or three of his students to whom he should communicate my disguise, who would watch the class and give me timely notice to withdraw should my disguise be suspected."[78]

By late May 1847, Blackwell had concluded that "if all the information which I am still collecting agree with what I have already received, I may sail for France in the course of the summer."[79] Some of her physician-advisers, she realized, would disapprove of a woman's heading off alone for Paris: "'You, a young unmarried lady,' they say, 'go to Paris, that city of fearful immorality, where every feeling will be outraged and insult attend you at every step; where vice is the natural atmosphere, and no young man can breathe it without being contaminated! Impossible, you are lost if you go!'"[80] But to their objections "that Paris was such a horrible place that I must give up my wish for a medical education," Blackwell replied in her diary "that if the path of duty led me to hell I would go there."[81]

Blackwell's acceptance three months later at Geneva Medical College in up-state New York and the promise of an M.D. degree obviated Parisian study plans, at least for the time being. "I fairly jumped for joy," she told her sister on receiving the news; "it seemed to me, that I was the luckiest mortal on the face of the earth, & that henceforth no difficulty remained."[82] Yet Blackwell did not relinquish the idea of studying in Paris. Her resolve was reinforced by her experience of hospital work during the long interlude between the first and second terms. Returning to Philadelphia after the close of the 1847–1848 winter term, Blackwell won permission to study in the Blockley Almshouse by political lobbying and by deftly playing on party rivalries among those who governed the institution.[83] But, as she discovered, gaining access to the wards did not necessarily mean gaining instruction. "I get very little from the physicians," she wrote to her sister; "they keep aloof, view me with suspicions, think I am stepping out of woman's sphere."[84] She later recalled of the young resident physicians that "when I walked into the wards they walked out," and that "they ceased to write the diagnosis and treatment of patients on the card at the head of each bed, which had hitherto been the custom, thus throwing me entirely on my own resources for clinical study."[85] Time at Blockley both made Blackwell realize how difficult it would be for a woman—even with M.D. degree in hand—to gain practical clinical experience and redoubled her appreciation of how critical such experience would be. "If I manage to succeed now, I shall entertain no fear of Woman's being able under favorable circumstances to study thoroughly & practise intelligently," she wrote from Blockley to her sister; "but I believe I shall have to go to France, before I can feel strong in knowledge."[86]

By the time she began the final term of medical lectures, Blackwell regarded study in Paris as an indispensable step in her education. "My plan for myself is this," she wrote in October 1848 to her sister: "after graduating as I presume I shall in January—to spend a year in Paris." The plan would require going into debt, borrowing over a thousand dollars. "This seems rather a formidable responsibility to incur," she acknowledged, "but I do it without the smallest hesitation or feeling of uneasiness—the experience & practical knowledge I shall thereby gain, are essential to me."[87] After graduation ceremonies in late January 1849, she returned to Philadelphia where, in addition to medical studies, she was also "rubbing up my French."[88] Her departure for Europe was precipitated by the suggestion of an English cousin visiting America that they make the Atlantic crossing together, and in mid-April Blackwell embarked for her tour of professional improvement abroad.[89]

Blackwell's studies in Paris (sketched in chapter 3) were to be chiefly at the Hôpital de la Maternité, the massive training school for midwives. Access to the other Paris hospitals she found greatly restricted. Nevertheless, the clinical experience Blackwell did gain convinced her that Paris offered American women physicians a singularly promising avenue to practical education. The stories she told after her return in 1851 became elements in an emerging women's advice network that drew on reports by American male physicians while underscoring the role gender played in determining opportunities for medical study in the French capital. Not long after she settled in New York, Blackwell told her sister of calls paid by two pioneer women physicians— Lydia Folger Fowler, the second woman in America to receive an M.D. degree, earned in 1850 from an Eclectic school in upstate New York, and Nancy Talbot Clark, who in 1852 had become the second woman to receive an M.D. from a regular school. Blackwell noted with satisfaction Clark's aspiration to study abroad and reported that they parted with Clark "looking upon me as her chief guide—and as we are the only two regulars, I gave her decidedly the right hand of friendship." Turning to Fowler's visit, Blackwell commented that "I believe I made a conquest of her too—but none of these women have any practical knowledge—I recommended the latter, who is lecturing on Midwifery to go to La Maternité for a year."[90] When later, in 1854, Clark made preparations to depart for Paris, Blackwell was distressed to learn that she had no interest in studying at the Maternité and took it upon herself to set Clark straight. "I believe I quite surprised and troubled her, by pointing out all the difficulties in her way, and showing how I had found all female medicine and surgery quite closed to me," Blackwell wrote to her sister. "She evidently thought she had nothing to do, but cross the ocean and step into first rate chances."[91]

Among the women medical students in the 1850s who accorded Elizabeth Blackwell's Parisian experiences a central role in deliberating their own educational course was her sister Emily. "I think you'll have to keep enough money for six months in the Maternité," Elizabeth told Emily; "I don't think you'll be able to do without that experience—not so much for the value of their treatment, as for the self confidence which acquaintance with such wide practice gives."[92] For Emily, who had just commenced her medical education, her elder sister's advice was a key ingredient in motivating her desire to study in Paris and shaping expectations of the experience to be had there. Thus in early autumn of 1853, in the same diary entry in which she recorded having just met the apprenticeship-trained physician Harriot Hunt for the first time at a women's rights convention, Emily made note of a day "spent quietly at home and while I sewed E. told me some of her Parisian experience."[93] Even after Emily left for Paris, Elizabeth continued to send detailed advice. If she managed to gain admission to institutions other than the Maternité, Elizabeth wrote, it would be wise "to avoid the more crowded Hospitals." Only a few weeks after Emily's departure, Elizabeth sent along the suggestion of her former medical teacher Daniel Brainard, just returned from Paris—namely, that she search out instruction at the Lourcine, the St. Louis, and the Hôpital des Enfants Malades, but steer clear of La Charité and La Pitié, both of them "thronged" with students.[94]

Emily Blackwell had resolved while still attending medical lectures that once she graduated she would head abroad for clinical experience. At the same time, her sister's experiences convinced her that if she wanted free access to the Paris medical world—not merely the cloistered life of the Maternité—she would have to make her way disguised as a man. "I must go to Europe next year and my plan for studying in disguise appears to me almost necessary," she wrote in her diary in summer 1853, between first and second lecture terms. "I certainly shall not otherwise obtain the opportunities I need." As she continued, "I have often thought that if I followed solely my own inclinations I should assume a man's dress and wander freely over the world throwing away the constant weary shackles that custom and poverty surround us."[95] Her application for a hospital assistantship was rejected, and she was unsure that she would graduate at the end of term; in October—on her twenty-seventh birthday—her diary entry made it clear that she expected Parisian study to be a turning point. "I am still on this side of the great epoch—my European visit," she reflected; "how young all my life on that side will look ten years hence."[96]

Only a few weeks after she received her M.D. from Western Reserve in Cleveland in 1854, Emily Blackwell left for Europe. The night before boarding the steamer she spent at the house of Nancy Clark, who saw her to the Boston dock "bringing me enough little biscuits &c in case I should be sick, to last me for provisions the whole passage."[97] Blackwell would go first to Britain, where the Edinburgh surgeon James Y. Simpson allowed her to follow his practice, but she viewed opportunities there always with a eye toward France.[98] When her application to study at the Edinburgh Royal Infirmary was finally turned down, she told her family that the decision "only makes my way a little clearer."[99] She was resigned to entering the Maternité, explaining, "I shall enter the Maternite at once, both because it will be the most disagreeable part of my visit, and because I shall learn to speak French and shall afterward be better qualified for my Campaign among the Drs." She hoped eventually to gain access to other Paris hospitals but realized that such opportunities would depend entirely on personal favor and influence.[100] As it happened, a string of family crises among the British Blackwells detained her in England for another half year, but with nearly every report of a new delay she wrote of her resolve to study in Paris.[101]

The plan of cross-dressing as the key that would spring every latch to the Paris medical institutions remained, to Emily's mind, a real option. The discrimination she experienced in Edinburgh left her "more & more struck with the immense difference it would make to me." Scarcely a week after she reached Edinburgh, a young American physician just graduated from Harvard, Horatio Robinson Storer, arrived in the city for a summer of medical study, and his effortless passage into all the Edinburgh medical facilities posed an infuriating contrast to the obstacles Blackwell encountered at every turn. "I, even when received with courtesy, am practically excluded from medical facilities," she told Elizabeth, whereas, in welcoming Storer, Edinburgh's medical men had "thrown everything open to him in the freeest most hospitable way."[102] Writing ten days later in her diary about the favoritism Simpson had shown Storer and the rejection she had just received from the Royal Infirmary, Blackwell complained, "I am weary of all this constant persecutions on all sides."[103]

Elizabeth wrote later that month cautioning that "disguise in France or elsewhere would by no means give you all you need; if the disguise were complete you would just be reduced to the level of the common poor student, and would be, I think, quite disappointed." She reminded her sister that at most of the Paris hospitals, students "crowded together in masses" and could "only see at a distance the most interesting cases." Still, if she could repeat her studies in Paris, Elizabeth wrote, "and if by putting on disguise I could get either an assistant's post or good visiting privilege, I would put it on."[104] Emily, for her part, was elated when at long last she was released from family affairs in Britain. "Now I am free," she wrote home in June 1855; "in a fortnight at farthest— I shall leave for Paris."[105]

No single motivation led Joynes, or Cabell, or the Blackwells to study in France, yet for all of them the leading attraction of medical Paris was the exceptional access it offered to practical experience. For a minority of medical travelers, though, this was a secondary incentive. A small number of Americans— perhaps no more than three or four dozen during the entire antebellum period—went to Paris explicitly to matriculate at the École de Médecine and fulfill the requirements for its M.D. degree. They came chiefly from Creole families in and around New Orleans, and expected to return to practices drawn from the Francophone population of Louisiana.[106] Some established Louisiana practitioners with American M.D. degrees hoped that Parisian experience might help them entice Creole patients away from their French-trained competitors.[107] But by and large, even those few Anglophone Americans who considered taking a French degree either decided that their time could be better spent or had that decision made for them. "I wrote to Papa to let me pass my examinations here," one young American wrote from Paris in 1837, "but did not get his consent, as the length of time required at this Medical School before the degree can be taken was longer than he wished me to remain in Europe."[108]

Americans could also be attracted by reasons beyond the medical advantages of Paris (and beyond the common desire for adventure). Some young physicians more interested in natural science than clinical medicine traveled to Paris principally to pursue such fields as comparative anatomy, chemistry, or bot-

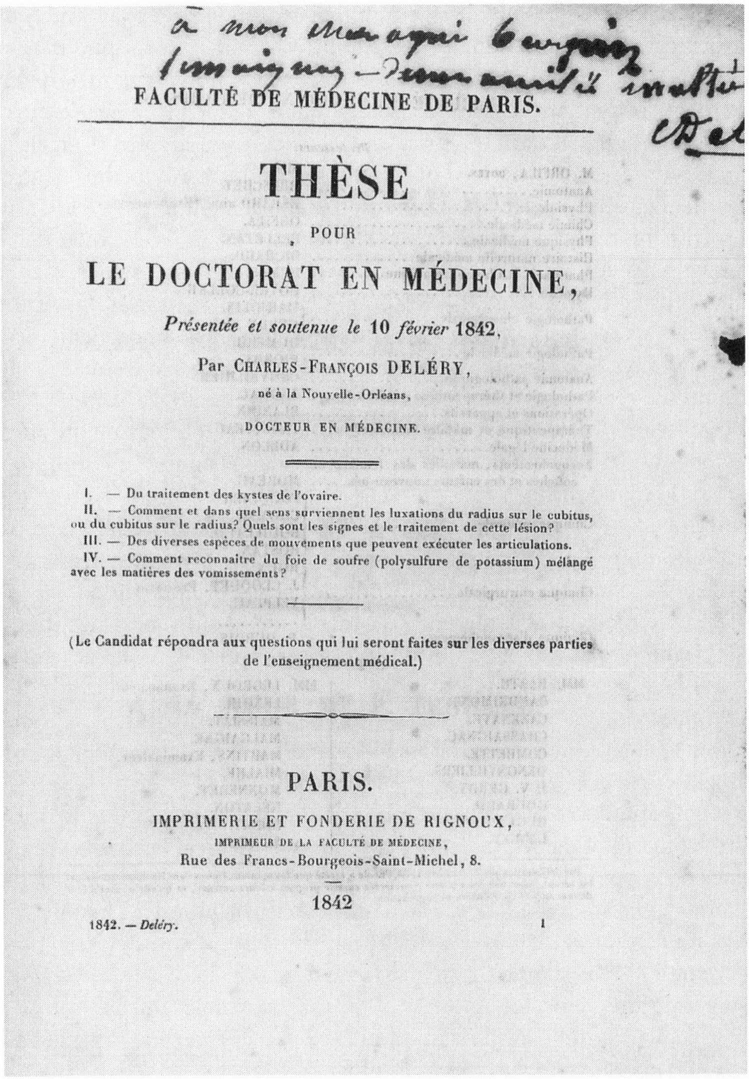

FACULTÉ DE MÉDECINE DE PARIS.

# THÈSE

POUR

## LE DOCTORAT EN MÉDECINE,

*Présentée et soutenue le* 10 *février* 1842,

Par CHARLES-FRANÇOIS DELÉRY,

né à la Nouvelle-Orléans,

DOCTEUR EN MÉDECINE.

I. — Du traitement des kystes de l'ovaire.
II. — Comment et dans quel sens surviennent les luxations du radius sur le cubitus, ou du cubitus sur le radius? Quels sont les signes et le traitement de cette lésion?
III. — Des diverses espèces de mouvements que peuvent exécuter les articulations.
IV. — Comment reconnaître du foie de soufre (polysulfure de potassium) mélangé avec les matières des vomissements?

(Le Candidat répondra aux questions qui lui seront faites sur les diverses parties de l'enseignement médical.)

## PARIS.

IMPRIMERIE ET FONDERIE DE RIGNOUX,
IMPRIMEUR DE LA FACULTÉ DE MÉDECINE,
Rue des Francs-Bourgeois-Saint-Michel, 8.

1842

1842. — *Deléry.*                                      1

Fig. 2.3. Thesis for the doctorate in medicine submitted to the Faculté de Médecine de Paris by Charles-François Deléry of "la Nouvelle-Orléans" in 1842. Of the hundreds of Americans who studied medicine in Paris during the antebellum period, only a few dozen, chiefly from Francophone Creole families in or near New Orleans, took a Parisian medical degree. (Thèses de Médecine, 3 vols., vol. 1, courtesy of Louisiana Collection, Howard-Tilton Memorial Library, Tulane University, New Orleans.)

any, as did some of their more established colleagues. Medicine, after all, was widely acknowledged as the best occupational choice for an American who wanted to cultivate science in a society that afforded few opportunities to take it up as a profession. One young man had decided to first earn his M.D. at

Harvard and then spend two years studying in Paris: "I feel every day that I have made a good choice," he wrote in 1845 to a friend. "There is so much of interest connected with the sciences, Botany, Nat-History, Comparative anatomy, &c which you'd not find in the Law, nor any other profession. Ah! it is a glorious study." The practice of medicine was "disagreeable," he admitted, but "the pleasures that a scientific man enjoy[s] in the profession far out balance any such objections."[109]

Young medical graduates ordinarily made study in the clinic the ostensible reason for their journey. Yet once they found themselves in Paris, other inclinations sometimes became clear. Gabriel E. Manigault, who as a child had toured France with his family, would recall in a memoir that while he was a medical student, it was seeing the management of a child's illness badly mangled that triggered his decision to study in France; as he explained, "It had always been my desire to revisit Paris after my medical studies in Charleston, and this incident confirmed me in the determination to improve myself by walking the hospitals."[110] Yet when in 1854 he set out for Paris, he carried with him letters of introduction from the South Carolina naturalist-physician John Edwards Holbrook to, among others, the herpetologist André-Marie Duméril at the Jardin des Plantes, as well as bottles of reptiles and fishes for its collection.[111] Although he would split his first year in Paris between work in the hospitals and in comparative anatomy, by the second year he abandoned medicine entirely and spent his time dissecting animals that died in the Jardin des Plantes and reassembling their skeletons.[112]

Others went for more personal reasons, and more than one young medical American was sent by his family in order that distance and the passage of time might erase the public's memory of a blemished reputation. A young Boston physician in Paris wrote home of the arrival of "John Warren whose conduct in Boston I have heard of having obliged him to flee the country"; while Edward Jenkins wrote from Paris worried that the community's memory of "my quarrel and other scrapes" might still be too vivid for him to seek a practice near the family home in South Carolina.[113] When Edward Cook's misconduct threatened to scotch his prospects for practice in Chillicothe, Ohio, the home of his socially prominent family, a medical friend suggested sending the young man to Paris and London "for the purpose of professional acquisition." "That he has been wild and rash and improvident is well known and thus has lost the confidence of an influential circle of friends in his native town," the Cincinnati physician Cornelius G. W. Comegys told Edward's father; "it is not at all too late however for him to redeem himself and earn a high position and add to the regards of his honored Fathers name. If he go abroad for the avowed purpose of a diligent study of his profession in the first schools of the world and in the mean time abandon all the defects that cling to him he will return at an age when physicians generally begin to get practice and being well known (for I propose to him to settle in Chillicothe) he will be sustained and by a class of people that will be an honor to him. I think he ought to stay at least two years and this is barely sufficient for him to go over the field of medicine and surgery." Comegys explained that Chillicothe was a strategic place for Edward to settle because "his absence and aims will be more widely known there than any where else and he would be consulted in rare diseases from the surrounding country when Physicians of less advantages would not be."[114]

Edward's father followed Comegys's advice but discovered that Paris was not the best place to send the young man for moral as well as professional improvement. When Comegys visited Paris the following summer, in 1851, he located Edward (and loaned him a hundred dollars) but found his situation discouraging. "I have regarded the trip to Paris as a means of changing Ed's career and leading him to that position which his natural abilities and family position open to him. I am sure that I can have no influence with him in the way of advice he neither sought or desired from me," Comegys told the father after returning to Ohio, "but I feel he was not diligent in medical observations."[115] Comegys asked Ruben Dimond Mussey, another Cincinnati physician in Paris, "to associate with him in his medical studies, so as to obtain a healthy influence over him." Half a year later, having heard from Mussey, Comegys informed Edward's father that matters looked grim. "I think it better that all should know the worst of his case. He is doing nothing in the present of medical knowledge & I now seriously fear he will not. I will now say that he did not while in Paris pay the least regard to my advice at any time and avoided my companionship." Comegys urged the father to exert political influence to have the American consul in Paris "search out Edward and see if he can save him or use any persuasion to get him to clean up his habits. His case is desperate and an extraordinary effort must be made or his speedy ruin is certain."[116]

Some physicians, of course, advised medical students *against* study in Paris. "The advantages afforded in Paris to young men who have not entered into practice," one medical editor visiting Paris wrote in 1845 to the readers of the *Western Lancet*, "are overrated in many particulars, more especially in relation to the practice of medicine."[117] Nearly all observers tended to agree that despite Parisian leadership in pathology and diagnosis, American therapeutic practice was superior to that of France (a perception explored in chapter 8). And many warned that while a seasoned practitioner would be able to distinguish between the good and the bad, study in the Paris hospitals placed the inexperienced recent graduate at risk of emulating misleading and dangerous models for the care of American patients. Especially as southern and western medical regionalism became more strident in the late antebellum period, the assertion that European treatment was inappropriate for American patients—like the argument that northern therapeutic teachings were ill-suited to the South and West—became increasingly common. "Instead of long pilgrimages to Europe for medical knowledge," one Ohio physician asserted in 1856, "we could here, with far less time and expenditure of money, give the student an American medical education on American soil; fill the west with a sound American medical literature, and with physicians far better qualified to treat the diseases of this country than any European school *can* develop."[118]

Nearly as common was the caution that Paris, a foreign city of doubtful morality, was a perilous place for young Americans to head off to alone. Louisville medical professor Austin Flint cautioned his students that despite its medical advantages, in Paris the young physician placed himself at risk of falling prey to "the temptations to pleasure and vice which meet him on every side." An older physician with greater knowledge of the world would be in a better position to recognize and resist Parisian seductions.[119] Here again, prospects for professional improvement in Paris were examined through the same lens used to scrutinize prospects within the United States, and Flint was echoing cautions about American cities. When Charles Caldwell returned from France to warn his pupils in Kentucky of the temptations of student life in "the contaminated atmosphere of Paris," he was voicing a judgment no different in kind or implication from that of a medical student from upstate New York who, studying in the City, wrote with repulsion of "the Sodom of New York."[120]

Young physicians contemplating a journey to Paris did not dismiss such warnings but assimilated them into their own expectations of the benefits and risks that lay ahead in France. In describing the kinds of knowledge they hoped to acquire, for example, they routinely stressed that they sought knowledge about disease, not medical treatment, which all agreed could be better learned in America. "I came to Paris not to study theories for I could study those as well or better at home—nor yet to study practice for the French practice is entirely opposed to the English and American schools," Henry Bryant wrote to his father in 1843, not long after arriving in Paris from Massachusetts, "but to study disease as it exists in the living and in the dead body."[121]

Equally, some listened attentively to warnings about Parisian snares to virtue. In 1833, George Cheyne Shattuck, Jr., studying medicine in Brunswick, Maine, wrote in his diary the cautionary words of Ruben Mussey, one of his professors. "He says that Paris is a place of abominations, and but few Americans who pass any time there escape being ruined," Shattuck recorded. "The French work from five in morning to five P.M. and then go to the opera or the brothel. The laxity of the women is astonishing. One gentleman was asked by his landlady if he had ever put a woman to bed and for how many he had done that office. A female lecturer on midwifery demonstrated on the live subject. An instance was mentioned of a young Canadian who went to Paris to study medicine, boarded, with a young widow, made love to her daughter and slept between them. His constitution was completely broken down."[122] Undeterred, Shattuck headed to Paris for medical study three years later; yet he had not taken Mussey's cautions lightly and on the eve of his departure recorded in the privacy of the same diary a prayer for moral resolve as he faced the dangers ahead.[123]

## PARIS AND THE SEASONED PRACTITIONER

Many of the Americans who sought professional improvement in Paris were practitioners who had already faced the trials of setting up practice, not fresh medical graduates. And they employed a somewhat different calculus in assessing the extent to which anticipated benefits outweighed costs. They too were warned that Parisian therapeutic practice offered a dangerous model for Americans, but were assured that as experienced practitioners, they would be able, as one physician in Paris told a Nashville medical editor, "to seize on the good and reject what is bad."[124] Older practitioners were also assumed to be less susceptible to the corrupting atmosphere of Paris than were younger students, but ordinarily had the added task of reassuring a spouse (and often in-laws) that their attention in Paris was closely riveted to medical affairs. More than this, while seasoned physicians were not so often dependent on others to finance the journey, the successful practice that generated independent means to pay for the trip usually came only to those who also had greater financial responsibilities, most especially to support a family.

Indeed, the most difficult obstacle the established physician had to overcome to make the journey was one that the new graduate was spared, namely, the danger of disrupting a practice that had taken time and labor to build. It was an understood reality of antebellum medical life that the physician who stayed too long away from home—for whatever reason—would, as one physician contemplating an absence of six months from Lowell, Massachusetts, put it, "almost entirely break up and destroy my professional interest in this city."[125] Young physicians paid some price for postponing the opening of an office and building of a practice. "It does not answer for a young physician to be long absent from home," a twenty-one-year-old Philadelphia practitioner wrote in his diary.[126] But established physicians, who knew that patients could not be relied upon to stay well in their absence, risked losing clients to competitors who stood eager to fill the gap. Some secured promises of loyalty from their patients before departing; "the families who employ me so far as I have yet consulted them offer to reëmploy me on my return," Comegys explained to a lay friend. "This is a matter of consequence," he admitted, "as I certainly would not sacrifice my business."[127] Others, such as a New York physician who wanted to study tuberculosis in Paris, took on a partner so that his practice would remain intact during his absence.[128] But there was no simple solution, and Ashbel Smith was typical in lamenting from Paris in 1832, "Were I not afraid that some one would step into my place in Salisbury [North Carolina], I would try to add a few months to my contemplated time of residing here."[129] It was not so much the expense of living in Paris as the loss of revenue from patients and the greater threat of undermining an established practice that compelled most older practitioners to settle for shorter trips to France—often months instead of years—than those their younger colleagues undertook.

Seasoned practitioners and new graduates sought similar kinds of professional improvement in Paris, principally experiential knowledge, but differences between their situations lent different casts to their motivations. One lure for both groups was the promise of adventure. For those who had already entered practice, however, the urge to travel sometimes grew not from youthful vigor but the realization that they were now harnessed to a medical life that was all too often relentless, repetitious, and exhausting. The satisfactions of a growing practice and growing family could be counterbalanced by the thought that these sturdy roots were likely to bind them to a place and to a routine they would pursue for the remainder of their lives. Settling down created a restlessness of its own. "We have a feint and distant contemplation of going to Paris together in a few years," a young physician practicing in Lowndesboro, Alabama, wrote in his diary in 1839, after receiving a letter from a former classmate who felt trapped in a rural Louisiana practice. "I have no idea of going no where out of the 'fenced ground' before I die. And live in such a large world too."[130] As it happened, he never made it to France, but for many, a journey to Paris, like a spell reattending a season of medical lectures or visiting a city hospital, provided one temporary and professionally acceptable escape.

Boredom was not the only aspect of starting practice that might lead a physician to Paris. Facing the realities of practice on their own, physicians confronted the limitations of their knowledge and abilities in a way fundamentally different from anything encountered during studentship. While some were complacent, if not smug, many physicians found this confrontation deeply disturbing. When in 1835 John Young Bassett was still attending lectures at Washington Medical College in Baltimore, a physician friend advised that "if by any favour of friendship or some new arrangement you can be examined this summer, reject the offer; aim at something higher than a mere diploma; go into the Almshouse or Hospital this summer & dont think of graduating until next spring."[131] He did graduate, though, and set up practice in Huntsville, Alabama. But far from being content, he experienced in practice a troubling realization of his responsibilities and inadequacies, and within the year Bassett set off for Paris. "Professional pride began to curdle in my stomach," he wrote in autobiographical reflections composed on shipboard, as he was returning from Europe, but then crossed the line out. "A desire to know more, to visit foreign schools & be acquainted with the great leaders in the profession took possession of me." He sought in Paris both the exhilarating sense of being in the midst of activity in medical science and a sturdier sense of professional competence. "But was I happy while in Europe?" he reflected on his return voyage. "No, & I didn't expect to be. I was not in search of happiness. I went as a pilgrim, as one doing a laborious duty."[132]

Practice, especially a country practice, could also bring the realization that opportunities for professional improvement of the sort that might bolster reputation and income had grown few. Most country practitioners were distant from medical schools and clinical institutions; but more than this, their professional routine tied them down and filled their days. Some clearly came to feel that if they were to change the prospects for their career and their family's future, they had to make some dramatic break away from that routine.

Robert Battey complained even in apprenticeship that "my time is so much occupied that I have little opportunity of gaining information except by daily practice."[133] A decade later, in 1857, with an M.D. degree in hand and established in Rome, Georgia, he again protested that there was little time he could call his own; his office was "a common rendesvous for everyone," he lamented, adding that "this feature of a country doctor's life is to me by no means pleasant and yet must be bourn as the law of custom."[134] When, several years later, he set out for Paris, Battey, like Bassett, framed his trip partly as an exercise of duty. "In my own short experience I have known what it is to feel human life leaning helplessly and even despairingly upon my feeble skill," he wrote in 1860 from Paris to his wife Martha. "Medical science has its foundations laid in *eternal truth* and if we but seek diligently the lights before us, we may enjoy the satisfaction of a daily growth in knowledge and experience—the consciousness of duty ever discharged to the best of the light given us."[135]

At the same time, Battey saw a trip to Paris as a calculated investment in his family's social and economic future. "There is obviously but one sure means of attaining such a professional status as will ensure me a handsome income for the use of our children," he wrote from France to his wife. "That means is knowledge of a superior order to that of my professional brethren—such a position will ensure me practice in the better classes of society who are able to pay promptly and able to pay also more liberal fees—it will secure me consultation practice which is more and most of all surgical practice." As he went on to explain, "You are aware that our physicians in the ordinary routine of practice can make nothing beyond a good living upon a large practice and by industrious labor—You are also aware that with our family of children to educate and settle in life—it behooves me to be making if possible something beyond a mere hand to mouth daily living—But how shall I do this? Not by working harder and riding more than they do." Articulating what many surely felt, he concluded that "there is a second inducement" for study in Paris: "I desire position—that I may be able to carry my wife and children into the front rank of society in the community in which I live—I desire to win for myself the esteem and confidence of the intelligent and cultivated that I may leave the legacy of an honorable name and worthy example for them to cherish and imitate."[136]

Physicians in city practice had equally strong if somewhat different incentives to travel. Unlike Bassett or Battey, they often had access to courses of clinical instruction; but so did their rivals. Having opened a practice, some realized just how slowly their ambitions were likely to be met in the ordinary course of things, and saw the trip to Paris, like dispensary work where they lived, as one means of accelerating their career. Comegys, having received his M.D. degree at the University of Pennsylvania, was optimistic about his prospects when in 1848 he settled in rapidly growing Cincinnati. But early in 1851 he resolved to travel to London and Paris for further study. "You will be perhaps taken by surprise by my announcing that I am making arrangements for going to Europe to spend six or seven months," he wrote to a lay friend, explaining that "the necessity of this for the proper discharge of those varied duties which I have assumed in society, I have no doubt about. Not only is this my own persuasion but also the general feeling of the profession and this is manifested by the now eminent practitioners of all city-communities having gone abroad for extended observations." He noted that competition in Cincinnati "has been brought to a very high pitch," asserting that "even the longest established and most estimable physicians have yielded a large and lucrative portions of their practice to homeopathy &c."[137] Comegys scheduled his absence during the healthy season to minimize the business he would miss, and did his best to guard his practice from competitors. He hoped that on homecoming he would stand a better chance of gaining a lucrative practice and perhaps even of filling a chair at one of the city's medical schools, a goal he achieved.[138]

Many of the practicing physicians who visited Paris, like Comegys, had not been long in practice and were finding the going difficult. Indeed, Kentucky physician Moses L. Linton, four years after receiving his M.D. from Transylvania, in 1839 used his bride's dowry to finance his trip to Paris.[139] Others left a flourishing business to embark on a journey they had longed to make for years. Augustus Henry Cenas, a New Orleans practitioner preparing to leave for France in 1830, explained to a medical friend that much earlier, when his ardent desire to study in Paris was nearly realized, "a trifling circumstance occurred to defer it—I then became entrammeled in practice, then marriage concurred to twist the chain," and it was only now, years later, "that I am able to put my wish in execution." He noted that "on reflection I am not sorry for the delay, for the length of time that I have practiced in this community has procured for me a name, and has established a kind of claim, that in the mind of the greater part of society would be greatly enhanced by a trip and sojourn of two years in Europe."[140]

For other older physicians, a trip to Paris was a professionally respectable sabbatical. Travel for health was well sanctioned by nineteenth-century medical thinking. It could be the functional equivalent of a vacation; but if combined with professional improvement, the break from practice was not only acceptable but admirable. "I am sometimes so overcome by my toils in seasons of sickness and in our summer heats as to feel that I am enjoying the Professional advantages of my situation at a very dear price," a New Orleans physician wrote to a Philadelphia medical friend. "I sometimes think it may be necessary for me after a while to relieve myself by a years absence and should it prove so I shall certainly put to the test your encomiums on Paris."[141] After the medical school in Davenport, Iowa, at which he was teaching was reorganized in 1851, Chandler B. Chapman took advantage of the career break to travel to Paris, partly to gain experience that he would put to use after his return by founding the Practical School for Anatomy in Madison, Wisconsin. But before deciding to go, he sought the advice of friends. "As regards your Tour to Europe," one wrote back, "my opinion is, the professional knowledge you would gain would not amount to much. I never have known anyone to come home from Europe much wiser than they were before they went professionally." But he urged that "if you have the means to spare, and can leave home, the time spent in traveling you never will regret. You would return home and enter your profession with double vigor."[142]

A good number of American physicians did make the trip as a kind of sabbatical, some engaging in serious study and some simply touring the famous medical sights.[143] Returning in 1856, Albany medical professor Alden March described his journey to a Boston medical editor as "a four months tour, through parts of France, Italy, Austria, Russia, Germany, Holland, England, and Scotland, which I was inclined to take with a view to improve my some what impaired health, by relaxation for a while from active and laborious professional life; and for general observation & improvement in the practical department of our profession." He proudly reported having traveled 11,580 miles in four months, "yet I made it my business to visit most of the medical institutions, Hospitals & Museums."[144]

For nearly all the American physicians who went to Paris, the journey was a special event, accorded an important place in their private and professional identity and routinely mentioned by their biographers. But as a step in professional improvement, study in Paris was imbedded in a process of medical education extended over years, not a discrete and routinized program of postgraduate education of a sort familiar to later generations.

The case of Anson Colman offers one concrete illustration of how deeply intertwined efforts at professional improvement—including study in Paris—were with practice as a physician. Colman was born in 1795 in Richfield Springs, New York, where he began medical apprenticeship at the age of seventeen. Around 1817 he attended lectures at the Fairfield Medical School in New York State, and with another of his preceptor's students he opened a copartnership in the town of Rochesterville, then a village of something over a thousand people that would later be known as Rochester.[145] Two years later he married a daughter of the town's founder and namesake, and the next few years brought practice, children, and participation in such projects as the organization of a county medical society. Then in the winter of 1824, six years after he had begun practicing medicine, Colman departed for Boston to attend another course of lectures. In a mode commonplace among physicians away for professional improvement—within the United States or abroad—his first letter reassured his wife, Catherine Colman, that he had seen nearly nothing of the city, his time being devoted entirely to medical studies. "The descriptions which I am able to give of Boston & its inhabitants must be very imperfect, for in truth, except Lectures, Hospitals, & operations, the sum total of all my knowledge is not worth relating," he wrote early in December, noting that "I find the advantages of the Boston Medical School & Hospital surpassing my most sanguine expectations."[146]

During the winter term, Anson and Catherine followed a pattern reproduced again and again by physicians studying in Paris and spouses left at home: they chided each other for not writing more often, reassured each other of their affection, and reaffirmed that the separation was a personal sacrifice made to advance professional interests on which their family's future depended. "I find that you are even more negligent than I am; else how could I be so often disappointed when I most expect & most need some token of remembrance from my dear Wife," Anson wrote to Catherine in mid-January. "You are situated in the very focus of all that is most interesting to me & have time to give full detail to the passing events. My situation is the very opposite; although situated in a delightful City with every thing around me which can conduce either to Professional attainments or Literary pleasures yet the mind unconsciously steals away even from these &[,] as if intent on indulging in thought more pure[,] contemplates with intense interest female worth, infant innocence, connubial bliss—But enough of this. I can when other objects are to be attained sacrifice present happiness to future & more permanent enjoyments."[147] Catherine replied, "Were it not for the hope I indulge of your future advancement in your profession, by attending strictly to your present advantages, and a belief that you are wholly occupied by the objects of your visit, I should be tempted to complain, and reject calm resignation to such apparent neglect. Do you know you left home two months ago and have not devoted your pen more than two hours to your wife[?]" She dismissed Anson's excuse for short letters, one physicians away from home commonly invoked, that he could write little that would have meaning for her because his mind was absorbed with medicine. "If you cannot spend time to gratify this native quality of the mind or do not feel willing to bring your mind and pen down to the capacity of a female *perhaps* that female taste and comprehension can *rise* to those subjects more congenial with your own," Catherine pointedly replied. "At all events she will try the experiment if you will write for her improvement, and fill your letters with something let the subjects be what they will, (those connected with your profession if you choose, Anatomy, Surgery, medical Jurisprudence or Chemistry, (you will now laugh). While writing on this subject let me remind you of an opinion you once gave in favor of females, which was that you believed they possessed capacities for intellectual improvement fully equal to the other sex."[148]

Anson returned to his family and practice at the end of term, then six years later, in 1831, again went east to attend lectures. He first visited New York, touring hospitals and taking in the opening lecture at a medical college, then proceeded to Philadelphia. Impressed by the vast scale of medical student culture in Philadelphia, he noted too that the older students, those already established in practice, naturally gravitated toward one another. "Students resort here from every part of America," he wrote Catherine in November, "many of whom are indicated by their premature gray locks and weatherbeaten features belong to the list of practitioners." He again pointed out how hard he was working, commenting that transcribing lecture notes in the evenings "makes my nights not much less laborious than the days," and cautioned Catherine not to expect him home between Christmas and New Year "unless the Professors should adjourn during that time; for whatever is going on at the medical Institutions here it is my determination to be present to witness."[149] By this point his ambition to study in Paris was clear, and he had found lodging with a French family, "rendering me every possible facility in acquiring a correct pronunciation of the french language." But his sense of isolation, he assured Catherine, was only intensified by the experience of hearing a foreign language spoken around him. "Here no wife, nor daughters, nor dear & sprightly boy are seen or heard—All, all are far away."[150]

At the end of the winter term Anson returned home, but in less than a year, in November 1833, he left for Europe, where he would visit both Paris and London. More perhaps than his studies in Boston and Philadelphia, his spending months alone in Paris seriously concerned his family. "I cordially unite with you my dear daughter in supplication and intercession to the great preserver of men," Anson's father wrote to Catherine, "that the same almighty power which could preserve a Joseph uncontaminated in the licentious court of Egypt, a Daniel and other pious Jews not only amidst the luxury and profligacy of a heathen court but in the den of the hungry and ferocious lions and in the midst of the heated furnace may be exerted to shield protect and preserve our friend incorruptible and uncontaminated in the midst of the luxury profligacy and infidelity that abounds in the metropolis of France." Skeptical that professional improvement warranted such risks, he concluded with the hope "that the same kind of providence may return him to his family and friends 'in health & purity of life' and that he may have no cause to regret the time and expense in acquiring professional science and that he will hereafter spend his days in domestic and professional duties."[151]

By now, for Catherine and Anson alike, the pattern of separation in the interests of his professional improvement was very familiar, though this trip would be twice as long as his earlier tours of study, some eight months. "Since I reached Paris I have been too much occupied to find time to write concerning any thing, not immediately connected with my Profession—Nor is it likely that during the few months alloted to my stay here I shall be able to be more punctual," he told Catherine in his first letter from Paris. His time in American cities had not entirely prepared him for the French capital, which he described as a "world *in* and *of* itself—This accumulation of every thing that is magnificent or mean—That is exaulted in intellect and refinement, or that is grovling, brutish, abandoned. In short of the widest extremes in every thing, daily and hourly, passing in rapid succession around the amazed beholder." But he dwelled on the professional advantages, which "more than equal my most sanguine expectations—In Surgury, in anatomy, diseases of the chest and of the Skin—In diseases & operations upon the eyes; in the various grades of venereal affections & in difficult obstetrical operations they are immense."[152] Catherine found the longer separation more difficult. She had thought she was pregnant again, but was not; as she wrote three months after his departure, "I have not had my monthly evacuation since you left—but *am not in the family way*." She proposed joining him in Paris and had put together enough funds to pay for the journey, but nothing came of that plan.[153] Anson returned to his family in July 1833, ready to enjoy the return on nearly two decades invested in his profession; he died from an aortic aneurism four years later, at the age of forty-two.

What fresh graduates and older practitioners generally shared was the perception that access to practical experience was the main reason to travel to France. A much smaller number of physicians, though, went to Europe for access of a different kind, access not to experiential knowledge but to anatomical models, pathological specimens, books, and instruments, which would enhance the facilities of the American schools they represented. These medical professors, traveling on their own initiative or, more often, sent by their school, usually stayed only a few months. Yet because they tended to be particularly vocal in relating what they had seen, their perceptions of the Parisian medical world were inordinately visible to the American medical profession. As professors, they had easy access to the lectern and to the pages of medical journals. More than this, telling others about their trip drew attention to both their professional stature and the purposes of their journey. Attracting notice to the tools of professional improvement they had brought back with them— specimens for a teaching museum, for example—advertised their school's pedagogic commitment and superior facilities. In the overcrowded marketplace, competition among schools for paying pupils was as vigorous as competition among practitioners for patients, and a trip to Paris was seen as a way to strengthen the reputation of practitioner and school alike.

Taking a step repeated at medical schools across the United States, the trustees of the Medical College of Ohio resolved around 1829 that "the best method of promoting the interests of the College was, that some individual well acquainted with its wants, should proceed to Europe, & having ascertained what articles might be purchased, to make such a selection as he thought proper." Together, the trustees and the faculty assembled a catalog of books, preparations, instruments, engravings, and wax models that they believed would help draw students away from the school's rivals, and selected an emissary to fulfill the commission.[154] Similarly, when in 1855 Henry H. Smith was appointed to the chair of surgery at the University of Pennsylvania, before lectures began he spent the summer in London and Paris, where he had studied for two years a decade and a half earlier, "to make every arrangement for obtaining a proper Cabinet to illustrate the surgical lectures," as he told another faculty member.[155]

Those who embarked on such a journey made sure their visit to Paris became widely known. After his return to Philadelphia, Smith's first performance as a new professor was an introductory address on "this tour of observation" in which he described medical Paris and told pupils about the cabinet of specimens he had assembled "for your benefit."[156] Students were made aware of not only their professor's absence but the aims of the trip. When Charles Caldwell was sent to collect a library for the newly established medical department of Transylvania University in 1821, a medical student wrote to his brother, "Dr Caldwell left for Europe on Monday[.] He goes to Europe for a three fold purpose to buy a library for the Medical Colledge, for his own improvement, and to visit the most important medical schools there, that he may be enabled the better to establish the school here."[157] Nearly eight months later he would again write that while Caldwell, expected soon, was still abroad, "1200 volumes of books, part of his purchase have arrived, and some very valuable apparatus for Chemical department."[158] Similarly, when Erasmus Darwin Fenner set off for Europe in 1859 to tour hospitals, in part to find models of clinical instruction to emulate at his New Orleans School of Medicine, his departure and aims were duly announced in the *New Orleans Medical News and Hospital Gazette*, that school's journal.[159]

Like travel for the improvement of the individual physician, a trip to Paris for the improvement of a medical school often is best understood in the context of the shortcomings that placed the school at a competitive disadvantage vis-à-vis its rivals. Just as some country practitioners regretted their relatively slim facilities for gaining extensive experience, so the faculty members of schools located in smaller towns were aware that they lacked the large clinical facilities and access to anatomical material city schools often boasted. When in 1839 the Faculty of Transylvania University sent Robert Peter to Paris, they were responding to the bitter rivalry between their Lexington school and the one nearby in Louisville. Fearful of losing the school's leading professor, the surgeon Benjamin Winslow Dudley, to the larger city of Louisville, one faculty member confided to his brother in 1836, "Should anything ever induce him to desert its fortune, it will be the difficulty which he experiences here of procuring subjects for anatomical demonstrations." He acknowledged that "this is in fact the weak point of our school and although we have very cautiously endeavored to keep the secret to ourselves yet it is beginning to appear to our disadvantage, especially in the eyes of those students who attend lectures here and in the Eastern schools." He went on to explain that "the limited population of this place, scarcely amounting to 6000[,] the extreme caution observed in the burial even of the black, the universal repugnance felt by the entire community against disinterments are among the causes which tend to embarrass the anatomical teachings of our school," adding, "It is this alone, I am sure, which would ever induce Dr. Dudley to leave us."[160]

When Robert Peter left for Paris in 1839 to collect "books apparatus and anatomical articles," then, it was to shore up Transylvania's weaknesses in the face of threatening competition.[161] "Our Med. school is in reality the second in standing in the Union," Peter boasted to his wife as he was about to sail for Europe.[162] By obtaining anatomical and pathological specimens in London and Paris, Peter hoped to compensate for the more intractable shortage of dissection material at Transylvania. Once in the French capital, of course, Peter found time for himself. Although early in his stay he would complain that "we have been engaged, the whole of our time, in business up to our ears," with that done, as he told his wife, "we shall now have some breathing time—or at least some time to see what is visible in Paris," and Peter would give himself over to a fuller exploration of medical Paris.[163]

## WHY NOT LONDON?

But again, why *Paris*? Why did American physicians bent on professional improvement abroad elect to go there in greater numbers and for longer stays than to the other cities they commonly visited, such as Edinburgh, Dublin, London, Heidelberg, Berlin, Vienna, Florence, and Rome? One way of isolating what was *singular* about the attraction of Paris is to turn the problem on its head and ask why American doctors generally decided against making some other city their principal destination. Why, in particular, not London? After all, most Americans included London on their medical itinerary abroad. Their stay there was by comparison brief and most gave the lion's share of their time to study in Paris. But in sorting out their options, they often wrote in their diaries and letters explicitly comparing the relative advantages of London and Paris, revealing in the process underlying assumptions about what made medical Paris exceptional as an educational emporium.[164]

Why, then, did Americans so consistently elect Paris over London as a place for medical study? In the extant historical literature the answer is regarded as obvious. Paris led the world in medical science, and therefore it was only natural that medical students should prefer it to London. Richard Shryock, expressing a view historians have almost uniformly shared, confidently asserted that the influx of foreign students into Paris should be ascribed to "the scientific supremacy of the French metropolis," and assumed that the migration of medical students to a particular center is a reliable index of its intellectual vitality. As Shryock wrote of American students, "Their presence in large numbers had long been an excellent test of the quality of such centers. Leyden, Edinburgh and London had been recognized in turn, before the work of Louis and Bichat brought Americans rather suddenly to Paris. Another generation would see them in Berlin, Munich and Vienna."[165]

In fact, however, there is surprisingly little evidence that would support this interpretation of the impressive shifts in migration. If we focus on what Americans valued about studying in London and Paris while in their midst, rather than relying on later recollections of these European experiences, it becomes clear that "the scientific supremacy" of France over England was not the most crucial consideration informing their choices about where to study. Instead, the most decisive factor was access to practical experience. What led Americans to chose Paris over London was the social structure of Parisian medical education more than the intellectual vibrancy of the Paris School, and, in turn, deficits in the social structure of London medical education far more than in the intellectual character of English medicine.

Americans who visited London between the 1810s and 1850s were dazzled by the medical world they found, both by its institutions and by the figures who peopled them. The great hospitals were far more expansive than anything in the United States, and Guy's, St. Bartholomew's, and St. Thomas's often elicited admiration every bit as awed as that lavished on La Pitié, La Charité, or Hôtel Dieu. Americans also reported with delight on the meetings of medical and scientific societies, where papers were read in their native tongue, and usually judged London's medical museums to be unrivaled. Henry Smith told his medical class at the University of Pennsylvania in 1855 that "in the elegant museums attached to their institutions, London surpasses both Paris and the United States."[166]

At the same time, American doctors in London were charmed by the great physicians and surgeons, men whose names were as prominent in the American medical literature as those of the Parisian stars, and whose minds Ameri-

cans gauged of equal caliber. "When ushered into the presence of the renowned, living representatives of HUNTER, COOPER, KEY, LISTON, and a host of
others, whose fame knows no limits but those of civilization, and no end but
the end of time," one doctor wrote home, "you can easily imagine that a modest man like myself experienced a feeling of extraordinary humiliation!" He
went on to say that "with time and observation this embarrassing spell happily
vanished,"[167] but other Americans insisted that English clinicians were the
finest in Europe. "While the London schools can boast of such enlightened
practitioners and teachers as Lawrence, Liston, Johnson, Blundell and Clark,
and can exhibit such examples of erudition and research as appear in Owen,
Willis and South," Joshua Flint, just returned from Europe, told students in
Louisville in 1838, "they will offer attractions to the medical student or traveller, unequalled by those of any similar institutions, on the other side of the
channel."[168] Americans relished the experience of walking the wards with the
famous London clinicians, attending their lectures, and witnessing their surgical operations. As portrayed in American accounts, in other words, its facilities, talent, and medical culture made London a serious rival to Paris.

More than this, visitors spelled out a whole host of reasons rooted in shared
culture and values as to why American students should prefer London over
Paris. Most obvious was a shared language. Many Americans arrived in Paris
knowing little French, and while most engaged a language tutor shortly after
arrival, as one American explained, "three or four months of one's time is
almost lost, which in England would be well employed."[169] Further, most antebellum physicians traced their professional heritage to Britain. A young South
Carolina physician who had devoted almost two years to study in Paris was
typical in insisting that he wanted to spend a few weeks touring London, Dublin, and Edinburgh before his return voyage, explaining in 1855 to his brother,
"I am unwilling to leave Europe without having seen the Hospitals and sights
of those cities, for you know that our Medical notions in America with some
few exceptions are taken from the English British Authors."[170]

Americans also dwelled on a shared Anglo-American morality. London was
regarded as a source of moral danger, doubly stigmatized by American suspicion of all large cities and by an overarching conviction that the Old World was
corrupt.[171] But most American physicians insisted that compared with France,
England could be relied upon for moral propriety, religious virtue, and relatively few temptations. "After considerable enquiry and no small opportunities
of acquainting myself with the subject, I am satisfied that this is one of the
most, if not *the most* sensual and thoroughly seductive city of either *ancient* or
*modern* times," one American doctor wrote from Paris. Shocked by what he
found there after visiting London, he affirmed that "those across the channel,
who speak our language, present a most striking contrast," and went on to say
that "I now see that the contempt which the English feel towards the French is
not altogether founded upon national jealousy. The two nations are separated,
morally, as far as the poles."[172]

American observers nearly all agreed, moreover, that the English surpassed
the French as healers. "As Englishmen," one St. Louis physician noted, "they

exhibit more common sense in their work than is seen among the more brilliant and perhaps more erudite men of the Continent."[173] Americans, of course, were confident that they were yet again better healers than the English, but English practice gave London the upper hand over Paris. Having spent eighteen months studying in the Paris hospitals, Joynes wrote in 1841 to his father in Virginia that a brief study tour in London would help "to correct the errors (if such there be) which the observation of the French method of practice may have instilled into my mind," and went on to explain that "in America, the English practice is looked upon much more favorably than the French, and as more nearly resembling our own."[174]

The legacy of imperialist exploitation that had provoked the American Revolution, on the other hand, left many Americans with a particular resentment against the English and bond with the French that persisted well past midcentury. Livid at British insistence on the right to stop and search American vessels, Joynes wrote in 1842 to his brother from Paris that "I long to see that intolerable arrogance & grasping avidity which distinguish the policy of Great Britain chased & humbled & nothing would delight me so much as a union of our Navy with that of France to give her a good sound beating." As he observed, "The French would be delighted to have an opportunity of 'bringing England's nose to the grindstone,' and it is to the United States that they look as their natural ally in such an enterprise."[175] None of the symbolism was lost on a doctor from Georgia who, in 1829, celebrated the 4th of July in Paris at a dinner presided over by General Lafayette that culminated in a ritual reading of the Declaration of Independence of the United States of America.[176]

In London, Americans were on the lookout for examples of English arrogance, condescension, and pomposity, and found plenty to write home about. Angered by the way British newspapers had reported on an address by the president of the United States, one American physician speculated that "nine tenths of the Editors have not read the message, but only abuse it because they are wont to abuse and oppose everything which is American."[177] In turn, Americans relished occasions to vent their annoyance by disparaging the more blatant shortfalls of British life: English climate and English food provided particularly easy targets. One Philadelphia physician, whose studies in France had already made him a disciple of the Paris School, found little to praise in England: "The atmosphere, physical and intellectual of the country," he wrote from London, "have reduced my poor brain, I sometimes think, to a condition but little differing from wet wool."[178]

Yet often Americans were surprised by what they found in London. "As you know I left N.Y. with strong prejudices against the English," John Stevenson wrote to his preceptor in 1818. "I expected to have been harassed, insulted, to have met all cold inhospitable, people climate and in short everything that was bad—but I found much on the contrary."[179] As an American physician who had just crossed from England to France wrote to another still in London, "Short and *prejudiced* as was my visit to England I look back upon those few days with high gratification.—My opinion of England & Englishmen is much more favorable than formerly.—And tho I cannot forget the wrongs our country has suffered at their hands, I trust it will not render me unwilling to acknowledge frankly all the good qualities I find the English possessed of."[180] However ambivalent Americans were toward their English heritage, cultural ties remained strong, and medical Americans still craved English approval and recognition.

Taken collectively, the travels of American doctors to London resembled a pilgrim's act of filial piety or a visit paid to an ancestral Home. They went seeking evidence of their profession's past as much as guidance for its future. London, one American medical visitor noted, "has been the theatre of action of the remarkable names that adorn the history of our noble science," and went on to report that "when I, for the first time, traversed the courts, museums, wards and operating rooms of those majestic hospitals, I felt that I was treading upon consecrated ground."[181] A Harvard medical professor, addressing the class in 1850, urged that every American who traveled abroad to study medicine should spend at least some time visiting "the land of his ancestors."[182]

The majority visited London as medical tourists. Accordingly, one physician writing home that he had seen Guy's and St. Thomas's reported in the same sentence on his visits to St. Paul's and the Tower.[183] Another, who spent sixteen days in London in 1847, recorded in his diary that on Wednesday he went to Westminster Hospital, Thursday to St. George's, Friday to St. Bartholomew's, and Saturday to King's College Hospital. The following week, before departing for Paris, he crowded in visits to University College Hospital and the museum of the Royal College of Surgeons.[184] Americans wanted to return home able to say they had seen the distinguished men and famous hospitals. As the Harvard medical professor James Jackson, Sr., advised his son, "It is well to see enough to talk about them—but more than [this] I shd not care for."[185]

Why, though, did most so briskly move along to Paris? The reports these American tourists made of medical London—its institutions, clinicians, and scientific culture—were remarkably favorable. And they made a good case for why the American student might actually be better off in London. Some invidious comparisons of English with French medical science were voiced as well: "As to the science of England and France, or rather Paris and London," Oliver Wendell Holmes wrote from Paris in 1833, "the Frenchmen have half a century in advance."[186] But this perception of the superior state of French medical science was *not* often cited by Americans at the time as a decisive reason to prefer study in Paris. Other things being equal, the advantages of a shared Anglo-American culture, language, and values should have tipped the balance in favor of London. Yet, overwhelmingly, Americans elected to study in Paris instead.

The single element pervasive in American accounts of Paris yet consistently missing from accounts of London was enthusiasm about free access to medical facilities and instruction. In Paris, the Philadelphia surgeon William Gibson reported after studying there in 1839, "the student revels from dawn to sunset, and, if he please, throughout the night, among lectures, dissections, demonstrations and preparations, until he is stuffed, crammed, and saturated with knowledge to such extent, as to leave no room for additional supply."[187] Comparable outpourings of enthusiasm by Americans in London are extraordinarily rare. "Above all," he concluded—explaining why medical Americans "should, almost to a man, take up their quarters, exclusively, in the French metropolis, and never think, afterwards of attending the lectures and walking the rounds of the English, Scotch, and Irish colleges and hospitals"—"I found that the regular course of lectures in the different hospitals and institutions, by men of the first eminence, were paid for by government, and *gratuitous*, as respected the pupil."[188]

Gibson's closing point—that the official course of instruction in the hospital wards and lecture halls of Paris came free of cost to foreigners—was one that American observers made persistently and emphatically. "We are under the special protection of the Government & the doors of establishments are open to us into which a native can not easily gain admission," Charles Jackson wrote from Paris to his sister in 1832. "This hospitality grew out of the policy of the great Napoleon who saw the advantages that would accrue to his Capital by encouraging the admiration of foreigners."[189] Such access to instruction without fees stood in bold contrast to the reigning perception of London. Commenting on the grim prospects of London for the medical student, one American physician wrote home in 1853, "The great expense attendant upon educating them in any part of Great Britain, is sufficient to keep all away from there," adding that "it is well so, for the climate would destroy a large percent."[190]

It was *access* more than scientific brilliance that chiefly decided Americans on the French over the British capital. Anatomy offered the most obvious example of restrictions on access in London, for the limited supply of cadavers was notorious and remained so long after passage of the Anatomy Act in 1832. "As for anatomical facilities, there is not a medical school, in any village in the United States, however small, which does not afford subjects for dissection cheaper and in great[er] abundance than either King's College, or University College, or any other College in London," one American wrote home in 1848. Comparing the experience of London students with his own recent experiences in Paris, he noted that "for what they were paying for a single lower extremity in London, they might have dissected in Paris, from the first of November to the middle of April, . . . and had their knives regularly sharpened into the bargain."[191] In Paris, government policies ensured a steady supply of bodies from the hospitals to the anatomy rooms.

Yet what principally drew Americans across the Atlantic was access to instruction from the living body at the bedside. It was a persistent source of wonderment to American physicians visiting Paris that they needed only show their diploma or passport in order to have a vast program of clinical instruction open up to them. In London, on the contrary, they found bedside instruction highly restricted, cursory, and exorbitantly expensive. "At Paris, I may follow 3 or 4 Hosp., at each having the same class of diseases grouped together[,] for 1/4 the money that it will cost me to be admitted to Guy's alone," one Bostonian wrote from London.[192] "What, in reality, are the hospital advantages of

London?" David Yandell asked rhetorically in a letter published in the *Western Journal of Medicine and Surgery*. "Great, very great. In comparison with those of Paris? Small, very small." He counseled American readers that "the attendance upon one single course of lectures in any one of the schools and any one of the hospitals, in London, will cost more than attendance during four years upon the lectures of eighteen professors and twelve hospitals in Paris."[193] And, as Yandell recalled of his attempt to follow Liston at University College Hospital, "it was not long before I began to experience that there was something wanting—that there were too many students about the beds of the patients; that I saw disease, but could neither feel [n]or hear disease; in a word, that my opportunities carried me to a certain point and there stopped."[194]

Americans also complained in Paris that the clinical lectures so freely open to them were woefully crowded, and that they had trouble understanding lectures delivered in rapid French. But it was not this official program of instruction by the famous professors but rather *paid private* clinical instruction that they principally relied upon. As chapter 3 will show, despite the social and intellectual transformations that marked French medicine between the 1810s and the 1850s, throughout this period it was such private tutelage that most powerfully attracted American doctors to Paris.

It might seem paradoxical that Americans dwelled so earnestly on the cost of clinical education in London when in fact they expected to pay for much of the instruction they received in Paris. This can be explained partly by the modest cost of clinical classes in France. But money was not the key issue, and in American rhetoric the *expense* of London medical education served an important symbolic function. What Americans saw as the mercenary ethos of the London hospital elite represented deeper flaws in the value system that underlay English medical education. As Jackson, Jr., complained in a letter home, "At Paris I am to study under the influence of men whose aim is *science*—at London, *gain*."[195]

Even if London had facilities that in some ways rivaled those of Paris, English medical polity, as Americans viewed it, fostered a closed rather than open system. The Paris hospitals were funded and controlled by the government, which employed clinicians to attend patients and teach and promoted access to the bodies of the sick and to their remains after death. By contrast, the London hospitals were private charitable institutions with lay boards of governors that vested medical control in a small number of socially elite physicians and surgeons. These practitioners tended to see the hospital as their private domain, guarding against poachers their privileged access to patients for teaching (a source of income) and for research (a source of eminence). "The American physician who arrives in London," Chandler Chapman warned after visiting both cities, "may be greatly disappointed. . . . The hospitals of London are well calculated to answer the end for which they were created, viz., to afford a temporary home for the sick poor, *and to get a great name* for the favored ones who have charge of them."[196] Charles Jackson wrote to his sister after crossing the Channel from Paris, "I do not care much about remaining longer in London than is necessary. I do not like the character of John Bull & moreover all their Institutions require the Golden Key whereas in France everything is free."[197]

The system of making appointments at the London hospitals embodied the mercenary, monopolistic ethos that, to American eyes, devalued the educational worth of that city's medical institutions. In Paris, as Americans noted, the appointment of clinical professors and *internes* was determined by *concours*, a democratic system of competitive examinations that tested merit. In London, by contrast, American observers asserted that more often than not, clinical appointments for students were sold as part of a lucrative enterprise. "The offices of dresser, house-surgeon and clerk, in some hospitals, are obtained by purchase," Yandell observed. "In Guy's hospital a dressership costs two hundred and fifty dollars per annum; in the London Hospital it commands one hundred and fifty dollars, as is also the case in the Middlesex Hospital."[198] Just as Americans pointed to *concours* as testimony to a French system that, whatever its imperfections, harmonized with meritocratic ideals, so they deplored the social and medical consequences of the English value system that gave hospital experience only to those who could pay.

The world of London medical education, then, as Americans depicted it, was a closed system, opened only a little by money or special favor. In 1837, as recorded in their minute book, the faculty of the Medical College at St. Bartholomew's Hospital "resolved to exclude strangers from attending the rounds and operations without permission, as such interfered with the comfort of regular students":[199] Americans saw clearly how this kind of attitude affected them. They recognized that the success of a medical visit to London depended upon the letters of introduction they could bring with them, but that in Paris such introductions were unnecessary, for admission to its medical world came by entitlement.[200] As Holmes wrote from London in 1834, "Without the personal interest of somebody it is impossible to see anything in this country."[201] Americans wrote proudly of a ward tour with Sir Benjamin Brodie or a breakfast with Sir Astley Cooper. The "professional gentlemen connected with the hospital[s], seem indefatigable in their attentions to visiters," one Boston physician reported from London in 1850. "This is gratifying to the tourist, whose very minutes must be economically expended." Yet the needs of the medical tourist were not those of the serious student; and the same physician went on to conclude that going to England for medical *study* was "preposterous."[202] One additional complaint about the London hospitals was that the patients were not French. In Paris, American students delighted in the assumption that the sick were there to be studied. By contrast, as Jackson, Jr., complained at Guy's, "The patients are Englishmen, & will not very readily submit to those in authority."[203]

It was precisely the kind of access to experiential knowledge afforded by private clinical instruction in Paris that was so persistently missing from American accounts of London. They could follow the ward rounds of the great clinicians but could not expect individualized bedside instruction from such important figures. The rules that governed private instruction in the London hospitals deserve closer historical study than they have received, as do the socioeconomic differences between lower-level clinical attendants in London, who often had to purchase their position, and Paris *internes*, who won theirs through *concours* (and who, Americans believed, often needed the modest sums they earned by private teaching). What is clear enough, however, is that if dressers and ward clerks in London regularly offered the kind of unofficial, private bedside instruction given by *internes* and *agrégés* in Paris, Americans showed little awareness of it.

The contrast between London and Paris is exemplified by the experience of Jackson, Jr. When in 1832 Jackson interrupted his studies in Paris to spend six months in London, forced there by his father's belief that in England there would be less danger from cholera, he complained bitterly that even though letters of introduction won him entrance to the hospitals, it was impossible there "to study *disease*, comme il faut." Instead of examining patients at the bedside and dissecting table, as he had in Paris, Jackson spent most of his time examining preserved pathological specimens at the museums of Guy's and the Royal College of Surgeons. He did learn there from the body, but the mediation between observer and disease was all too apparent. The single experience in London he valued most was the opportunity to study the pathologist Robert Carswell's colored pictures—visual representations of pathoanatomical lesions Carswell had prepared in Paris. The irony was not lost on Jackson. Nor was its message: however grand the hospitals of London, and however imposing its clinicians, that city did not afford the same access to the body Americans so celebrated in Paris.[204] To a striking extent, the comparisons American observers made between London and Paris were seconded by *English* observers, especially those reformers discussed in chapter 6. As one English critic charged in 1835, echoing Jackson's complaints, "While the French physician is pursuing science, the English physician is hunting fees."[205]

American doctors went to Paris primarily for experiential knowledge, but after returning they more ardently told a story of the French empiricist departure that became the linchpin in their program to reform American medicine. With this shift in storytelling about Paris came a new story about London. In order to mount their crusade against rationalism, they first needed to reconstruct medical history to create its dominance, and in this project British medicine provided the necessary foil. It was not London, known as a place where students learned by walking the wards, but rather Edinburgh that was widely identified with rationalistic systems; yet in reform polemics, the distinction between Scottish medicine and English medicine was easily blurred. What emerged was a wider demonization of British medicine as a bastion of the rationalism reformers held responsible for many of the American profession's ills.

Occasionally American physicians still abroad spoke of their abhorrence for the rationalistic bent of British medicine. "I can't express to you the low esteem in wh. I hold the English as Pathologists, as Men *who really know and understand the nature of Disease*," Jackson, Jr., wrote his father from Paris in 1833, having returned there after his stay in London. He was particularly incensed over a book by his medical host in London, Francis Boott, "in wh. he attempts to support a priori opinions by badly observed & half-proven facts." Holding Boott's epistemological misdeeds to be typically British, Jackson went on to denounce all "the London wld-be Pathologists."[206] From Philadelphia, Alfred Stillé wrote in 1843 to Shattuck in Boston about a new treatise by William Prout on the stomach and renal diseases, describing it as "a valuable work" but "overrun with those absurd hypotheses which an English medical Author seems to consider essential to the completeness of his work." Shattuck, who, like Stillé, had become a devoted disciple of Paris medicine a decade earlier, would have approved of Stillé's conclusion that "the English are wonderful metaphysicians."[207]

Those American doctors who had studied in Paris and consecrated themselves to French ideals sometimes were critical of English medical science when they visited London. But it was after they returned home that invidious contrasts between the intellectual characters of English and French medicine became commonplace and shrill. The social structure of English medical education not only led Americans to prefer Paris over London as a place to study but, by fostering that choice, fundamentally informed the way Americans came to depict the intellectual character of English medicine.

Over time this story of English stagnation and French vitality influenced other Americans setting off for medical study abroad. And certainly it is *this* contrast between London and Paris that has most captured the attention of historians. But if we look at how Americans abroad *at the time* compared London with Paris, not at the retrospective representations that American disciples of the Paris School created partly for their own polemical purposes, it becomes clear that the intellectual character of English medicine had relatively little to do with their decisions about where to study. Even Pierre Louis, who came to emblemize for his American disciples the chief achievement of French medicine—its empiricist departure—was sought by Americans in the first instance as a conduit to practical experience in the clinic, not as a sage mentor investigating at the cutting edge. The migration of American physicians to Paris was testimony above all not to the intellectual vibrancy of Paris medicine but to realities of access.

# Errand to Paris

"To delineate the localities I have visited, and describe the emotion I have felt," Ashbel Smith, newly arrived in Paris in the winter of 1832, wrote home to North Carolina, "would be to write an enormous book—which nobody would read."[1] Smith was right on both counts. To map the Parisian medical world even at a single moment in time was a daunting task; Heinrich Ludwig Meding's two-volume *Paris médical: vade-mecum des médecins étrangers* (1852–1853) ran to over nine hundred pages, and it said nothing about how the territory it charted was perceived or experienced by foreign students.[2]

This chapter sketches in broad strokes what it was like for an antebellum American to make a tour of professional improvement to Paris. As a Charleston physician studying in Paris in 1852 wrote in his diary, "As this is not a Guide Book, I have no idea of forcing myself into minutiae."[3] By identifying patterns in the diverse ways Americans pursued study abroad, however, one can begin to see what, collectively, they most valued. Medical study was also imbedded within a wider matrix of the mundane and exhilarating social realities of life in Paris, and that broader context matters in understanding what the journey meant to an American physician. Subsequent chapters explore the ways Americans perceived the methods, ideas, institutions, practices, and values of French medicine; how they sought selectively to transport these elements to their own country; and the meaning they found in them for American medicine. Here, the aim is to unfold the experiential basis for American representations of the Paris School.

## PASSAGE TO FRANCE

"I leave home to day & for a very long absence," George Cheyne Shattuck, Jr., wrote in his diary in April 1836, ready to set sail for France, where he would spend the next four years. "The future is unknown but I must press on to meet it & then trust to God." The twenty-two-year-old son of one of Boston's most eminent physicians, Shattuck had just received his M.D. from Harvard. "I think I can say that I am not seeking my own immediate gratification & pleasure in my proposed enterprise & should prefer to settle down at home, & enjoy the good which a kind providence has assigned me." Having been given a bon voyage party two days earlier by another Boston physician and having said his farewells, Shattuck wrote as a benediction on his journey: "May I feel deeply that my opportunities are great blessings for the use of which I shall be deeply responsible."[4]

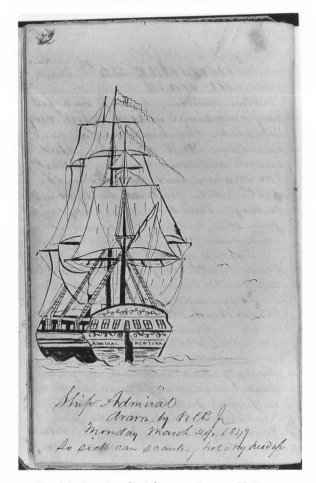

Fig. 3.1. Crossing the Atlantic to Paris in 1847, one
American sketched his own vessel, the *Admiral*, onto a
page of his diary, which recorded daily life on shipboard.
(William E. Bartlett, Jr., Travel Journal, 1847, MS 2511,
entry for 26 Mar. 1847, courtesy of Manuscripts Division,
Maryland Historical Society Library, Baltimore.)

The voyage across the Atlantic by sail could be trying. Bad weather could
mean days waiting in port to depart, while the crossing itself took from a couple of weeks to a couple of months. Steamships came to offer a faster alternative, though initially there was reason to worry that safety was traded for the
faster journey. In 1839, for example, Robert Peter found his desire to return
from Paris by steam at odds with his wife's concern for his well-being. "Let us
sum up this part of the argument by supposing (what is not true) that the
steam is twice as dangerous as the sail vessel.—eh bien! The steamer crosses in
13, 15, or 19 days in all weather—The sail vessel goes to America, which is

always the long passage, in 24, 30, 40, or 60 or even 90 days." Thus, reaching the conclusion he wanted, "the sail vessel is 3 *times as long* as the steamer, in making the passage—and, consequently the danger is greater on the sail vessel."[5] Through the 1850s some Americans chose a slower sailing vessel "in preference to steaming it."[6] By that decade, though, an eleven-day crossing like the one Gabriel Manigault made in 1854 on the Cunard steamer *Europa* was not uncommon.[7] Steam travel made the journey less arduous and encouraged the growing number of Americans who went to Paris in the 1840s and 1850s.

Most travelers set out on their voyage alone. Morton Waring boarded his ship for Le Havre at ten o'clock at night: "I sailed from Charleston So Ca on the 1st of June 1856," he wrote in his diary; "it was then for the first time that I ever left home." Conscious of his new freedom, this young physician was also apprehensive when the next morning "I awoke a[t] seven o'clock to find myself far away at sea out of sight of any land."[8] Other physicians made the journey together, or, as became increasingly likely, encountered other Paris-bound medical travelers on shipboard. One medical tourist who visited Paris in 1857 even boarded the ship with an entourage of a dozen family members.[9]

Seemingly the central shared experience of all who sailed was seasickness. Waring reported that shortly after departure he was "taken Sick and remained so for eight days not knowing and caring still less for that which was being transacted about me."[10] Storms or iceberg sightings broke the sameness of the days; Francis Peyre Porcher reported that his vessel "got in fields of ice and had to steer amid & with it 300 miles to the South. . . . A tall ice berg at sea like an old castle shining in the sun light is one of the most impressive objects one can behold—one of these was large as a mountain."[11] Crossing in 1854 on the steamship *Arabia*, recent medical graduate Emily Blackwell wrote home of "the appearance of a whale which went spouting by this morning, creating quite a sensation on the deck."[12] These Paris-bound passengers filled most of the days, however, by studying medical books, reading novels, and working on French grammar.

For a significant minority the voyage was a working one. John K. Kane, Jr., found himself caring for a passenger with epilepsy during his crossing in 1857. "The doctor of the ship is very young and is only making his first trip he only graduated last spring," Kane explained to his family. "He got very much frightened and not knowing what to do called me in."[13] Henry Bryant, on the other hand, signed on to care for passengers on his 1843 crossing. "We had about two hundred steerage passengers big and little, and I had my hands full of practice from the time I came on board the ship," he told his father. "I never saw such a horrible condition as they were in all my life—It was as bad as any slave ship could be—and used to make me sick as a dog when I went down to make my daily visits." Out of fifty cases ranging "from belly aches to Fevers," he noted with pride that "not a single death occurred though Captain Brittain says he never went across before without a death."[14] Philip Gooch had eighty steerage passengers under his charge in 1846. "Most of them have been misinformed as regards life in the U.S. and are now returning to Ireland after an

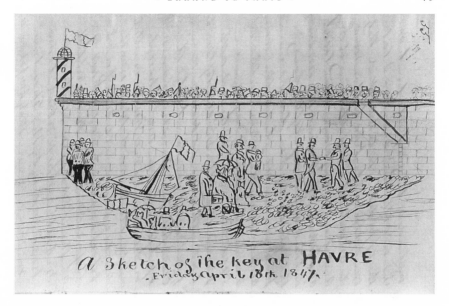

*a Sketch of the key at HAVRE*
*Friday April 18th 1847.*

Fig. 3.2. One American's depiction in his diary of landing in Le Havre after thirty-seven days crossing the Atlantic. (William E. Bartlett, Jr., Travel Journal, 1847, MS 2511, entry for 26 Mar. 1847, courtesy of Manuscripts Division, Maryland Historical Society Library, Baltimore.)

absence of a few months," he noted in his diary. "O! what a mess—all grades and conditions of humanity—Some misers, some wretches, & some well informed, honest poor devils." Gooch was not so fortunate as Bryant, however, and reported the death of a consumptive girl whose body "was committed to the deep."[15] Working the return trip also proved an appealing option for young physicians who, like Edward Jenkins, had overspent their budgets; as Jenkins wrote to his brother from Paris, "I propose to cross as Surgeon of an Emigrant Ship, which will save me the sum of one hundred & sixty dollars (the price of passage in the Steamer from Liverpool to New York)."[16]

Some Americans crossed directly to France, but as many landed in Liverpool. Most of the latter paused at least briefly in London and some lingered in Britain for serious study before crossing the Channel. Few remained in Le Havre more than a night, and almost no one found the port town captivating. Yet Americans strove in their diaries and letters to record emotions and reflections of an intensity fitting to commemorate their passage into France. Charles Jackson, his ship anchored off Le Havre, made resolutions about how he would conduct himself in the world he was about to enter. "I shall never tempt the quicksands of pleasure which are not those of rectitude & honor," he told his sister. "I shall always direct myself as in the presence of my relatives & friends whose eye could follow & whose censure condemn error & praise & encourage truth."[17] Levin Joynes, delayed a day in Le Havre while his papers were put in order, took nationalistic satisfaction in the celebration he witnessed of the

4th of July. "There were thirty six American vessels in port and their sailors had a grand procession through the streets with a band of music, and the American flag, floating alongside the tri-color of France," he told his father. "I felt very proud of my country."[18]

After clearing the customshouse and resting for the night, the traveler proceeded to Rouen, where almost everyone who left any record wrote of seeing with their own eyes the spot where Joan of Arc was burned.[19] Raised with the historical sensibility of the New World, they were somewhat in awe of the physical sites of European history. From Rouen, usually leaving late at night, they traveled the remaining eighty-five miles to Paris by *diligence*, a kind of articulated horse-drawn stagecoach that Georgia physician Louis Alexander Dugas described as "three carriages stuck together & placed on 4 huge wheels."[20] "By dint of much cracking of whips & many vociferations on the part of the driver," Joynes told his father, the *diligence* moved ahead toward Paris. "Having passed through many ancient towns, and some very beautiful country I entered Paris through a fine avenue of trees & with Napoleon's triumphal arch in full view. I shall not attempt in this letter to give you any account of this great city, where wealth & poverty, splendor & misery, science & ignorance are so strangely blended."[21]

### "ICI A PARIS"

"Is it possible[?]" New York physician Willard Parker asked in his diary on reaching Paris in 1837. "Am I in the gay city of Paris—known the world over for its gaity—its debauchery—for its science. The City to which I have looked with so much longing in relation to my profession. Thanks be to God. I am in the very same city."[22] Arrival often elicited a sense of disbelief. As the newly arrived Bostonian James Jackson, Jr., wrote to his father, "I can hardly yet persuade myself that I am in a world like that I have left behind me, so different is this great city fr. anything wh. I had ever conceived."[23] Dugas echoed the same point. "Is it possible?" he wrote to his brother shortly after arriving in 1828. "I can scarcely realize [it] myself, so much does it seem a dream to me."[24] What these Americans shared was the sense of having crossed into a different world. "Behold me," Robert Peter wrote to his wife on his arrival, "at the centre of civilization," and proceeded to try to convey some sense of his emotions of being "*ici a Paris*."[25]

What the newly arrived American did next varied according to connections, confidence, objectives, and temperament. Some plunged headlong into medical studies. "I arrived here yesterday & took lodgings in the *Place Pantheon* & entered my name as a private pupil," John Young Bassett reported home, "& expect for the next six months to see nothing but the Hospitals."[26] Others, with equal determination, set out to explore the cultural and social pleasures of what one described as "fan-faired Paris, the city of gaiety, fashion and vice."[27] And still others, intimidated by the scale and unfamiliarity of Paris, for a while, as Waring put it, "kept very quiet."[28] Jenkins admitted that "at first I was so much annoyed by the many inconveniences which arose from my ignorance of the language; and my dislike to many of the French habits; that I found it almost impossible to do any thing but brood over my imaginary misfortunes; and wish myself at home."[29]

The examples of how two medical Americans charted their course during their first several weeks in Paris exemplify the ways new arrivals oriented themselves to Parisian life, entered its medical world, and settled into a routine. The first, Henry Willard Williams, was still a student when, in 1846, at the age of twenty-five, he set out for Paris. While working as secretary and publishing agent for the Massachusetts Anti-Slavery Society, the Boston native had attended medical lectures at Harvard, though not taken his M.D. degree. Williams, unmarried, sailed from New York in April, glad that he had opted for the slower crossing by sail; "there is a beauty in a ship which a steam boat can never possess," he observed, and that first evening before retiring to his cabin he reflected on "the beauty with which we swept on our course, our full sails swelling proudly in the moonlight." Soon, though, he fell prey to seasickness—"I looked as if I was going to die"—and, once he had recovered, boredom. He discovered a Dr. Treadwell among the other passengers but complained that "even my comrade in Medicine is not very much a comrade on ship board, though he will be as a fellow student when we are in Paris." Williams did, however, begin the regular correspondence to his three sisters he would continue throughout his three-year stay in Europe, letters he asked them to save so that in later years he could "call back to memory" his experiences abroad. After a three-week crossing he landed in Le Havre, and full of reflections on how exertion in France might change his future, he made his way to Paris.[30]

Williams found lodging at the Hôtel de Seine in St. Germain, the Latin Quarter or student district on the Left Bank, and with Treadwell began exploring the city—crossing the river for the review of the troops at the Tuileries Palace, for example. "I intend to delay a few days longer the commencement of my studies, for I find that they will be in a *new* world, from the circle of which it will be difficult to escape when I am once within it," he told his sisters, writing after a second day of sightseeing that "another *year* of *events* has seemed to pass over me since I left off writing last night."[31]

At first, Williams explained, he would take his medical work slowly "as it is not quite safe to be so much in the air of a hospital till habituated to it, and I have many things to see and learn yet, in other quarters." He was keenly aware of social freedom unlike anything at home: "I might stay here three years and nobody but my landlord and the police know of my existence. No one knows me; no one cares anything about me, and I need care for no one else." But he resolved to turn to his studies soon. "I regard the ten days I have been in this country as altogether an episode—a digression from existence; but I expect now to return once more to active life," he told his sisters. "I never had so much of existence concentrated in a year."[32]

A week after reaching Paris, Williams reported that "today for the first time I entered the Hospital, Hotel Dieu, and the Ecole de Medicine." At seven in the morning he followed the ward visit of surgeon Henri-Louis Roger, then the medical rounds of Pierre Louis. At nine he heard physician Léon Rostan lecture, then left the hospital for breakfast. Williams next tried the lectures given throughout the day in the amphitheater of the École de Médecine, where he complained that the oak benches were hard and backless and the students kept their hats on. He was unsure about how to choose among all that was on offer, noting that "at the same hours as at Hotel Dieu the visits and lectures are made at the other hospitals, and it is difficult to know which to neglect among so many excellent ones." But what most confounded him was the French language, for the gap between reading words in a book and comprehending sentences uttered by native speakers was wider than he had bargained for. "One professor I listened to for an hour today without understanding a single sentence," he wrote of that first day, deciding on the spot to spend his time "attending for the present those Professors whom I can best understand." Private medical lessons would have to be deferred "till I know more of the language."[33] By the following evening he was even more frustrated. "Today I have neither *learned* nor *enjoyed* anything," he reported. "I am not enough settled to know what books to get, or even what lectures to attend, and I have spoiled my temper and lost my patience by trying to read my French Grammar. I can remember *facts* well enough, but words, words, words. . . ." That morning he had heard Philippe Ricord's lecture at the Hôpital du Midi and another at the École: "The last I could make nothing of and did not feel in the mood to stay."[34]

"This is certainly a very *blue* time with me," Williams complained several days later. "I have recalled myself from the total abandonment to enjoyment in which I indulged for the first week, but I have not yet been able to settle my fixed course of study. Consequently I feel uneasy and dissatisfied." He had, though, made arrangements for a private tutor in French and was trying to be optimistic. "At present I mean to arrange my pursuits in nearly the following manner," he told his sisters: "I shall attend the Hospital Hotel Dieu one day, and La Charité the next from eight to ten; lectures [at the École de Médecine] from eleven or half past ten till three, then my French lesson for an hour, then sometimes a lecture during the hour before dinner which we have, when at home, at five o'clock and after dinner which occupies an hour, I intend to stroll to the Garden of Luxembourg." Still, he admitted that "there is very little danger of my doing much in the way of study at present until I become accustomed to the language and life."[35]

In another three weeks, Williams had settled into a routine. "I go to the Hospital regularly, take regularly the same quantity of coffee, and eat the regular number of feet of bread at breakfast, pursue the same studies, eat almost the same dinner and take the same walk to the Garden at twilight." He was beginning to grow comfortable reading French, though still not understanding or speaking it; but he attributed that deficiency to the fact that all the residents of

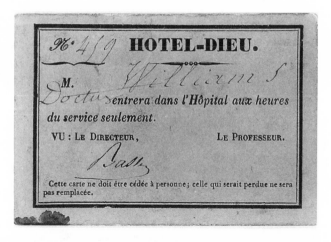

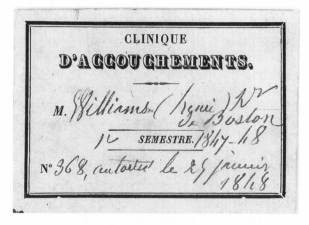

Fig. 3.3. Tickets to the official course of clinical instruction
were granted to foreign physicians without a fee. These
admitted Henry W. Williams to the Hôtel Dieu and the
Clinique d'Accouchements in 1848. (Henry Williard Williams
Papers, courtesy of Francis A. Countway Library
of Medicine, Boston.)

his hotel spoke English, and hit upon the plan of moving into the house where
his language tutor lived and only French was spoken.[36] Another couple of
weeks would find him more contented, reflecting that "I am enjoying the privileges which I had dreamed of rather than hoped for. . . . I know that in some
respects these are the happiest days of my life." And he boasted to his sisters
that "I yesterday understood an entire French lecture, perhaps as well as if it
had been English."[37] Late in June he wrote that, emboldened by improvements
in his French, "next week I commence a private course on Diseases of the Eyes,
which I expect to follow an hour each day for five days of the week, during
three months." He had also realized that limiting his studies to a few institu-

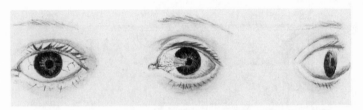

Fig. 3.4. Henry W. Williams used skills gained in the drawing lessons
he took in Paris in 1846 to preserve the pathological observations
he made in the French clinic, and returned to Boston with a
collection of colored pencil sketches of diseases of the eye.
(Henry Williard Williams Papers, courtesy of Francis A. Countway
Library of Medicine, Boston.)

tions was the best way to economize time, and resolved for the present to follow ward rounds only at the Hôtel Dieu. "I am satisfied it is best to follow one Hospital regularly and then go to another, rather than run about to different ones each day of the week."[38]

Over the next couple of years, Williams sampled widely from the medical instruction Paris offered. Perhaps reflecting the fact that he had not yet earned an M.D. degree, he attended more of the didactic lectures at the École de Médecine than most of his compatriots.[39] A letter of introduction from Henry Ingersoll Bowditch helped win free access to Louis's wards at the Hôtel Dieu, where he reveled in the opportunity to hone his skill studying chest diseases by auscultation and percussion.[40] By October 1846 Williams was spending most of his time studying diseases of children, particularly at the Hôpital des Enfants Trouvés. He complained that his change of residence had placed him two and a half miles away from the morning *clinique* at the Hôpital Necker—"une longue promenade, et il faut que je vais à tres bonne heure," as he told his sisters, for by November he had begun writing all his letters to them in simple French. But the same move placed him closer to his winter's work at Clamart, the dissecting rooms where he would spend four to six hours a day.[41] Late in the spring of 1847 he began a seven-month grand tour of the Continent, exploring as he went the medical cultures of Vienna, Cologne, Milan, and Florence.[42] He returned to Paris in time to witness the February 1848 revolution, the abdication of the king, and the creation of "la Republique Francaise."[43] Williams followed another private course on diseases of the eyes, then proceeded in late spring to London, where he studied briefly before embarking for home.[44]

The private course Williams had begun as soon as his French was up to it—Julius Sichel's class on eye diseases, which he started in July 1846—set the trajectory his career would follow for the next half century. By attending Sichel's clinical lectures, demonstrations, and operations for an hour five days a week, and by reading on eye diseases at the library of the École de Médecine, Williams had told his sisters, "I hope to be 'tres habile' in three months."[45] He also took drawing lessons in Paris and would return to Boston with carefully colored depictions of the pathologies of the eye he had studied abroad.[46] Before leaving Paris, he collected books and surgical instruments to be shipped home;

"the box is marked H. W. Williams, M.D., Boston," he told his sisters, and included "the most lovely little case of eye instruments you ever saw."[47] It was only after his return, in 1849, that he actually received his M.D. from Harvard, where later he would become the school's first professor of ophthalmology.

Abel Lawrence Peirson offers a second example, in this instance an American intent on making good use of a brief round of medical tourism. Peirson had received his M.D. from Harvard three decades before Williams, and at the time he departed for Paris in September 1832 he was thirty-six years old, married, a father, and well established in Salem, Massachusetts. The first nine days of the voyage he was "very, very sick" but wrote to his wife that favorable winds meant "we have now the prospect of being in Paris in less than one month from the time we parted in Boston Square." He discovered that another passenger was willing to tutor him in French; "I think you would be awed at my attempts to parley vou."[48] He landed in Le Havre, traveled by *diligence* to Rouen, then on to Paris ("the only feeling was admiration & the only *notion* magnificence," he reported on entering the city), and settled into a hotel near the Place Vendôme.[49]

Peirson was soon visited by "the young American doctors, who went into exatories on seeing us," including Henry Bowditch, Mason Warren, and James Jackson, Jr. With such welcoming medical advisers, "I could not possibly be better situated. The only great drawback to every comfort is, that I cannot understand french & a great evil it is."[50] The following morning at seven he was off with Jackson to Louis's rounds at La Pitié, where they stayed till noon. "If I were to tell you how much I am delighted with the opportunities I found here, I should go in to raptures," he wrote home. "I can only say that for studying diseases of the Lungs, it is all I wish. By *special favour* we (J.J. & I) are allowed to visit here any hour we please. Tomorrow at 7. I commence operations again at the same hospital & in the same course of the day I begin a course of private instruction on diseases of the skin at Hospital St Louis wh. I shall follow daily for [the] time I spend here wh. I fear will be only one month." He also planned to see operations by the "great surgeons." "So you can see I have begun in earnest," he finished his report of the day, "& God be thanked for the opportunities with wh. I am surrounded."[51]

The next morning, 23 October, at seven o'clock Peirson and Jackson were again at La Pitié, where they spent three hours studying pulmonary diseases with the stethoscope and an hour "making a call on M. Louis, with whom I am delighted." From there they went together to the Hôpital Saint Louis, where Peirson stayed two hours and made arrangements for lessons three times a week on diseases of the skin. "The rest of our time was consumed in walking from one of these places to another, wh. are widely separated," Peirson reported.[52] Over the next several days he continued his studies at La Pitié and the Saint Louis, and visited the Hôtel Dieu long enough to see Guillaume Dupuytren operate. "I have not yet seen any of the wonders of Paris [and] I am afraid after I get back I shall be found to be very little of an accomplished traveler," he wrote; but in fact he managed to attend the opera with friends, visit the Jardin des Plantes with Jackson, and stroll through the garden of the

Tuileries. "Today I have been occupied as usual, & I think them very profit-ably—especially at St. Louis, where we made the itch the theme of our study!" he began his daily letter entry on the 27th; "I think this lesson alone is worth all the fee I am to give the 'interne' who shows us the cases." That evening he attended a meeting of the newly founded Société Médicale d'Observation, headed by Louis. The following morning, like every other morning, he was at La Pitié at seven, and that evening "at 6 I dined with my four american friends—Drs. Bowditch, Ware, Green & J. Jackson—We had a real yankee dinner & a most agreable time."[53] The dinner marked one week since his first step into a Paris hospital.

Guided by other Massachusetts physicians who already knew the medical ways of the French capital, and aware of his limited time abroad, Peirson had moved immediately into the Paris medical world and briskly into a fixed routine. He kept to much the same schedule throughout his stay. Yet he also found time to see the Hôpital des Enfants Malades (where he "met with many interesting cases of skin disease, wh. was the principal object of our visit"), to purchase anatomical specimens and arrange to have them shipped home, and to visit the military surgeon Baron Dominique-Jean Larrey at the Hôtel des Invalides. As his departure approached, Peirson resolved that "the rest of the week I shall pass in going to several Hospitals I have not yet seen, & if I can find time, I mean to visit the gallery of the Leouvre, for fear I should be asked if I had seen so famous a place."[54] Peirson left Paris scarcely a month after he had docked in Le Havre, setting off for four months touring in Italy. He returned briefly and "commenced my old round at la pitié,"[55] then left for a fortnight in London, where he busily toured its medical sights.[56] Back in Paris for a final four days, he revisited La Pitié, La Charité, the Saint Louis, and the Hôtel des Invalides. "As we draw near the end of our visit every thing is getting hurried & disturbed," he recorded.[57] One day away from landing in the United States, he acceded in his letterbook to a remark his wife had made in one of her letters, that he had "seen a great deal more of the world than I had any right to expect to."[58]

Divergent as the experiences of Peirson and Williams were, once they gained their bearings both of them fell into a daily pattern of study that—with enor-mous variations in the detail—most Americans pursued. The morning's work began at one of the hospitals, where at seven o'clock the student followed the physician or surgeon on candlelit ward rounds, listened to his subsequent clin-ical lecture, and then perhaps witnessed operations or autopsies that he per-formed. Leaving the hospital at ten or eleven, the student returned home for breakfast or went to a restaurant. The afternoon's activities were more varied and might include lectures at the École de Médecine, dissecting (or performing operations on the dead body) at the École Pratique or at the Clamart, French lessons, or private courses in the clinic. This structured plan of study ended with dinner, the second meal of the day, at five or six in the evening.

The cases of Peirson and Williams also exemplify certain themes central to the usual experience of American physicians negotiating this new world. Language was a problem for most Americans, who ordinarily knew some French before

they left the United States but discovered once abroad that difficulty understanding spoken French slowed their way. "If the words pronounced by the speaker
were given me in a book, I could read them without any difficulty," Philadelphian Robert Harris wrote pathetically after a week in Paris, "but as they come
from the mouth of a Frenchman, they are so much blended together and curtailed of their syllabic sounds that one cannot tell where one word ends and
another begins."[59] Accordingly, like Williams, nearly all medical Americans who
planned to remain in Paris for any length of time engaged a private French tutor
and made language lessons an integral part of their weekly routine.

Another key step in orientation was getting a sense of which among the
many options for medical study were most worthwhile. Like Peirson, probably
the majority of Americans could count on counsel from compatriots already
settled into the Parisian medical world. The American medical community in
Paris was constantly in flux, but its accumulated experience was passed along
from year to year by word of mouth. Just as Peirson relied on other Massachusetts physicians, Manigault looked to fellow South Carolinians; arriving in
Paris in 1854, he wrote that "I soon hunted up Dr. Gaillard Thomas in the
Latin Quarter and made inquiries about the proper lectures to attend and hospitals to visit."[60] Others, like Williams, were initially on their own, at least until
they started to meet other Americans in the hospitals or in their lodgings. But
in addition to advice gleaned before departure from teachers and medical journals—which by the 1840s and 1850s abounded with practical directions—
information was available from a number of guidebooks. General guides, especially *Galignani's Guide to Paris*, which Austin Flint described in an 1854 letter
from France as "that indispensable companion of the stranger in Paris," included accounts of the medical school, hospitals, and dissecting rooms.[61] More
than this, guidebooks for the foreign medical student, such as Meding's,
mapped *Paris médical* in meticulous detail.[62]

Newly arrived American also had to acquaint themselves with the geography
of the city and the ways it constrained their options. Maps of medical Paris
could be found in guidebooks, and at least one American physician, Frank
Hastings Hamilton, had a map made to accompany an article he sent to the
*Buffalo Medical Journal and Monthly Review* in 1846.[63] As Americans soon discovered, the vicinity of the École de Médecine was the city's medical hub. It
was there in the Latin Quarter, one visitor noted, that "the greater number of
the hospitals, the École de Médécine and its Museum, the Clinical Hospital of
the School of Medicine, the Museum of Dupuytren, are situated, where all the
medical students and many of the professors, private lecturers, demonstrators,
medical booksellers, instrument makers, medical artistes, anatomical workers
in wax and papier maché, preparers of natural and artificial skeletons and other
varieties of surgical and anatomical specimens, reside."[64]

Yet the American visitor soon discovered that the medical spaces of Paris,
even if they had a center, were widely dispersed. The Hôtel Dieu, located next
to the Cathedral of Notre Dame on the Ile de la Cité, was only a short stroll
north from blocks where the École de Médecine, the Hôpital des Cliniques,

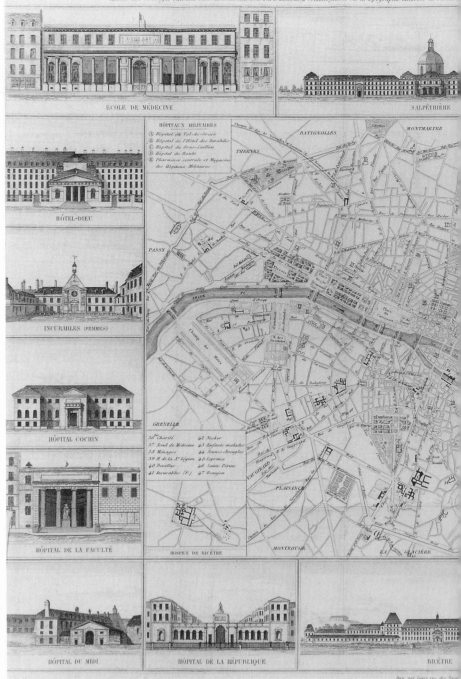

Annexe aux ouvrages suivants du Dr HENRI MEDING: Paris médical (2 Volumes). Essai sur la topographie médicale de Paris M.

ÉCOLE DE MÉDECINE

SALPÉTRIÈRE

HÔTEL-DIEU

INCURABLES (FEMMES)

HÔPITAL COCHIN

HÔPITAL DE LA FACULTÉ

HÔPITAUX MILITAIRES
A) Hôpital du Val-de-Grace
B) Hôpital de l'Hôtel des Invalides
C) Hôpital du Gros-Caillou
D) Hôpital du Roule
E) Pharmacie centrale et Magasins des Hôpitaux Militaires

GRENELLE

36 Charité                42 Necker
37 Acad. de Médecine      43 Enfants-malades
38 Ménages                44 Jeunes-Aveugles
39 H. de la XIe légion    45 Lespérance
40 Devillas               46 Sainte-Périne
41 Incurables (F.)        47 Bensçon

HOSPICE DE BICÊTRE

HÔPITAL DU MIDI

HÔPITAL DE LA RÉPUBLIQUE

BICÊTRE

Imp. par Louis rue des Sao

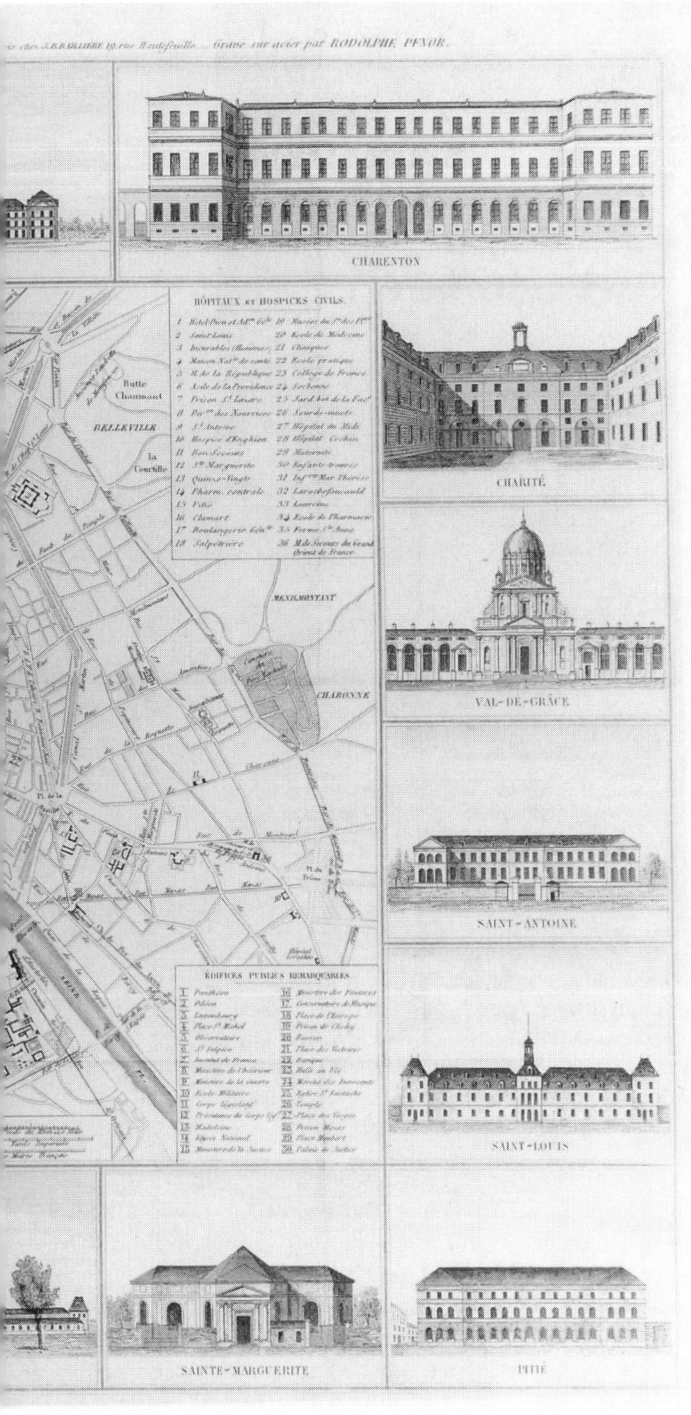

CHARENTON

HÔPITAUX ET HOSPICES CIVILS.

| 1 | Hôtel-Dieu et Ad.on Gle | 19 | Succur.du 1.er des P.tes |
| 2 | Saint-Louis | 20 | Ecole de Médecine |
| 3 | Incurables (hommes) | 21 | Clinique |
| 4 | Maison Nat.le de santé | 22 | Ecole pratique |
| 5 | H. de la République | 23 | Collège de France |
| 6 | Asile de la Providence | 24 | Sorbonne |
| 7 | Prison St Lazare | 25 | Jard.bot.et de France |
| 8 | Dép.t des Nourrices | 26 | Sourds-muets |
| 9 | St Antoine | 27 | Hôpital du Midi |
| 10 | Hospice d'Enghien | 28 | Hôpital Cochin |
| 11 | Bon-Secours | 29 | Maternité |
| 12 | Ste Marguerite | 30 | Enfants-trouvés |
| 13 | Quinze-Vingts | 31 | Inf.rie Mar.Thérèse |
| 14 | Pharm. centrale | 32 | Larochefoucauld |
| 15 | Pitié | 33 | Lourcine |
| 16 | Clamart | 34 | Ecole de Pharmacie |
| 17 | Boulangerie Gle | 35 | Forme 1.re Sem. |
| 18 | Salpétrière | 36 | Mde Sœurs du Grand Orient de France |

CHARITÉ

VAL-DE-GRÂCE

SAINT-ANTOINE

ÉDIFICES PUBLICS REMARQUABLES.

| 1 | Panthéon | 16 | Ministère des Finances |
| 2 | Pélion | 17 | Conservatoire de Musique |
| 3 | Luxembourg | 18 | Place de l'Europe |
| 4 | Place St Michel | 19 | Prison de Clichy |
| 5 | Observatoire | 20 | Louvre |
| 6 | St Sulpice | 21 | Place des Victoires |
| 7 | Institut de France | 22 | Banque |
| 8 | Ministère de l'Intérieur | 23 | Halle au Blé |
| 9 | Ministère de la Guerre | 24 | Marché des Innocents |
| 10 | Ecole Militaire | 25 | Eglise St Eustache |
| 11 | Corps Législatif | 26 | Temple |
| 12 | Présidence du Corps Lég. | 27 | Place des Vosges |
| 13 | Madeleine | 28 | Prison Mazas |
| 14 | Square National | 29 | Place Royale |
| 15 | Ministère de la Justice | 30 | Palais de Justice |

SAINT-LOUIS

SAINTE-MARGUERITE

PITIÉ

Fig. 3.5. Guidebooks for the foreign medical student in Paris often included a map of the city, situating the leading hospitals and other sites of medical instruction. (From Henri Meding, *Paris médical: vade-mecum des médecins étrangers*, 2 vols. [Paris: J.-B. Baillière, 1852–1853], vol. 1, after p. 352.)

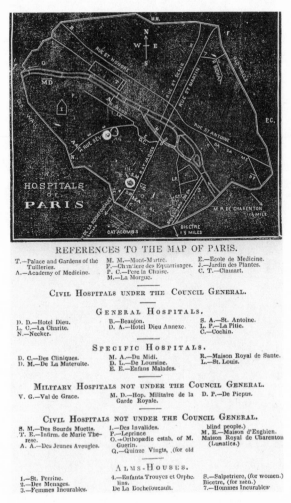

REFERENCES TO THE MAP OF PARIS.

T.—Palace and Gardens of the    M. M.—Mont-Martre.    E.—Ecole de Medicine.
     Tuilleries.    F.—Chamiere des Equarrisages.    J.—Jardin des Plantes.
A.—Academy of Medicine.    P. C.—Pere la Chaise.    C. T.—Clamart.
     M.—La Morgue.

CIVIL HOSPITALS UNDER THE COUNCIL GENERAL.

GENERAL HOSPITALS.

D. D.—Hotel Dieu.    B.—Beaujon.    S. A.—St. Antoine.
L. C.—La Charite.    D. A.—Hotel Dieu Annexe.    L. P.—La Pitie.
N.—Necker.    C.—Cochin.

SPECIFIC HOSPITALS.

D. C.—Des Cliniques.    M. A.—Du Midi.    R.—Maison Royal de Sante.
D. M.—De La Maternite.    D. L.—De Loursine.    L.—St. Louis.
     E. E.—Enfans Malades.

MILITARY HOSPITALS NOT UNDER THE COUNCIL GENERAL.

V. G.—Val de Grace.    M. D.—Hop. Militaire de la    D. P.—De Picpus.
     Garde Royale.

CIVIL HOSPITALS NOT UNDER THE COUNCIL GENERAL.

S. M.—Des Sourds Muetts.    I.—Des Invalides.    blind people.)
T. E.—Infirm. de Marie The-    P.—Leprince    M. E.—Maison d'Enghien.
     resc.    O.—Orthopædic estab. of M.    Maison Royal de Charenton
A. A.—Des Jeunes Aveugles.      Guerin.      (Lunatics.)
     Q.—Quinze Vingts, (for old

ALMS-HOUSES.

1.—St. Perrine.    4.—Enfants Trouves et Orphe.    S.—Salpetriere, (for women.)
2.—Des Menages.      lins.    Bicetre, (for men.)
3.—Femmes Incurables.    De La Rochefoucault.    7.—Hommes Incurables·

Fig. 3.6. Reports on medical Paris sent home by American physicians abounded in American medical journals and in this instance from 1846 included a map locating the hospitals of the French capital. (From F. H. Hamilton, "Notes of an European Tour" [Paris, (1846)], *Buffalo Medical Journal and Monthly Review* 2 [1846]: 396–409, p. 409.)

and the École Pratique were clustered together. But from there it was a long walk to La Pitié or the Clamart, both near the Jardin des Plantes, still on the Left Bank, and longer to the Hôpital Saint Louis or Hôpital Beaujon on the Right Bank. Peirson's comments about how much time it took him to walk from La Pitié to the Saint Louis, or Williams's gripe that one of his hospitals was nearly three miles from his residence, echoed routinely voiced complaints.[65] As another American wrote home, visiting more than one hospital in

a day "is more of a feat than an advantage."[66] Geography, like language, structured and constrained the student's options.

Geography certainly made deciding where to live more difficult than it first
appeared. On arriving, Americans generally went first to a hotel on the Right
Bank, and those, like Peirson, on a short visit might well go to the Hôtel
Meurice and remain there.[67] After a few days, however, most moved across the
Seine to lodgings such as those Williams found in the Latin Quarter.[68] This
placed them closer to the École de Médecine and many of the hospitals, yet
even then, as Colman complained, to attend the candlelit ward rounds at seven
each morning "it is necessary to have the *garçon* of the hotel where we lodge
call us up at a quarter, or at fartherest half past six and then to hurry on our
clothes as fast as we can upon a cold brick floor, hasten down stairs and plunge
into the narrow, dark and crooked streets, wending our way as fast as possible
to the hospital." While the Hôtel Dieu was nearby, other hospitals, as Colman
noted, "are situated in various & remote parts of the city; *and Paris you will
recollect is of no mean size.*"[69]

It was not uncommon for Americans to move to be near the site of their
current medical pursuits. "You will perceive that my address is changed," Jenkins wrote to his brother, explaining that "I have taken new lodgings to get
into the neighborhood of the Dissection Rooms."[70] Henry Bryant, on arriving
in December 1843, went first to a Right Bank hotel. Two weeks later he told his
father of his impending "emmigration from the fashionable to the studious
world," writing after the move that "I am on the other side of the river in the
midst of dirt[,] hospitals and medical students."[71] A month later he wrote
again that he had found lodging with a family back on the Right Bank near the
Madeleine in order to study with Jean-Nicolas Marjolin and Louis at the
Hôpital Beaujon, far from the École de Médecine. "I shall be about three miles
from my medical friends in the Quartier Latin so I shall not talk much English
with them," he told his father.[72] While these new quarters placed him only ten
minutes from morning rounds at the Beaujon, at two in the afternoon "I am
obliged to cross the river in order to be in time for the lecture which I attend
at the Hotel Dieu at three. From the Hotel Dieu I manage by dint of hard
scrambling, to get back in time for dinner at half past five."[73] His moves would
continue, as would his fretting about distances. "You say that you think the
Garden of Plants is a place where I should find much profitable ammusement,"
he wrote his father in midsummer, "but you do not remember that in Paris it
is a little different from Boston—it is about three quarters of an hours walk
from my room."[74] By the following January he was also dissecting in the after-
noons at the Clamart, on the other side of the river, noting that "a walk from
my room there [is] about five miles and takes me about an hour and ten minutes of my top speed"; the following month Bryant once again was contemplating a change of lodging.[75]

It is the eclecticism of the plans of study pursued by Williams and Peirson
that exemplifies the broader experiences of American physicians sorting out
how best to use what medical Paris offered. To be sure, like them most Ameri-

cans, as they became oriented, tended to narrow their focus. Even by the 1820s, while Americans generally studied both internal medicine and surgery, they tended to concentrate their attention on either one or the other. Elisha Bartlett wrote from Paris in 1826 that he would "devote nearly all our time to [the] study of Anatomy and Surgery, for which expressly we are here," while James Lawrence Cabell wrote in 1837 that "I shall not meddle a great deal with Surgery."[76] By the 1840s and 1850s, as chapter 9 will explore, a more special-ized focus, such as Williams's interest in diseases of the eye, would grow in-creasingly common. As Flint noted in 1854, the visiting American "must select the branches which he desires to pursue," for "without definite ideas on this point, the mind would be likely to be confused, and perhaps discouraged by the multiplicity of advantages."[77] What all American physicians in Paris shared was the need to be very selective. However clearly guidebooks presented the available options, there was no standard blueprint for a tour of professional improvement in France. Nevertheless, as the next section shows, even though each American student patched together a quilt that was distinctly his or her own, persistent motifs begin to reveal what collectively they most valued out of the varied medical experiences Paris offered.

## The Paradise of Parisian Medical Life

"Here I am in Paris in accordance with a desire which possessed me for years," Ashbel Smith wrote home in 1832. "When in America I sighed as you know after opportunities for improvement; here on the contrary I have only to regret that I can avail myself of but few comparatively of the almost innumerable facilities which this metropolis affords. Yet science displays its cabinet and Instruction opens its halls *gratuitously* to all who ask knowledge[.] I have not time in the 24 hours."[78] All this tallied up to the medical component of what Oliver Wendell Holmes called "the paradise of Parisian life."[79] Inventories of what was on offer abound in the letters Americans wrote home, in the contem-porary medical literature, and in the writings of later historians. Erwin Ack-erknecht, having cataloged the facilities for medical instruction in Paris, con-cluded that "a review of the teaching resources of Paris in the first half of the nineteenth century makes it easy to understand why, for several decades, it became the Mecca of medical students from all over the world."[80]

Smith's enthusiasm, however, was tempered by a telling note of frustration that other Americans shared. "This *is* a grand city certainly," Williams wrote from Paris, noting that "a man must be an idiot not to learn something, for he has nothing to do but *absorb*"; yet he admitted that he felt "discouraged" by "the utter hopelessness of being able to *absorb* more than a small portion of that which is offered to me."[81] Out of all the opportunities for gaining medical knowledge and experience Paris afforded, American soon realized they would have to choose only a small sample. As Flint put the matter, "it is entirely out of the question for the medical student to avail himself, at one time of more

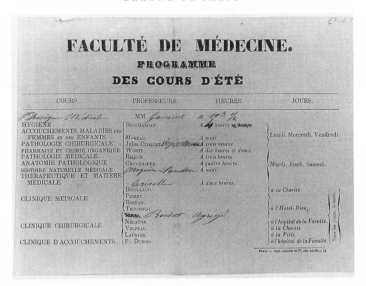

Fig. 3.7. Schedule of the official course of didactic lectures at the
Faculté de Médecine in the early 1850s. (William Joseph Holt
Papers, courtesy of Manuscripts Division, South Caroliniana
Library, University of South Carolina, Columbia.)

than a fractional part of the opportunities constantly offered for prosecuting
the medical and collateral sciences."[82] Plainly it is not enough merely to inventory the resources available to the foreign student: to understand the educational "paradise" the Paris School represented to Americans, we must look at
how they actually used these vast resources. Diverse though their choices were,
clear patterns emerge that in some ways were remarkably durable from the
1810s through the 1850s.

The didactic lectures that made up the official course at the École de Médecine, to begin with, were never foremost in their attention, despite the fact that
these, like most public instruction in medicine, were underwritten by the
French government and freely open to them. To Americans, who in the United
States had to purchase a ticket for each course of medical lectures they attended, it was a source of endless marvel that they could attend lectures by
medical professors "who," as Samuel Gridley Howe wrote home in 1830, "are
the most celebrated and the best in the world, who lecture on every subject,
and whose lectures are *gratis*."[83] Thus James L. Kitchen, who had paid to attend Nathaniel Chapman's Philadelphia lectures, which he recorded in his
class notebook, two years later in Paris used blank pages of the same bound
volume to preserve his notes on lectures by René-T.-H. Laennec and François-
J.-V. Broussais, which he attended without any fee whatsoever.[84] The schedule
of lectures was published and, as Holmes noted, "the whole walls round the
École de Médecine are covered with notices of lectures, the greater part of them
gratuitous."[85] Yet, as Alexander Wilcox wrote from Paris in 1845, after ward

visits in the morning "those who are studying the rudiments of medicine go to the school; but this institution is very little frequented by the Americans, who generally devote themselves to clinical studies."[86]

Even those Americans who did not yet have an M.D. ordinarily had attended a course of medical lectures before traveling to France, one factor that diminished the appeal of lectures at the École de Médecine. As important was the fact that no part of instruction was so mediated by language as didactic lectures. Furthermore, one American noted, "the American and foreigners generally, have not time to avail themselves of these public lectures; for the course on one branch alone is often protracted through three or four years."[87]

What took place in the lecture theater was nevertheless part of a spectacle not to be missed. Most Americans wanted to return able to say that they had seen the famous professors in action, and therefore included lectures at the École on their sightseeing rounds; "a great number of the lectures we attend but a few times— merely as a matter of curiosity and to see the professors," Bartlett told his sister.[88] Americans reveled in the sight of students from many nations drawn to the same hall, not least of all because it affirmed that they were at the center of things medical. When Alabama physician William B. Crawford wrote in his journal that the room for Mathieu Orfila's lecture was so crowded he could not get in, it was partly in complaint but partly in testimony to his own presence at the hub.[89] "The course of lectures this winter at the *Ecole de Medicine* is attended by about 1,600 students of all ages, and all nations from Ethiopia to Lapland," M. M. Rodgers wrote from Paris in 1851, and proceeded to describe the English, Americans, Scots, Germans, French, Italians, Spaniards, Greeks, Turks, Malays, and Africans who filled the amphitheater.[90] It was a heady experience. Yet, except for the handful of Americans who sought a medical degree in Paris, few spent a large share of their time in the lecture hall of the École.

Nearly all American physicians who passed much time at all in Paris, on the other hand, spent some significant portion of it at the dissecting table, and a number regarded this as the core of their Parisian experience. Their letters recounted government policies that ensured a steady supply of bodies from the hospitals to the anatomy rooms, and they widely shared the conclusion Hamilton voiced that "it is this enlightened policy which renders Paris the greatest school of anatomy in the world."[91] Kane confessed (and bragged) to his parents that perhaps he was spending too much time at the dissecting table—"I am the first man in the dissecting rooms every morning and the doorkeeper complains that I always keep him waiting in the evening"—"but," he explained, "I never have had such advantages for the study of it and I feel that I never shall have them again."[92] Absorbed in anatomy, and with growing aspirations to teach the subject, he wrote that "I have been hard at work all day[,] I might almost say all week for my dreams for the last week have been so filled with the various muscles nerves &c which form the face and neck down that I can hardly be said to have stopt work even at night."[93]

Arrangements for anatomical dissection varied widely over time. Early in the century anatomy rooms were scattered through the city, but after these were

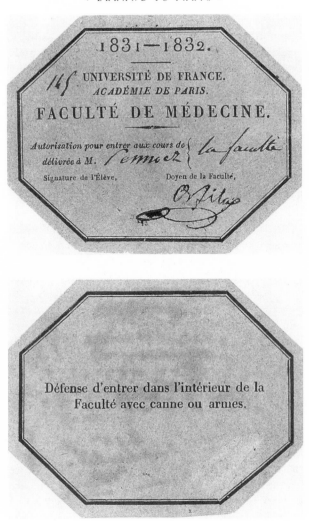

Fig. 3.8. Front and back of ticket admitting Philadelphian
Caspar Wistar Pennock to lectures given by the Faculté de
Médecine. Americans readily obtained such tickets—this one
signed by Mathieu-J.-B. Orfila, dean of the Faculté—without
any fee. (Courtesy of Francis A. Countway Library of
Medicine, Boston.)

suppressed as a public health nuisance, the activity was officially restricted to
only two sites: the Amphithéâtre des Hôpitaux, a newly built establishment
opened in November 1833 to replace the dissecting facilities that had been
closed down, and the École Pratique. Controlled by the faculty of the École de
Médecine and conveniently located near it, the École Pratique could accommo-
date some two hundred students at a time, though its rooms were, as Ameri-

cans complained, "very badly kept . . . dirty, damp, and wet."[94] The newer and much larger Amphithéâtre des Hôpitaux, usually known as the Clamart after the site on which it was built, was controlled by the hospitals and located near the Jardin des Plantes, and Americans generally concurred that it was "the best conducted and most comfortable dissecting establishment in the world."[95] "To this place, 'Clamart,' the carts, employed for the purpose, bring every morning the unclaimed dead of the various hospitals," Moses L. Linton observed in 1840. "When they arrive, and the bodies are deposited in a central hall, a bell is rung to summon the students to what would appear to the uninitiated a melancholy market."[96]

While the cost of dissection varied, Americans persistently judged the fees to be very modest, reporting in the 1850s that thirty francs, or six dollars, bought an unlimited supply of bodies and the demonstrator's aid for the entire winter.[97] "There is not the least prejudice existing here against dissections & even the patients themselves do not seem to mind it, tho' they are aware of their fate, for more than two-thirds of the dead are carried to the Ecole Practique or *Clamart*," Bassett wrote in 1836 to his sister in Alabama. "The other day an old woman bade me *adieu* as we passed her bed without calling & I stopped to ask her if she was going out. She said, yes, she was going to the *Clamart*," Bassett wrote, expressing the universal assumption that patients who died in hospital would be dissected, "& I told her we might meet again."[98]

Though dissection sometimes was possible during warm weather (and in other years prohibited), it was generally regarded as a winter pursuit. "I have been at work at the Dissecting room of the Ecole Med. almost incessantly," Charles Jackson told his brother-in-law in the winter of 1830, writing again in early March that "we are still 'cutting up' the Frenchmen-women & children but the warm weather now approaching will soon order a retreat. Even now they decompose as fast as they appear."[99] Winter dissecting posed annoyances of its own, though; "it is any thing but amusing in such cold weather as we have had," Bryant told his father, "as you can easily imagine when I tell you that I was an hour the other day with my hands covered with Blood &c— which froze as it run out on the table."[100]

Practice at performing surgical operations on the cadaver was another advantage of free access to bodies. "As regular dissections are prohibited during the summer months, all the subjects that are brought to the rooms are given to the young men to practise operations upon," Stewart observed in 1843.[101] Particularly after the Clamart opened, Americans widely expected anatomical dissection there in winter and operative surgery in summer to be among the chief advantages Paris offered the foreign student. "In the course of a few weeks I have become an expert and rapid operator," Holmes, working at the Clamart, told his parents. Holmes and a Swiss student had

bought a few cheap instruments together, and began to make ourselves operators. It is an odd thing for anybody but a medical student to think of, that human flesh should be sold like beef or mutton. But at twelve o'clock every day, the hour of distribution of subjects, you might have seen M. Bizot and myself—like the old gentlemen one sometimes sees at a market—choosing our day's provision with the same epicurean nicety. We paid fifty sous apiece for our subject, and before evening we had cut him into inch pieces. Now all this can hardly be done anywhere in the world but at Paris,—in England and America we can *dissect*, but rarely operate upon the subject, while here one who knows how to use his hands, and who gives his attention exclusively to the subject for a time, may, as I have said I have done, become an expert operator in a few weeks.[102]

What in 1847 one British visitor described in his journal as the "magnificent opportunities" for dissection exemplified the free access to the body Parisian medical polity afforded, and perhaps chiefly accounted for what another British practitioner referred to in 1836 as "the immense number of medical students . . . daily flocking to Paris."[103] Nevertheless, unlike the British, who often traveled to France principally for dissection experience that was exorbitantly expensive at home, Americans relished the convenience and economy of dissecting and operating on the dead body in Paris but seldom regarded this as sufficient to warrant the journey.[104]

Access to clinical instruction was a different matter. American hospitals of any substantial size existed only in the largest cities, and even in these patient populations were tiny and student access meager compared with what the hospitals of Paris offered. Indeed, whereas in the United States most physicians learned by observing the private, domiciliary practice of their preceptors, in Paris American students saw practice *only* in large public hospitals. And this vast program of hospital instruction came without fees or hindrances. A recurring theme in American accounts in Paris was amazement that what they had been told was actually true—that they could freely follow the renowned professors on their morning ward rounds, listen to the lectures they delivered in the hospitals, and witness their performance of operations and autopsies. "Admission to the hospitals during the hours of service is obtained without difficulty by any who are, or assume to be physicians," Flint reported. "A person who bears a medical aspect passes without any question being asked, but if stopped by the *concierge*, he is readily admitted on stating that he is a foreigner and a physician, or he is directed to the *bureau*, where on showing his passport, he receives a free ticket of admission, unlimited in time."[105]

Yet as a vehicle for acquiring the kinds of clinical knowledge and experience that Americans most sought, this official system of clinical instruction presented serious limitations. One major difficulty was that all of the professors at the various hospitals of Paris made their teaching rounds of the wards at the same hour of the morning, which meant that the student could follow only one each day. "My greatest difficulty in employing my time is the selection of courses," Cabell, recently arrived in Paris, lamented. "There is so much offered & so much that I would like to undertake that until now I have been skipping from place to place, unable to give the preference to any one."[106] Colman, describing his routine in 1833, wrote home that "I spend the mornings at the

Hospitals which I attend—say from half past six, or seven in the morning until eleven or twelve—This time is occupied 1st in attending the rounds of the wards to see the cases, new, and old, which are under treatment, 2 in witnessing the operations which are performed in the amphitheater of the hospital . . . 3d Then there is a lecture on the important cases which have been observed during the rounds in the wards—Perhaps after this comes a *Post Mortem* examination." But like many of his fellows, he went on to complain that this meant rounds before sunrise: "We usually see from one hundred & fifty to two hundred, or even more of the patients by candle light."[107] Further, Harris complained, instruction at the bedside often was superficial. "As the physicians go to the hospitals every day, they do not say much about a patient except the first time of visiting him; and as the examinations are made in the consultation room before the patient enters, the students have but little opportunity of studying what is to them very important, the commencing examination and treatment of the cases."[108]

Language posed another problem. Hospital teaching was more accessible than were didactic lectures; as one American rightly noted, "bedside instruction in Paris is the most profitable and fortunately the most easily understood by the student."[109] Still, catching brief comments during ward rounds and absorbing the lectures that followed in the amphitheaters could prove daunting. This difficulty of understanding French lecturers encouraged Americans to concentrate on the clinical information they could acquire directly by looking and seeing. "Time is not wasted following *Velpeau* through the grand (everything is grand here) wards of *La Charite*, nor in hearing him lecture," Bassett told his wife, "tho I did not understand one half or more than one half of what he said—but I understood his operations."[110] So too Jenkins, who, describing the official course of morning instruction at the hospitals, wrote home that "I have been attending three of them on different days of the week," went on to confess, "I have merely followed the Surgical portions which in my ignorance of the language is easiest comprehended."[111]

Seeing, however, much less touching, was not that easy, for ward visits were notoriously crowded. Witnessing for the first time Dupuytren's morning visit, Peirson wrote to his wife: "Two hundred pupils follow him to [the] bed side of each patient. How much they must learn!"[112] It is unclear to what extent his irony was intentional, but others were more explicit about the difficulty even of glimpsing the patient under such circumstances. "The number of students around the bedside is always immense and consequently it is difficult to hear or see," a Canadian observer appraised things in 1846, "and as for the use of the stethoscope it is almost impossible, the patients having the option of allowing you to examine themselves or not, excepting during the visit of the physician, which is of course very hurried."[113] "Velpeau says very little at the bedside," Wilcox reported in 1845, and "owing to the number who follow this surgeon, it is impossible for many to receive much instruction during the *visit*, and this must be at the expense of a degree of pushing and scrambling."[114] Competing for space with French students, at the bedside and in the lecture hall, was a perennial cause for complaint. "There was jamming, sq[u]eezing, bullying, cursing, and, what is so common among French students, *black-guarding* as we style it," David W. Yandell typically griped.[115]

What Americans wanted most from the Paris Clinic was the chance to exercise their senses, but, as Yandell noted, "beyond a certain, and that quite limited number [of students], seeing becomes a thing quite impossible; and unless the student himself can see, hear and feel the patients, it is quite clear that he will walk the wards of the hospital for many a long day before he can become a diagnostician or practitioner. Merely breathing the atmosphere of the hospitals is far from being adequate." The American student crossed the Atlantic in order to "auscult, and percuss, and *touch* for himself," yet the realities of official hospital instruction by the professors afforded little opportunity for such an education of the senses.[116]

Most Americans did devote many of their mornings to the regular ward visits and lectures, but they favored hospitals remote from the vicinity of the École de Médecine and therefore least crowded by French students. The Hôpital Saint Louis "is so far from the quarter occupied by students, that very few frequent it," a New York physician wrote from Paris in 1849. "Thus far I have observed that Americans compose the greater part of the students who walk through this hospital, so far distant. It is the same at the Hôpital des Enfants Malades, and Hôpital Neckar."[117] Bryant noted in 1843 that the inconvenient Right Bank location of the Hôpital Beaujon meant that "the opportunities of studying are according to my view much better than the regular or rather other hospitals." The institution had imposing clinicians, Louis and Marjolin, but, as Bryant explained to his father, "It is not so much however the names of the men that makes me prefer it as, from its being so far from the head quarter of medical students, you are able to make the visit all most alone few if any medical students going the rounds—You are thereby ennabled to examine each patient as much as you please."[118]

Americans likewise gravitated toward certain French clinicians because their language habits made their instruction more accessible. When F. Campbell Stewart visited Paris in 1847, he was pleased to note that when Archille-Louis Foville showed him about La Salpêtrière, "he chiefly spoke in English, which he had at perfect command," and that Paul Dubois "speaks English with facility, which makes his communications with Americans and English the more agreeable."[119] Americans routinely sought out the Baltimore-born Paris clinician Ricord, surgeon-in-chief at the Hôpital de Vénériens du Midi from 1831 to 1860, and delighted in thinking of him as their countryman; Ricord even served a term as president of the Anglo-Parisian Medical Society.[120] Appealing as this was for the medical tourist, however, the regular clinical courses remained in French, and therefore what mattered was the *way* particular clinicians spoke that language. Dupuytren, Linton noted, "speaks too rapidly to be understood by foreigners, and hence is not so much followed by them as Velpeau, whose enunciation is slow and distinct."[121] Accordingly, as another American noted, "the best seats in Velpeau's amphitheater have the name of

*American* seats, as they are always filled by the Yankees, who have gone and occupied them long before the lecture commences."[122]

Americans were also drawn to particular subjects—especially midwifery—that afforded experience little available in the United States. The *clinique d'ac-couchements* Dubois gave at the Hôpital des Cliniques, for example, persistently attracted an American following. "Every student who visits Paris should attend here one or two months at least, if he desires to acquire a practical knowledge of midwifery," the author of one American guidebook recommended. "There are, on average, two deliveries during each day in the year, and I have seen as many as four women in labour at the same time in the 'Salle d'Accouchements.'" He explained that "when a woman is taken in labour, notice is given to the initiated, by means of a lantern suspended from the porter's lodge, and the first two students who arrive are entitled to assist in the delivery; and in many cases to accomplish it themselves; those who arrive afterwards are accommodated with seats around a railing, serving as a partition between them and the patient, with those who are engaged about her. All, however, have an opportunity of seeing what is going on, and witnessing the birth of the child."[123] One American noted in his diary that another student came by his room "to tell me that the Caesarian Section wil take place at 3," writing: "I went to the Clinic where I saw the operation performed very successfully well by Dubois alone. There were 300 people in the room."[124]

To some extent, though, Americans attended the official program of clinical instruction for the same reasons they attended lectures at the École de Médecine. Seeing the great hospitals, following the famous physicians on their morning rounds, witnessing the famous surgeons operate—it was all part of being at the center of things. It was not growth in medical knowledge alone that led Waring after his first visit to the Hôpital Saint Louis to write in his diary: "it was a delightful morning. felt as if I was almost transported to fairy land."[125] The language Americans used in describing such clinical lessons commonly included vividly detailed attention to the physical staging of the room, how the orator's voice sounded, how he dressed, and the character his physical presence conveyed. Such reports betrayed an underlying sense of clinical teaching as spectacle, a relished sense of the sheer theatricality of seeing the medical lions perform. Like their visits to the renowned professional sites and figures of London, attending such hospital instruction was partly medical tourism. After returning to Kentucky in 1854, Flint told his medical class that in Paris the visiting American "may gratify his curiosity by visiting, on different days, different hospitals, or different wards of the same hospital, but there is little advantage in this beyond the mere gratification of curiosity."[126] Yet, as Flint had noted while still in Paris, "Curiosity, of course, leads the medical visitor in Paris to see most of them."[127]

There was, however, another form of clinical instruction, namely, *private* lessons. Arrangements varied considerably, but typically four or five students arranged with an *interne* to admit them to his wards at hours when they were otherwise shut to students. In return for a fee, the *interne* would point out interesting cases, allow the students to examine the patients, and answer questions. "Though the lectures are given publicly & the hospitals open in the morning during the visits of the attending physicians, they are not attended by the students during other parts of the day, except under these circumstances," Cabell told his uncle. "The *Internes* or medical assistants who reside in the Hospital & prescribe for the sick in the absence of the Professors, generally make an evening visit through their wards giving clinical instruction to a small class, these numbering generally limited to 4 or 5, on the payment of 30 francs a month from each."[128]

Courses of private instruction became for the majority of Americans the most valued core of their studies in Paris, and this pattern persisted from the 1820s through the 1850s. Private tutelage circumvented many of the obstacles that diminished the usefulness to Americans of regular hospital teaching. It compensated for their imperfect command of French: instead of gaining knowledge mediated by the remarks of the professor, they could systematically look, listen, and touch, learning through their own sensory experience and the guidance of an *interne* they employed. And it assured them space and time at the bedside. As one American described it, "Form a class of four, or even two, and offer an *interne* five dollars per month each, and the doors of the hospital turn noiselessly on their hinges, . . . the patients are your own, to be examined at your leisure, and the *interne* at your side to assist, direct, and instruct you."[129]

There were at least two quite different types of proprietary instruction, often conflated as *private classes* in the minds and reports of visiting Americans. On the one hand, as Porcher reported in 1853, "Each Interne or Chief of the Cliniques of any note, has his private class of four or five at the Hospitals, who, for twenty-five to fifty francs per month, enjoy the privilege of making visits and examinations, and of studying, auscultation and percussion with him during the evening."[130] Cabell explained in 1837 that "during the visit of the attending physician in the morning, there being generally a large crowd, it is just possible to see the patient & to hear the remarks of the physician, but hardly ever practicable for the student to examine for himself. For this reason the *Internes*, who are graduates of two, three, four or five years, limit their classes to so small a number. Most american students are in the habit of taking thus a course at one hospital on diseases of the Heart, another on those of the lungs, another of the eyes & another of the skin, while some add to these a course on surgery & midwifery &c."[131] Such an arrangement became an established albeit informal institution, and two decades later Chandler Chapman described a nearly identical system by which *internes* managed to "add to their small income by giving instruction to private classes."[132]

For a physician such as young Henry Bryant, son of an affluent Boston merchant and trader, even individual clinical tutoring could be arranged. "When I followed Barthage at the Hotel Dieu I had some opportunity to study but there were four others," he wrote to his father in 1844, going on to describe his new arrangement with Louis's *interne* at the Hôpital Beaujon. "With Cossy I am alone and have all the advantages concentrated on my single self that the five enjoyed at the other side of the river." The *interne*, Bryant explained, "does not tell me that the patient has this and that but asks me to examine them and then asks my opinion. If I am right he tells me so and explains anything that is strange if not he tells me where I [have] been mistaken and I examine the patient again till I find what I ought to."[133] Such individualized attention certainly helped Bryant when he took the further step, unusual for an American, of entering and winning the competition or *concours* for a position as *externe* at the same hospital.[134]

The other kind of private class had a more formal structure and defined focus, most often but not always clinical. Private, for-fee classes, often given by *agrégés* or junior members of the faculty, were offered on such topics as diseases of the lungs, skin, or eyes; diseases of children; the use of the stethoscope or microscope; physiology; legal medicine; pathological and surgical anatomy; and "touching" in midwifery. "Paris abounds in private teachers," one American physician reported in 1848. "Private instruction can be obtained on any subject. Magendie's assistant delivers lectures on Physiology; Blandin's assistant on Operative Surgery; Paul Dubois' assistant on the *Toucher*; the keeper of Dupuytren's Museum on Pathological Anatomy. The price of these tickets varies from six to ten dollars. Then there are Sichel's, and Desmarre's, and Tavignot's clinics on diseases of the eye, a clinic on diseases of the ear, etc. etc."[135] Lists of such courses appeared in the guidebooks and were posted in the vicinity of the École de Médecine.[136]

The distinctive advantage of these courses was the union of access to the body with individualized instruction. For example, while the official course of instruction in midwifery, for which Americans paid nothing, let them watch the professor demonstrate physical examination of pregnant women, in paid private courses the students performed examinations themselves. Such private courses on midwifery—*touching* courses, as they were called—represented par excellence hands-on access to the female body. "A course of Touching," Charles Jackson explained, gave the student experience at systematic "examination by touch [of] the state of the mouth of the womb &c during all periods of Pregnancy."[137] As Jackson wrote to his brother-in-law in 1829, "We attend a course Midwifery of Touching a course of examinations in wh. P[re]g[nant] females are brot into be examined in all stages of the gestation & the lecturer first examines or touches, explains the state of things as he finds them to us[.] we then severally & in succession make the examinations while the Professor sits by our side to direct & explain everything. This course is worth the expense of crossing the seas as it is peculiar to France & french women as you may well suppose."[138]

Another American, who took the *agrégé* Charles-M.-E. Pajot's private *cours d'accouchements* a quarter century later, described much the same plan. "It continues from three to four months, and each pays the small sum of twenty-five francs, including the use of the *toucher*." Trying to re-create the scene for readers of the *Charleston Medical Journal and Review*, he wrote: "It is a small room, filled with students and graduates of medicine, native and foreign. We have now arrived at that portion of the course devoted to the examinations, and M. P[ajot] has before us four women in different stages of gestation, and one not *enciente*, which allows of comparison. Each student in turn, touches and explores carefully the latter, under the immediate direction of the chief, and then proceeds alone to examine the others. One of these informed one of us, that she received two francs for the use of her person on each occasion, and that she sometimes attended more than one room of a similar nature."[139] It was access Americans relished, but to which they also grew accustomed; thus Waring wrote as a matter-of-fact daily entry in his diary, "Touched at Pajots then went to dinner."[140]

Just as arrangements with *internes* provided special access to the living body, so other private courses on normal, pathological, and surgical anatomy combined access to cadavers with the expertise of Parisian instructors. Students could take a public course on operative surgery at the Clamart or École Pratique, paying only the nominal sum for their material, but for an additional fee they might engage an *agrégé* to give individualized guidance in performing surgical operations on the dead body. "It is true that the courses are all public but they are crowded," Bassett reported; therefore, "I have found much advantage in employing private instructors & paying them." He went on to describe the course he had arranged: "Six of [us] engaged *Mons. Chassaignac*—he is a juge [agrégé] to the Faculty—and one of the best anatomists in France—to give us private instruction in Surgery. We perform all the operations two or more times ourselves under his eye." Like his touching class on midwifery—which Bassett judged "taught to perfection"—such a course extracted the full measure of experience possible from hands-on access to the body.[141]

Most Americans made both kinds of private course central parts of their Parisian studies. Wilcox, who studied in Paris in 1844–1845, reported to the *Western Lancet* that the private courses he took during his twelve-month stay included "Cazeaux on obstetrics, Sichel on the diseases of the eye, Desmanes on the same, Barth on pathological anatomy, Louget on the nervous system and on vivisections, and Ripbail on bandaging." In addition, he arranged regular clinical visits with *internes* during the afternoon. In this way, "I took one course on auscultation at the Beaujon, in the service of Louis; two on surgery at La Charité, in the service of Velpeau; and two at this hospital, in Rayer's service. Besides these, I had a course on the diseases of the skin, at Saint Louis, in the service of Devergie; one at the Children's Hospital, in the service of Baudeloque; and one at St. Lazarre, on syphilis in women, and the exploration of diseases of the neck of the uterus, by means of the speculum, and their treatment."[142]

Americans recognized that their experience of the Paris School was very different from that of its French students. "It is a fact well known here, that much the larger proportion of the amount of fees paid for the private courses, and to *internes* for clinical instruction at the hospitals, comes from foreigners," a Louisville journal editor noted as a footnote to a letter from Paris published in 1854, "and especially from the American students and practitioners who visit Paris for medical improvement."[143] Cost was one factor, for, as another American observed, though "this is the very best clinical instruction that one can acquire," such courses "are tolerably expensive, and hence are not enjoyed but rarely by others than the English and Americans."[144]

Some young Americans sorted out the realities of Parisian clinical education only slowly as they went along, then had to explain them to family at home paying the bills. "The expenses attending the studies here are few," Jenkins wrote in 1853 to his elder brother in South Carolina not long after arriving in Paris. "There are besides the regular lectures others given by younger but talented and prominent men which being more practical are attended by foreigners whose time is generally short. The expenses attending vary from five to eight dollars."[145] Five months later, however, he had come to realize how crucial such private courses were, and drafted another letter, asking his brother to send money:

> The idea of the freedom of expense in pursuing the study of Medicine is an egregious error: at least to the student whose time is comparatively limited. It is very true that the Lectures at the College of Medicine and at the various hospitals, are with some few exceptions free to any who chose to attend, but the student who has but one, two or even three years can not afford to follow the professors, with very few exceptions, through their very diffuse lectures. To us the practical information at the bedside is what is needed; to obtain which one has to pay pretty considerably. The Lectures on the diseases of children which I have been taking has cost me ten dollars a month. The lectures I refer to are given by the young Physicians engaged in the hospitals. . . . These young men when still "Chefs de Cliniques" that is assistants of the Professors having charge of the Hospitals, give private courses of lectures at the bedside. The expense attending these are considerable. To give an example, I expect to pay for lessons on the single subject of *Auscultation*, a thing not much known in America except by name, during the course of the year the sum of seventy two dollars.[146]

Jenkins was portraying the Paris School in a way that would persuade his brother to forward the additional funds; but at the same time, he was expressing what most Americans realized from the outset, namely, that paid private instruction was what best warranted the voyage across the Atlantic.

The small sorority of women physicians who made the journey from the United States to Paris before 1860 faced a vastly more complicated situation and were compelled to take on the formidable task of discovering for themselves how to gain access to the experience that made the French capital a Mecca for medical men. "There is certainly no city where a student (a *man*) can study to such advantage," Elizabeth Blackwell wrote from Paris in 1850 with pointed irony to the *Boston Medical and Surgical Journal*; "it fully deserves its reputation."[147] In published guides for the foreign student, ordinarily it was an unexamined assumption that the reader would be male. Negotiating a woman's way into the Parisian medical world meant first and foremost finding or creating openings to instruction that were not reserved for men. Like their male counterparts, the few American women who traveled to France for medical study in the 1850s—and the many who followed after the Civil War—came seeking access to experiential knowledge of the body. But medical women's experience of the Paris Clinic was governed by different rules and assumed a different character.

When Blackwell arrived in Paris in May 1849, her aim was to gain practical experience in surgery and in obstetrics. She "launched boldly into the sea of Paris," Blackwell wrote home shortly after reaching the city, "with a map in my hand and hope in my heart." Although she worried that her French was inelegant and her vocabulary inadequate, Blackwell brought a letter of introduction from a Boston physician and soon had her first medical interview, with Pierre Louis. "I told him frankly of my earnest desire for hospital and practical instruction," Blackwell later recalled, and "after a long conversation he most strongly advised me to enter La Maternité, where in one most important branch I could in a short time obtain more valuable practical knowledge than could be obtained anywhere else."[148] Reluctant to commit herself to the Maternité, the immense lying-in hospital and residential training school for midwives housed in a former convent, Blackwell spent June attending lectures at the Collège de France and the Jardin des Plantes, seeing the sights of Paris, and unsuccessfully petitioning for permission to follow clinical instruction at the hospitals. When she applied to attend the lectures of Dubois and Armand Trousseau at the École de Médecine, an application also turned down, Trousseau suggested that disguising herself as a man would be the only way to overcome the entrenched policies of gender discrimination.[149] Resigned to the conclusion that "entrance into La Maternité would be the most direct first step in obtaining the practical instruction needed," Blackwell decided to follow Louis's advice in studying obstetrics, and to later renew her campaign for access to the other hospitals and practical instruction in surgery.[150] The next four months at the Maternité, however, constituted nearly all the clinical instruction that she would receive in Paris.

By stepping through the gateway of the former convent at the end of June, Blackwell, as she wrote home, "said good bye to the world, and shut myself within the high walls of the Maternité, where no echo of the busy universe is allowed to penetrate."[151] Even before entering the "strange gloomy life" there, Blackwell knew she was giving herself over to what she described as "strict imprisonment."[152] The Maternité was quite unlike the other hospitals of Paris, and the regimented routine of pupils at its École d'Accouchement bore little resemblance to the life of male medical students studying at other clinical institutions. Closed to male students, it was a place of training for *élèves sage-femmes*, young women largely from the provinces who, after closely supervised studies in the capital, would return home to practice as midwives. The institution was governed by strict rules designed to cloister its pupils from the life of the city outside. Into this institution the twenty-nine-year-old Blackwell entered, not with the standing of a physician doing advanced clinical study or even a medical student, but with that of a midwife-in-training.[153] And neither

Blackwell's petitions nor those of the American consul succeeded in winning exemption from the rules. "The physicians of Paris, as far as I can judge, are determined not to grant the slightest favour to a feminine M.D.," Blackwell wrote to her mother the day after she entered the institution. "I could not obtain from any persons connected with the Maternité the smallest modification to suit the very different status with which I enter from the young French *sages-femmes*; but I was determined to enter on whatever conditions."[154]

Accordingly Blackwell, together with the other *élèves*, slept in a dormitory of sixteen beds; rose at 5:30 to begin a supervised daily schedule that included not only lectures and ward service but communal meals and communal baths; and received visitors only at prescribed hours in the chaperoned parlor. She "blessed Heaven" that she was Protestant, which excused her from morning and evening prayers, vespers, baptisms of newborns, and all the ministrations of "the great fat, red-faced priest" and "his sensual-looking worship."[155] And, like the other pupils at the Maternité, for nearly four months Blackwell was not permitted to leave the confines of its walls. Only in late October did she have "my first day of freedom," a day spent with her sister Anna, then living in Paris. "How gay and free and delightful the city seemed to me after my four months' imprisonment," she wrote home, "four months shut up within the high boundary wall of the institution, with the sky above the tops of tall houses only visible, and all life concentrated in a single subject!" As the rules demanded, "punctually at eight o'clock the recluse retired again from the vanities of the world."[156] When fourteen months later and in England Blackwell spent an evening with Bessie Parkes, seated by the fire recounting the story of her hard-won medical education, Parkes was moved and appalled. "Such a tale!" Parkes in turn wrote to Barbara Leigh Smith, who would become a lifelong friend of Blackwell's; "the physical hardships of 4 months in the Maternity hosp at Paris sleeping in a dotorie with 30 coarse girls & women & learning to be midwives, whose noise & vulgarity were beyond description—(Think of *that* my dainty darling)."[157]

In exchange for her confinement, however, Blackwell gained access to clinical experience surpassing anything she had hoped for. She found much of the instruction given by the *aides-sage-femmes* too elementary but regarded the lessons—like the fact of being cut off from other English speakers—as an effective means of improving her French. And, like other American doctors, she found French treatment of patients deplorable: "With all the instruction they have received, the very first principles of humane treatment seem too often neglected," she commented in her journal. "They are still ignorant midwives with their mischievous interference," and their management of birthing women left her "disgusted."[158] The lectures and clinical instruction given by the *médecin-accoucheur* Paul Dubois and his *interne* were more rewarding. Most of all, as she wrote to her mother, "nature is always here in great abundance to be studied."[159] At the time of Blackwell's visit, 5,786 parturient women were admitted to the Maternité annually, and of them 382 died while in the institution.[160] Blackwell's free access to the wards and *salle d'accouche-*

*ments* gave her a more extensive field for making observations than she could have had anywhere in the United States and fuller opportunities for obstetrical study than any of her male compatriots experienced elsewhere in Paris. Dubois, she noted one day in August, detained her after lecture to say that "he wished I would stay a year and gain the gold medal; said I should be the best obstetrician, male or female, in America!"[161] Dubois reiterated his encouragement a month later, and when Blackwell pointed out that there were other branches of medicine she wanted to study while abroad, "he replied that anything else I might learn elsewhere as well as in Paris, but that the opportunity of seeing all that was remarkable in three thousand deliveries in that space of time could be met with nowhere else in the world."[162]

By October, Blackwell had decided to extend her stay at the Maternité to half a year. But early in November the plan was curtailed abruptly when water accidentally splashed from the diseased eye of an infant into her own, leaving Blackwell very sick and, eventually, blind in one eye.[163] Ironically, and perhaps not coincidentally, it was only after she was incapacitated by the accident that Dubois visited and left her overjoyed by, as she wrote in her journal, "understanding for the first time the justice of my determination to obtain a full medical education, and obliged to confess that I was right in principle."[164] She took satisfaction in writing that she had "received permission from Government to visit the hospitals," but the slow recovery from her accident drained most of her energies for the next six months.[165] Blackwell "employed a *répétiteur* who drilled me in anatomy and smuggled me into the dead-house of La Charité at great risk of detection, where I operated on the *cadavre*," she later wrote, describing this difficult period to her sister Emily, and "I once made the rounds of his wards in the Hôtel Dieu with Roux, heard his lectures, and saw his operations."[166] She gradually accepted that her impaired vision unfitted her for surgery, and when in May 1850 an English cousin won permission for her to enter St. Bartholomew's Hospital as a student, she welcomed this chance for clinical study in London.[167] ("A sensible, quiet, discrete lady—she gained a fair knowledge (not more) of medicine," James Paget, who kept private notes on the performance of all his students at St. Bartholomew's, wrote of her.)[168] Late in her life, appraising her studies at the Maternité, Blackwell reflected that "my residence there was an invaluable one at that stage of the medical campaign, when no hospitals, dispensaries, or practical *cliniques* were open to women."[169]

Nancy Talbot Clark declined at first to follow Blackwell's example when she traveled to Paris for medical study in 1854. After she received her M.D. in 1852, Clark had told Blackwell that she would like "some time hence" to go abroad for study with her younger sister Emily Blackwell, and in late spring 1854, Elizabeth wrote to Emily, "If you go into the Maternité for three or four months would you object to her entering at the same time? Would her companionship be unpleasant in any way?"[170] Clark, however, made it clear that she was not inclined to pursue intensive obstetrical training. "She is quite contented I see with a midwife practice in that department—the entire absence of science," Elizabeth told Emily with disgust; "this is evidently the natural tendency of present women—instinct and habit, not intelligent thought."[171] Though Clark may eventually have studied at the Maternité, she spent several months following the official instruction at other hospitals—a step facilitated by the fact that Clark, a widow, was always accompanied by her physician-brother Israel Tisdale Talbot, a graduate of a homeopathic college in Philadel-phia who just before leaving for Europe had received a second, regular M.D. degree from Harvard. A Charleston physician who encountered Clark at Dubois's clinical lectures noted that she was invariably observed in her brother's company, adding in a letter to an American journal that "Mrs. C., lately applied for the dissections at 'Clamart' but this very properly was refused her."[172] Emily Blackwell told her family that "my own impression is that though Mrs. Clark got inside many hospitals and received a good deal of per-sonal courtesy her visit to Paris amounted to very little."[173] For her part, when Emily finally reached Paris—dressed, in the event, as a woman, not disguised as a man—she did not limit her studies to obstetrics but did follow her sister's path into the Maternité, which for American women physicians would remain the central institution for Parisian studies at least through the mid-1860s.[174]

What most Americans wanted above all else from medical study in Paris was practical instruction and experience: that much female and male doctors had in common. Their clinical pupilage in Paris, moreover, informed a shared per-ception that the access to experiential knowledge to be had from the bodies assembled there was vastly greater than anything available in their own coun-try. Yet American physicians' experiences in France, no less than their medical educations in the United States, were profoundly structured by gender. Whereas men found in Paris an educational "paradise" that was incomparably open and freely entered as a matter of entitlement, women found a largely closed system, opened a bit by special favor or special sacrifice. It was emblem-atic of this difference that the entry fee Elizabeth Blackwell paid to acquire extensive clinical experience was, as she self-consciously described it, "my lib-erty." Much as she valued what she gained from her residence at the Maternité, she characterized it as "my prison life."[175] Her representation of herself, in a letter written to her mother from the institution, as "the Voluntary Prisoner" contrasts starkly with the images her male counterparts depicted of their un-checked freedom in Paris.[176] The very suggestion of cross-dressing as a strategy to win clinical access, a plan proposed to Elizabeth and considered by Emily, required a language of disguise, artifice, and calculated deception that stood in blunt opposition to the celebration of openness, freedom, and effortless enti-tlement in men's discourse on access to the body in the Paris Clinic. Neverthe-less, after the Civil War the promise of more open clinical experience would draw a growing number of American women physicians to Paris.

While it was the human body that most fully captured the attention of med-ical Americans in Paris, in varying measures they also explored wider fields of scientific instruction. "I crossed the Seine, and went into the room of the Insti-tute, where the Academy of Science holds its weekly meetings," Bartlett wrote home on his second visit to Paris, in 1846. "Amongst the many brilliant and great reputations with which the room was soon crowded, I will mention only a few—Isidore Geoffroy St. Hilaire; the surgeons Roux and Velpeau; Dutrochet; the chemists Gay-Lussac and Thenard, whose names are as inseparably linked as the Siamese twins; Mirbel, the botanist; Biot, the astronomer; Flourens, one of the perpetual Secretaries; Baron Charles Dupin; and last, but certainly not least in this illustrious catalogue, the great astronomer *Arags*."[177] For an American with growing aspirations to contribute to natural science it was an exhilarating sight affirming that even though he would have to return to the scientific periphery, for the moment he stood at the center.

Especially in the late 1840s and 1850s (as chapter 9 will explore) American physicians devoted increasing amounts of their time in Paris to courses on topics such as microscopy and experimental physiology, taught by figures like Charles Robin and Claude Bernard. Yet by that time, Americans had been writing home for decades expressing their frustration that the plethora of medical opportunities left them little time to take advantage of instruction in the collateral sciences. "So much of my time has been ocupied this winter at the dissecting room that I have been unable to attend much to the course of publick lectures which are at the Sorbonne Garden of Plants, College of France School of Mines &c &c upon subjects of Science," Charles Jackson lamented in 1830. Still, among his other activities Jackson attended Georges Cuvier's winter course on the history of natural history.[178] The shifting roster of lecturers was vast, and most Americans made attending some of their performances part of their Parisian experience. Samuel Wigglesworth, for example, followed Broussais's lectures on "phrenology as applied to Medicine" in 1836, writing home to Massachusetts that at its opening "the amphitheater was crowded more thickly than you ever saw Fanueil Hall on Caucus night," while Porcher attended a course at the Sorbonne on "French Dramatic Literature."[179]

Medical museums were recurrently deemed weak in Paris, though one American judged in 1846 that the recently established Musée Dupuytren "is one of the first places in Paris which the medical tourist should visit."[180] The museological strength of medical Paris was instead the immense collection of living specimens displayed in the wards. Thus Robert Peter wrote of his visit to the lunatic asylum Bicêtre in 1839: "Saw Dr Ferris go around the wards and heard his lectures, illustrated by skulls of idiots and by living specimens, which were interrogated in order to show the extent of their intellect."[181]

Natural history museums, on the other hand, especially the complex at the Jardin des Plantes, persistently attracted Americans, mostly as occasional visitors but sometimes as committed students. "This Garden is in fact a great school of natural history: some twelve or fifteen of the most eminent scientific men in Paris give courses of gratuitous lectures here, which are attended by crowds of students," Joynes wrote to his father, describing the collections in botany, mineralogy and geology, zoology, and comparative anatomy. "The museums of which we boast, even the best of them, sink into insignificance by the side of the mammoth ones at the Garden of Plants." As Joynes enthused,

"What a feast is here presented for the student of natural history! If he desires to pursue any single branch of science, the most ample means are afforded for perfecting himself in it. The cabinets are constantly open to him, a rich library upon the spot contains all the works he may wish to consult, and a professor, or perhaps two or three, are constantly labouring for his instruction, and yet all this is *gratis.*"[182]

Here again, most Americans felt their limited time abroad hopelessly inadequate to the opportunities they found. "When I came here I had intended to study Nat Hist at the garden of Plants but I found that I could not study both that and medicine," Bryant wrote home; "I gave it up—I have not been there but twice since I have been in Paris."[183] So too Manigault reported in 1856 taking Francis Turquand Miles, his former anatomy professor from South Carolina, to the Jardin to meet Louis-Pierre Gratiolet, "who agreed to let him dissect any dead animal that was not otherwise wanted, as Dr. Miles had a taste for that kind of study." Miles, Manigault noted, "was much pleased with Gratiolet and would have liked to know him better, but he could not continue going to the Garden, as it interfered with his medical studies."[184]

Confronted by the limitations of time and the imperative of choice, Manigault, after spending his first year in Paris at the hospitals, deserted medical study altogether and gave his second year almost entirely to work at the Jardin des Plantes. Arriving in Paris in 1854, having just received his M.D. in Charleston, Manigault brought a letter of introduction to André Duméril, professor of herpetology, from the Charleston naturalist and physician John Edwards Holbrook, who himself had studied at the Jardin in the early 1820s. Encouraged to visit the comparative anatomy laboratory whenever he wished, Manigault spent more and more of his time dissecting and assembling skeletons, noting that winter was his season of opportunity because the animals "die in quantities as soon as the leaves begin to drop, or in other words, as soon as the cold weather commences, and sometimes there are so many on hand that some have to be thrown away."[185] Manigault later explained in his autobiographical recollections that "from the commencement of my studies in medecine I had always felt a repugnance for its practice," and in Paris "gradually, while thinking over my plans for the future, [I] abandoned the idea of practising physic."[186]

Jeffries Wyman—who had received his M.D. from Harvard in 1837 and in 1840–1841 lectured on comparative anatomy as curator of the Lowell Institute in Boston—was even more committed to natural history than Manigault when he set off for Paris. And, like Manigault, while Wyman spent time at the hospitals, his real passion was the Jardin des Plantes. At the start of 1841 he reported to his brother Morrill that he was "visiting the Hospitals in the morning & attending lectures during the rest of the day."[187] But he soon gravitated to the Jardin, where he studied at the museum—"surrounded by 'all creation' in a convenient space"—and took lectures from, among others, Achille Valenciennes, Isidore Geoffroy Saint-Hilaire, Pierre Flourens, Étienne Serres, and Alexandre Brongniart. "I make Natural History the main object of my visit here," he told his friend, Boston physician and naturalist David Humphreys Storer, in August. "The greatest object of attraction as I have already stated is the museum which is unquestionably far superior to any thing of the kind in the world."[188] By October Jeffries informed Morrill that he had moved from the Latin Quarter to a room near the Jardin "& nearly opposite the entrance of La Pitié," noting that "I intend to follow Lisfranc at La Pitié every morning, which I shall have sufficient time to do before the lectures commence in the Garden."[189] Preparing to leave Paris six months later, Jeffries felt satisfied that he had used so much of his time "diligently studying Nat[l] History." Yet, he reflected, "I sometimes think that it would have been more wise to have confined myself entirely to medicine as it is a matter of great uncertainty whether Nat[l] Hist. will ever give me a living."[190]

Most American physicians in the French capital, however, forced to make choices about how to spend their limited time abroad, focused their energies on exercising the singular access Paris gave them to the human body. And while various pedagogic contexts enabled them to learn from the body, it was through private courses that they were best able to exploit what Paris had to offer. From a professional point of view, through the 1850s paid private instruction in the wards and dissecting rooms represented "the paradise of Parisian life" to two generations of American medical migrants.

### IN "A LAND OF STRANGERS"

"Almost every moment of my time is occupied in professional pursuits or in the study of the French language," Samuel Wigglesworth wrote from Paris to his father in 1836, "so that you may judge I have as yet had little time to see the sights and wonders of Paris."[191] Statements such as this abounded in the reports Americans sent home, affirmations of how hard they were working and how single-mindedly they were absorbed in medical improvement. Ashbel Smith made the same point with better evidence: "In attendance at the hospitals, one which commenced at 6 A.M.—in seeing them perform surgical operations on the living—in repeating these operations, myself, on the dead body; in dissecting—in hearing lectures on the various sciences, medicine, &c I am engaged at least 8 generally 10 hours daily."[192]

But what of the remaining fourteen to sixteen hours? Even the devoted student was likely to spend as many waking hours outside the medical world as within it. Smith, at least, was moderately candid and went on to say, "I have roamed to a *certain extent* through every class of society from balls *honored* by the presence of the king, to 12½ cent parties where one may exchange his ticket of entrance for 3 dances or 2 bottles of beer."[193] The time medical Americans spent in lecture halls, hospital wards, and dissecting rooms was only one part of their Parisian experience; and their other hours—the focus of this section—would color the ways they perceived Paris, remembered their time there, and understood its place in their lives.

At night, back in their room at a pension or lodging house, one nodal point in the weekly routine was writing about Paris. Antebellum diaries, like letters, were not necessarily thought of as private documents, and on homecoming a travel diary in particular might be circulated among family and friends. What Americans inscribed there were selective representations both of Paris and of themselves. Yet the pages reveal much about their affective lives. A persistent theme was awareness of being an outsider, with the dual sense of exclusion and superiority that might bring. Writing also prompted reflection on what it meant to be American, just as it catalyzed one stage in the construction of self in which the transforming power of Parisian experience was counterbalanced against a growing valuation of ties to home. A young man such as Waring, who had never before been away from home, could leave a document at once remarkably banal and compellingly self-reflective. "These are notes taken by Morton N. Waring in Paris AD 1856," he began his travel journal. "If in after years like some weary Traveller, I am permitted to turn to this memoir of my pilgrimage, it will lull the care worn spirit of a drooping life, by the thoughts of my Boyhood & Sunny dreams, but if Death's autumn gale shall detach my leaf from Life's Oak, there will come after me some who might find pleasure in perusing these notes, to while away the restless moments of a tedious hour or think of Morton."[194]

The letters themselves often began by recounting what set the act of writing them apart from the ordinary flow of things: taking pen in hand, calling to mind the last letter received, turning thoughts homeward. Writing served an important professional function, for, as chapter 4 will show, one way of transmitting French medicine to America and advertising one's absence in France for professional improvement was sending letters home for publication in a newspaper or medical journal. But it served an important cognitive function as well, for self-consciously reflecting on what one had seen and experienced and then putting those reflections on paper were key elements in the process of distilling a complex set of impressions into a simplified, streamlined, tellable story. It was in significant measure through the process of letter writing that American physicians began to construct *their* Paris School—imposing order and structure on disparate observations and perceptions and beginning to assign meaning to them.

An even more pressing epistolary duty was owed to family. A few married physicians made the journey with their wives, but most of the former were medical tourists—studying, perhaps, but for weeks or a couple of months rather than years.[195] Usually the married man made the journey alone. Regular letters were expected, though few wives, and few husbands, felt that their partner wrote often enough. Their correspondence, which ranged from moving expressions of longing to perfunctory formal exercises, played out feelings of freedom and loneliness, reproach and regret, empathy and indifference, guilt and defensive resolve. In these letters, representations of self and of one's engagement with life in Paris depended very much on not just who was writing but to whom. In his guarded letters to his sister-in-law, for example, John

Young Bassett did not present the same image of Paris and his activities there as in letters to his wife, Isaphoena.[196] "Why are you so sad?" John wrote to Isa the day after he arrived in Paris. "Do you think you alone suffer from our separation? You who are not separated from your friends, nor your dear little children, & from your husband but for a short time—did I say a short time, it is beginning to be a long time with me already."[197] Four months later: "Beare up for a while, I will soon be with you to pet and quarrel, and I am sure you will wish me in France again many a time, but I wont go."[198] For her part, Isa urged him not to wait to send long epistles, but to write frequent, short letters— "sort-o-howdy's," she called them.[199] If their correspondence did good work in sustaining the bonds between them, ultimately it was inadequate. Isa had to cope with the overheard gossip of neighbors in the Alabama town where they lived saying he had left her, while John intensely missed his toddlers, worried they might not remember him, and found himself in Paris "continually conjuring up dangers."[200]

The young, unmarried physician ordinarily was also expected to write fortnightly or monthly to his family, usually with the understanding that a letter to one member would be passed around for all to read. Perhaps the most consistent message young men sought to convey to their parents (or uncles, brothers, or whoever was paying the bills) was that they were studying terribly hard. Reinforced by the protest that they had been so occupied in the hospitals that they had yet to see anything of the city, this was also the most commonly invoked excuse for short or tardy letters. Holmes, more inclined to parody convention than to follow it, closed one letter to his mother and father by saying that "bad correspondent as I am, you must contrive to prevent any of my dear friends and relations from getting outrageous, by the customary phrases, 'much engaged in his profession,' 'time entirely occupied,' and the rest."[201] It is striking how seldom parents wrote with admonishments to work hard; instead, preoccupied with the health of their physician-child, fathers and mothers much more often wrote urging them not to overexert themselves.

Such anxiety about the possibility of illness far from home in what one Paris-bound American called "a land of strangers" was not unwarranted.[202] Medical study—days spent breathing hospital air dense with disease-producing miasmas—was seen as a dangerous activity.[203] And accidents were common. "I have lost an eye," Elizabeth Blackwell wrote from France in 1850 of what she had diagnosed as ophthalmia. "While at the Maternité, I attended an infant afflicted with the disease, and as I was syringing the eye, a drop of the water spirted up from his eye to mine."[204] Blackwell was told she would be completely blind, but gradually she regained sight in one eye; she lost the use of the other eye, however, and had it replaced with an eye of glass.[205]

Cutting on the dead body equally involved risk, as nineteenth-century medical Americans recognized. A prick of the finger by the knife might be tersely mentioned as a routine diary entry, but it threatened the possibility of serious illness. "I came very near getting into trouble the other day by dissecting," Bryant wrote to his father about his work at the Clamart.

> I had a little bit of a sore on one of my fingers and not wishing to get a dissecting wound I covered it over with a bit of sticking plaster—after I had finished as it was very dirty I took it off—and then on looking for my instruments found that somebody had taken my sponge and dirtied it—without thinking I took it and squeezed it and the blood &c run all over my hands—after I got home and was sitting very quietly reading in my room I was taken with a regular chill afterwards with a high fever and great pain in the arm pit—I thought at first I was done for and should probably have at least a phlebite with any quantity of abcess in my arm pit at the least—I had a most tremendous fever all night did not sleep a wink all night and was very sick in bed all day.

He recovered in a few days but reflected on other incidents among his fellow students earlier in Boston and now in Paris: "I have no doubt that out of a hundred persons dissecting there would be at least one dangerously sick, and probably one death in the same number each season."[206] Seven months later, Bryant received another dissection wound, this time from a saw wielded by another student. Pain, chills, vomiting, and apprehension ensued, and Bryant "went to bed determined to let operation alone for the future provided I got well in time to recommence."[207] The consequences of such a wound could be fatal. "Je suis allé il y a peu de jours à l'interment d'un Médecin Anglais, qui est mort à la suite d'une piqure anatomique," Williams reported to his sisters of a fellow student who had accidently cut himself at the dissecting table, "mais j'ai été tres fortuné à cet égard moi même." He concluded optimistically, "Avec un peu de soin il y a peu de danger."[208] Letters sent home by American physicians reporting a death among their number—from whatever cause—could not help but deepen the anxieties of their families; and many surely would have agreed with Shattuck who, writing from Paris to his mother that "a medical student from Philadelphia died yesterday [of] an illness of four days," noted that "a death in a strange land is peculiarly melancholy."[209]

Families shared other worries as well about the American alone in Paris—"removed so far from the influence of home and friends, and without the wholesome restraints of social associations or even public opinion," as Flint put it.[210] "The gardens—the opera—the cancan—and the thousand and one places of amusement to be found in the gay metropolis—to say nothing of that somewhat fabulous combination of graces and soft inclinations, the *grisettes*," one physician wrote home, "take all these into consideration, and then require a man to throw aside his moral straight-waistcoat for the time, and substitute the loose luxurious dishabille of genteel depravity, and it is not surprising that people inclined to a life of *abandon* should find Paris a delightful place for the gratification of the propensity."[211] Frances Peter wrote from their home in Kentucky to her husband Robert in Paris saying, "I dislike the idea sometimes of thinking that you are now in the most profligate capital in Europe—where you will meet with so many temptations to idleness and dissipation and I wish myself with you again and again."[212] When Martha Battey sent a similar message to her husband Robert, suggesting that perhaps he should return to Georgia, he wrote back, "It is not wise to make your picture of home bondage too dark and strongly marked—least peradventure my heart might satisfy itse[l]f with the gay pleasures and social freedom of 'La belle Paris' and the opportunity never offer to bring your fancied iron rule."[213]

American physicians in Paris generally were agreed about the condition of French morals and mores—Parisian indulgence, as one put it, "in vice, license & excess"[214]—but differed widely in assessing its lessons. Some were repelled by what one called "this vile old Babylon," while others were charmed by a city that put on "one of the most brilliant shows in the world."[215] For many, the spectacle of Parisian life was a new experience to be savored. Writing in 1840 of the forthcoming ceremony marking the reinterment of Napoléon's remains in French soil, Joynes told his sister that "it will be an occasion such as has never been witnessed before, and never will be again. I shall consider it an *era in my life*, to have witnessed it."[216] At the same time, many maintained that the French passion for spectacle fostered show at the expense of something sturdier and more authentic. "You would never know that there was such a day as Sunday here except by your almanack," Joynes wrote to his mother, echoing an observation on French religious life that disapproving American Protestants made again and again.[217]

Yet Americans did not merely observe the life of Paris; to varying extents they engaged in it. They visited the Louvre and Notre Dame, made short excursions to Versailles and Alfort, and planned longer tours through the Continent, just as they witnessed fêtes, attended theater, went to church services, and, when it was rumored that the guillotine was about to be used, hurried through the streets to watch. Some took lovers or visited brothels. They bought medical books and surgical instruments for themselves and pathological specimens, skeletons, and libraries for medical schools at home. And they bought hats, china, bracelets, and prints to take home with them as presents.

They could not help but notice political events unfolding in the streets of Paris, most violently in the revolutions of 1830 and 1848, though they generally expressed their own political sympathies in words rather than actions. "I arrived at the Place Victoire just as the National Guard was charging upon the people," Bowditch reported of the uprising of 1832. "I, being, not much of a warrier, fled most rapidly over barricades & down narrow streets till I found myself fairly lodged in utter darkness, by the shutting of a door, through which I had entered with a crowd of other brave spirits."[218] Ashbel Smith, writing from Paris the same day as Bowditch, kept aloof from the fighting but reported to a friend that "I make the most of it in the study of gunshot wounds."[219] Charles Jackson, who was away touring England at the time of the revolution of 1830—"I missed the revolution in France!" he wrote home sulkily after returning to Paris—took advantage of the same circumstance, following a course at the Hôtel Dieu with Dupuytren "on Gun Shot & Sabre wounds with plenty of illustrations from the late Glorious Revolution of July."[220]

Not all stayed so aloof, however. The Crimean War in particular captured their attention. In 1854, Jenkins seriously considered taking a commission as a surgeon in the Russian army—partly out of sympathy with the Russian cause, partly because he needed the money, and principally, as he explained to his brother, because of "the amount of practical knowledge which the position would give one the opportunity of acquiring."[221] He decided against this course but noted that two acquaintances signed on. Some twenty Americans then studying medicine in Paris did join the medical staff of the Russian army, and half of them were killed during their service. William Joseph Holt, a South Carolinian who entered the fray, had received his M.D. in Georgia before making the journey to Paris in 1852. He studied there for two years until, as he wrote in his diary, "on the 19th, July, 1854, I left Paris for Brussels, with the intention of consulting with Count Chreptowitch as to enlisting in the Russian Service as a Surgeon."[222] Holt went on to serve at Sevastopol during the siege, leaving a detailed account of his exploits in his diary, and returned home with extensive experience in military medicine—experience he soon would put to use as surgeon in the Confederate army.[223]

In Paris, most Americans studying medicine did become part of a community. There was a large Anglophone population in the city, bound together not least of all by *Galignani's Messenger*, the English-language morning newspaper, and by Galignani's reading room. Yet the interaction of medical Americans with the British residents of the city, even British medical students, was meager. Many discovered that being in France intensified their awareness of being American. "The poor English are much hated here," Dugas wrote in 1828 to his mother, "& as I am always taken for one, I continually hear myself called as I pass, rost. Bif, diable d'Anglais, Goddam, &c."[224] Bryant tried to identify himself as non-English by growing a beard. When visiting England on his way to Paris, he told his father, he had found that his beard "attracted a great deal of attention so I cut it off and endeavoured to render myself 'tout au fait' Anglais"; but he reported from Paris that "a shaved face was as rare here as an unshaved one in England." As he explained, "Every body, who saw me immediately took me for an Englishman from the smoothness of my chin. I therefore determined to allow that beautiful addition to my personal attraction to sprout again and at present it is in a perfect shoe brush state."[225]

Medical Americans often became involved in the flourishing American community of Paris—what one physician, assessing "the American colony" in 1855, called a "seething cauldron" of intrigues and rivalries.[226] Politics sometimes brought Americans together, at least for symbolic action. After the revolution of 1848, for example, as Williams reported to his sisters, "Les Americains iront aujourd'hui, en masse, feliciter le gouvernement provisoire. J'irai avec les autres, car si'il faut avoir une procession, il vaut mieux de la faire aussie nombreuse que possible."[227] Celebrations on each 4th of July also drew members of the community together for a "fête Americaine," as did parties periodically held by the ambassador. Holmes, however, may have expressed the sentiments of many when he wrote to his parents of the recent "American ball": "I did not go to it; first, because I did not want to—and second, because I did not choose to spend seventy-five francs for a parcel of folks of whom I knew little more than that they were raised on the same side of the water as I was."[228] American physicians regularly visited acquaintances from home who were passing through the city, but medical study distanced them physically from most of the American community. "The number of Americans in Paris is astonishing," Wigglesworth noted in 1836, but, writing from his residence in the Latin Quarter, he observed that "the Americans whom I have seen on this side of the river are all physicians or students of medicine."[229]

More cohesive was the student community medical Americans formed themselves. This community was far from inclusive, and, particularly as the American medical student population of Paris grew in the 1840s and 1850s (and as tensions stemming from regional politics intensified at home), students from Massachusetts and others from South Carolina tended to form their own circles. At the same time, in Paris physicians from different parts of America met, shared experiences, and forged bonds that would hold together a lasting network after their return. They took meals together, shared cadavers at the dissecting table, and spent evenings talking in each other's rooms. They advised one another about studying in Paris and touring in Europe. Charles Jackson, in 1832, even put together a course for his compères, most likely American and English. "I gave a course of lectures at the Hopital St Antoine on Surgical Anatomy which gave me a little reputation among the foreign students," he wrote home. "This course was given to a few friends attached to the hospital & served to give me an opportunity of reviewing my anatomy previous to my departure——The students furnished me with as many subjects as I required & sometimes I used 4 or 5 bodies per day."[230]

Social interactions with French men and women, especially of their own socioeconomic class, were few. Except for cases in which Americans had letters introducing them to French acquaintances of their circle at home—a good number of travelers in the 1820s and early 1830s brought such letters to Lafayette, for example—their interactions with the nonmedical French tended to be with landladies, landlords, and shopkeepers, not their social peers. Residence in the Latin Quarter fostered this situation, for medical study, as one noted, placed them among "the poor and destitute, the student, and of that class, known only in Paris—the grisette."[231] Williams was not alone in complaining that he had "no opportunity of speaking to any of the other sex, except in the stores, which are mostly in their hands, or by chatting with the grisettes on an afternoon, in the Gardens of the Luxembourg."[232] Nevertheless, like others Williams was fascinated by "the class termed grisettes," which, as he understood it, encompassed "all the young mantua-makers, tailoresses, shop girls, &c," and also "the young girls with or without a particular profession, whose principal business is to assist the students in disposing of their time and money. *Most* of the first class belong to the second, but not all. They have temptations to mischief in the different manners of French society, and in their own poverty and miserable compensation."[233] As another American physician who visited Paris in 1844 reported, "A student can live on the most intimate terms with his *grisette*, in many of the hotels, without giving offence to landlord or landlady. *Grisettes* visit their rooms, when they please. The student and his *grisette* often dine together at a restaurant, and at many of the houses I presume there would be no sort of objection to them dining at the *table d'hote*. I would not advise that any young man be sent to Paris to improve his morals."[234]

Interactions with *medical* Frenchmen outside pedagogic settings also were quite limited. Americans and Britons alike noted that professional letters of introduction met with gracious attention in England were only lightly regarded in France.[235] Only a few French clinicians cultivated the company of Americans, as Louis did by inviting many of them—Wood, Holmes, Jackson, Bryant, Williams, and Stewardson, among others—to dinners at his house. Williams enjoyed discovering that another guest at the small dinner party he attended was Victor Hugo, who was related to Louis by marriage, and called the evening "a perfect bijou," and Bryant wrote home describing the entire menu, concluding that "I had rather dine with Louis than with the King."[236]

Louis's Société Médicale d'Observation, organized in Paris by a small band of French, Swiss, and American students in 1832, with Louis as perpetual president and Gabriel Andral and François Chomel as officers, was made up of physicians consecrated to his program of rigorous observation and numerical analysis of signs and symptoms in the living patient and physical lesions at autopsy. A small and intense group in which each member in turn prepared a medical report, which then was criticized by the rest, the Société met weekly as a forum for honing skills in clinical observation and analysis, and usually counted a few Americans among its members. "Our object is the *exact study of disease*," as Jackson, Jr., a founding member, described the society to his father.[237] "At this moment America is not represented in the 'Society of Observations of Paris,'" Louis wrote to Bowditch in 1846, "however I hope that a friend of Mr Williams' will soon enter, and it only rests with Mr Williams himself as soon as he is familiar with French to become one of us. I hope this may be soon, for as long as the society is without Americans, it seems incomplete to me."[238] The Société produced lasting relationships between Louis's French pupils François-Louis Valleix and E. Rufz and a number of his American disciples.

Interconnections among members of the Anglophone medical student community were formalized in 1837 when the Parisian Medical Society was founded by, among other Britons, the Scottish physician John Hughes Bennett. The society had its own quarters, including a reading room, and held regular meetings. For a few years, between 1848 and 1851, it shared facilities with the German medical students' organization, the Verein deutscher Aerzte in Paris, founded in 1844. From the late 1830s through the early 1850s, a number of Americans became members and even officers of the society, which, as one reported, was open to virtually anyone willing to pay the hefty membership fee of thirty francs.[239]

Americans founded their own organization, the American Medical Society in Paris, in 1851, only a few years after the first national medical society—the American Medical Association—had been founded in their own country in 1847. Indeed, the Paris group was recognized by the AMA as an *American* society, entitled to send delegates to annual AMA meetings. Like its British counterpart, the American society established a library and reading room and held regular evening meetings. For Americans who arrived in Paris during the 1850s it was an institutionalized source of the kind of advice that hitherto had been passed along informally from experienced students to newcomers. Its membership was open to all orthodox graduates and students—those, as the constitution put it, of "the regular medical profession." The society also facilitated interactions among American physicians from different parts of the United States: a roster of 114 active members for 1851–1854 was drawn from twenty-nine states and the District of Columbia.[240]

ONE AMERICAN IN PARIS

Perhaps the best way to display how medical activities were tightly interwoven with life outside the hospitals is through a closer look at one American's Parisian experiences. Philip Claiborne Gooch was in most respects an unremarkable representative of the young American physicians who set off to Paris for professional improvement. Born in Richmond in 1825, in 1845 he received his M.D. from the University of Virginia. While a student he began keeping a terse but frank diary, and even though there may have been little in his medical or social life to distinguish him from his peers, the record he left of his daily routine is exceptional. "To keep a diary or an accurate journal, requires more industry, method, regularity, etc., than I possess," he wrote in his first diary in 1845.

> But still I have found that with little trouble I have recorded many little events and little particulars about big events, etc., which I should have otherwise forgotten. I have never kept a diary useful to anybody else or one which would permit any one else to read. So should I die suddenly, or this book fall accidentally into the hands of any one, by all that is right, by my memory, by honor and everything else, I hope and beg that it may be immediately committed to the flames. I only expect herein to devote some two or three lines to account for each of Gods days which pass, and when I get married and be settled in a state of "nothing to do," or am at sea, or in prison, then I may fill pages with reflections, dissertations, etc.[241]

In September 1846, Gooch, age twenty-one, sailed for Europe, working his passage as ship's surgeon. Docking in Liverpool, he traveled directly to Edinburgh, where he remained studying medicine for the next eleven months. There he observed practice at the Royal Infirmary and attended lectures by William P. Alison, Robert Christison, John Goodsir, William Thomson, and James Simpson, among others. He was especially taken with Simpson's lectures on midwifery and the arguments Simpson made for the "necessity of medical aid in delivery."[242] Skeptical of surgical anesthesia, Gooch wrote in January 1847, after seeing three operations using the new practice at the Royal Infirmary, "The failure of the ether pleased me very much."[243] But scarcely a week later he had to report, "Had my skepticism shaken in 'Ether'-ism today by an operation by Wm. Miller."[244] Impressed, two days later he inhaled ether while a friend wielding forceps painlessly extracted his tooth. "I reckon everything claimed for ether is true—I will investigate it myself," he vowed.[245] Gooch left Edinburgh in mid-September for Manchester, then London, where he spent three weeks. In London he played medical tourist, visiting half a dozen hospitals and the famous figures who had charge of them, then crossed the Channel to Le Havre and on to Paris, where he arrived at the end of October 1847.

Gooch spoke some French when he arrived, but found he could not follow lectures and immediately made arrangements for private French lessons.[246] During his first several months, he pursued the kind of eclectic medical course most of his countrymen followed. He attended *cliniques* at the Hôtel Dieu, La Charité, and the Hôpital du Midi; dissected at the École Pratique; and registered, after six weeks, for Sichel's private course on diseases of the eye and, after ten, for Dubois's instruction on midwifery. In mid-December he attended a meeting of the Parisian Medical Society "where I heard and joined in a foolish debate on the Ether discovery."[247] He was elected a member of the society a week later, usually went there several times a week to read, and in mid-January delivered a paper on "Fevers and Their Treatment."[248] At the same time, he established a circle of a dozen or so friends—young American and English physicians and students, like himself. With them he played cards, billiards, and backgammon; got drunk; studied medicine; visited brothels; and went to meetings of the Parisian Medical Society.

By the start of 1848 Gooch had grown comfortably integrated into both medical and social worlds, an adaptation to Paris exemplified by the fact that starting on New Year's Day of 1848, he wrote his journal entirely in rather bad French. On one typical Wednesday in January, Gooch's medical activities—attending Dubois's *clinique d'accouchements* and a meeting of the council of the Parisian Medical Society—were followed by playing billiards with Shannon until midnight then returning together to his room "where we drank two bottles of cognac and talked until 7:30."[249] The diary entry for the following day began:

> Thursday 27th. We went with Kingsley to the l'hopital Lourcine. Shannon was very drunk and very insulting on the street and after some business with K he drank coffee in a café for poor people and I went in the hospital where I saw 75 women examined with the speculum. Rose, Shannon and Kingsley went skating and I went to bed until 6 when I dined. at 8 Daniell came and we went to the prado where I danced like three Parisians. At 1:30 he left while I chatted.[250]

Over the next week he continued to read at the society's room, follow Sichel's private course, and attend Dubois's *clinique*; as one diary entry on the latter read tersely, "Went to the hospital clinic and touched the women."[251] He also spent a good deal of time playing billiards, won thirty-five francs one evening and fifty-five another playing cards, and, at one dinner, was "very drunk. I broke the glasses, etc."[252] Another evening, in the company of several friends, Gooch sought out Eppes and, as he wrote, "We went together to his woman's place but she was busy and we went to 15 rue Mauvais garçons (and we were) with the women."253

In February, his routine was briefly disrupted by political events. "I am in a state, like the city, of incertitude," he wrote on the 21st. "Perhaps tomorrow at this time (8 P.M.) the peace which exists now will be replaced by the uproar of a Parisian riot—perhaps Odilion Barrot will have the place of Louis Phillippe, or he will have paid with his opposition colleagues, for their patriotism, by the loss of his head. There are now many new regiments in Paris, and the officers are thrown in every section dressed like bourgeois as if they were citizens from the provinces." He described the repressive system of surveillance by the secret police and closed his entry: "I am very quiet."254 Yet several days later he could write exuberantly: "The National Guard is completely with the people. The king has left for some chateau. The Tuileries have been taken by the crowd, and I was there—on the throne and on the bed of His Majesty." He noted that "many citizens are dead. But the Municipal's are forced to retreat. Long live the Republic."255

For the time being he stopped going to the hospitals and, unlike some of his friends, embraced rather than avoided the life of the street. " 'Bonjour citoyen' everybody says. I was enrolled as a French citizen (8th county) and went to the Hotel de Ville where I saw 89 of the dead in one room. All the fortifications of Paris are with the people now. I saw everything with the red badge of liberty and took souvenirs from the Municipals from their hats and horses. Spoke with McIntosh and Eppes who are very much afraid, and Scott who does not want to go out."256 The following day: "24 batallions of the National Guard were called—mobile—and I am very willing to go with them. I went to Rose's and Shannon's who came to dinner with me. We went to Ganahl's. His woman was in bed, but we talked until 11."257 After a few days, Gooch returned to his work at the École Pratique, and, the following week, "I attended the meeting of the Americans who went to the government to offer their congratulations, etc. There were more than 275 of us. Everything is as it should be."258

Daily life was again peaceful, but not dull. When Armstrong, one of their number, "received letters commanding his departure from Paris, from his father," some twenty-six members of the Parisian Medical Society dined together to see him off. At the dinner, Gooch reported, "I found seven kinds of wine around my plate. Afterwards we went to the Baroness's. She was at the party, Castellane Street, where we also went. Found many Parisian lionesses, princesses, etc. playing Asuquenette. We resisted the temptations of the evening and went to Brent's where Shannon was a little talkative, and left from there at 2:30, and I went to bed."259 Some days were more fully occupied with medicine than others; thus 5 May:

> I got up early. Went to l'hopital Lourcine, where I saw many cases with the speculum, to l'Ecole practique where I began a course on operative surgery—afterwards to la charité to begin a course on auscultation. Dine at the Restaurant. Showed the rooms [of the society] to an American who has been here for only three days and

who does not understand a word of French. Read the newspapers and went to bed at 11.[260]

A couple of weeks later, though, the full daily entry read:

Tuesday, May 23. I went to my classes. I pricked my finger at l'Ecole practique.

Wednesday Gooch went to classes as usual, and, in the evening, to a discussion on typhoid fever at the medical society. But his finger, which on Thursday he cauterized himself, was troublesome. Friday he again tried to go to classes, but "I was so sick that I had to come back to my place and go to bed." As Gooch recorded, "I was very delirious and with terrible fever all night. In the morning of Saturday 27. I found my tonsils very swollen and I questioned then all this constitutional upheaval. I called Mr. Velpeau to see me and take out my tonsils. He came at 2, but refused to do the operation because of the intense inflammation which existed. Scott came and applied 20 leeches, the strongest and the largest that we have seen. They sucked very well and the blood flowed all night."[261] Severely ill from his dissection wound, Gooch was hardly alone; on Sunday, he was visited by "Drs. MacKenzie, Powers, Noel, Ganahl, Ron Hume, Shannon, Eppes, Upson, Scott, McIntosh, Victor." He regained his health, but scarcely two weeks after the first accident wrote: "To the class at l'Ecole practique, where I made some very pretty operations on a subject—a woman, the most beautiful woman I have ever seen. I touched my finger with a knife."[262] This time, though, no illness ensued.

In late June politics again crowded out all else from Gooch's attention. "I no longer have confidence in the French. They fired on the barricades and raked the streets with cannon, but at 11 it was all over and consternation prevailed everywhere," he wrote on Friday, June 23 of the riots he had seen. "I have a cold from talking in favor of law, order, and the Republic."[263] On Saturday he wrote that "the streets are full of bayonets and one cannot pass, even officers, without the watch-word,"[264] but by morning "the rioters are 100,000 or more strong" and all had changed. "You could not go out, but I found a way to go everywhere. I showed a waiter's apron and instruments, bandages, pins, lint, etc, etc, and I went to la Charité, where there were only 35 or 40 wounded. I looked at all of them and talked with some representatives of the people, who have adopted (the assembly) the wounded and the widows and the orphans as 'enfants de la republique.' I went to Rose and Shannon's. I found Manigault who has not been able to return home for three days. . . . I went to Scott's and McIntosh's who begged me to return home, but there was still fighting near l'hotel dieu I went there. I saw many barricades and troops. I was told 'you cannot pass, etc.,' but I did so with no difficulty." Gooch spent several hours at the Hôtel Dieu before returning home. "The struggle is over. The insurgents are all defeated."[265]

Returning to his medical work that summer—at La Charité, the Hôtel Dieu, La Pitié, the Hôpital des Cliniques, and the medical society, of which he was now an officer—Gooch revealed in his diary that, like many of the men in his circle, he had formed an attachment with a young women, a *grisette*, Clementine: "My woman dined here and came back to supper and to sleep," he wrote on a Sunday early in August, for example.[266] He was angry to discover several days later that she had another lover, and told her so, but she apparently ignored his pique. The same day Dufour, a fellow medical student who was ill with varioloid and could not leave his room, sent Gooch on an errand to deliver two hundred francs to his *grisette* Anna.[267] The group discussed among themselves what should be done about the problem of another of their number, "Champy and his woman whom he cannot pay."[268] Gooch wrote home that summer to his mother in Virginia, "I have now got the hang of Paris & the french so I am now profiting by everything here."[269]

Perhaps Gooch was aware that his private diary was growing in some ways more intensely private than it had been when he had begun making daily entries as a student in Charlottesville, and that, unlike the travel journals of most of his peers, his was not suited for circulation among family members after his return home. At this juncture, he bought a new bound volume and in a large hand wrote in English on the cover: "Journal of the most private nature of Phil Claiborne Gooch. 'Kill me, but don't read this book.'" And as his first entry in the new volume (inscribed, like all the daily reports, entirely in French), he wrote:

23 rue Racine. Paris. September 1st, 1848.

Eh bien! Behold the beginning of another volume of my "Journal," dignified with that name. But since it is only for my eyes—to assist my memory I do not care what will be thought of it if it is read by some other person. But if it were to fall by accident, or bad luck, some of these days when I am dead in the hands of my family or of a swine who would like to meddle with me or with my affairs—I beg them to stop here. But if one persisted in reading it he will have my *curse* [ma *malediction*] whether I be in hell or elsewhere.[270]

Gooch continued to pursue his medical studies with undiminished vigor, but at the same time his private affairs and those of his friends became more complex and more taxing. Several days into the new volume, he wrote, "Scott is very sick—cold, fever and gonorrhea (which he caught from the first woman since his return—and what is more, she was his woman)."[271] He spent some of the next morning tending Scott and later returned to his room to study Orfila on toxicology.[272] Over the next couple of weeks he periodically attended morning rounds at La Charité and the Hôtel Dieu, followed Sichel's private course, and, late in the month, bought a set of surgical instruments and (after getting Scott's advice on the matter) started dissecting at the Clamart. At the end of that same week, on Saturday morning, he was awakened at six by his friend Theodore Champy, desperate because he somehow had engaged himself to fight a duel; Gooch spent the next few hours soothing the offended opponent, forestalling the duel, and catching the end of morning rounds at the Hôtel

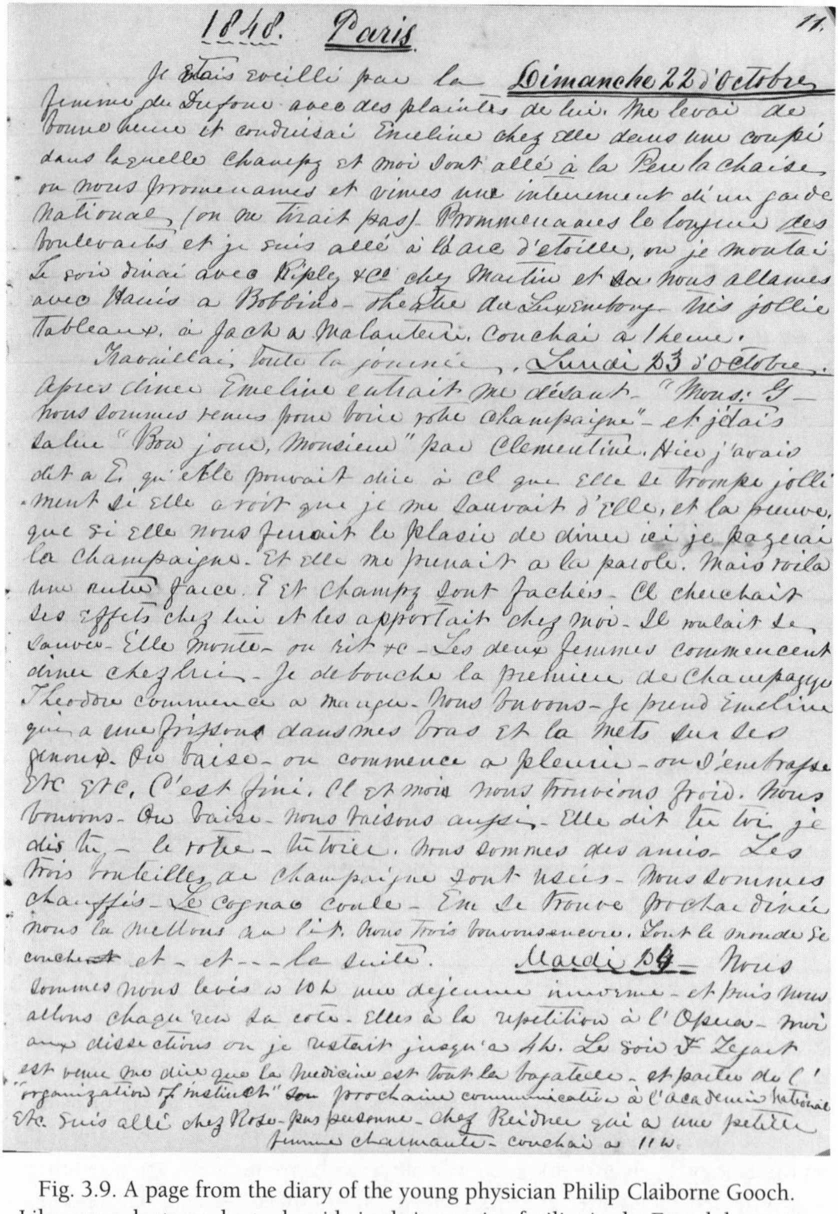

1848. Paris 11.
Je étais eveillé par la Dimanche 22 d'octobre
femme du Dufour avec des plaintes de lui. Me levai de
bonne heure et conduisai Emeline chez elle dans une coupé
dans laquelle Champz et moi sont allé à la Pere la chaise
ou nous promenames et vimes une interrement d'un garde
National (on ne tirait pas). Promenames le longue des
boulevards et je suis allé à l'arc d'étoille, ou je montai
Le soir dinai avec Ripley &c chez Martin et de nous allames
avec Harris a Bobbino — theatre du Luxembourg. Très jollie
tableaux. à Jack a Malanterie. Couchai à 1 heure.
Travaillai toute la journée, Lundi 23 d'octobre.
Apres diner Emeline entrait me disant — "Mons: G —
nous sommes venus pour boire votre champaigne" — et j'étais
salué "Bon jour, Monsieur" par Clementine. Hier j'avais
dit a E. qu'elle pouvait dire à Cl que elle se trompe jolli
-ment si elle croit que je me sauvait d'elle, et la preuve,
que si elle nous ferait le plasir de diner ici je payerai
la champaigne. Et elle me prenait a la parole. Mais voila
une autre farce. E et Champz sont fachés — Cl cherchait
ses effets chez lui et les apportait chez moi — Il voulait se
sauver — Elle monte — on rit &c — Les deux femmes commencent
diner chez lui — Je debouche la premiere de champagne
Theodore commence a manger — Nous buvons — Je prend Emeline
qui a une frissons dans mes bras et la mets sur ses
genoux. On baise — on commence a pleurir — on s'embrasse
Etc Etc. C'est fini. Cl et moi nous trouvions froid. Nous
buvons — On baise — nous faisons aussi — Elle dit tu toi je
dis tu — le votre — tu toie. Nous sommes des amis — Les
trois bouteilles de champaigne sont usées — Nous sommes
chauffés — Le cognac coule — Em se trouve prochaidiné
nous la mettons au lit. Nous trois buvons encore. Tout le monde se
couche et — et — — la suite. Mardi 24 — Nous
sommes nous levés a 10 h une dejeuner inorme — et puis nous
allons chaqu'un sa coté. Elles à la repetition à l'Opera — moi
aux dissections ou je restait jusqu'a 4 h. Le soir F Lejart
est venu me dire que la medicine est tout la bagatelle — et parler de l'
"organization of instinct" son prochaine communication à l'academie National
Etc. Suis allé chez Rose — pas personne — chez Reidner qui a une petite
femme charmante — couchai a 11 h.

Fig. 3.9. A page from the diary of the young physician Philip Claiborne Gooch. Like many doctors who took pride in their growing facility in the French language, Gooch began in 1848 to write his Paris diary entirely in simple, often very poor, French—a practice he continued after returning to his native Virginia. (Philip Claiborne Gooch, Diary, 1 Sept. 1848–16 May 1852, Philip Claiborne Gooch Diaries, courtesy of Division of Archives and Manuscripts, Virginia Historical Society, Richmond.)

Dieu; then, as he wrote in closing that Saturday's entry, "I worked all day at Clamard."[273]

Clementine, it seems, had left him, but one day as he was coming back to his lodging (a week after stopping Champy's duel) "little (formerly my) Clementine saw me. She got off the omnibus and arrived here five minutes after I entered, saying to Ch[ampy] and his girl [Emeline] (who came back after all yesterday about midnight) that I had run away from her, etc.!!! She made me nervous, it is true, but I waited until she left, and I went to Clamard, where I dissected until 5." That evening he played billiards with Scott, then went home and talked with Champy until one in the morning.[274] Gooch left Paris briefly, touring Belgium and the Netherlands, and returned to find that Clementine was now staying with Champy. Gooch, for his part, began to spend time with Champy's erstwhile companion Emeline, who arranged a reconciliation between Gooch and the estranged Clementine:

> I worked all day. Monday, 23rd October. After dinner, Emeline came in telling me, "Mons. G[ooch]—we came to drink your champagne"— and I was greeted "Bon jour, monsieur" by Clementine. Yesterday I told E[meline] that she could say to Cl[ementine] that she is very much mistaken if she believes that I ran away from her, and the proof, that if she would give us the pleasure of dining here I will pay for the champagne. And she took me at my word. But there is another farce. E[meline] and Champy are mad. Cl[ementine] got her things at his place and brought them to my room. He wanted to run away. She comes upstairs—we laugh, etc.—The two women begin to dine with him. I uncork the first bottle of champagne. Theodore begins to eat. We drink. I take Emeline, who has the shivers, in my arms and put her on her knees. We kiss—we start to cry. We embrace, etc., etc. It is finished. Cl[ementine] and I are cold. We drink. They kiss. We kiss also. She says tu toi. I say tu—the votre—the familiar form. We are friends. Three bottles of champagne are empty. We are warm. The cognac flows. Em[eline] is drunk. We put her to bed. The three of us drink some more. Everyone goes to bed and— and————what follows.[275]

In the morning, Gooch reported, "We got up at 10. An enormous breakfast, and then each of us goes his way, the girls to the rehearsal at the Opera, me to dissections, where I stayed until 4."[276]

Two weeks later, Gooch packed his things for the journey back to the United States, leaving Paris on 12 November, the same day he recorded in his diary the proclamation of the Constitution of the French Republic.[277] From Liverpool he again worked his passage as ship's surgeon and made his way to his family's home in Airfield, Virginia. Within the first three years after his return, Gooch, twenty-three years old at the time of his homecoming, would successfully establish himself in medical practice, be elected to head the Richmond Board of Health during the 1849 cholera epidemic, found and edit a medical journal (that served as a platform for proselytizing for French ways), and be elected secretary of the American Medical Association. He died of fever in Richmond in 1853.

## Becoming a Disciple

Americans often sought for signs within themselves that they were being transformed by their experience in Paris. A growing command of French or growing deftness in negotiating Parisian life offered mundane but reassuring indicators of change. Holmes, for example, took enormous satisfaction in the increasing ease with which he made his way. "I feel now as if I had known Paris from my childhood," he wrote to his brother scarcely three months after arriving in the city. "I am as much at home, day and night, in the streets as in Boston, or almost so."[278] Several months later he told his parents that "I acquire every day the little practical matters of experience which teach one how to make the most of such a city as Paris."[279]

A deeper transformation, though, and one key to propelling the French impulse in American medicine, was the process of becoming a disciple of the Paris School. During their time in Paris the American physicians who studied there laid claim to a new tradition and, with it, acquired a new sense of their own heritage. The professional and personal meaning that heritage held for them must be understood within the context of American social relations and their identity as American physicians. Implicit in all their efforts to portray and disseminate French medicine would be a pattern of patronage and obligation that undergirded American assumptions about the relationship between teacher and pupil, preceptor and apprentice, master and disciple, and, in a largely male professional culture, often father and son.

Discipleship both ordered the relationship between past and present and conferred identity. The student assumed responsibilities to his preceptor and the tradition he represented, including the obligation to practice in accordance with its teachings, to defend them, and often to pass them along to others. Being one's father's son was a measure of who one was, in medicine as in society. Nevertheless, while many young men during the antebellum period did learn medicine in the first instance from their fathers or uncles, by this time the kinship bonds more often were metaphorical.

By the second quarter of the century, social and professional changes had loosened the relationship between master and pupil. Within medicine, as schools increasingly took over functions once served by apprenticeship, individualized interactions between preceptor and apprentice were partly supplanted by less personal interactions between professor and medical class. Students began to see themselves as disciples less of their preceptors than of their professors. When James Norcom, a North Carolina physician who had studied at the University of Pennsylvania and remained devoted to his "old master Rush,"[280] gave his sons the names Benjamin Rush and Caspar Wistar after his professors in Philadelphia, he was expressing filial relationships that to him were very real. Discipleship to a famous professor such as Rush created a new web of alliances among the many students spread across the country.

Many medical Americans, no less than the rest of their compatriots, felt uneasy about the fact that their lineage was traced most convincingly to Britain. Professional allegiances to Edinburgh, for example, coexisted in the New Republic with strident calls for cultural independence; and some would take great satisfaction in the symbolism of the redirection of Americans studying medicine abroad away from Britain. Antebellum American physicians did not doubt the special relationship between their culture and that of Britain. Yet many of them welcomed the prospect of forming new allegiances that would create a new professional lineage.

To some extent, Americans placed themselves in an apprentice-preceptor relationship with the Paris clinicians by the very act of going to France to study. Young physicians especially were inclined to cast their relationship to the French in terms of mentorship that were familiar, and, in the unsettling context of a foreign country, perhaps reassuring. What that formal relationship scarcely begins to express, however, is the way that many of them ardently embraced the role of disciple—with all the loyalties and obligations it implied—and made that role an important part of their professional self-definition. For some who had only weak ties to their father-preceptor at home, this step was relatively easy; for others whose devotions were strongly in place before they left America, it was a source of considerable dismay. But in either event, many of the Americans who traveled to Paris assigned French medicine a central place in their lineage, one that bound them to a new tradition and conferred upon them a special identity as its disciples.

Most of these Americans never formed close personal ties to any particular Parisian mentor; the object of their admiration was an abstract model of the Paris School. But some came to regard a single mentor as an embodiment of the Paris School and projected onto a single person the broader ideals that claimed their commitment. Nowhere was this more fervently expressed than in the American discipleship to Pierre Louis, a devotion that William Osler depicted toward the end of the century in an essay on Louis's American pupils, of whom he listed thirty-seven.[281] These disciples made Louis more than any other figure stand for the Paris School in American eyes, leading Williams, who in 1846 had just met Louis, to describe him as "perhaps the most celebrated man of the age in the Medical Profession."[282] Yet Williams's perception was unmistakably American rather than French, for Louis never enjoyed the prominence in France that he gained in the United States. At first glance Louis seems an unlikely candidate for what Holmes rightly spoke of as "idolatry."[283] And even Williams complained that Louis, "though never anything like rude, never takes any notice of those who follow him day after day."[284]

The process through which Louis's most ardent American pupil, James Jackson, Jr., came to regard himself as a committed disciple offers one exemplar of how Americans became attached to their French mentors and displays some of the conflicts that discipleship could arouse. When Jackson arrived in Paris in May 1831, fresh from studying with his father, James Jackson, Sr. (Harvard medical professor, a founder of the Massachusetts General Hospital, and one of the most eminent physicians in the United States), he like most Americans was eager to sample widely all that Paris offered. His cousin Charles Jackson visited his room soon after his arrival to describe the options for medical study and "held out to me a bill of fare, wh. I may say almost crazed me,"[285] and James split up his time following various clinicians. He especially admired Gabriel Andral's *clinique* at La Pitié and within two months wrote to his mother that he had left his old boardinghouse for a room in the building where Andral lived, a move he hoped might aid him (once his French improved) in getting to know the eminent clinician.[286] His main complaint was that ward rounds were too crowded and French students too pushy. "It is extremely difficult to get near the beds when there are many Frenchmen in the room," he told his father. "It has more than once happened to me that just as I was laying my head upon a patient's back to examine him by auscutat[n] a french head wld. slip between mine and that same back occupying the place whence I had intended to reap instruction—this knock upon the h'd wld. very likely be accompanied with the French man's ever-ready Pardon, Mons." Jackson also attended Louis's *clinique*, which he judged "very good but again not very remarkable—I have heard better in Boston and in Paris."[287] His admiration of Andral grew, but he spent increasing amounts of time in Louis's wards chiefly because access to the bedside was easier there. "You will perhaps ask what right I have in Louis' ward when I have been so boastful of my privilege to follow Andral," he wrote his father, but explained that "Louis happens to have just at present the greatest number of interest[g] cases."[288]

Access to bedside instruction continued to be Jackson's chief preoccupation. At Louis-Benoît Guersant's *clinique* at the Hôpital des Enfants Malades, he complained that "the crowd is too great to learn much," but made private arrangements with an *interne* to visit the wards in the evenings.[289] Several months later, in October, he complained about the crowds at the Hôtel Dieu, noting that "I have got a ticket to Hotel Dieu but do not expect to use it a great deal—it is almost impossible to gain knowledge there." Dissatisfied with a private class on the use of the uterine speculum attended by over eighty pupils, Jackson approached the surgeon Armand Velpeau for advice, but he suggested no better alternatives.[290] Jackson later told his father, "I have made two or three efforts to follow Chomel at Hotel Dieu—but it is impossible to do so with advantage—one may hear the Clinique to be sure and a very good one too, but he cannot see the patients."[291] He was pleased that Louis had lost the *concours* for the "chair of Clinique" at the Hôtel Dieu and noted that his vote would have gone to the winner, Jean-Baptiste Bouillaud. "My reason for being satisfied with his rejection is that he will give a Clinique at La Pitié during the winter wh. I shall be able to attend." Jackson had come to admire Louis's skill at auscultation but looked forward to his *clinique*—"very exact, but not very eloquent"—principally because it would be uncrowded.[292] Louis, Jackson told his father after the *clinique* had started, "is perhaps as good, as exact an observer of *facts* as Andral but does not compare with him in force of mind, in imagination, in genius."[293]

By the start of 1832, Jackson's devotion to Andral had intensified, and he even told Jackson, Sr., that "his opinions are on many points so like y'r own that I find in him as it were a second father." In two new and preeminently French fields, pathological anatomy and auscultation, Jackson suggested that Andral's teaching even had the advantage over that of his Boston father.[294] All the while, Jackson continued to follow Louis. Over the seven months since his arrival the young American's French had improved—which mattered, for Louis spoke no English[295]—and he reveled in each small sign of approval Louis gave him. "Vous êtes bien habitué à l'auscultation," the teacher remarked one day after Jackson had interpreted sounds heard in a patient's chest, leading Jackson to write his father, "In very truth my heart leaped for joy."[296] Jackson continued to praise Andral but proceeded to make plans to leave Paris to study in Edinburgh and, later, in Germany. The overriding problem with Andral was that he was "too popular for any one to derive as much fr. him as if he were less so."[297]

A turning point in Jackson's relationship with Louis came in early February 1832, when (in return for the grand sum of a thousand francs, some $230) Louis agreed to give private lessons on auscultation to Jackson and Philadelphians Gerhard and Pennock. Elated, Jackson postponed his planned visit to Edinburgh and resented anything that drew him away from his new studies. He acknowledged that he should attend Broussais's *clinique*, for example, but wrote that "it is like tearing a heart-string to leave La Pitié—since my happy arrangement."[298] Within a few weeks he regretted his earlier assessment of Louis: "I did not do Louis justice—I did not then know half his merit." He still maintained that Andral had a better claim to genius, but insisted that "in clinical instruction Louis is the superior—of this I am now convinced—Andral has delighted me I almost love him, but Louis has taught me more." When Louis disclosed later that month the plan to create his Société Médicale d'Observation, "a select corp" that Jackson proudly noted would include him, Jackson was again deeply flattered.[299] He felt part of an exclusive inner circle that would spearhead a new departure in medicine, and for the first time referred to Louis as "*my master*."[300] Late in March, also for the first time he compared Louis—the "father," as he put it, of the numerical method—with his own father. Still, "I feel more gratitude towards Louis than any one else in Paris—for I have learned far more from him and he treats me with marked kindness and attention—but I admire Andral more and esteem him as a man of higher qualities of mind."[301]

The arrival of cholera in Paris the following month—when Jackson was compelled to chose between duty to his father to leave Paris and duty to remain and investigate the disease in a Louisian fashion—was another turning point. By lingering in Paris he disobeyed his father and did so out of loyalty to Louis and his new program. Writing from Le Havre, finally on his way to London, he told his father of his ardent commitment to Louis ("I blush with shame and yet with joy and pride as I write his name") yet reaffirmed his allegiance to "my three masters in Medicine, yourself, Andral and Louis (I love to couple you and I *love* you all . . . )."[302] During the ensuing six months in Britain, he pined for Paris: "Tho' in London, I am as it were, still in Paris; for my scenes are all Parisian," he wrote, noting later, "I sigh for Paris."[303] Reflection on what he had left behind strengthened his growing perception of himself as a disciple of Louis.

Returning to Paris and to La Pitié in October, Jackson told his father, "you are the only living man who will welcome me again with more warmth & sincere feeling than did Louis," reporting that "I love him more & more daily." Louis, he wrote, "is almost your rival in my breast, so much does he treat me like one belonging to him."[304] During the next few months, the son's letters were filled with affirmations of his affection and loyalty: "I am *your own son* medically as well as naturally," he wrote in December, clearly feeling there was reason to put into words what always before had been left unsaid.[305] Yet he was now intellectually and emotionally ready to give himself to Louis. He put aside the idea of going to Germany, a plan his father had at long last approved, and set forward an impassioned proposal, suggested by Louis, for putting off practice for five years and devoting himself entirely to medical investigation. He acknowledged to his father in March, "You'll think me close upon Rebellion."[306]

During his final months in Louis's wards, Jackson spent "8 hours a day, living, breathing, studying, investigating the morbid phenomena themselves."[307] Louis was the "Father of Pathology as a Science," and by this time Jackson had fully embraced his role as an acolyte in this new faith. Before he left Paris to return to Boston (to set up practice, for his father had vetoed Louis's proposal), he persuaded Louis to sit for a portrait that the young man could take back with him to America. "You are to see it on one condition only," he told his father, "viz: that you go & do likewise, that while my French Father ornaments one side of the mantle piece, my dear Father may the other."[308] The portraits would be a physical expression of his divided allegiances: his two medical fathers; the older tradition of Anglo-American medicine and the new French departure; his two lineages. Finally leaving Paris in mid-July 1833, he wrote to his father, "In two hours I am out of Paris. I will not attempt to describe to you the agony it gives me to quit Louis; he is my second father & God knows that's a name I of all men cannot use lightly. I may not persuade you to look upon him with my eyes exactly as a scientific man but in your Heart he must have the share of a brother for he almost shares my affection with you."[309]

Jackson's transformation in Paris—his growing discipleship to Louis and all he represented—was gradual and uncalculated. Access to clinical instruction was what drew him to Louis over Andral, and Louis's willingness to offer a course of paid private instruction clinched the deal. The young man was flattered by approval from the French clinician, whose initial aloofness may even have enhanced the satisfaction Jackson felt in his encouragement and, eventually, affection. Like the other American disciples of Louis, Jackson did not claim genius for Louis and understood this to be part of their mentor's appeal:

Louis offered a pathway for attaining medical truth that required only diligence and direction—not innate brilliance.[310] Nor did his program require the ingenuity of the system builder. As with the relationship of Americans to the Paris School in general, Jackson became Louis's devoted disciple for reasons quite different from those that had attracted him in the first place.

Jackson was in some ways unusual: certainly he was both exceptionally articulate and exceptionally young. Yet the broad patterns of his growing discipleship recurred in the lives not only of the other American followers of Louis but of many of the other American pupils of French medicine. By representing Louis as father of the numerical method and "Father of Pathology as a Science," Jackson expressed a view of Louis as progenitor of a new medical tradition, a view crucial both to the way they understood their heritage and to the energy with which they disseminated his teachings. For Jackson as for others, the contradictions in his dual lineage were not neatly resolved but could be managed by his retaining an allegiance to both at once—by his passing along the established tradition of medicine his American father represented while simultaneously urging the new departure his French father had instigated. In the American context, preaching the Louisian gospel fulfilled a responsibility that discipleship imposed while serving the interests of their careers. The Paris School, for those Americans who had studied there and could claim to have been transformed by the experience, had become the Old School, and their identity as its old boys brought expectations of both privilege and duty.

## "Mais Tout Cela N'est Pas 'Sweet Home'"

Leaving Paris could be emotionally difficult, notwithstanding the attractions of home. "I can hardly conceive that more than 2½ years have elapsed since I left my native land," Charles Jackson wrote as he prepared to depart. "Stationed in the richest garden of science I have been able to pluck some of the fruits & flowers which surround me & hope to be able hereafter to make the seed of knowledge planted in me of some use to my friends & my country."[311] Still on shipboard but soon to dock in New York, he reflected that "I now land on my native shores with the feelings of exalting pleasure, mingled with regret, that I have forever turned my back on the celebrated schools of Europe & that too at a moment when—I was making the most rapid progress in Professional learning."[312] The pleasures of life in Paris were hard to give up, one Philadelphian lamented as he prepared to leave, especially convinced as he was that "our life at home is like our city, a parallelogram no eccentric or sudden curves in it, no excitement."[313]

Some American physicians were able to extend their stay beyond the period envisioned at the outset, and a few sought to remain permanently. David P. Holton, who had received his M.D. in 1839 from the College of Physicians and Surgeons in New York, put the American consul in Paris to a great deal of effort in 1856 to obtain for him formal permission to practice in France.[314] Jenkins managed to stay in Europe for two years and wanted to remain two or three years longer, but spent his time in Paris always under the threat of being called back to South Carolina—first to take charge of the planting to enable his brother to study law, and later because the fall of the cotton market in 1854 severely depressed his family's finances. "I am sure that the advantages I have derived from the visit to Europe will be worth to me far more than the sum it has cost, but, I fear, that the embarrassment to which the furnishing of that sum has, and will give rise, will render those benefits very dearly bought," he told his father.[315] Most who considered lingering found themselves pressed to return home—by their families, by their finances, or, for those medically established before departing, by fear of losing their practices.

Homesickness, perhaps feigned by some but not by all, counterbalanced the enticements of Paris. "I dont believe you all who know how anxious I was to be off to Paris have any idea how glad I should be to be home again," Kane told his parents in 1857.[316] "But what makes me so home-sick?" Dugas wrote to his sister in 1829. "I look forward with anxiousness to the day of my departure for the new World, not that [I] really dislike this, but because I am completely tired of being a wanderer and unsettled."[317] Reviewing the cultural life he so relished in Paris, Dugas nonetheless wrote to his mother, "Mais tout cela n'est pas 'sweet home'!"[318]

Leaving Paris turned the thoughts of American physicians to the future and the course they would take on reaching their native land. At the same time, looking homeward prompted reflection on the time spent in France and the meaning of that experience. "Once more and for the last time, I have returned to my own solitary chamber, drawn close the window curtains and set myself down, not to read, scarcely to reflect, but excited by the preparations for my departure," Anson wrote to his wife Catherine Colman on the eve of his departure. He dwelled on the thought "that this time and these scenes are passed by—gone for ever—that Paris will be to me, ere to morrows sun shall have brightened her tallest spire but in remembrance." He was ready to leave, having "sent off my boxes of books Anatomical preparations and instruments." But, unable to sleep, he spent the night writing letters, assured that sleep would come "when the memory and the imagination are not excited and goaded on by what has passed, or what is expected or hoped for in the future." As Anson reflected on his experience, he wrote that "it is true I shall never return; but I shall have gathered such hints, and shall bring back with me such aids to study and investigation, as will, I hope, render the few months that I am now spending abroad the most important to me in my whole life."[319]

## CHAPTER 4

# Contexts of Transmission: Duty and Distinction

"THE Physician has alas! but little occasion to distinguish himself," Samuel Henry Dickson, long a medical professor in Charleston and more recently in New York, lamented in 1848 to his nephew, warning the young medical student not to expect much reward for intellectual attainment. "The Community concern themselves very little with the merits or demerits, and we are too practical or too prejudiced to award the palm correctly." Therefore, Dickson advised, "it is well for us when we can [to] substitute for Ambition a strong sense of duty."[1] Perhaps the caution was prudent. Yet for the American physicians who studied in Paris, duty and ambition to a remarkable extent coincided in their proselytizing for the Paris School.

The Americans who made the journey to France were crucial to the passage of French medicine to America, but they were not passive conduits through which the lessons of Paris flowed. They actively chose to take up some of what they witnessed in Paris and to urge it on the medical profession in America. Therefore understanding their choices and why they so energetically acted on them is critical to comprehending the transmission of French medicine.

We know surprisingly little about how professional knowledge moved in antebellum America. Transmission was seldom an unproblematic matter of replication, and like all cultural transmission, that of medical ideas and practices from France to the United States involved transformation as well. After their return, the work of the American physicians who had studied in Paris in investigating disease, reforming professional knowledge and institutions, and caring for patients became powerful forces for reconstructing American medicine along the lines of French models (or at least American interpretations of those models). In all of these instances, however, disseminating French medicine was subordinate to other professional purposes, an important and often intended outcome produced during the pursuit of some other explicit aim, be it healing a sick person or revealing truth. Chapters 6–8 will explore how French medical ways were selected and reshaped as they were transported to America. There, the focus will be how French medicine was expressed in American programs for medical investigation, practice, and professional reform. Here, the focus is more narrowly on the vehicles of transmission—such as letter writing, artifact collecting, translating, journal editing, and teaching—that Paris-experienced American physicians used to promulgate French medicine. A close look at the vehicles of transmission and the dynamics of their operation will begin to clarify the way a body of ideas, techniques, and ideals made the journey across the Atlantic.

The social context to which American physicians returned induced them to make their allegiance to French medicine and the mission of transmitting it central components of their private and public identity. Other physicians, in turn, protested against the Frenchification of American medicine. Yet far from impeding dissemination, such resentment intensified the significance a proclaimed commitment to the Paris School held for those who had studied in France. In urging Parisian lessons on the rest of their profession they found the exercise of duty and bids for professional distinction—their sense of obligation and the interests of career making—to be in reassuring harmony.

## TRANSMISSION FROM PARIS

Americans in Paris were keenly sensitive to what they felt was an obligation and special opportunity to record their impressions of medical Paris while still in its midst and to relay them to America. The letter writing that occupied so much of their time abroad was not only a means to tell family, friends, and colleagues about their routine but also one of the best methods for conveying Parisian medical ways to the profession in America. The medical content of letters varied widely, according to the writer and the recipient. Like medical students at American schools, those studying abroad complained to nonmedical kinsfolk that because medicine occupied all of their attention, they really had little to say. "If you were only a Doctor I could write to you all the wonderful cases that I see," Henry Bryant wrote from Paris in 1844 to his father, "but as you are unfortunately not you must excuse the poverty of my letter."[2] Yet Bryant apparently concluded that Parisian medical matters would interest his father, and proceeded to fill his letters with all but the most technical detail. Medical men were less likely to discuss professional matters in letters to their mothers, sisters, and daughters than in those to their nonphysician fathers, brothers, and sons. But when writing to the latter group, or to their wives, often they provided a rich description of the Parisian medical world. Friends and neighbors no doubt heard much about the family member in Europe for professional improvement, and this was one way Parisian medicine came to the attention of a broader American public, while occasional requests that family letters be shown to former preceptors assured that they also reached medical hands.

Letters written to other physicians provided a more direct channel to the American medical profession. Just as students commonly reported to their preceptors at home about the new theories and practices they encountered in the medical school classroom, those studying in Paris wrote back to their mentors in America. Physicians who sent their sons or younger brothers to Paris expected regular reports providing a vicarious view of French medicine. When James Jackson, Jr., set off in 1831, it was understood that every other week he would send a full report to his physician-father. The father, too, wrote regular letters (nearly a hundred of them), partly to further his son's education through a continuing dialogue on his medical experiences, but also to advance the father's knowledge through myriad questions about French medical ways.

Letters to medical classmates and colleagues provided firsthand accounts of Paris to Americans who could not make the journey themselves. "I thank you for your promptitude in answering my letter, and for the interesting accounts you have given me of your Hospital visits and doings generally in Paris," Joseph Winthrop wrote from Charleston to Gabriel Manigault. "The cliniques on Auscultation & Percussion, to which you refer, must be very interesting & instructive, and I am very glad that you are becoming acquainted with subjects of so much importance in the accurate diagnosis of chest-afflictions." Winthrop went on to describe his own efforts at dissecting, adding somewhat morosely that he found it "difficult to keep up a systematic course of study."[3] The demand for correspondence could be pointed. "I heard some time ago that your son George was in Paris," Thomas Lincoln wrote to the Boston physician George C. Shattuck, Sr., "but have not since heard of him and have never heard from him. I am willing to believe that it is because his leisure is so small in his present situation that he is not inclined to squander his time by writing to old acquaintances, but it seems as if he might remember that I never was in France and probably never can be, and that almost any thing which should befall him there would interest me."[4]

Especially eager to receive news from Paris were Americans who had completed their studies there and were back home. Familiar with the French medical world, they were interested in new developments. "I take some pleasure in writing to a man who has been on the pavé of Paris," G. Roberts Smith wrote from Paris in 1834 to William Wood Gerhard, who had only recently returned to Philadelphia. When he wrote to "the 'set'" at home who had not experienced Paris, Smith continued, "I cannot describe things to them 'con amore' because I know they do not enter my feelings."[5] Several months earlier, Thomas Stewardson had written to Gerhard reporting that the last volume of the Paris clinician François-J.-V. Broussais's *Examen* had just appeared. Realizing the value of fresh news, he added that "as you will not probably see the work for some time after you receive this I will transcribe 2 or 3 sentences as a specimen."[6]

The professional information transmitted in such letters was in some ways private and conveyed meanings that only a few could appreciate. Yet the boundaries between private and public were often blurred. Like much nineteenth-century correspondence, letters physicians sent from Paris sometimes were published in local newspapers. Josiah C. Nott, who was abroad in Paris and other cities in 1859 to collect materials for a new medical school in Mobile, sent home detailed reports on his progress for the *Mobile Daily Register*.[7] Levin Joynes told his father in Accomack, Virginia, "I am gratified to hear that Dr Dunbar found my letter of sufficient interest to be brought to the notice of his class, and I wish that my letters in the 'Visiter' were better worth the space they occupy." His professional studies, he explained, meant that his was "necessarily a sort of hop-skip-and-jump correspondence, and is sadly deficient." Yet he clearly took satisfaction in their publication, writing to his sister that "I receive the 'Visitor' regularly at present," and noting that "the last two of my letters that I have seen look much better than the preceding ones."[8]

The leading forum for publishing letters sent home was the medical journal. Letters from abroad were a regular feature of medical journals in the 1820s and 1830s, and grew increasingly common with the proliferation of journals in the 1840s and 1850s. Accounts of medical cases, institutions, practitioners, and practices were often accompanied by abstracts of Parisian medical society meetings and the contents of new books. Thus with one letter recounting his observations of cutaneous diseases at the Hôpital Saint Louis, Austin Flint also sent his translation of a chapter from Alphonse Devergie's recent treatise on skin diseases.[9] Letters, which editors often solicited from physicians preparing to depart for Europe,[10] provided original copy that was perennially in short supply, and their publication served their authors as well. "In candor," Alden March digressed in a letter to a medical journal describing how well European practitioners had received him, "I fear I have laid myself open to the charge of advertising myself."[11] When John Collins Warren noted in an 1837 letter to the *Boston Medical and Surgical Journal* that his report on the numerical method was based on "private conversations I had with Louis," he not only conveyed privileged knowledge to its readers but also displayed his own privileged access to that knowledge.[12] So too in 1840 the editor of a Louisville medical journal amply rewarded Moses L. Linton for his contributions by identifying him in a preface to his letters as "one of the most gifted and promising young physicians in Kentucky, now on a tour of professional improvement. Dr. L. has industry, a noble ambition, a true love of science, and describes accurately and elegantly, whatever he sees."[13]

The broader professional context of letter writing as a vehicle for transmitting French medicine is clearly illustrated by the case of David W. Yandell. After graduating in 1846 from the Louisville Medical Institute, where his father was one of the leading professors, Yandell traveled to Paris and London for further study. Over the next two years he sent his father, Lundsford P. Yandell, an extensive series of letters, which the senior Yandell then published in the *Western Journal of Medicine and Surgery*, which he coedited with Daniel Drake. "Our Foreign Correspondent," as the elder Yandell styled his son, proceeded to fill nearly four hundred pages with "such novelties as I see in the hospitals, and meet with in the European journals of medicine,"[14] including his own observations in the Paris hospitals, the Clamart, and the museums; comments on the French debate over ether anesthesia, the training of veterinary surgeons, and medical reform; and summaries of papers given at the Academy of Sciences, recent journal articles, and clinical lectures. As soon as the last report appeared, the younger Yandell republished these letters as *Notes on Medical Matters and Medical Men in London and Paris* (1848).[15] For the senior Yandell, an aggressive promoter of his son's career, his son's epistolary labor neatly served multiple professional purposes.

Nor was Yandell singular in turning his letters into a book. Augustus Gardner, after receiving his M.D. from Harvard, traveled to Paris in 1844 and published a long series of letters home, first in the *Newark Daily Advertiser* and later as *Old Wine in New Bottles: or, Spare Hours of a Student in Paris* (1848).[16] And James Jackson, Sr., in the most widely republished set of medical letters from Paris, after his son's death collected together his correspondence in *A Memoir of James Jackson, Jr., M.D., with Extracts from His Letters to His Father; and Medical Cases, Collected by Him* (1835).[17]

Other physicians drafted their Parisian observations as books in the first place. William Gibson, professor of surgery at the University of Pennsylvania who had visited Europe several times, noted that he had long been in the habit in lectures of telling students about the medical people and places of Britain and France, but that there was not time in the crowded curriculum to do the topic justice. To fill this gap, he explained, he published the journal of his most recent trip as *Rambles in Europe in 1839. With Sketches of Prominent Surgeons, Physicians, Medical Schools, Hospitals, Literary Personages, Scenery, Etc.* (1841), which he hoped would appeal to students, colleagues, and the public.[18] Ferdinand Campbell Stewart, who left for Paris in 1837 after graduating in medicine from the University of Pennsylvania, published his notes after his return as *Eminent French Surgeons, with a Historical and Statistical Account of the Hospitals of Paris; together with Miscellaneous Information and Biographical Notices of the Most Eminent Living Parisian Surgeons* (1845). He saw the volume principally as a "student's guide, for such of his young countrymen as might be disposed to visit that city for the purpose of completing their professional education," but he too hoped the volume would interest the general reader.[19] Cornelius Comegys was among those who considered writing such a guide, telling a friend in 1852 that he hoped it would sell, but never completed the project.[20]

These letters and books informed American physicians about French medicine but served other important functions as well. For Americans in Paris, reports sent home advertised the fact that they were gaining experience out of the ordinary, warranting special confidence in their skill. They were also proselytizing for the distinctive banner under which many of them elected to launch their careers. Telling others about Paris medicine was for many physicians a way of fulfilling obligations that the privilege of going abroad to study conferred, and, even more, an exercise of the duty to preach a new gospel of medical truth.

Letters were not the only physical artifacts sent home; others included French books, wax anatomical models, dry and wet anatomical preparations, pathological specimens, apparatus such as stethoscopes and microscopes, drawings and prints, and surgical instruments. A skeleton procured in Paris might betray little about its French origin, but most of these exports carried with them messages about the context in which they were produced. No instrument symbolized symptom-lesion correlation more clearly than the stethoscope, for example, and for the first generation of Americans who obtained the then-novel instrument it represented both the Paris School and the epistemological approach that made French medicine distinctive. "I forward you a stethoscope as you desired," John Bell wrote from Paris in 1822 to Usher Parsons, who had been in that city three years earlier, not long after René-T.-H. Laennec first announced his new invention, "& would have accompanied it with a Memoire upon its application to the study of certain states of pregnancy lately written, as well as the other works you desired but unfortunately I have not yet rec$^d$ a remittance from home which will allow me to make the purchase without inconvenience. The value of your stethoscope is increased from the circumstance of its being examined & used by M. Laennec."[21] Interest in new instruments for physical examination stimulated demand for information on how the French used them. "I wish you would ask Rose's if they have such things as speculums in Philadelphia," Nott wrote in 1833 to a friend from Charleston. "It is an instrument the French use for examining the interior of the Vagina and Rectum. I do not know how they are constructed," Nott admitted, but asked "do enquire about these & let me know S[outh] C[arolina] price."[22]

Surgical instruments similarly served as vehicles to which ideas and practices were attached. The Paris surgeon Jean Civiale's instrument for lithotrity (crushing bladder stones rather than cutting for them as in lithotomy), for example, drew enthusiastic American attention to his operative techniques. Samuel Brown, a medical professor at Transylvania University in Kentucky, arrived in Paris in 1824, only a few months after Civiale had performed the first successful lithotrity. "This morning waited on M Civiale with a letter of introduction & was met with singular politeness," he wrote in his diary. "He instantly shewed me all his Instruments. . . . He exhibited many fragments of calculi which he had extracted from different patients *without any pain*. In short he convinced me of the efficacy of his instruments in breaking down & removing all calculi from the smallest to the greatest & most liberally & kindly invited me to be present at all his operations whilst I remained in Paris—Since the discovery of vaccination nothing so interesting to humanity has been made known." That evening Brown reflected, "This has been one of the happiest days of my life. I shall devote myself to this important subject & I hope to transport it to my country."[23] The following day, he paraphrased his diary entry and appended a description of the operation in a letter to the Philadelphia physician René La Roche (who was engaged to his niece), adding, "I hope to take this important art home to my country with a complete set of Instruments which are by no means complicated. This alone will pay me for the voyage."[24] Many of those who in later years visited Paris also sought to watch Civiale operate and to take his instrument home with them. Trying to justify spending seventy-five dollars for the instrument, Louis Alexander Dugas wrote from Paris to his mother in Georgia that "introducing it into our country I believe renders a great service to humanity, for it is a marvelous thing."[25]

Pathological preparations and models, expressions of the primacy of pathological anatomy in French medicine and the ready access to specimens that Paris afforded, were also shipped back in large numbers for the museums of American schools and for private cabinets. Revisiting in 1853 a Paris model-

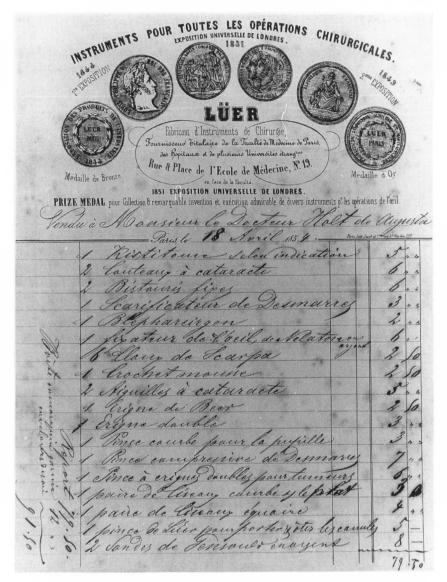

Fig. 4.1. An invoice for surgical instruments purchased in Paris by a Georgia physician in 1854. Along with books and pathological preparations, instruments were among the most common medical artifacts Americans took home with them. (William Joseph Holt Papers, courtesy of Manuscripts Division, South Caroliniana Library, University of South Carolina, Columbia.)

maker he had frequented some years earlier to make "large purchaces" for his pathological museum, George B. Wood was pleased to learn that other Americans had patronized the same shop "apparently stimulated thereto by my example."[26] Several months later, Wood made arrangements for Paul Broca to prepare pathological specimens for him and to make "25 original photo-graphic pictures of the diseased structures of the bowels, lungs, and brain, to be sent to Philadelphia before the end of the year" in return for 625 francs or about $125. "I intend them for my pathological museum," Wood noted in his diary.[27]

Judged by sheer quantity, what American physicians bought above all in Paris were books. French medical texts supplemented the teachings of the Paris clinicians, and Americans could study them at leisure after they returned. Such volumes could also introduce the formal teachings of the Paris School to other physicians unable to leave the United States. Even Americans who admitted to a shaky knowledge of French packed at least a few books in their baggage, and later on many commissioned colleagues headed to France to buy more books for them.[28] "You may possibly be astonished at the number of books that I have bought for myself," Robert Peter wrote sheepishly from Paris to his wife, preparing her for the crates about to arrive on their doorstep in Lexington, "but buying books with me was always a very seductive thing."[29]

The transmission of physical artifacts was motivated by intellectual curiosity and the well-being of American patients, but surely by more than that alone. For practitioners, new instruments might provide an edge over competitors in recruiting patients. For professors, French specimens and books enhanced the claims of their school to pedagogic excellence, its ability to attract students, and thereby the reputation and income of the professors. "We have a great many fine books and a great deal of excellent apparatus and anatomical and other models," a Kentucky medical professor sent to Europe to collect materials for his school wrote back toward the end of his tour in 1839. "Transylvania will shine."[30] Access to books and preparations could help win paying students for the private instructor as well. Justifying to his father the expense of paying the Paris-experienced Gerhard for a private course on diseases of the chest in 1839, Joynes, studying in Philadelphia, explained that Gerhard "has also offered me the use of any book I may want from the library of the Hospital free of cost, as he has the privilege of admission into the library: without this kindness of his, I should have to pay for the use of the books."[31]

Parisian trophies could also draw attention to Paris-returned physicians. Caspar Wistar Pennock, for example, was cultivating men in a position to help make his career when he sent back materials from Paris for the Philadelphia Almshouse. "This Board, feeling highly gratified with the attention manifested by Dr. Caspar W. Pennock (late resident student in this house) in the valuable donation which has this day been made, in his name, of numerous plans, publications and manuscript documents relating to the Hospitals of Paris," the Board of Guardians resolved at a meeting in 1831, "request their President to convey to him their acknowledgements for the same; & to impress to him, their sincere desire, that the useful investigations in which he appears to be engaged, may result successfully to himself and beneficially to his fellow man."[32] Within two years of his return from Paris, Pennock would be appointed attending physician to the Almshouse.

Along with such benefits, books, specimens, and instruments would provide visible and perhaps comforting souvenirs of Parisian medicine in America, tangible emblems of the commitments Americans had taken up and sought to express in their native land. American anatomical and pathological museums, for example, were partly rooted in British medical traditions; yet during the antebellum period specimens collected in Paris became a core of many private cabinets and of the pathological museums at medical schools that were important instruments in teaching. Such collections were physical expressions of the emphasis on visual display of pathoanatomical lesions that was central to Paris medicine, while the specimens preserved in glass jars presented observers not only concrete lessons in morbid anatomy but also exemplifications of labor at the dissecting table—a virtual autopsy. Collections assembled in museums were an evocative remembrance of Parisian experiences that at the same time captured in miniature the pathoanatomical enterprise of the Paris Clinic.[33]

Even though Americans often spoke of the particular benefits they expected their transmission of French medicine to bring, during their time in Paris they rarely reflected self-consciously on the motives that drove them to relay French ideas, methods, and artifacts. Transmission was an objective of the journey more often taken for granted than articulated. Preparation for the homeward voyage was among the few occasions that routinely urged Americans to take stock of what they would transport with them. A few other events, however, gave Americans immersed in Parisian studies a special opportunity to convey home the messages of the Paris School and prompted deep reflection on the meaning of that task.

The coming of Asiatic cholera to Paris in 1832 was one such event. New to Europe and dramatic in the sudden way it killed, cholera captured the attention of the American physicians studying in Paris as it did the attention of Parisians. Moving from India westward, the cholera pandemic reached Vienna some months before it invaded Paris. Charles Jackson, who had traveled to Vienna in September 1831 after study in Paris, was openly pleased by the unexpected opportunity to witness the new disease, which officially appeared in Vienna the day after he arrived. "I have had occasion to see a disease, which does not occur with us, & which perhaps you may never have an opportunity of observing," he wrote with obvious satisfaction two weeks later to Jackson, Jr., still in Paris. "Knowing the interest you take in whatever concerns the medical profession, I am sure you will receive with pleasure the few observations I have been able to collect," and he went on to give a grim depiction of the besieged city.[34]

Freshly committed to French methods of investigating disease, Charles Jackson was quick to take advantage of his situation. "When I first learned of the existence of the cholera," he told James, "I obtained permission to visit the Allgemeines Krankenhaus (general Hospital) where a large number of cholera patients were treated." Charles went on to describe in detail the symptoms of the disease based on observations "which I have made myself by the bed side of the patient." He noted that treatment was uniformly futile, and underscored his conviction that the disease was not contagious. "The people here however think otherwise & I have to keep secret the circumstance of my visiting the Cholera Hospitals." While he had already assisted at the dissection of one cholera victim, and would later publish some three hundred autopsy reports he collected in Vienna, Charles told his cousin that "I dare not yet form an opinion[.] I have given you all the facts I can pick up & intend to go again & again until something turns up to warrant a lexicon."[35]

James Jackson, Sr., in Boston, was chiefly concerned by the movement of cholera toward Paris and his son. "What are you to do if the cholera reaches you," he began a letter to James late in November, advising him to "fly" if possible: "I w$^d$ not stay any where for the sake of studying the disease."[36] When in March 1832 cholera did reach Paris, it proved fully as savage as had been rumored, and would claim 18,402 victims within 189 days.[37] James, however, saw it as a splendid opportunity to put into practice ideals of clinical and pathoanatomical investigation to which he had increasingly been drawn. "I lament to tell you that Cholera, wh. was yet a little doubtful when I last wrote (3 days since) is now reigning in Paris," he wrote to his father on 1 April. "But you are anxious for me—you suffer because I still remain here," he acknowledged. "We are in the city where we may see a dis. of the most frightful nature, wh. will in all probability soon reach our own dear country," James continued with a righteous sense of mission. "We are bound as men and phys$^{ns}$ to stay and see this dis.—as a Phys$^n$ you know it and feel it—as a father, you dread it. For myself I confess, I shd. be unwilling to return to Amer. and not have at least made an effort to learn the nature and the best treat$^t$ of this destroyer of life. I feel bound to remain."[38]

James promised he would leave for the relative safety of London if cholera threatened the better classes of society, but disobeyed. "I anticipate a hard thought from you, when you see me still writing fr. Paris," he told his father, but admitted he was spending his days studying cholera.[39] He began a detailed chronicle of the epidemic, which he sent only after he was safely out of Paris. "My dear father, it is not that I have forgotten to whom obedience is due nor that I wld. willfully disobey," he explained in his first entry, "but that my duty, my interest, my love of medical investigations, my desire to improve this opportunity of studying almost alone and side by side with the greatest Pathologist of the age a disease wh. has engaged the attention and baffled the research of many of the most celebrated in our profession—it is that I wish to send you some exact observations, exact both as to symptoms and morbid appearances; that . . . in fine, . . . this wonderful and dreadful malady so engages and fastens my attention that I can think of nought else."[40] James's resolve became even firmer when Gabriel Andral offered him the chance to study the disease with him in La Pitié. "It seemed as tho' he had imparted to me a new feeling I may almost call it a new 'besoin' so essential have I since found and still find it to satisfy and yield to it," he wrote in his chronicle. "Never had I or shall I again have a similar opportunity."[41]

This was a turning point for James. He still spoke of his duty to his father, but from this time onward his letters were filled with reflections on his duty as a medical investigator. Through his studies of cholera, he hoped to transmit to America a knowledge of a deadly disease threatening to cross the Atlantic and thereby to validate the French medicine to which he had consecrated himself. "I almost weep to write you again fr. Paris," he opened another letter to his father. "It is now the first moment of my life that I have been placed between two duties each strong, each binding and where my great difficulty is to decide wh. is the most so. But I have decided—as I know against y'r present wishes." He challenged his father, asking, "Were the dis. about you wld. you fly? You cld. not, for the public wld. look to you. You wld. not, for y'r sense of duty wld. prevent you."[42]

At the end of April, James finally left for London. There he copied the observations on cholera cases he had made in Paris, and sent them to Boston for his father to publish as a book, which he hoped might "show the Boston public the enemy in his true colors."[43] Jackson, Sr., not only obliged but encouraged James to go back to Paris once the cholera had passed, rather than returning to the United States.[44]

Neither Jackson, Jr.'s course nor the sense of opportunity and obligation that animated it were unique. Other American physicians in Paris also decided to remain to investigate cholera. After studying the disease for five weeks in Vienna, Charles Jackson returned to Paris where he assisted in the autopsies of cholera victims in François Magendie's department at the Hôtel Dieu.[45] Ashbel Smith remained in Paris to study the disease and prepare a treatise on it, writing in June to Jackson, Jr., in London that he was "laboring at the Cholera which I hope to finish for the next packet."[46] And Gerhard and Pennock continued to study cholera in Louis's wards and autopsy room even after Jackson, Jr., had left for London, and sent home a book manuscript on the disease. "The American physicians who remained in Paris during the epidemic," they explained early in May in a summary of their observations for the *American Journal of Medical Sciences*, "did not aspire to the honour of representing their profession—belonging to the youngest classes of it, they could pretend to nothing more than their own instruction, and would only be useful as interpreters of the Parisian pathologists."[47] But that opportunity to act as interpreters presented a chance to serve their country without leaving France and to display to their compatriots both their courage and the power of Parisian medical ways.

Begun with high expectations, this enterprise ended in some disappointment. Applying French methods to studying the new disease failed to either dispel its mysteries or reveal how it could be vanquished. At the end of summer, Gerhard lamented to Jackson, Jr., that cholera had proven intractable, writing that "its pathology is evidently beyond the reach of the scalpel and is perhaps too deeply concealed for me ever to discover." And despite their ambitions of finding an effective therapy, "I have yet to learn that medicine is of *any* service in proper cholera." Nevertheless, Gerhard tried to reassure Jackson, and himself, that they had chosen the right course. "I was so long in a state of painful suspense whether I should immediately return to America or remain longer in Europe," he admitted. "As soon as we had heard of the appearance of cholera in Canada, Smith, Janeway, and Mutter left Paris and sailed in the first ship. Pennock and myself were extremely anxious to return, especially as the letters we received from both our families, seemed to prefer such a course, but we were unwilling to take so important a step until we should be assured that the cholera was really extending towards the United States: finally the question was settled by the unpleasant news that it had reached both New York and Philad[a], and the consciousness that we could not arrive in time to be of essential service."[48]

Their early hopes, however, are in some ways more revealing than the temporary discouragement that ensued. In the same letter in which he regretted their failure to identify an effective therapy for cholera, Gerhard looked forward to the therapeutic triumphs he predicted in Jackson, Jr.'s future once he introduced the numerical method to his father's wards at the Massachusetts General Hospital.[49] To physicians such as Jackson, Jr., Charles Jackson, Pennock, and Gerhard, cholera represented an opportunity to impress upon physicians in the United States the promise of French medicine. They hoped that their own investigations in Paris would disclose important pathological and therapeutic truths that would vindicate their allegiances and bring recognition at home for their achievements. Especially at a moment when their country was threatened with invasion by a devastating disease, they longed to present the knowledge that would bring salvation. But more even than this, they hoped to use studies of cholera as a vehicle for transmitting a broader program of French medicine—to convert the American medical profession en masse by the sheer demonstrated power of French methods to shield their country from the impending epidemic. In some respects cholera was a special case and here as elsewhere prompted people to articulate much that ordinarily remained unsaid. But the response of some American physicians in Paris to the disease clearly points to a broader pattern, for it displays the duty they felt to transmit French medicine to their country—a duty that was in no way inconsistent with the practical rewards that an enhanced professional reputation could simultaneously bring them.

## RETURN AND IDENTITY

The prospect of homecoming often fixed the minds of those returning on the uncertainty of their professional future. Some, especially established older practitioners or recent graduates from established medical families, had a good idea of the professional pathway awaiting them; others capitalized on the experience gained in Paris in applying for medical school or hospital positions; and still others began seeking advice on where they might best try to set up practice.[50] "What am I to do when I get there," Levin Joynes wrote from Paris to his father in Accomack, Virginia. "Where am I to begin my career[?] I know just as little as the man in the moon." He went on to say, "I should not be aston-

ished however, if I were to commit the folly of going to work upon the ague &
fever in Accomack."[51] His most immediate apprehension, however, was "the
influence of miasmata on my return to our feverish region" after two years of
"uninterrupted health" in Europe, a concern common to Southerners returning to malarial districts.[52]

These Americans were well aware that the medical world they were leaving
was vastly different from the one to which they now returned. "I have seen
some Americans, who, after staying a year in Europe, spoke of it in such enthusiastic terms of admiration and of their own country with such indifference,
that they seemed to dread the idea of returning to spend their lives in our
unrefined, half-witted & democratic community," Joynes wrote from Paris to
his father.[53] He elsewhere inquired about a medical friend who had returned
from Paris to his practice: "Does he seem pleased to get back to his old habits,
or does he feel like a bird returned to his cage, after being permitted to fly
almost for an hour with a string tied to him?"[54] Some looked to the Americans
who had already returned home for reassurance. "Ye Gods. I *feel* my Parisian
existence oozing away," G. Roberts Smith wrote in 1834 to Gerhard, who was
back in Philadelphia. "You have made the plunge, and assure me it is not very
painful; cependant, I fear it."[55] With sober resignation, Dugas told his mother
in Augusta, Georgia, "I sincerely hope that when at home, I shall never be
thoughtless enough to think myself unhappy merely because I may then experience less happiness than I momentarily enjoyed in seeing the great things of
the world!"[56]

Once in America, these Paris-returned physicians, especially the first generation, were remarkably confident that they had brought back an important
message. Yet often too, they felt isolated and bored. John Young Bassett, who
returned to Huntsville, complained that he had no clinic for research, no colleagues who cared about what he had learned abroad, and no access to books.[57]
Even those who returned to the most active centers of medical enterprise in the
country bemoaned the lethargy they felt in Boston, New York, and Philadelphia in the wake of Paris. "I know of but little new in Boston," Shattuck wrote
to Thomas Hun in 1839, the year they both returned from Paris. "Je vois
toujours mon petit chemin. Of one thing I can assure you," he added sardonically: "Boston & Paris are somewhat different, in many respects so. We have
neither the large hospitals, nor a great number of cultivators of science, nor a
Grand Opera. . . . Still we exist."[58] Stewardson, still in Europe, wrote to Gerhard shortly after the latter arrived home, "I saw your letter to Rufz and Louis
and am sorry to find that Philad[a] is so dull in an intellectual point of view."[59]

Nostalgia for what had been left behind was perhaps inevitable, and many
longed for the exciting sense of being at the hub that they now could recapture
only in memory. "What have we not missed in Paris!" Samuel Parkman, just
returned to Boston, sighed to Hun, who was back in Albany after six years of
study in France.[60] "I received a charming letter from our dear little doctor," one
acquaintance of Holmes had written to another in 1833, when Holmes was in
Paris, noting that Holmes reported having "refreshed himself with making love

to a pretty Grisette."[61] Holmes's poem "La Grisette," written in 1836, a year after he returned to Boston, surely embodied one strain of his nostalgia.[62] Two years later Eleanor Shattuck reported to her brother George, still in Paris, that "yesterday Dr. Wigglesworth & Dr. Holmes dined here, after dinner Holmes read us a description he had written of the Medical Professors of Paris." After noting that Holmes was a man of talent but "dreadfully conceited," she went on to say, "both of them spoke in the highest terms of Paris, said they would rather live there than [any] other place in the world & how discontented it made one feel to come back here after having been there," and cautioned her brother, "I hope you will not come back with such feelings."[63]

Some Americans recognized that by returning with French affectations, or by pining too openly for Paris, they risked arousing ire. "It is no advantage to a young physician to return home from Europe with the reputation of being imbued with *French ideas* either of medicine, of morals, or of dress," Joynes wrote from Paris to his father.[64] More commonly, it was the family at home that warned those abroad to shed their "French puppyisms."[65] "In order to appear like a man of sense, returning from so long an absence, passed in a foreign land speaking a different language, it is requisite on landing that you remember never to use a french word, but confine yourself to your own language, otherwise it has the appearance of affectation & is usually met with ridicule," Henry Bryant's father wrote to him in Paris.[66]

Many nevertheless did return with a French manner in more than just medicine. "They say I have returned quite *Frenchified*," John Green wrote just after his homecoming in 1848, insisting that "of this I am totally unconscious."[67] Jenkins quipped in a letter from Paris that "I shall endeavour to retain a sufficiency of my native tongue to enable me to make myself understood by my friends on my return." But he told his mother with obvious satisfaction that he had become "too much of a Frenchman" to fall in line with "the exclusive ideas" of his native South Carolinians. "The fact is that the French manner is so very different from ours, and so very attractive that one is entirely unable to resist it's influence."[68] Another American physician in Paris, having just received a letter from the recently returned Gerhard, wrote to congratulate him on "the admirable manner in which you have dropped the 'Parisien' and turned American," though in the case of Gerhard, who clung tightly to Parisian conceits, the congratulations were somewhat misplaced.[69]

One of the most blatant expressions of nostalgia was the inclination of Paris-returned Americans to use French. There was evident appeal in an idioglossia that harkened back to their experience in France, whether expressed in correspondence to each other or in the deployment of French medical terms, as in Laennec's descriptions of sounds heard through a stethoscope. "For the honour of America, I am glad to say they are comparatively few," one physician in Paris observed, "[who] have in a measure forgotten their native tongue, or at least pretend so."[70] Yet after returning, they often used such salutations as "Cher et savant confrere" and "Illustre Professeur et chere confrere" and sprinkled their letters with French phrases.[71] Nor did they use French simply in

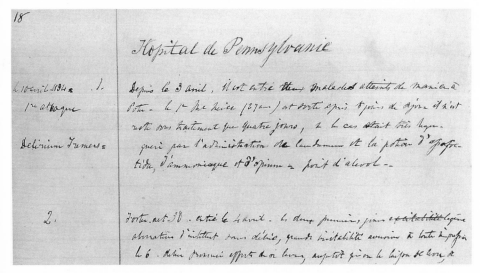

Fig. 4.2. Opening lines of a page from William Wood Gerhard's "Journal Medical." While studying in Paris, the Philadelphia physician had begun to record his autopsy reports in French, a practice he continued at the Pennsylvania Hospital after his return, heading the new section "Hôpital de Pennsylvanie." (William Wood Gerhard, Journal Medical, 11 Mar. 1833–17 Mar. 1839, entries starting 10 Apr. 1834, courtesy of Historical Collections, Library of the College of Physicians of Philadelphia.)

lighthearted ways. When Jackson, Jr., within a year after his return home, realized in 1833 that he was dying, he wrote to Gerhard that "mes Plaques de Peyer ont été inflamméés depuis cinq semaines," imagining within his body the pathognomonic sign of typhoid fever—lesions of the Peyer's patches of the small intestine—that Louis had identified.[72] For Gerhard's part, after returning to Philadelphia he continued to make autopsy reports at the Pennsylvania Hospital in the same bound journal he had used to record autopsies the previous year in Paris, but headed the new section "Hôpital de Pennsylvanie." Months after his return, Gerhard inscribed into the volume, for example, the "Autopsie de Richard Hughes, 24 heures apres la mort," and proceeded to write this report, as he did many others, in French.[73]

For these physicians, their Frenchness went hand in hand with a sense of superiority to the masses of the American medical community. Alfred Stillé, inspired partly by his clinical studies in Philadelphia with the recently returned Gerhard, left in 1836 just after receiving his M.D. from the University of Pennsylvania for more than two years in Paris; but on returning he found the intellectual climate of his native city discouraging. Skeptical of the support a Pathological Society would attract from his fellow Philadelphians, Stillé lamented in 1842 to Shattuck, "I do not believe that it will flourish; the true spirit of scientific research in pathology can hardly be said to exist here."[74] Such perceptions of intellectual sloth led many physicians who returned from Paris to disparage the rest of the profession in America, which neither shared their enlightenment nor seemed sufficiently ready to honor it. In another letter to Shattuck, Stillé bemoaned the "large number of young men who might have made good citizens as farmers, tradesmen, or mechanics" but who had trained as physicians instead, only to "plod along as stupid routinists" ignorant of the high standards of medical learning to which he believed the profession should aspire. "How little our professional brethren seem to esteem those requisitions," he lamented. "They scarcely look beyond the narrow sphere of their daily ministrations to regard the high source from which their duties spring, or care to penetrate beyond palpable results into the mysterious & wonderful recesses of Nature & Disease."[75]

What made matters worse is that when returning physicians were drawn into interactions with those who had never left home, the latter were often skeptical or openly hostile to the pretensions of Parisian medicine. As one practitioner typically sniped at a Cincinnati medical society meeting, he was "rather inclined to think that the *European trips* of some of the professional brethren had made them somewhat dissatisfied with such old names as quinsy."[76] Even a committed disciple of Parisian medicine could find the superior airs assumed by a young physician fresh from Paris overbearing. Elisha Bartlett, for example, teaching in Lexington, complained in 1847 to a friend about an annoying physician who had just moved to town, "a young fellow recently from Paris—pompous, vain, boasting, illiterate and ignorant! The latter genius and myself have crossed each other's teeth two or three times."[77]

Resentment stemmed from a variety of sources, ranging from fear of economic and intellectual competition to cultural nationalism. Every time a medical writer celebrated the advantages of Parisian training over that received by "the homebred man,"[78] the implicit assertion of superiority was clear. As the number of Americans who traveled to Paris grew, criticism of both French medicine and the Americans who proclaimed allegiance to it mounted. Most stinging were criticisms voiced by physicians who had themselves visited Paris, often as tourists. Even if they had only briefly made the rounds of the major medical sights, they spoke with the authority of people who knew firsthand what they were talking about. Joshua B. Flint, in an introductory address he composed on shipboard as he returned from a short trip to England and France, told students at the Louisville Medical Institute in 1838 that "multitudes of young men, in the enthusiasm of their new doctorate, and with a commendable ambition to render their education complete, at no small expense of time and means, hurry to the 'School' and hospitals of Paris, with hopes of augmenting their professional resources, which I am quite sure are seldom realized." These deluded young men, he went on, "mistake bustle for progress, and novelties for improvements, and fancy themselves adding to their stores of healing knowledge, when they are only substituting the seductive and impracticable subtleties of their new masters, for the sober, rational, available instructions of their native schools."[79] Charles Caldwell, another Louisville professor, was less lenient in a letter from Europe to the *Western Journal of Medicine and Surgery* in 1841, noting that "it is regarded as an important feather in the cap of a young physician, in the United States, to have passed some time, and expended his money, in attendance on schools and *amusements* in Paris." In his judgment, "in most cases, it is not only *useless*, but *injurious*— and too often productive of absolute ruin."[80] Caldwell returned with what one of his students described in his class notebook as a "contemptible opinion" of the Paris hospitals as a place for an American to study.[81] Underlying such criticism was the broader and increasingly common attack on French medicine discussed in chapter 8 for being indifferent to aiding sick people and dangerous at the bedside.

Such assaults—voiced in medical journals, society meetings, and classrooms—made those who valued their time in Paris cling to that experience even tighter as a significant part of their personal and professional identity. They were bound to one another by shared commitments, friendships, and memories, and a consciousness emerged of their identity as a group apart from the masses of their profession. In the face of widely voiced denigration of what defined that special identity, they closed ranks. Clearly reflecting the extent to which a shared past could define group identity, Stillé revealingly referred to those Philadelphia physicians who had studied in Paris as, collectively, "*Parisians.*"[82]

A network developed based only in part on friendships forged in Paris. As Stewardson was about to return to America in 1834, he wrote to Gerhard, "I anticipate the enjoyment of your society as one of the greatest blessings in store for me in my native city," and added, "I probably should never have known you thoroughly had we not been at Paris together and my ardent wish is that the friendship there begun will last as long as we do."[83] Stewardson then asked Gerhard to use his influence in helping him win a post as intern at the Pennsylvania Hospital. In the mid-1830s, both men were among the leaders of a virtual takeover of the College of Physicians of Philadelphia by a group of young, Paris-experienced fellows of the institution, a local coup they commemorated by electing Louis a foreign associate member.[84]

The ties connecting physicians who shared Parisian experience extended between cities and across regions. Back in America, they exchanged letters reaffirming their shared identity and exchanged publications exemplifying their common faith. They distributed books for each other, wrote supportive reviews of those books, and exchanged pathological specimens. They collaborated in translating French medical texts, writing books, and editing journals. They sought each other as colleagues on medical school faculties and, when applying for teaching and hospital positions, looked to each other for letters of recommendation and well-placed private words. Some visited each other's homes, and in time their families exchanged letters as well. In confronting the realities of American medical life, they could sometimes turn to each other for reassurance and support.

This was a large and uneven network, tightly woven between some individuals, especially of the first generation to study in Paris, and tied only by loose threads to others, but it also extended outward to draw together people connected in no other way than through their shared Parisian experiences and commitments. It reached physicians who had taken up the French medical faith but had not made the journey to Paris in person, and, through correspondence and letters introducing travelers, it reached some practitioners in France and Britain. "You will probably feel surprised at being addressed by one who is an utter stranger to you," a young Paris-experienced English practitioner wrote to Jackson, Sr., "but I think the name of *Louis* will be a passport to your acquaintance."[85] George B. Wood, meeting Henry Ingersoll Bowditch for the first time when both were traveling in New England, found the latter aloof until Bowditch realized that they shared Parisian medical experience and acquaintances. Once that was known, Bowditch took Wood in hand, showed him around Boston, and as a parting gift presented him with a copy of his recent translation of Louis on typhoid fever.[86] This sense of fraternity was one expression of the role French experience had in defining the way Paris-returned American physicians thought about themselves, a part of their personal identity.

The intellectual and social strife of the American professional context urged the American "Parisians" to make their allegiance to French medicine a part of their *public* identity as well. The act of describing medical Paris and asserting its significance took on a very different complexion when performed in America than it had in France. In proselytizing for Parisian medicine—especially in the face of hostility—American devotees were making a professional statement about where they stood and who they were. Publicly proclaiming that one had been to Paris and had seen there the direction the American medical future should take was a political act. As personal memory of Paris was made public in this way, the possession of this memory and allegiance to what it stood for became part of the returned physician's professional persona. One consequence was that urging Parisian medical ways came even more to be imbued with both a strident sense of mission and defensiveness.

Yet because there were enormous differences in the circumstances to which Americans returned, their French experience gave rise to diverse meanings in their professional and personal identities. They did not come home to form a homogeneous group with a devotion to French medicine giving uniform definition to their aspirations. Like members of other groups within American society bound together by ethnicity, gender, class, political allegiance, or religion, their lives—even their professional lives—did not take definition from any one category alone. Northerner and Southerner, nationally prominent professor and overburdened community practitioner, woman and man, established professional leader and ambitious recent graduate, affluent urban physician and struggling country doctor: these were dualities that shaped their individual identities in ways at least as powerful as the shared experience of Parisian study. Professional, social, and political points of conflict among them worked against the cohesiveness stemming from a shared past. While in Paris, the Virginian Philip Gooch complained in his diary of the behavior of "The Damn 'Yankee' Coles," deriding Coles for penny-pinching, a common regional stereotype.[87] And while a Massachusetts acquaintance urged Bassett to emancipate his slaves, the Alabama physician asserted defensively that "I am a slave holder (a *small one*), and feel at liberty to remain so, until the laws of the Country, my own conscience, or my neighbors order it otherwise."[88]

The ways in which they could demonstrate their Parisian commitments also varied enormously according to circumstance. Some—as professors, editors, writers, and professional leaders—were enabled by talent, labor, luck, patronage, and birth to find platforms for developing their careers and intellectual allegiances to the fullest extent possible within the constraints of American society. The more limited options available to others tended to pull them out of the Parisian network. Many of those who returned from Paris in the late 1850s found their aspirations, and ultimately their lives, curtailed by the Civil War. Others elected to make their careers outside medicine. Manigault, who studied in Paris in the mid-1850s, returned from two years in France to take charge of his father's South Carolina plantation Silk Hope, which gave him time to cultivate his leading passion, natural history. When the Civil War broke out, he joined the Confederate forces (as a soldier, not a surgeon), was captured, and during Reconstruction became curator of the Charleston Museum; but by choice he never practiced medicine.[89] So too William Walker, a native of Nashville who studied in France after receiving his M.D. degree from the University of Pennsylvania in 1843, decided in the Paris hospitals that medical practice was distasteful and that some other career would better suit him; he turned first to law, then to journalism, and then to leading a series of invasions and foreign-sponsored "revolutions" in Latin America, where in 1856 he was inaugurated president of Nicaragua and, in 1860, died before a Honduran firing squad.[90]

Others, unlike Manigault and Walker, were deeply attached to medicine but simply unable to construct a career in the overcrowded medical world of antebellum America. John Christopher Faber was in 1837 living on the Rue de Rivoli in Paris, spending his time studying medicine, and writing his sister in Spartanberg, South Carolina, that life seemed "very agreeable."[91] By 1840, he had settled in Charleston and could tell his sister that workmen were busy preparing his office; "my books are all safely housed, I have procured me a little furniture and soon I shall be lord of my mansion." He recognized that "for the first few years I must content myself with little practice, but otherwise I cannot fail to find employment for which I shall be compensated"; but a year later he was still waiting for "a few patients."[92] After another eight months he was hired to assist Eli Geddings in the surgical department of the Medical College of South Carolina. "Along with doctors Holbrook and Ogier[, I] have engaged to examine a private class on two branches of medicine and with the preparation of a Lecture to be delivered before the medical society and attention to the *precious few* cases in practice which may become mine," he reported, "I will be kept quite busy."[93] Patients still did not appear, but Faber's other activities both filled his time and seemed to be leading him into the channel to professional eminence.

By the middle of 1842, however, having tried "every honorable means to procure a decent practice," having exhausted his bank stock, and having run up a substantial debt, Faber was compelled to look for some other way to make a living. "Hard necessity," he wrote to his sister, "has forced me to relinquish my profession to which with heart & soul I am devoted." Resigned to become a schoolmaster—"hard's my fate!"—he lamented that although "I was never made for a school room," at least it would pay.[94] Geddings, Thomas L. Ogier, and John Edwards Holbrook, Faber's Charleston colleagues, all of whom had medical experience in Paris, went on to successful careers and played important roles in the dissemination of French medicine in America, but the aspirations Faber had formed abroad were now at an end. "Had *one friend* been found to relieve me at a time when I felt that something must be done to discharge pecuniary obligations, the hand would have been cheerfully seized," he told his sister, "& it would have prevented me from abandoning a profession which next to life was dear & in the acquirement of which so many years of hard toil, so many a sleepless night has been spent." He added sardonically that while "most of my professional Brethren will be leading but a precarious life, at all events *mine is certain.*"[95]

Confronted with the realities of the American context, ideals and resolutions formed in Paris frequently were derailed. Few Americans were able to shape careers that bore much resemblance to those pursued in the Paris Clinic. For many of the first generation, commitments made in Paris did remain central to their identity through the end of their lives. But by the 1850s, rapid growth in the number of Americans who annually made the journey rendered the experience of having studied in Paris less and less distinctive. Some of these younger travelers did see their time in Paris as special, but many would come to take it for granted.

Despite such wide diversity, what remains striking is the extent to which a shared Paris experience created bonds among American physicians that, while by no means dissolving the barriers among individuals, went far toward transcending them. The link between Parisian experience and the public and private identity of some American physicians would be a key factor in propelling the dissemination of French medicine in the United States.

## DISSEMINATION, IDENTITY, AND CAREER BUILDING

While in Paris, American physicians had been motivated by both duty and career interests to transmit French medicine back to their own country. That dual motivation persisted in driving them to proselytize for the Paris School after their return. But the more calculated their efforts became, the more memory was transformed into polemic. In Paris, merely writing down an account of one's daily routine and posting it home helped spread the French gospel, but the matter was not so simple after a return to St. Louis or New York. Distanced from Parisian wards and dissecting rooms, Americans more self-consciously selected from their recollections particular aspects of French medicine to hold up as models for the rest of their profession to admire and emulate. The vehicles by which French medicine was conveyed changed as well. Letters, specimens, and books all moved within the United States as they had moved across the Atlantic, but for Paris-returned physicians these were no longer the most powerful conduits for conveying the messages of French medicine to a broader audience.

The peculiar professional situations of the Americans who had studied in Paris and the institutional vehicles they used to amplify their voice gave them an influence far out of proportion to their numbers. This grew in part from their sense of mission. But it stemmed equally from the complex interaction between the dissemination of knowledge and career building. Those who studied in France were as a group the physicians most likely on their return to occupy positions of influence in their profession. Because many of them began with socioeconomic advantages, often boasting a distinguished medical parentage as well, they could count on influential support in their bid for professional distinction. Those who had less advantaged origins had already shown special initiative and perseverance in mustering the resources that took them to Paris, and that ambition often persisted after they came home. The Americans who had studied in France, in other words, were far more likely than the average practitioner to have careers that empowered their opinions—on French medicine or anything else. At the same time, the activities they used to urge Parisian medical ways—writing and translating books, contributing to and editing medical journals, presenting addresses at medical society meetings, serving as medical school professors—all helped further their own careers. Proselytizing for French ways and career building were mutually reinforcing.

Translating writings by the French clinicians was the most direct way to convey the formal content of Paris School teachings to other American physicians. Some of the translations that appeared in America were made by British practitioners, then pirated by American publishers. In fact, what may have been the most widely disseminated French medical treatise in America was the English physician John Forbes's 1821 translation of René Laennec's *De l'auscultation médiate ou traité du diagnostic des maladies des poumons et du coeur* (1819). Holmes later noted correctly that Forbes built his career on this translation.[96] While other British translations also gained wide circulation in America, a strikingly large proportion of the translations into English of writings produced by the Paris School came from Americans.

Of course one need not have gone to Paris to translate texts by Parisian writers. Forbes had not made the trip across the Channel, and the patient records he kept during the years when he was beginning to use Laennec's new instrument reveal that it was a formidable struggle for him to sort out the clinical meaning of the sounds he heard through the stethoscope, despite his translation of Laennec's words on the subject.[97] Indeed, Russell Maulitz has shown how Forbes transformed Laennec's treatise in the process of translating it.[98] F.-J.-V. Broussais's *De l'irritation et de la folie* was translated into English in 1831 by Thomas Cooper, English-born but compelled to emigrate to America in 1794 because of his radical thinking, which embraced sympathy with the French Revolution and passionate materialism. Cooper, a political philosopher and teacher who had some training in medicine, was drawn into the Jeffersonian circle after he settled in South Carolina, and the materialism of Broussais's treatise more than its medical content enticed him to translate it.[99]

Even before significant numbers of Americans started to make the journey to Paris, some translations appeared from American pens, often wielded by practitioners with no Parisian experience. In January 1805, the enterprising Charles Caldwell wrote from Philadelphia to Lemuel Kollock, a leading Savannah physician, "From the first of November to about the eighth instant, I was very zealously engaged in the translation of a French treatise on Surgery, by the celebrated Dessault, late of the Hotel-Dieu in Paris. The work is now ready for the press and will be published with all possible dispatch. Proposals will, in a few days, be forwarded to your care." Aware that Pierre-Joseph Desault's *Journal* had already appeared in translation, Caldwell dismissed it as "little more than mere catch-words, from which the author lectured, and from which the present work was composed."[100] Caldwell, an aggressive advocate of a domestically produced American medical literature—the cultivation of which he had only months earlier described to Kollock as a patriotic duty[101]—saw no inconsistency between that purpose and translating a French work. His avowed aim was to place a useful work in the hands of the American profession, not to promote some wider program of French medicine. "The Dr still continues industrious," another Philadelphia physician wrote to Kollock about Caldwell two years later. "He has lately given a Translation of another French Author. *Alibert on Malignant Intermittents*."[102] Boston physician George Hayward's plan in 1819 to publish his three-volume translation of Xavier Bichat's *General Anatomy*, which appeared in 1822, elicited advance subscriptions from some 154 physicians in a dozen states.[103]

With the influx of American doctors into Paris, however, translating took on a different scale and more expansive purpose. From the 1820s onward translations of French medical works rapidly proliferated. Most were produced by Americans who had studied in Paris, and, more often than not, produced relatively soon after their return from France. Translating suited these young physicians in a number of ways. It put to good use their knowledge of French medicine and language skills. It was also a way of making professionally constructive use of their time at a stage in their careers when most were eagerly searching for professional responsibilities rather than overwhelmed by them. And for these practitioners, as for Caldwell, it drew attention to their industry, promoting their careers. At the same time, translating was one means of calling attention to the teachings of the Paris School and making them accessible to practitioners and students who could not read the texts in French. What was most distinctly new about the translating enterprise from about 1820 onward was this latter aim of using translation as a vehicle to promote a broader program of French medicine.

It was commonplace wisdom that translating, like the pursuit of natural history, was a professionally respectable way for young practitioners to spend

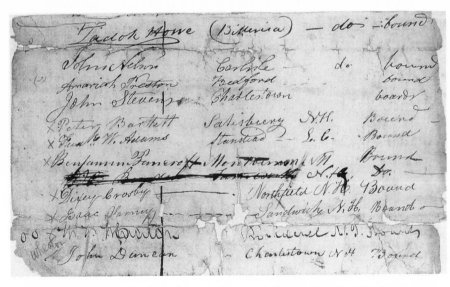

Fig. 4.3. Opening lines of an advance subscription list circulated in 1819 for George Hayward's proposed translation of Xavier Bichat's *General Anatomy*. Among the earliest subscribers on a list of 154 names are James Jackson, Jacob Bigelow, and Edward Augustus Holyoke. (Courtesy of Francis A. Countway Library of Medicine, Boston.)

some of the abundant leisure time on their hands while they awaited their first patients. Often, that was a very long wait indeed. "My professional business has been almost nothing during the last month, not more than one visit a day," Stillé wrote to Shattuck in 1842, over two years after his return from Paris. But, he noted, his time was "pretty well occupied in other ways"; he was keeping up with activity in Paris by reading recent French medical works, had just finished a long review for publication, and, as he added in a later letter, was "engaged in translating a part of Gabriel Andral's essay on blood, entitled 'Hematologic Pathologique.'"[104]

Some young practitioners were explicit about the professional incentives that prompted them to translate. Dugas, while still in Paris, had written to his mother, "I am busy now translating a French work on medicine and if I can succeed I shall begin another, until I have enough experience to *compose* one. In this way," as he told her, "on se fait connaitre a bon marche."[105] Samuel Parkman, recently returned to Boston, was in 1839 "settled in an office," but, far from establishing an active practice, the most he could tell his "cher confrère" Thomas Hun was that he had "had several patients who I suppose would pay if I only knew how to ask them for it." Part of his free time was devoted to cultivating a cabinet of specimens, whereas for the rest, "my leisure hours I am employing in translating and shall very probably commit the bêtise of publishing a book." As he explained, "Il faut gagner une reputation, and as I cannot gain it at present upon my own labors, I may ride in upon the back of somebody else."[106]

Translating might bring modest financial rewards, but these were not the rewards that mattered most. The young English practitioner William Baly explained to his mother the motivation that he, like young Americans, tended to take for granted. In 1836, having recently returned from study in France and Germany and put up a plate announcing himself as surgeon, he wrote with annoyance to his mother, "I have *not* had a patient, at least a profitable one."[107] A month later, still waiting for patients, he described his plan to translate Johannes Müller's *Handbuch der Physiologie*. "You will of course understand that it is not pecuniary gain that I expect from this," Baly explained, "it is rather the good that may arise from any credit it may gain me & from its being known that I am acquainted with German Medical works."[108] So too Philadelphia physician John Hooker Packard, who within a few years of returning from Paris published a *Treatise on Fractures* (1859), his translation of Joseph-François Malgaigne's work, told his uncle two years later, "I am sorry to say that your kind wishes for the success of my translation are not likely to be fulfilled, so far as its rapid sale is concerned"; but he went on, after discussing his application for a post at the Pennsylvania Hospital, to assure his uncle that "its publication has certainly been of advantage to me."[109]

Translating, then, served functions in some respects akin to dispensary work: it displayed laudable professional devotion and enterprise, gave evidence of professional experience, and, by doing so, attracted attention. It was a form of distinction that, like medical publishing in general, might draw public notice and thereby paying patients. It could also help win a hospital or teaching post. Translating a French medical work was special, however, in that it not only helped promote the ways of the Paris School but proclaimed the identification of the translator with French medical expertise.

Translating a medical text and finding a publisher were only first steps in making the work known. Equally important was to ensure that the translation was well noticed and reviewed. After all, the extensive summaries of translated texts that appeared in journals reached the hands of more physicians than ever took up the published book itself. Authors actively labored to get editors to publish reviews and to secure favorable reviewers. After receiving a complimentary letter from Holmes on his recent *Philosophy of Medical Science* (1844), Bartlett wrote directly to Holmes asking him to review it for the *North American Medical and Surgical Journal*.[110] In 1828 John Bell wrote to the editor of the *North American*, René La Roche, to "announce the publication of a second edition of Broussais's Physiology." Bell noted that his translation was a "work of some labour, since I made free with the text & added many notes, and a preface of sixteen pages, and an index."[111] In 1838, John Dix Fisher wrote to Isaac Hays, editor of the *American Journal of the Medical Sciences*, "I have been translating Professor Andral's notes contained in the last French edition of Laennec's work on the Diseases of the Chest. An new american edition of Laennec—(Forbes' edition)—to which are added Andral's notes as translated by myself—and also some remarks on *cerebral auscultation*—has been printed and will soon be published by Sam$^l$ Wood & Sons of New York." Fisher, who had studied with both Laennec and Andral, added, "You will have a copy, as soon as any one of them may be completed—I hope you will notice the work, and even should you find fault with the translation I beg you will not lash me *too* severely."[112]

Of the various ways that Paris-returned Americans might have kept up with events in France, translations and imported new works were particularly important. The common appearance of these titles in library and estate inventories of antebellum American physicians provides one indicator of their dissemination.[113] Another way of keeping up with events in France was correspondence, not just among Americans but also between Americans and Parisian mentors. These exchanges, far from routine, were nonetheless significant. Thus Civiale wrote from Paris to La Roche in Philadelphia soliciting the "coopération de mes confrères" in collecting information for his surgical research and providing La Roche with a blank form to fill in with information from other Americans in the interests of "la science & l'humanité."[114] And Paul Eve wrote from Nashville to a Paris physician, "Avoir la bonté, s'il vous plais, de me donné ce que vous avez de nevelle dans nôtre science."[115]

There is little evidence that many individual American doctors subscribed to French medical journals. In part, this was because many of them could use the collections of medical schools or societies, which did often include French periodicals on their subscription list.[116] More than this, Americans simply did not need to read French journals in order to feel that they were abreast of the latest news from Paris: for that, they could turn to American journals. When Alden March drafted a prospectus for the *Albany Medical and Surgical Records* in 1830, he quite typically noted that "in common with other medical journals ... we shall devote a portion of our sheet to a brief analysis of foreign & domestic medicine, carefully gleaning every thing most worthy of preservation."[117] American journals borrowed a considerable proportion of their copy from exchanges with foreign periodicals and disseminated French medicine through new articles, translated ones, letters from abroad, and reviews.

The proliferation of American medical journals during precisely those decades when Americans began to go to Paris in large numbers was a critically important factor in the visibility French medicine attained in the United States. In 1812, one supporter of an Albany journal, bemoaning the sparsity of subscribers in his vicinity of western New York state, told the editor that "the fact is, our physicians are a set of plodding, mean, lowlive Blockheads with a *few* exceptions."[118] However, the number of medical periodicals published in America, modest in the New Republic, mounted rapidly during the 1820s and 1830s, and the founding of new journals accelerated further during the 1840s and 1850s. Many of these were established in the newer regions of the West and South, but the number published in the Northeast multiplied as well. Lack of support led many new journals to fold, yet an imposing number survived. Without this vigorous growth in medical journalism, the dissemination of French medicine in America would have been considerably slower, more modest, and far less evident to the vast majority of American physicians.

A large proportion of these journals were edited by physicians who had studied in France. This was true of older and established journals, particularly as the Paris-returned Americans themselves grew older and established, but especially of the multitude of fledgling publications. Editing a journal, after all, was another vehicle ambitious physicians could use to affirm their intellectual leadership and advance their careers. In composing their journals, editors who had studied in Paris were also well placed to draw upon the broader network of American "Parisians."

The growing prominence of French medicine in antebellum journals partly depended on the initiative of contributors, and the multiple motivations that led Americans abroad to send letters and reports for publication also encouraged them after their return to submit articles that showed the imprint of their French commitments—be they case histories, accounts of the medical geography of their region, pathological reports, or broader statements on medical reform. "In Paris I witnessed . . ." is a remarkably common phrase in contributions to medical journals from this period, one often imbedded in the case history of a patient with typhoid fever or in an essay on the treatment of internal inflammation. Using it was a way both to recall and to display the author's Parisian experience. Writing reviews of recent French books, like translating, was a way of keeping up with recent Parisian thought and exhibiting one's identification with it. Many contributions were unsolicited. Thus T. Romeyn Beck wrote in 1820 to John W. Francis in Albany, editor of the *Register and Encyclopedia* and his former preceptor, describing an article he planned to submit, and added "I will likewise send you, a translation of the Introduction to Bichat's Anatomie Generale." He went on to say, "Should it be well received and any curiosity excited to see a remainder of the book I think I shall (with health & leisure granted me) set about to translate it."[119]

Editors were as enterprising as contributors in making French medicine prominent. When La Roche was in France in 1828, he spent considerable time gathering materials for the *North American Medical and Surgical Journal*. "Your boxes of books & your papers from Nice have arrived safely," a coworker on the *North American* wrote to him from Philadelphia. "Several of them have been translated & two or three will appear in our October No."[120] Editors also solicited reviews of French works. "Your letter respecting a Review of Esquirol on Insanity I have rec^d, but I am unable to procure a copy of the work here," the Paris-experienced alienist Amariah Brigham wrote from New York in 1838 to Isaac Hays, editor of the *American Journal of the Medical Sciences* in Philadelphia. "There has been but one copy imported here which I saw a few days since—but did not buy it because most of it, is contained in the *Dict sciences Medicales*. When I rec^d your letter I hastened to the Book-Store but found it had been sold—Consequently I shall not be able to notice it, in your next number—but if you will send me a copy (I will pay for it) I will prepare a Review of it for the following number."[121] Editors also sometimes urged authors to take recent French writings into account in their articles. In a letter sent to inform Hays that he had finally finished his promised paper on epidemics, Joseph Mather Smith, a professor at the College of Physicians and Surgeons in New York, wrote in 1834, "I thank you for your [torn] reference to Andral's article on that subject. . . . I have read it, and have also consulted the other French Dictionaries."[122]

A commitment to proselytize for French medicine sometimes was among the many incentives that intersected in the creation of a new journal. Especially early in the century, journals were launched partly in the name of cultural nationalism, as a forum for cultivating American literature that demonstrated independence from Europe (a medical independence that paradoxically the philosophy of the Paris School sustained by what Americans took to be its insistence on empirical observation of local circumstances). Equally, many of the journals founded in the South and West sought to serve distinctively regional cultural interests, most boldly expressed by southern separatist attempts to free the region from its dependence upon northern institutions, including literature. Medical societies sometimes saw establishing a journal as one way of stimulating intellectual life in a profession notorious for its apathy, as well as a way to promote reforms. A medical journal was also seen as enhancing the power of a school to attract students. The faculty of the Medical Department of the University of Louisville resolved in 1857 "that a Medical Journal published under the auspices of the Faculty would contribute materially to the prosperity of the School," and established a committee to undertake the project.[123] Such an enterprise would simultaneously advance the professional and economic interests of the professor-editors.

Some of these more general patterns in the founding of a medical journal can be illustrated by the activities of the young Virginian Philip Claiborne Gooch during his first few years back from study in Paris. Two months after returning to his home in Airfield, near Richmond, in February 1849, Gooch announced the opening of his practice, and while he began to attract patients, they remained distressingly few. He did win professional recognition, however. At the beginning of June, when cholera broke out only three months after he had started practice, Gooch was elected secretary of the Richmond Board of Health.[124] "I am stopped at every step and asked for news of the cholera," he wrote a week later.[125] His diary entries over the ensuing months display his active engagement in the social and medical life of the community. He attended church and was active in the Freemasons; overcame a good deal of "humbug" in order to perform an autopsy; and took advantage of a medical friend's imminent departure for Paris to send a letter by him.[126] Early in March 1850, he wrote, "Everything upset by the thought that I must give an address before the alumni of the Medical College here, next Saturday, and I have not begun to write it!!! What horror!!!"[127] He also recorded his attendance on an increasing number of patients. Still, by the end of March he would write: "I am very distressed. Broke and $300 in debt."[128] Throughout this period, Gooch continued to record the events of his life, including his attendance on patients, in the same bound journal that he had used to record his activities in Paris, and, moreover, continued to record them in French.

On 9 November 1850, Gooch, twenty-five years old, wrote in his journal of a new professional enterprise: "I decided to establish a medical journal in Richmond."[129] The next day he drafted a circular, which solicited subscriptions to the projected *Stethoscope, or Virginia Medical Gazette* and spelled out its objectives. The aim of the new journal was "to aid in the advancement of medicine as a science, and its votaries throughout the state of Virginia; to aid in drawing into active usefulness the great fund of information and talent which is now dormant; to collect and diffuse all the facts which Medical science is rapidly developing, both in our own country and abroad; . . . in short, to promote the universal interests of our science." Gooch stressed that "arrangements have been made at great expense, to give a full digest of the contents of our own as well as of the Medical journals and transactions of England and the Continent of Europe."[130] From this point onward, interspersed with his other social and professional activities are notes on his work for the journal: collecting subscriptions (three dollars, sometimes delivered in person); collecting copy; receiving the first exchange journal (the *Boston Medical and Surgical Journal*); reading proofs; fretting over having enough material for each subsequent issue; and seeing the first number in print, writing, "I have done well."[131] It was demanding. But Gooch found evident satisfaction in the completion of each number, in being able to write in his private diary (still kept in French), "Le Stethoscope est fini."[132]

The founding of the *Stethoscope*, in many ways typical of the multitude of local medical journals that proliferated during the late antebellum period, had its origins in a number of forces. Gooch's immediate career interests—winning public and professional recognition and patronage—provided one stimulus. Another came from southern sectionalism, and one prominent theme in the new journal was the need to cultivate a distinctively southern medicine. Urging the necessity of southern medical schools for southern students, for example, an editorial that appeared in 1852 called for making a school in Richmond "the great medical Paris of America."[133] At the same time, the journal not only became one vehicle for disseminating French medical ways but also grew out of Gooch's identification with French medicine. Printed under the masthead was a motto chosen from Broussais: "Medicine is enriched by facts only."[134] Perhaps most telling is the title, for it was not by happenstance that Gooch selected a name for the journal that identified it with the Paris School. His choice apparently attracted criticism from some who thought it implied too exclusive devotion to auscultation, to which Gooch replied that his journal was to be no more exclusive in its focus than the London *Lancet*;[135] Laennec's instrument, however, was manifestly French.

Several months before he resolved to start the *Stethoscope*, Gooch had applied, unsuccessfully, for the position of professor of obstetrics and the diseases of women and children at the University of Missouri, and the letters gathered in support of his candidacy provide one indicator of how his career and experience abroad were regarded by other, sympathetic physicians. "The Dr has not only availed himself of the best instruction, which this country could afford, but for some years past he has had an opportunity of attending the Lectures of several of the ablest obstetricians of Europe," wrote one Richmond practitioner. "With such advantages, combined with the zeal and industry which belongs to him, his appointment will I am sure give entire satisfaction." Another wrote, "Dr Gooch's canon of Study in the various European hospitals particularly those of Paris and Edinburgh is known to me to have been one of constant & devoted assiduosity, referring principally to the peculiar branch of Study & Science, which he now desires to illustrate by lectures." Having dealt with his qualifications as a physician, most of Gooch's sponsors went on to testify to his standing as a gentleman; as one physician wrote smugly, "In all other relations, of Family, morals, and character, I need only say to you that he is my friend."[136] Nearly all of those who wrote letters on Gooch's behalf stressed his experience in Europe as the distinguishing professional factor in his bid for a professorship.[137]

Many of the physicians who studied in Paris did become medical school professors at some point in their career—by one historian's probably inflated estimate, one in three.[138] In the long run, their use of these positions as platforms for teaching French ways would be the most important route by which the medicine of the Paris School became integrated into American medicine. Medical schools, like medical journals, proliferated during those decades when the influx of Paris-returned Americans was growing large—trebling between 1800 and 1820 and trebling again between 1820 and 1860.[139] Many of these started up in the South and West, and the prospect of faculty positions in these schools was one factor pulling Paris-experienced physicians from the eastern seaboard to these newer regions. By midcentury, at many American medical schools most if not all the faculty members had studied in Paris. The multiplication of schools did not standardize antebellum medicine. But their enormous proliferation during the very decades when large numbers of physicians returned from Paris eager for professional distinction was important in moving the Parisian commitments of a relative few into the training of the next generation.

Drawing upon Parisian recollections in lectures, professors exhibited to students the value they attached to French ideas and practices and to their own experience abroad. Through lectures, introductory addresses, and social interactions, if a particular professor had spent time studying in Paris, students were sure to hear of it. "Dr Locke has returned from Europe & has already begun his course of Lectures to the Med. Class—He is rich in new chemical facts," a Cincinnati medical professor wrote to a friend in 1837; while a Boston physician reported that John Collins Warren "gives a fine course of lectures this winter. He goes into the subject of comparative anatomy and amuses the students with anecdotes of persons & things he has seen in Europe."[140] After Caldwell returned with books and apparatus he had been sent to collect for Transylvania University, a student there could write in 1822 that the overall "improvement" of the school "since last winter, has been manifest and gratifying."[141]

Textbooks could also be used to draw attention to their French origins. Usually the selection of texts was the prerogative of each faculty member. In reply to an inquiry from Comegys in 1852, asking if the school would adopt his contemplated translation of books by two Paris clinicians, the dean at the University of Pennsylvania was encouraging but informed him that "the adoption of text books for the chairs was left to the Professors respectively."[142] Gerhard persuaded Jackson, Sr., in 1834 to recommend his forthcoming translation of Louis on pulmonary consumption to Harvard medical students. "No work on the same subject is equal in value to this," Jackson wrote back. "I shall recommend this work to the pupils of our school in such terms as the above, having a sincere desire that they should study it." But, he continued, "they are poor, many of them, and will not get it at once. Ultimately however I should think that large numbers, say 200 in three years, would be sold in this market." Jackson went on to suggest two other eastern professors who probably would recommend the text, and added, "I think that, with care, the profession in the S. and western schools can be made to do the same."[143] Pupils sometimes read French medical books in apprenticeship before they attended lectures,[144] but use at a school placed a textbook in the hands of a much larger readership.

Students could themselves disseminate French medicine while still in school. Just as students in Paris reported on the medical forefront, students attending lectures at American schools regularly wrote home describing their lessons to medical kin and preceptors. Samuel Brown, a medical student at Transylvania, in 1821 sent his brother—still a medical apprentice—detailed advice about the course of reading that he should pursue. For physiology, instead of the Edinburgh physician William Cullen's text he suggested that "Richerand or Bichat would be the works I prefer—Bichat on Life is a work of uncommon genius & great utility in the study of the causes of disease."[145] So too as students became practitioners, they used medical societies (often unwittingly) as forums for disseminating the French medical lessons they had been taught. In the early antebellum period, some medical societies even served an explicit educational function. So long as societies held licensing power, de facto or de jure, they were in a position not only to examine candidates but to issue lists of the books each student was expected to know. In 1822, Bichat was the only French author on the list of the Massachusetts Medical Society,[146] but by 1836 nine out of the thirty-three required books were translations of texts by Parisian authors, including treatises by Velpeau, Laennec, Pierre-Augustin Béclard, and two each by Bichat and Louis. (Added to the published list was a note explaining that Louis's *Researches on Phthisis* would be required once a translation had been published in America.)[147] Even after societies lost this formal function, their meetings continued to provide an important forum for some physicians to recall their Parisian experiences.[148]

It is more difficult to say how aware American patients were of the ascendancy of the Paris School. Accounts of American doctors studying in Paris that appeared in newspapers no doubt drew some notice, but perhaps the strongest evidence is the remarkable number of ill Americans during the antebellum period who themselves made the journey to consult with Parisian physicians and surgeons.[149] In any event, for American doctors it became virtually impossible from the 1820s onward not to notice the rising prominence of French medicine in America. In 1827, several Philadelphia physicians could write to La Roche, "It has been resolved by a number of your professional friends to offer you a public dinner previously to your departure for your Europe, as a testimony of their respect for your professional and private work."[150] By 1842, however, Franklin Bache would complain to George B. Wood, "It is proposed to give a complimentary dinner to Dr. R[andolph] which will take place in about a week at a country place on the Schuylkill. This may be very well, for he is certainly a good fellow, but still we could not afford, [in] these hard times, to give a dinner to all the clever Doctors who might return from a tour in Europe."[151]

However much the American medical profession was aware of a growing French influence, and however much disciples and critics alike dwelled on the Frenchness of what was transmitted from Paris, as the dissemination of French medicine proceeded many of the ideas and practices Americans took up became less and less identifiably French. Indicators of French influence in the content of instruction at antebellum medical schools, for example, are very easy to find. The notes on lectures that students took abound with references to French ideas, institutions, practices, and clinicians.[152] The same is true of the M.D. theses students wrote, which ordinarily were regurgitations of what was heard in lectures and read in the school's library.[153] Yet one of the most striking things about the various elements of French medicine as they appeared in these contexts is the extent to which their Frenchness gradually became muted—much less distinct than in, say, letters sent from Paris or in translations.

This diminishing distinction is important, for it indicates the extent to which French medicine, as it came to be presented to students at antebellum American schools, was intermeshed into the broader body of medical lessons. From the viewpoint of students trying to learn what they were told in the classroom, it would have been very difficult to sort out what was French and what was not; moreover, trying to do so would be pointless. What was taught, at least as students perceived it, was no longer French medicine; it was simply medicine, the established canon that as aspiring professionals they were expected to master. Once these young graduates moved into practice, they took French medical ways with them without necessarily knowing the national origins of the knowledge and practices they employed. As American physicians soon preoccupied with their workaday routine, they had literally made French medicine their own. It was in this way above all that French medicine was made part of the texture of American medicine—that much of French medicine in fact became American medicine.

# Telling a Historical Story

OF ALL the messages American physicians transmitted home from Paris, the one that most distinctly characterized their program for American medicine was the animus against speculation and for the empirical pursuit of truth, against rationalistic systems and for knowledge rooted in the collection of observed facts. Most antebellum American intellectuals would have claimed this cluster of commitments as their own, and would have readily affirmed that they and these reform-minded physicians were marching together under the banner of Baconianism. In fields ranging from natural science to religion, appeals to Baconianism were pervasive.[1] This was by no means strictly the philosophy of Francis Bacon's *Novum Organum* but a rather more flexible collection of attitudes toward knowledge for which Bacon had come to stand. More often than not those Americans who invoked Baconianism felt little need to define it, but all could agree that it stood for an allegiance to empiricism and fact and hostility to speculation and hypothesis. Antebellum medical writings abound with homage to Bacon. Yet, unlike most American intellectuals of the period, Paris-returned physicians overwhelmingly reembroidered the familiar banner of Baconianism with a different insignia, one that was unmistakably French.

Why did these American physicians make Baconianism French? Some of the answers seem self-evident, chief among them the fact that to those who studied in Paris, the epistemological stance they took up *was* French. The precise meaning of their version of Parisian empiricism, like that of American Baconianism, was assumed more often than defined. Yet what they had witnessed in Paris was a medical world informed by the sensual empiricism of the French idéologues and a postrevolutionary attitude toward medical knowledge informed by the thought of John Locke, Étienne Bonnot de Condillac, and Pierre-J.-G. Cabanis. This empiricist tradition had Baconian roots, but in selecting an emblem under which to march they found special appeal in something distinctive that they had experienced firsthand. As disciples of the French school, they saw themselves as having received truth directly from the masters, which they could never claim with Bacon.

Another part of the explanation for these physicians' choice to depict their commitment to empiricism as quintessentially French rests in the fact that many of them not only returned to make their Parisian experience a central part of their identity but returned to a country profoundly ambivalent toward Britain, not least of all in the wake of the War of 1812. Cultural nationalism was at work here, for as comparison with the English illustrates, there was nothing inevitable about the American interpretation of Parisian empiricism. English medical practitioners who studied in Paris generally acknowledged the soundness of the attitude toward knowledge they witnessed there but saw in it nothing essentially new. They tended to praise French medical empiricists by congratulating them on being good Baconians, recasting Parisian empiricism as part of an older English epistemological tradition. The American disciples of French medicine, by contrast, could have called their program Baconian but chose not to. They did not seek to diminish Bacon by stressing the Frenchness of their campaign and often spoke of him with reverence, nor did they stigmatize him merely for being English; but the credit due Bacon was not the point. To some Americans, there was considerable appeal in hoisting a new and distinctly non-British standard, one they could march under confident in the clarity of their mission.

More than this, the representation by American physicians of the medical empiricism they encountered in Paris as something distinctly French grew from the way they viewed and wished to portray medical history. They depicted the Paris School as a turning point, an epistemological break with the past that inaugurated a new medical era. It was a revolt against two millennia of epistemological delusion, but one that at the same time could be presented as a return to a much earlier, authentic Hippocratic empiricism. Both the Frenchness and newness of the Paris School helped make it a distinctive banner under which Americans could rally their own reform movement. Representing their epistemological position as a radically new French empiricism rather than as yet another expression of Baconianism was essential to a historical narrative they relied upon to define the meaning of the Paris School and to clarify their role as its emissaries. Telling a historical story that situated the Paris School at an abrupt disruption in the course of medical thought helped validate the importance of the program to which they had consecrated themselves while it underscored the promise of the newly launched battle against medical systems. Even though most American physicians did not take up their account of history intact, and often neglected to stress the role of the Paris School that its disciples so celebrated, the campaign against the spirit of system that this account of history was designed to propel became perhaps the most powerful intellectual impulse in antebellum American medicine.

The importance to these physicians of telling and retelling this story stemmed from the professional place occupied by history in nineteenth-century medicine. At least through the first two-thirds of the century, much of the professional definition and authority that later physicians would derive from science came from history. It was medical history and the values it displayed that validated the regular physician's regularity, confirming participation in a learned tradition and identity as a professional. History placed physicians in a continuing lineage and affirmed the links with the past that gave them legitimacy. Especially at a time when a multitude of alternative healers were competing successfully for recognition and clients, recounting a historical story that displayed two millennia of enduring tradition was a tool orthodox physicians used to set themselves apart.[2]

Much of professional argument, moreover, was cast as historical polemic. This form of history making was much more than the kind of culturally enhancing but detachable framework for presenting medical ideas that it would become in many twentieth-century texts: it *was* medicine. Engagement with classical texts was not merely a leisure activity for the cultivated physician but engagement with a living tradition—not an antiquarian pursuit but a medical one. History played a prominent role in transmitting and defending a medical position, whether it was a matter of conveying the established canon to students in a classroom or introducing a new idea to colleagues at a society meeting. By the final third of the century, the professional place of medical history was already changing markedly. Indeed, the Americans who studied in Paris were part of the last generations to accord medical history the professional stature (and function) it had held for centuries.

The particular account of history constructed by the American disciples of the Paris School served them in two leading ways. First, it provided the most important vehicle they had for urging the ideas and ideals of French medicine on the rest of their profession. Second, it helped them understand the place in history occupied by the Paris School and by themselves. This understanding, in turn, clarified and empowered their identity as those responsible for transmitting French medicine to America. The Paris School, as presented in this historical narrative, provided a new reference point for an American medical profession seeking to re-create a past for itself, a vision of the past that affirmed the importance of the mission its disciples had embarked upon and gave them a chart by which to square their course. Critics would dispute this narrative and present an alternative historical account of their own. But the American Parisians held fast to their version of history as the linchpin of their broader program, for it at once explained the past, gave meaning to the present, and offered a plan for the future.

## DISCIPLESHIP

The historical narrative told by Americans committed to the Paris School situated them in relationships to both a long professional past and a parentage they sought to celebrate. The cultivation of Pierre Louis as a professional father by his American pupils *after* they returned to the United States exemplifies broader patterns in the ways discipleship governed the construction of historical accounts.

Just as Paris-returned Americans in general formed a network after their return, so Louis's followers created a smaller, tighter group held together by their special medical parentage. They kept up an active correspondence discussing their researches, trading news about their careers, assessing new books and reviews to gauge the progress of Louis's reputation in America, and reaffirming their shared faith. Not long after returning to Boston, James Jackson, Jr., wrote to Caspar Pennock in Philadelphia, anxious to show him his portrait of Louis and, equally, to ask Pennock, "Y-a-t-il d'hommes a Phil$^e$ qui connaissent même a moitié les mérites de notre Louis[?] Y-en-a-t-il qui en parlent et qui ont lu ses ouvrages[?]"[3] Some of them kept up a correspondence with

Louis or with his Parisian disciples such as François-Louis Valleix and E. Rufz, and reports on Louis's research, health, or medical society were passed along through the wider network.[4] They also wrote letters of introduction to Louis for American travelers to Paris whom they saw as potential converts.[5] Thus in a single letter to Louis in 1848, William Gerhard could introduce George Wood, a Philadelphia physician visiting Paris; relate news of the recent activities of his confrères Pennock and Thomas Stewardson; and tell Louis of his own investigations "à l'hopital de Pennsylvanie."[6]

They drew upon their association with Louis as a claim to distinction—in applications for clinical and teaching posts[7]—and promoted his example in the clinic, in the classroom, and in their writings. Interpreting Louis for the American medical public was a task they possessively claimed as a right. "My friend Gerhard was engaged in translating Louis' Phthisis: he had finished nearly ¼ of it & a young man fr. N. York, whose mind & acquisitions are not at all equal to the work proposed to Louis to do the same thing," Jackson, Jr., wrote to his father from Paris in 1833. But, he continued, "I wld. rather lose my right hand than that my dear master's work shd. be translated by one who wld. murder it."[8] Jackson, Jr., resolved to collaborate with Gerhard on the project and beat the interloper into print. However, the larger aim of translation, as Gerhard put it, was to "render of immediate utility the results of the *master* as well as increased the taste for this kind of study."[9] There were, of course, other aims as well, as one physician recognized when he congratulated George C. Shattuck, Jr., on his 1839 translation of Louis's treatise on yellow fever. "Your first appearance in public under the august shade of Louis['s] reputation has been of service to you & has made you more generally known than you otherwise as a young physician could have hoped for"; and he added, "I hope it has also brought you the solid remuneration of practice."[10]

The celebration of Louis by this core of proselytes could arouse resentment both in those opposed to Louis's teachings and in others who felt excluded from an elite fellowship. In 1847 David W. Yandell took satisfaction in noting, correctly, that "Louis is not the great man in Paris that he is in the United States."[11] Yet that made it all the more frustrating for someone like Henry Bryant, who clearly wanted to join Louis's inner circle when he arrived in Paris in 1844 and followed Louis in the wards, but found the French clinician less than welcoming. Piqued, he wrote home that Louis was "very irritable and very frequently has a blowing up with some of his subordinates." He asked his father to get letters of introduction to Louis from Shattuck and Jackson, Sr. "I do not know how much of a favour it would be considered," he said of approaching Jackson, but added that "you need not have any diffidence in asking Dr Shattuck—as he gives letters to all the students who wish them whether he knows them or not."[12] When Bryant's Boston acquaintance Warren arrived in Paris six weeks later, however, Bryant found the entering wedge he needed. Only a few days after Bryant had called on Warren, he reported to his father, "M. Louis told me this morning that he had seen Dr. Warren and asked me if I was a friend of his," a connection that led to an invitation from Louis to dine with him at his house; "you can imagine I am very well satisfied with myself," he told his father.[13] Bryant nonetheless added, "It is true that he always befriends the Americans and it is very right for him to do so as they have been making his reputation."[14]

For his American disciples, Louis embodied a new faith to be venerated, proselytized for, and defended. Writing to Shattuck in 1844 about the creed that bound them together, Alfred Stillé made a brief nod to Bacon and then proceeded to affirm, "Louis, I maintain, was the first to give any thing like development to the inductive system." Stressing the newness of the numerical method, he asserted that "it has demonstrated many errors which *seemed* to repose upon well observed facts, and many more which were sanctified by tradition & the voice of authority. Nevertheless men are, and were, slow in admitting its superior accuracy. The advocates of *rational* investigation, and the defenders of pure observation, are thus opposed; they are at war."[15] As Louis came to be mythologized, the depiction of him as father not just of the numerical method but of a new era in the history of medicine became increasingly prominent.

## HISTORY: REVOLT AND RETURN

As Americans who had studied in France were drawn into professional interactions after their return, their claims for the importance and newness of the Paris School became more systematic and stylized, and nowhere more so than in their presentation of history. Glossing over all subtleties, their account of medical history was this: Since the collapse of the classical Greco-Roman world, Western medicine with only a few notable exceptions—Vesalius, Sydenham, Morgagni, and Hunter—was dominated by rationalism and speculation, only worsened in the Enlightenment by the reigning spirit of system. The Paris School that emerged in the wake of the French Revolution marked a break, a valiant revolt against the dogma and speculative embellishment of Old Regime medicine. But it marked a break only with the medical errors of the past rather than with medical tradition itself, for to some extent it involved a return to Hippocratic observation of nature. With liberation from the spirit of system in sight, and with the empiricist pathway to truth revealed, it was now up to the acolytes of the Paris School to carry on the good fight and establish a new medical order. The pivot upon which this historical interpretation turned was the French empiricist revolt.

In private writings, this version of history was tacit knowledge there was no need to spell out. In public rhetoric, however, it was a story that in part or in full they told again and again. Professional rituals such as introductory addresses at medical schools offered particularly strategic occasions to recount this historical narrative. But because history telling was such an inbuilt part of ordinary professional argument and persuasion, it often appeared in didactic lectures to students, in textbooks, and in technical contributions to medical journals as well. Already common in the 1820s and 1830s, as the number of committed disciples of French medicine grew this account of history became commonplace during the 1840s and 1850s, and some would continue to repeat it through the end of their lives. Told initially to persuade students and colleagues, over time it increasingly functioned as a form of righteous action, an affirmation of a shared creed recited less to convert the unenlightened than to reassure the faithful.

The French revolution in medicine, as these Americans told the story, represented a fresh start in reconstructing medical knowledge. "A BICHAT, a BECLARD, a BROUSSAIS, have been given to the world; ignorance and error are now trembling, tottering, falling!" one physician told members of a local South Carolina medical society in 1837. "The flimsy theories and unphilosophical writings of many from the time of HIPPOCRATES, to the present, are now being exploded and consigned to the depository of the antiquary."[16] Echoing this view, a Boston physician asserted flatly that "disease has never, until quite recently, been investigated." Direct empirical observation was just beginning to expose the "incomprehensible mysticism and absurd speculations of the closet dogmatists upon the nature of disease."[17]

Early in the antebellum period, this kind of historical claim was often made to assert the freshness and importance of what was just appearing from Paris. Reviewing in 1831 a translation of Gabriel Andral's *Treatise on Pathological Anatomy* gave a New York physician the occasion to sketch the broader historical context in which he believed the work should be placed. "Scientific pathological anatomy," he began, "has created a distinct era in our profession and is destined to form the ground-work of modern medicine, freed from loose conjecture and ingenious hypothesis." This new departure "hardly dates beyond the labours of the present French school of contemporary writers." He regarded Broussais as "the efficient pioneer in subverting that vicious mode of considering and investigating disease which had been so long consecrated by time and authority . . . [who] furnishes us with the first well-digested example of philosophical induction applied to the investigation of disease, by strictly connecting the morbid alterations of structure found after death with the various symptoms the disease exhibited in its progress, from its commencement to its termination." Suggesting that "we might go one step further back," he noted that Xavier Bichat had established the foundation for this method of investigating disease. However, "If we go further back we shall find little to compare with the science of the present day."[18]

By midcentury, such historical claims were more reflective but no less intent on identifying the Paris School as a new departure. In 1848, Stillé used the preface to his *Elements of General Pathology* as a forum for reaffirming his Parisian faith as the foundation for a new medical order. "The theories which ruled the world successively, have disappeared one after another, like succeeding fashions in equipage and dress, while many of the *facts* recorded two centuries before the Christian era, recur in the daily walks of our profession, precisely as the Father of medicine inscribed them on his tablets," he began.[19] But the great observers, Hippocrates "as well as all his successors, until very recently, preferred to communicate the general results, rather than the elements of their experience, in the form of aphorisms, or short, pithy maxims, which were easily remembered by their pupils." A more rigorous use of observation was required, Stillé insisted, and "it became necessary, therefore, that the moderns should apply themselves to the *natural* history of disease, and build up the science anew, from its very foundations, by slow and gradual labour. Thus it is, that nearly the whole domain of pathology, such as we now possess it, is of very recent acquisition."[20]

Stillé gestured approvingly to Bacon but denied that Bacon's method had instigated a new departure in medicine. "It is somewhat remarkable, that although these precepts were promulgated more than two hundred years ago, and many physicians since that time have professed to guide their inquiries by the Baconian philosophy, yet not until within twenty or thirty years has any one carried them into literal execution."[21] Louis, he argued, was the first to develop this method in medicine by not merely asserting but acting on the conviction "that the science of medicine is founded *alone* upon the observation of facts, to the *entire exclusion* of all hypothetical reasoning." Stillé noted that "from the beginning of time to the present day, the same material phenomena have been presented to the senses, but in medicine, with comparatively little profit, until a recent date": it was the Paris School that had revealed a pathway to lasting change.[22]

What such disciples of French medicine as Stillé sought to convey by presenting history this way, and what others took away from their words, were not necessarily the same. It was fully possible to take up the call to battle against speculation without embracing the proposition that the Paris School marked the critical turning point between the old medicine and the new, and many Americans followed this course. The program for reevaluating established medical knowledge was part of a broader movement in American thought. Not only professionals but educated Americans in general spoke much about the error of blind allegiance to authority and the importance of making independent judgments. This was expressed among intellectuals by the proclaimed allegiance to Baconianism and became even more widely pronounced with Jacksonian calls for all American men and women to exercise their democratic duty by making up their own minds about everything that concerned the social, political, and natural worlds. In the medical profession as elsewhere in American society, rhetorical allegiance to independent thinking was routine. "Blind devotion to authority is an obstacle to the acquisition of knowledge," Lundsford P. Yandell told a new class of Transylvania medical students in 1825, echoing preceptors throughout the country, Paris-experienced or not.[23] Even calls within medicine for empirically determined fact were expressed in rhetorical conventions that, as chapter 7 will explore, had much wider social and political resonances.

Much of the account of history that the American Parisians promoted was widely taken up by the American medical profession, even if others assigned a less radical role to French medicine in instigating change. This was most force-fully expressed in a campaign against speculative systems of pathology and therapeutics, which came to represent a wide spectrum of the profession's in-tellectual and social ills. The disciples of the Paris School spearheaded this assault and were the most strident champions for the empiricist crusade against systems—orthodox and antiorthodox—and all that they stood for. As they urged the messages of the Paris School on their colleagues and students, and as this French influence merged with broader American attitudes toward knowledge and authority, the assault on system became one of the most force-ful impulses in the American arbitration of medical knowledge.

The wider dissemination of the empiricist campaign against system is evi-dent in antebellum M.D. theses, in which students, reproducing the depiction of medical history they had been taught, presented the battle against systems as the leading intellectual campaign of their era. In the antisystem M.D. theses that proliferated, ordinarily the first task was to display the long-standing op-pression of medicine by systems, persisting through the present. "System-mak-ing is a characteristic of the times," one medical student at Transylvania began his thesis in 1841. "The marks of this fondness for theorizing are nowhere more plainly perceptible than in the history and progress of Medical Science. Scarcely does one fair fabric of hypothesis and conjecture crumble into dust, ere another superstructure, composed of the same flimsy materials, rises upon its ruins."[24] The following year, another student at the same school wrote, "In looking back over the history of medical science; we observe nothing that has exerted a more baneful influence upon the curative art, or therapeutic applica-tion of medicines; than the many systems that have been established."[25] Each student then went on to catalog the dire consequences of system building, chief among them ineffective practice and a block to progress. The evils of antiorthodox medicine were likewise attributed to system building, for not only Cullenism, Brownianism, and Cookeism, but equally Thomsonianism, hydropathy, and homeopathy were brought forward as examples of the absurd systems of practice to which unchecked speculation could lead. Even confront-ing only the systems of regular physicians, another thesis writer complained, the medical student could well feel overwhelmed by what he called "the gush of speculation."[26]

Such gloomy lamentations were often but the start of what took the form of a jeremiad. Identifying evil and loudly deploring it provided a springboard to pleas for reform. There was satisfaction in having at last recognized a pattern repeated over the long course of medical history. "New systems have arisen from time to time, ever since the healing of the sick was resolved into a science; but comet like they have feebly blared for a season and passed away; leaving their boasting admirers like Pharoah's army, engulphed in the dark waves of oblivion," wrote one Albany student in 1850.[27] So too another student urged, "From time immemorial, each age has had its favorite cherished theory, and with the age, its offspring died." One lesson, he continued, was to realize that "error, though aged and venerable, is not the less an error, and the keen scalpel of science should ever be ready to expose, and remove the deformity."[28] Similarly, a medical student in South Carolina urged that "'the spirit of system' . . . has greatly retarded the progress of medicine"; but while he held that "the spirit of system is a propensity belonging to the human mind," the modern recognition that the medical profession faced "no greater enemy" offered hope in the struggle to overcome it.[29] The persistent message was that in recognizing the spirit of system as seductive and dangerous, the nineteenth-century physician had finally come to understand that facts rather than speculations provided the only sturdy foundation for the medicine of the future. Thus a Transylvania medical student who dedicated his 1848 thesis to his teacher Elisha Bartlett concluded that instead of the fanciful system building of the past, "ours is a sterner and less pleasing duty. It is the allotted task of our age to remove the crumbling relics of a false philosophy."[30]

This campaign against the spirit of system, pursued by students and by the professors who imparted it to them, was propelled largely by the Paris School. Yet American physicians influenced by French teachings were perfectly at liberty to take up what they found helpful in Parisian medicine and make it their own without drawing attention to its French provenance. At the same time, nothing compelled them to assert that what they adopted from France was particularly novel, much less revolutionary. In England, Russell Maulitz has shown, the secure and conservative elite, even those who had studied in Paris, could take up elements of French pathology and assimilate them into long-standing English medical and surgical traditions. Practitioners on the margins of professional power and eager to promote change, on the other hand, were more likely to stress the Frenchness of new pathological teachings.[31] So too many conservative Americans took part in the ongoing reform of medical knowledge while glossing over the role of Parisian lessons. At a meeting of the Medico-Chirurgical Society of Cincinnati in 1847, one physician could "congratulate the profession upon the evident approach of a new era in medicine," explaining that "it was plain that the dicta of the schools were loosing their influence, and that the thinking men in the profession were coming up to the investigation of truth after the true Baconian method."[32]

Yet compared with the English, what is striking about the Americans is how receptive they tended to be not only to the epistemological message of the Paris School but also to the notion that it was fundamentally new. Those Americans who studied in France more uniformly and energetically celebrated the newness of the Parisian medical ways than did their English counterparts. They were also more inclined to draw attention to the place of the Paris School in history as an epistemological turning point. And they were more likely to make discipleship to French medicine an important and visible part of their identity.

The putative newness of the Paris School and the epistemological break with tradition it was made to stand for had a powerful appeal for physicians self-conscious of the newness and cultural potential of their own nation, liberated, as many saw it, from not only the Old World but the burden of its past. Just as Americans saw their country forging a new social and political order, so the radical empiricism of the French revolution in medicine offered a basis for creating a new medical tradition, and its newness enhanced its symbolic value. Citizens of the New Republic contrasted the intellectual despotism of the Old World with the freedom of thought of the New. Thus a Virginian studying medicine in Edinburgh in 1805 could complain that one would be branded "a damnable heretic" for openly considering Brunonian doctrines. "How different is it from our School," he wrote home, identifying this British posture in medicine "with that political principle which says that the mass of mankind must have some one to think for them."[33] Similarly, an American physician wrote from London in 1839, "Here improvement is checked and cramped by old forms and old customs, that they cannot shake off.—With us we have no such thing, we look at things without prejudice,—try all things reject the worthless or useless and improve upon the good."[34] Perceptions such as this encouraged confidence in American destiny, the conviction that Americans, of all peoples, could bring to fruition the new departure in medicine. "The day of personal authority and universal sway in our science has passed," one student from Alabama optimistically claimed in his 1857 thesis, "and the great American principles of free thought and free speech, prevails."[35] History, medical and civil, combined in giving American physicians a special mission. "It rests with ourselves to take a national position, as regards the science of medicine," Austin Flint, writing from Paris, asserted in 1854, "in keeping with the political importance of our republic."[36]

In the account of history that the Americans who had pledged themselves to French medicine urged, then, there were wide-ranging professional and cultural reasons to stress the newness of the Paris School. Without contradiction, however, they used history to reveal continuities between features of Parisian medicine they admired and a thread of truth that extended backward in time. The crusade against the spirit of system, according to this depiction of it, was in some respects a return to Western medicine's classical roots; and for the American disciples of Parisian medicine, as for some among their French medical heroes—such as Cabanis, Philippe Pinel, and Laennec—Hippocrates especially represented a usable past.

Hippocrates was to be admired for freeing himself from the speculation regnant in his time and for providing a model of empirical observation of fact that distinguished him from the centuries of speculative theorists that ensued, from Galen onward. "Although the science at his day was in its infancy, and himself entangled in the labyrinthian maze of speculation and hypothesis, yet notwithstanding this he deemed all our knowledge in medicine, to consist in the observance of actual phenomena and their generalization," an Albany student wrote in his 1840 thesis.[37] At the same time, "Hippocrates has left us a masterpiece which excites our surprise and admiration, when we remember the remote age in which it was written," a St. Louis medical professor told his class in 1845, proposing that to understand the reasons for such lasting success his students need only recognize "with what care that great man avoided the delusive guide of imagination."[38] Another physician held up the writings of Hippocrates on epidemics as a model of the empirical revelation of enduring truths: "He is here the historian of nature, and his descriptions will continue true to the end of time."[39] That the products of empirical observation had survived intact testified to the durability of fact, contrasted with the frailty and ultimate transience of speculations.

Invoking the example of Hippocrates was a way of blunting the unsettling radicalness of the claim that the science of medicine was in its infancy. But it also provided one way of proclaiming a new departure in medicine without denying a longer lineage that was an important source of the profession's identity and confidence. It retained what was good from the past—"those glorious principles handed down to us from Hypocrates and other Fathers," as one medical student in Nashville put it[40]—while positing a revolution that not only overthrew past errors but continued full circle to restore something important that had been lost, that is, Hippocratic observation of nature.

This theme of return, like depictions of the empiricist revolt against established authority, was rooted not only in a particular understanding of the medical past but also in broader conventions in American thought and rhetoric. Indeed, it has been suggested that the theme of return was the one unifying motif that recurred in all of the diverse movements for social change during the Jacksonian Era.[41] Just as social reformers demanded change not only in the name of progress but also by calling for a return to a more authentic, simpler, ancestral American past, so medical reformers seeking to dispel the spirit of system sought both to break with the past and simultaneously to return to an older, purer, ancestral past represented by the most revered of the medical fathers, Hippocrates.

These coexisting themes of revolt and return are exemplified by the thought of Elisha Bartlett. On the one hand, in his empiricist manifesto *An Essay on the Philosophy of Medical Science* (1844), dedicated to Louis, Bartlett gave the fullest account by any American of the philosophy of the Paris School and its place in the wider history of medical knowledge. Erwin Ackerknecht regarded the book as "the only systematic formulation of the philosophical approach of the great Paris clinical school," and claimed for Bartlett the title "the philosopher of the Paris clinical school."[42] In Bartlett's text, as in his lectures to students, he assailed rationalism and urged in its place close, empirical observation of fact after the Paris model.[43]

Medical hypotheses and theories, Bartlett argued, "have ever impeded the progress of the science which they professes to promote. Not only so, but they have almost always acted injuriously upon the practical applications of the science of medicine."[44] He insisted that "so far as medical science has any just title to the appellation; and so far as medical art possesses any rules, sufficiently positive to be worth anything, it is owing, exclusively, to the diligent, unprejudiced, and conscientious study of the phenomena and relationships of disease. The sole tendency of every departure from this study,—the sole tendency of every attempt to refer these phenomena to certain unknown and assumed conditions, for the purpose of rendering them *rational*, has been to hinder the progress and improvement of the science and the art. So has it ever been, so will it ever be."[45] He cataloged the systems that had reigned, each in its turn, and underscored excessive reliance on rationalism as the fundamental flaw that characterized all of them, denouncing Cullenism, Brownism, Rushism, Broussaisism, "and all the host of other so called rational *isms*."[46] Pathological systems were "*a priori* abstractions, under the misnomer of laws, or principles," and it was not merely deluded but dangerous to deduce therapeutics from them.[47] In the place of such system building he proposed "a pure philosophical empiricism."[48]

Bartlett's critics and admirers alike agreed that his was a radical book. Critics denounced him for slighting Bacon and accused him of being "blinded by his ardor to demolish speculative theories."[49] Supporters, many among them physicians who had studied in Paris, applauded his single-minded zeal. The Paris-experienced Alabama physician Josiah Clark Nott reviewed it as "the most remarkable medical book yet written in this country," one that "tears off the veil which has ever been thrown over false science and exposes it in all its deformity." By undermining the "hypothetical explanations" and "baseless visions" of rationalistic systems, Bartlett had shown that "Galenism, Cullenism, Brownism, Rushism, Broussaisism, like Cookeism and Thompsonism now stand only as monuments of the fallacy and madness of human reason; because they are hypothetical explanations of facts, and not legitimate deductions from them."[50] Stillé made a similar appraisal of the book privately in a letter to Shattuck, recognizing in Bartlett's arguments "those of my own medical creed, & of yours, & of all of us who have been brought up in the school of that 'Prince of medical logicians' Louis." Bartlett, Stillé continued, "has settled the question whether a priori reasoning can discover new truths in medicine. His work should be considered a sufficient answer to hypothesis-mongers of all sorts whether within or without the medical profession. Its style is clear, correct, and logical; it shows a thorough mastery of his subjects, a love of truth for its own sake, and a certain dignified inflexibility becoming one who has undertaken to call to account the worshippers of idols."[51]

Yet, like the other American physicians who shared his Parisian faith, however stridently Bartlett asserted the radical newness of Parisian epistemology, he also pointed back toward Hippocrates as an earlier prophet of the Louisian faith. Bartlett's celebration of Hippocrates as progenitor of the empiricist program was especially clear in an introductory address he delivered in 1852 at the College of Physicians and Surgeons in New York, later published as *A Discourse on the Times, Character and Writings of Hippocrates*. His address opened with inventive and richly detailed scenes of the Greek physician at the bedside, tableaux calculated to evoke a distant time and place. But Bartlett soon turned the attention of his listeners to Hippocrates, or, rather, to what Bartlett imagined Hippocrates would have said had he been invited to speak at such an occasion: "the Valedictory Address to the graduating class of the school of Cos, at the term of the first year of the 95th Olympiad." He would have begun "by warning his hearers against the subtle and dangerous errors of superstition" and perhaps of "the system of his Cnidian neighbors," Bartlett suggested. "He would speak of the great revolution that had so recently taken place in the Greek mind, even then only partially accomplished." Then, Bartlett continued, "he would have warned his hearers against the seductive but dangerous influences of the philosophers," those whose systems were based on "empty hypothesis and idle speculation" rather than "observation and experience," and "he would have shown that they had accomplished nothing, and that in the very nature of things they could accomplish nothing, for the real advancement of knowledge." Hippocrates, in other words, unmistakably was cast as the first sensual empiricist and was made to look as distinctly Parisian as possible. Indeed, in speaking by proxy for Hippocrates, Bartlett used language remarkably similar to that he used in his own *Philosophy of Medical Science*.[52]

But lest the slower members of his audience fail to draw the connection between past and present, Bartlett went on to spell it out. Hippocrates, in the first volume of Littré's translation, *Ancient Medicine*, had exposed the errors of the "speculative philosophers," those whose "system . . . consisted in vague, shadowy, hypothetical, *à priori* speculations and conjectures." As Bartlett put it, "The true character of medical science, and of these *à priori* hypothetical systems, could hardly be more clearly and succinctly stated, more logically argued, or more happily and forcibly illustrated, than it is in this Essay. And this is the very question that still divides medical opinion—that is unsettled to-day, as it was when this Essay was written; dogmatic rationalism, on one side—simple, philosophical empiricism, on the other." Framed this way, the French empiricist revolt against system appeared no less a revolution, but a revolution that could claim return to reassuringly antiquated and venerable beginnings.[53]

## A MALLEABLE HISTORY

The theme of return was an important corollary to the account of medical history used to propel the campaign against the spirit of system. It made the story more complex without diminishing claims for the newness of the Paris School or the importance of the French empiricist revolt. The broad narrative, however, was not told with a single voice even by those who shared a common discipleship to French medicine. While it uniformly urged the animus against systems, it could be made to serve a variety of other ends. Further, even though the overarching structure of the narrative persisted throughout the antebellum period, elements of the historical account changed over time.

Readjustments made in the face of changing circumstances can be seen clearly in the transformation between the late 1820s and the early 1840s in the American portrayal of François-J.-V. Broussais. Early in this period, he was brought forward as a paragon of the French medical revolution and exemplary system-basher. But as his reputation changed both in France and in the United States, Broussaisism came to be widely regarded as the preeminent model of a rationalistic system and its attendant evils. As this transformation proceeded, the place assigned to Broussais in historical accounts was turned on its head.

Broussais's own revolt against established medical doctrines had indeed been radical, and no one said so more brashly than Broussais himself. Published in 1816, just at the time when large numbers of foreign students were arriving in Paris, his *Examen de la doctrine médicale généralement adoptée* was an assault against all medical doctrines that had come before, but most especially against Pinel, whom Broussais denounced as an ontologist. In Broussais's assertively antiontological, "physiological" conception of disease, he insisted on a shift in medical attention from symptoms and essentialism to lesions and localism. He denied the existence of specific diseases and held that overstimulated bodily functioning led to anatomical lesions (almost always expressed as inflammation of the gastrointestinal tract). This was the process that most diseased conditions shared, he asserted, one to be treated chiefly by local depletion using leeches.[54] What many found most appealing in Broussais was his unsparing condemnation of all earlier systems of medicine and their builders, "those obscure & purely speculative logicians, who follow in the treatment of human infirmities, the chimeras of their imaginations, rather than the real disorders which are presented to their senses."[55] By the third edition, published between 1829 and 1834, his *Examen* had expanded to some 2,200 pages, a wide-ranging history of medicine that analyzed each system of the past in turn only to denounce it.[56]

In America as in France, Broussais drew considerable attention, much of it captured less by his particular views on pathogenesis and therapy than by his programmatic empiricism and localism. By the mid-1820s, the various vehicles that brought French medicine to the American profession all were at work transporting Broussais's teachings. Philadelphia physician Isaac Hays, who shared the enthusiasm for Broussais of his mentor at the University of Pennsylvania, Samuel Chapman, not only published *History of Chronic Phlegmasiae or Chronic Inflammations* (1831) and *Principles of Physiological Medicine* (1832), his translations of Broussais's treatises, but also used the pages of the *American Journal of the Medical Sciences*, which he edited starting in 1827, as one forum for urging Broussais's doctrines. The claim that Broussais had inaugurated a new era became common. "Of all the systems of medicine yet proposed, that of BROUSSAIS is the only one strictly conformable to the Baconian principles, and therefore erected on an immoveable foundation," one physician asserted in the *American Journal* in 1831, noting that "the medical doctrines of Broussais are founded on observations made at the bed-side, and in the dissecting-room."[57] The South Carolina physicians and brothers William Blackstone Nott and Josiah Clark Nott were so committed in their allegiance to Broussais's teachings that the former christened his eldest son John Broussais Nott.[58] In New Orleans, Creole physicians who had received their medical degrees in Paris were particularly devoted followers,[59] and Anglophone Louisiana physicians, such as Edward Hall Barton, also became proselytizing converts.[60]

Not all physicians were convinced that Broussais's doctrines were particularly novel, much less true. "I am still engaged in examining the new doctrines of the French School of medicine," a North Carolina practitioner wrote in 1832 to his son, a medical student in Philadelphia, "and the farther I advance in the examination, the more am I convinced that there is but little that is new in them, & that what is new, much is erroneous"; and he proceeded to explicate the similarities between Broussais's ideas and those of John Brown and Benjamin Rush.[61] Some practitioners also criticized blind allegiance to Broussais's rules of practice, as did one Louisiana observer who complained that the profession there was "mostly wedded to systems and riding hobby's," citing in evidence the numerous "followers of Broussai."[62] Nevertheless, other translations of Broussais's works appeared in multiple editions,[63] American physicians in Paris attended his lectures and reported on them,[64] American students and practitioners bought his books,[65] and professors incorporated his ideas into their lectures.[66]

As late as 1837, the year before Broussais's death, John P. Barratt, a South Carolina physician, asserted that the Broussaisian revolution was leading medicine to a new age,[67] but by that time Broussais's reputation had plummeted in the eyes of most Parisian and American physicians alike. His fall from grace in France during the 1830s was partly propelled by assaults from a younger generation of Parisian clinicians, Louis among them. "Broussais is bellowing & grunting about diseases of the Heart," Jackson, Jr., wrote from the amphitheater of the École de Médecine in 1832. "I am not here to listen to him, but have simply come in to the last ½ of his Lecture in order to secure a good seat at Andral's wh. will follow it. You cannot conceive of the feeling of disgust wh. I have for this man Broussais & his mode of studying Medicine—it is c̄[um] infinite pleasure that I see the benches empty during the hour of 2 to 3 (his Lect.) & full again fr. 3 to 4, when Andral holds the chair." To Jackson, as to Louis, Broussais's antisystem rhetoric had proven to be merely groundwork for the building of a rationalistic system of his own. "The idea of the *World*'s being so long deceived about this man is to me quite inconceivable—happily, henceforward, Pathology is not to be studied, à la Broussais i.e. à priori."[68]

Just as Louis was a leading antagonist of Broussais in Paris, so Louis's disciples led the assault in America. "The day before yesterday the last volume of Broussais' examen appeared, in my opinion a glorious day of triumph for Louis," Stewardson wrote from Paris to Gerhard in 1834. "I bought the work only yesterday and have as yet read only a part of his examination of Louis but I have read enough to justify me in saying that it is miserably weak . . . base and mean."[69] Jonathan Mason Warren seconded this perception, writing the following day from Paris to his father, Boston surgeon John Collins Warren, that Broussais had written "in the spirit of a man grasping for this fallen system and will serve only to place Louis at the very head of the Morbid Anatomists of the age."[70] Six months later Stewardson reported that "Louis has written an answer to Broussais which I read a few days since—It is a masterly performance and altogether worthy of its author."[71] Louis's rebuttal, the culmination of a long-standing feud, was as fierce as Broussais's own polemics, and the fact that Louis dedicated his *Examen de l'examen de M. Broussais relativement à la phthisie et à l'affection typhoïde* (1834) to the memory of Jackson, Jr., won a special place for the volume in the eyes and hearts of American readers.[72]

By the mid-1830s, the overall American appraisal of Broussais was decisively turning. "The masterly 'examination' of medical doctrines, by Broussais," a Louisville medical professor told his students in 1838, "was only introductory to a new system of his own, which, under favor of an imposing name, and the eloquent advocacy of its founder, rose into the ascendant with unexampled rapidity." But "its fall was not less rapid and signal," he continued, noting that Broussais "now lectures to empty benches, where, ten years ago, disciples crowded to his instructions by thousands."[73] Denouncing Broussais in words that might once have been used to praise him, a Transylvania medical student insisted in 1835 that unlike Broussais, "we are not forced to resort to idle hypothesis, or vain speculation, to explain the phenomena observed in disease; but rest our explanation upon the facts observed."[74] Broussaisism continued to recruit some followers, and Broussaisist ideas continued to appear in class-rooms;[75] but no longer was he pointed to as a hero of the medical revolution. By his death in 1839, Broussais's "physiological doctrine of disease had already passed through its complete revolution," an American obituary observed. "As a system, the physiological doctrine can scarcely be said to exist; very few of these ultra adherents can now be found, except amongst the French army surgeons, and in some parts of the tropical regions of America."[76]

By 1840, the collapse of Broussaisism was celebrated by American physicians not just as the end of yet another misguided system but as the end of the system-building impulse in medicine altogether. "Since the downfall of Broussaisism, no other exclusive system of medicine has been favored," Moses Linton wrote from Paris in that year. The "spirit of speculation," he argued, finally had been dispelled; "he does not understand the signs of the times, who looks for the establishment of an exclusive system."[77]

In the historical narrative that proclaimed the campaign against the spirit of system, Broussais thus came to be redefined—from a father of the revolution to father of the last medical system. This latter role preserved for him a central if unenviable place in the historical account, for during the 1840s and 1850s Broussaisism, like Cullenism, Brownianism, Rushism, and Hahnemannism, was one of the models most commonly cited by Americans to exhibit system building and all its evils. Broussaisism, instead of marking the dawn of a post-revolutionary era, was a final episode in the revolutionary struggle. The story persisted fundamentally intact; only Broussais's role was recast.

The same broad historical narrative that proclaimed medicine's liberation by the empiricist spirit of the Paris School could also be adapted to the circumstances and needs of particular groups within the American medical profession. One powerful variation on this story is displayed by the antebellum southern drive for regional medical separatism. Leading southern physicians, many of whom had studied in Paris, found in the account of the revolt against system both support for their intellectual and political aspirations and a framework for defining their medical program.

Especially from the 1830s, and intensifying in the 1840s and 1850s, the call for empirical observation of disease that was a hallmark of the French impulse throughout the United States was echoed in the American South by a call for empirical observation of *southern* diseases. The starting premise was that only direct observation of concrete individual patients, at the bedside and at the autopsy table, could generate valid knowledge about morbid natural history. Therefore, southern physicians reasoned with a logic entirely in keeping with French precepts, authentic knowledge of the diseases of the American South could be derived only from close study of the peoples of that region pursued within the context of its peculiar environments. A South Carolina physician who, in 1848, enthusiastically reviewed Elisha Bartlett's *History, Diagnosis and Treatment of the Fevers of the United States* (1847), went on to note that the natural history of "our remittent and congestive fevers of the South" had yet to be written. "Much original work remains to be done by those residing in malarious regions before a complete history of their fevers can be written. Their Louis has not yet appeared."[78]

More than just calling for the study of southern diseases, however, this logic demanded the rejection of all rules for their diagnosis and treatment that had not stemmed from direct observation—demanded, in other words, the overthrow of northern American and European authority over southern medicine. Overturning rationalistic systems and overturning northern authority, both misleading in southern practice, were projects that in the eyes of many southern physicians went hand in hand. Rejecting "fashionable dogmas" and "hypotheses" would be the first step toward preparing his treatise on fevers, one Memphis physician told a Philadelphia editor in 1857, and in the process such a work "would open the eyes of southern practitioners, and confirm them in the disposition now manifested by many, to cut loose from and declare their independence of, all northern and European authors on this subject."[79] Expressing a similar animus against established authority, a New Orleans physician urged in 1856, "The day is coming when the folly of treating the diseases of negroes by books written by authors who have never seen a negro, and know nothing of his anatomical and physiological peculiarities, and who have never been in a cane or cotton field, or in a negro quarter, will be apparent." That, he continued, "will prepare the way for seeing the folly of treating white people, in a Southern climate, by the remedies found most appropriate for the same people in a Northern climate."[80] Signaled by a revolt against authority in favor of empirical observation, an Atlanta physician asserted in 1855, "a new era has dawned upon the profession of Medicine in the South."[81]

Like the broader narrative about the overthrow of systems, this southern story of revolt also invoked a theme of return. And as in the broader narrative the return was to be to Hippocrates, depicted, however, to highlight not just his allegiance to observation but also his standing as a model southern physician. During the 1850s, the most strident leaders of the movement for southern medical separatism—such as Samuel Cartwright, Erasmus Darwin Fenner, Josiah Nott, and Alexander Means—used the theme of return in an account of history that was yet another way to call for overthrowing northern authority. "Hippocrates lived in a southern climate, presenting diseases similar to our own, and his practice points out the true treatment of southern diseases," one physician told the annual gathering of the Medical Association of the State of Alabama in 1855.[82] Constructed from observations of southern climates, constitutions, and diseases, the principles of this medicine were matched to southern needs and were still suited to many of the needs of the American South. But just as Hippocratic observation of nature had been subverted by centuries of speculative system making, so Hippocratic knowledge of southern diseases had been corrupted when medicine moved northward after the fall of Rome. As an Atlanta professor told an entering class of medical students, "the floods of vandal barbarism poured down upon the doomed city, from the plains of the North, and bore off upon their dark and turbid bosom, almost every trace of learning and refinement." The looted remnants of superior southern medicine were taken to cold climates and there were distorted to meet northern needs.[83] When medical dominance finally passed to Edinburgh, "a new nomenclature was there made to embrace the new order of diseases observed, new theories invented, and a new practice adopted to suit the diseases of that little hyperborean corner of the globe," as Cartwright put it.[84] The systems developed by "Cullen and his followers . . . became quite too frigid for the ardent temperament and more relaxed system of our 'Sunny South.' "[85] Adherence to Cullen's system, therefore, or to the authority of any northern teacher, led the southern physician to practice in ways fundamentally unsuited to the realities of his region.

The message of this story was clear. Hippocrates was the archetypal southern physician, for, rather than relying on established wisdom he observed for himself southern diseases, peoples, and environments, developing morbid natural histories and therapeutic strategies appropriate to southern patients. Southern physicians, in turn, needed to follow the Hippocratic example, recognize the distinctive character of southern medicine, and liberate themselves from northern and European systems. What those who advocated this return to Hippocrates envisaged was nothing less than a Greek Revival medicine, confluent with other streams in antebellum southern culture ranging from architecture to politics yet informed by the epistemological lessons of the Paris School.

The account of history put forward by the American disciples of the Paris School, like the southern variation on it, was designed not only to persuade and reassure but also to promote action, and chapters 6–8 explore the work it stimulated. The point here is that this particular account of history, first articulated by the disciples of French medicine to help them understand the meaning of the Paris School, provided the conceptual framework for the crusade against the spirit of system, and, as parts of the account were taken up by other physicians, a context for the leading movement by regular physicians in antebellum America to reform medical knowledge.

## Counterhistory

To this history there was also a counterhistory, one that instead of celebrating the Paris School sought to expose its evils and to denounce the revolutionary changes claimed in its name. Challenging all that the disciples of French medicine held dear, some American physicians asserted that the Paris School represented nothing really new. More than this, they charged that its program to reform medical knowledge was misdirected and dangerous. To them, French medicine represented not a source of salvation for American medicine but one of corruption. As they deployed their own account of history, a fight was on for the past with the future at stake.

The treatment of Louis in this alternative account illustrates the broader treatment of the French school by critics. In 1844, for example, the English-born physician Robley Dunglison delivered an introductory address to his class at Jefferson Medical College in Philadelphia that accused Louis's program of misdirecting practice and endeavored to strip it of all meaningful claims to newness. Dunglison began by tracing medicine from Hippocrates through the Alexandrians and, after noting the extreme positions represented by the Dogmatists and the Empirics, suggested that "in all ages, from the periods to which allusion has been made downwards, there have been physicians, who pretended to be guided solely by a rigid attention to observation, and others who have indulged in the wildest and most visionary hypotheses, despising all observation." He proceeded to say that "the closest approximation to the ancient sect of Empirics is the modern French *School of Observation*," and quoted from Bartlett's *Philosophy of Medical Science* to exemplify the stand of that school.[86] "Yet schools of this kind have existed in all times," he asserted, "and, from the first moment that a medicinal agent was prescribed to the present day, physicians have professed to be observers and 'to have but one aim and object, to ascertain the actual constitution of things.'"[87]

Dunglison then turned to "the distinguished head of this modern school—if it may be so termed—the indefatigable and philosophical Louis."[88] Dunglison denied that the numerical method represented anything new and dwelled on "the heresy of trusting implicitly to simple observation," urging that doctors must instead employ "a wise combination of dogmatism or rationalism with empiricism—to employ the language of the ancients."[89] He underscored his argument by noting, as did many critics, that from Louis's work "not a particle of therapeutical information is added to what we already possessed on the subject," and concluded that "a glance at the history of medicine exhibits, that the science has suffered more from faulty observation than from faulty theories."[90]

Joshua Flint made similar points using a different strategy when he gave an introductory address to his Louisville medical students in 1838. Having just returned from a brief visit to Europe, he used the occasion to discredit Paris as a place for Americans to study medicine, to denounce French therapeutics as feeble, and above all to disparage French medicine as dogmatic, asserting that "their systems are equally remarkable for their multiplicity and transitoriness."[91] Flint began with an exposé of the rise and fall of Broussaisism, noting with satisfaction that Broussais's tirade against all the speculative medical systems of the past had proved to be nothing more than ground clearing for a new system of his own. He then turned to "Laennec and his pupils," who maintained "the exclusive precision of their own method with as much pertinacity as if Hyppocrates, Sydenham, and Morgagni had never lived," as he put it. "And now we are in the midst of another 'epoch,' as they are fond of terming their successive dogmas—the 'school of observation,' par excellence, better known as the 'numerical system.'"[92] He affirmed that "the method of observation is certainly good—indispensable; but it is a desperate push for originality to claim it, or its application to medical studies, as the invention of any modern master."[93]

"Neither is this numerical system, as some claim for it, a return to the Hippocratic method of medical investigation," Flint insisted. "The sage of Cos, indeed, employed observation, but always with a view to some specific conclusion, and not in the *omnium-gatherum*, irrelevant manner of our modern fact gatherers."[94] Flint went on to reassert his "reverence for the method of the Novum Organum," urging medical students headed abroad to chose the less "dazzling and seductive" lessons of British teachers over the French, and insisted that "the *numerical system*" was "hindering the progress of rational medicine."[95] He concluded by noting that "not long since, a large portion of the élite of our profession had realized a charm in *Broussaisism*," and warned that "a similar infatuation has since doomed another body of ardent and promising young men, to the tread-mill of *Numericalism*."[96]

Instead of seeing in the Paris School liberation from systems, in other words, these critics regarded it as the source of new ones, such as the defunct system of Broussais and the ascendant one of Louis. Flint insisted that Louis, far from being a modern Hippocrates, was "head of a sect," and told his students that he spoke in order to "counteract this propensity for system-worship, and to overthrow the idols it has set up."[97] Dunglison also called Louis the head of both a "school" and a "system."[98] Other critics, such as Cincinnati medical professor Leonidas Moreau Lawson, not only denounced this "system" but insisted more sweepingly that "modern medicine admits of improvement, but not revolutionary changes."[99]

Assertions such as these led the American disciples of French medicine not to rewrite their account of history but to reaffirm it more stridently than ever. In 1840, for example, the New York medical professor Martyn Paine published a two-volume work, *Medical and Physiological Commentaries*, which, in the appraisal of Louis's Boston pupil Henry Ingersoll Bowditch, had as its main object "a violent attack" on the numerical method and on Louis in particular.[100] Paine, for his part, proudly affirmed that he undertook his denunciation of Louis "in protecting my brethren, from Hippocrates to the present time, against his almost universal scorn and derision,—in demonstrating the fallacy of the assumption that 'medicine is now in its infancy.'"[101] Not long after it was published, John Hamilton, a Dublin practitioner sympathetic to French medicine who had just been given the book to review, wrote to Shattuck alerting him to this assault on his mentor. "I shut the book & refused to review it," Hamilton wrote, noting that Paine "seems mad on the subject of philosophy" and "would bring us back to the old dreaming theoretical days . . . & as for the Baconian philosophy he despises it, looking on facts as things only calculated . . . to quench the fire of genius & to contort the reasoning powers." Hamilton told Shattuck that "I looked on you when here as an out and out disciple of Louis," and encouraged him to refute Paine's charges. "He seems to think this attack on Louis very necessary as a great many young American physicians came to America imbued with Louis notions greatly to the disservice of medicine in their native country," Hamilton explained. "This is so personal to you that I think you ought to call him out[.] He therefore hopes by his 'Observations' on the writings of Louis, to un-numericalize them."[102]

Bowditch took up the defense instead, leading Louis to write expressing his gratitude and reaffirming the newness of his program. "As to numeric analysis," Louis told Bowditch, "if it has been tried before me, it was done by instinct and never in any other way, no one else ever formulated a law by which to arrive at the knowledge of the truth. Besides the numeric analysis occupies physicians only since yesterday, if one may say so, it is an entirely new thing."[103] Bowditch's rebuttal to Paine in the *Boston Medical and Surgical Journal* and subsequent exchanges between them, like the attacks on Louis made by Dunglison and Flint, were voiced in very public forums. And certainly the strident rhetoric deployed in such contexts came partly from the fact that in defending the Paris School and the place they had assigned it in history, the American Parisians were also defending a tradition in which they had rooted their identity.

Yet just as discipleship was a significant part of their private identity, their defensiveness was expressed in their private rhetoric as well. When Lawson sent Bartlett a copy of an introductory lecture trouncing Louis in 1846, for example, Bartlett wrote back a detailed rebuttal of what he regarded as a misrepresentation of Louis's work. Then, acknowledging to Lawson that there was "fundamental disagreement between our views of the nature and character of medical science," he proceeded to lecture him on the broader errors of his vision. "You sneer at the medical philosophy of such men as Louis, Andral, Chomel, Grisolle, James Jackson, Oliver Wendell Holmes, and so on, and so on," Bartlett wrote. "I cannot refrain from asking you one very simple question. *If Louis's conclusions are wrong, will you have the goodness to inform me and your readers, in what way, by what process and method, this error can be shown and demonstrated*, unless it be by following *precisely* the method which he followed. If you can show *any other way* of getting at the truth in this and all similar questions, I will quit the banner of Bacon and Louis, and range myself under those of Aristotle and Martin Payne."[104]

The American disciples of French medicine deployed and defended an account of history that affirmed the role of the Paris School as the start of a new and singularly promising era in medicine. Some other Americans brought forward a counterhistory that both denied the newness of the Paris School and disclaimed its promise. Most antebellum American physicians, however, took up a position somewhere in between, optimistically embracing the account of history that proclaimed the campaign against the spirit of system to be a distinct product of their times while often glossing over the French origins of this impulse and moderating the radicalism of its most aggressive proponents. Those American Parisians who propagated their distinctive account of history, even if they could not control the way it was retold, to a large extent attained the end they sought: the campaign against the spirit of system had become a central theme in antebellum American medicine.

# "They Manage These Things Better in France": Polity and Reform

THE ACCOUNT of medical history that the American disciples of the Paris School related to propel their campaign "against the spirit of system" conveyed a highly selective and peculiarly American image of French medicine. Out of the complex and changing realities of the Parisian medical world, Americans persistently tended to select its characteristic epistemological stance—strident empiricism and equally strident antirationalism—as its most prominent feature. There was nothing inevitable about this particular way of depicting French medicine, however, as English comparison shows, for the English instead tended to stress French medical polity (a term used at the time), that is, the social and legal organization of the French medical profession, its institutional arrangements, relationship with the state, and rewards system, as well as the value system that undergirded all of these.

The differing images the Americans and the English presented were products of a process of selection begun in Paris. What those who made the journey perceived as most noteworthy were those features of Parisian medicine that most powerfully resonated with implications for the medical profession in their own countries, whether they judged these implications to be desirable or threatening. The letters and diaries of the English and Americans in Paris spoke of broadly the same things; but there were important national differences in emphasis. These medical migrants then returned to tell stories about what they had witnessed and what it meant, stories that they and some of their colleagues who had not traveled to Paris in person repeated and elaborated into vivid and remarkably durable images. Both the Americans and the English told stories rooted in the realities of the Parisian medical world, but they selectively highlighted certain of its features and glossed over others. American and English representations differed so much in emphasis as to constitute two nationally distinct models of Parisian medicine and its significance. These broad national differences in constructions of the Paris School are especially clear in the rhetoric of reform, for in both countries it was in the context of professional reform that images of French medicine were most boldly deployed.

This chapter and the next—on French medical polity and epistemology respectively—explore the ways that elements of French medicine were appraised and selectively taken up, and how they acquired meaning in programs to reform medicine in America and in England. Certain aspects of French medicine found concrete expression in English and American ideas, institutions, and practices, but the aspirations of reformers matter here as much as the fulfill-ment or failure of their schemes. A comparative perspective discloses patterns in the French impulse in American medicine that a focus on the United States alone would leave undetected.

## ENGLISH REFORMERS AND FRENCH MEDICAL POLITY

Medical communication across the Channel did not cease during the Napole-onic Wars, but after Waterloo, as English awareness of the medical vigor of Paris intensified, an exodus of medical students to Paris commenced that con-tinued through midcentury.[1] By 1835 William Baly, recently arrived in the French capital after completing a hospital dressership in London, could report to his mother in Lynn Regis that "300 English students [are] here every year" to study medicine.[2] Some traveled to Paris to master French medical ways, but for most Parisian study was a means of gaining extensive anatomical and clini-cal experience, often difficult to acquire at home. A young practitioner seeking a commission in the Army Medical Department in 1845 noted in his diary that the director general in London had told him "that a journey to Paris and a course of study there was the best thing I could do in order to forward my views as a candidate for a commission."[3] Many returned with certificates testi-fying to the instruction they had followed and expertise they could claim.[4] Some Englishmen even complained that French study was forced upon them by the growing esteem in which the public held it. "My object in coming here," one medical student wrote from Paris in 1830 to his former preceptor in Bris-tol, "was, that the idea entertained by the world in the present day is that a man can scarcely be able to practice his profession unless he has completed his education in this metropolis; and as I am . . . to be dependent on the opinion of the public and they choose to humble themselves in this way my only course is to sail with the stream."[5]

From the outset, it was exceptionally free access to experience that most drew English medical visitors to Paris. John Green Crosse, a Norwich surgeon, traveled there late in 1814, during the brief interlude of peace between the abdication of Napoléon and his return from exile in Elba. "I find immense opportunities of gaining information without any expence—the medical schools are upon a surprizing scale, & the matter in w$^{ch}$ they are conducted is admirable," Crosse wrote home in January 1815.[6] He noted that the professors at the École de Médecine were paid by the government and "y$^e$ lectures are free to every one," so that the visiting foreigner "can reap all the advantages of this school without a farthing of expence." In anatomy, "the only expence of dis-secting is what you pay for the bodies, w$^{ch}$ are procured from y$^e$ hospitals & cost you about six or seven shillings each."[7] Crosse described rooms near La Pitié that "hold between forty & fifty dissecting tables each—& above four hundred pupils dissect there—*all* the cadavers from Hotel Dieu are carried thither for dissection—so that, so long as the Hotel Dieu is not without *pa-tients*, there is no doubt but the *physicians* and *surgeons* will supply this school *plentifully* with *dead bodies*."[8] The organization of the Paris hospitals as teaching institutions particularly captured his attention, and he noted that "upon the whole I think the English Surgeon, who spends a short time here, will have much less pleasure from witnessing y^e practice of the hospitals, than from observing the way in which they are conducted to render them schools for y^e education of students."[9] These arrangements Crosse deemed worthy of emulation. "I assure you," he wrote home, "there are many things that might be transferred with advantage to y^e London Schools, particularly in points that have relation to the education of Medical Students."[10]

Several months later the young Exeter surgeon John Haddy James arrived in Paris, and his depiction closely matched Crosse's account. After serving as a medical officer in the British army at the Battle of Waterloo in June 1815, James was quartered in the French capital during its military occupation. Regimental duties placed only meager demands on his time, and he spent the better part of six months studying medicine. In his diary James underscored the access foreigners enjoyed to the city's medical institutions. "The whole of the Hospitals, & the whole of the public collections in Paris, whether at the Jardin des Plantes, at the Hopital de la Charite, or here [at the École de Médecine] all belong to the same general plan.—and every facility is offered to every Student & Stranger, to see & consult every thing," he observed. "Public Lectures are given at the expence of Government, on every branch of the Science, but principally on Surgery & Anatomy." Students had ready access to the dissecting rooms and "the price of the bodies is only 5 Francs." The same was true of the medical museums, where "all those [whose] object is science, have free admission to examine every specimen, of every kind, the whole is open to them."[11] The "essential difference" between Paris and London was money, he wrote home from France, for "the System of things at Paris, renders it much less essential here."[12]

By dwelling on free access to knowledge and experience and the social system that facilitated that access, Crosse and James were contributing to what through midcentury was the most prominent English representation of the Paris School. This was a depiction highlighting French medical polity—the mode of managing affairs and principles of organization that prevailed in the Paris Clinic. Americans equally celebrated free access to practical experience, but the workings of the Paris School that made that access possible chiefly interested them as an explanatory frame for the opportunities they enjoyed as students. That was the point of the contrast they drew—described in chapter 2—between the open French system and the closed one of London: Paris was a better destination for study abroad. English observers, however, were preoccupied with comparing the polity that encouraged the flourishing medical culture of Paris with that of their own country, and especially London—partly because they brought with them to France a nationalistic expectation of cultural and institutional parity if not superiority and partly because they saw in this Parisian model powerful possibilities for explaining and remedying professional ills in their native land.[13]

English students in Paris did voice many of the same complaints that Americans articulated about medical, logistic, and moral impediments to professional improvement. While instruction in the wards was freely open, for example, the English perennially complained about large crowds and pushy Frenchmen. "French students push their way more rudely than English.—for which numerous 'Pardons' are poor return," the twenty-five-year-old Leeds surgeon Thomas Pridgin Teale wrote in his journal. Describing a surgical procedure at the Hôpital des Cliniques, he protested that "the plan of operation is villainous as students and internes all crowd a round, the operator can hardly move his elbow, and none but those close can see."[14] And even enthusiastic visitors complained that *cliniques* at the major hospitals all were held at the same hour of the morning, that French therapeutic practice was so inert it was hardly worth studying, and that the French language made it hard to grasp just what professors were trying to say.[15]

Partly to get around such difficulties, in 1827 one enterprising British physician, Dr. Caldwell, offered a plan of organized, supervised medical study in Paris that spared his compatriots the trouble of negotiating their way alone. "Many young gentlemen who come to Paris, not knowing much of the language, and being strangers to the customs of the place, lose much valuable time for want of having their studies directed," Caldwell suggested in a broadside, "and finding their situation while they remain in many respects irksome and unpleasant, relax their exertions, get connected with society injurious to their morals, and return to England without having fully availed themselves of the beneficial opportunities here presented to them." Caldwell promised students "such society and domestic comforts as to render their situation advantageous and agreeable." Students "are directed in the various branches of Medical Science, connected with the Hospitals and University; receive Anatomical Demonstrations combined with Physiology, and enjoy regular Conferences on Medical and Surgical subjects, etc." His broadside underscored the fact that lectures at the École de Médecine and attendance at the hospitals (including "the situation of Dresser") were all free of expense, and that subjects for dissection cost only a few francs. Caldwell appended a testimonial—garnished with the names of such Parisian luminaries as Chomel, Dupuytren, Andral, and Orfila—affirming that "*with regard to* INSTRUCTION AND MORALITY, STUDENTS *and their* FAMILIES *will find in* DR. Caldwell *all the* SECURITY *desirable*."[16]

As English travelers sent home reports—widely circulated by the medical journals that proliferated in England during the first third of the century—and returned themselves, French techniques, concepts, and institutional models were selectively taken up and put to a variety of clinical and social uses. In pathological anatomy, for example, Russell Maulitz has argued, the Bichatian tradition of tissue pathology was transplanted and transformed: the English domesticators of French pathological anatomy, as he put it, "domesticated a dog until it became a cat." It was fully possible, moreover, to take up aspects of Parisian medicine without acknowledging their origins or concluding that French ways held promise for wider programs of reform, a tack taken by some among the English elite.[17] At the same time, as Adrian Desmond has shown, ultraradicals in English medicine, those blocked from the strongholds of power, could embrace a French product such as the new philosophical anatomy (comparative anatomy in the Geoffroy Saint-Hilaire tradition) and make it a key ingredient in their broader leveling campaign.[18] Above all, at home the preoccupation with French medical polity intensified and took on powerful political meaning.

From the 1810s through the 1840s, the French medical model was most vigorously deployed in England in programs to reform polity, including the organization, institutions, and values of the medical profession. The particular judgments passed on this endeavor varied wildly across a socioeconomic and political hierarchy. "'They manage these things better in France'"—an 1837 editorial in the radical reformist journal *Lancet* began, borrowing a familiar cliché from novelist Nicholas Sterne—"may well serve as a text for the observations we are about to make." The writer then drew an invidious comparison between "the well-ordered administration of the Parisian hospitals and the pernicious system, by which the utility of our own hospitals is so considerably diminished." Focusing on *concours* as an embodiment of the wider order of things in Paris, he asserted that "*there*, place is obtained by merit;—*here*, by money or by intrigue."[19] Conversely, the editor of the conservative *London Medical Gazette*, displaying perhaps better appreciation of Sterne's irony, retorted to such enthusiasm by stating, "'They manage these things better in France,' is the alpha and omega of their argument, as still they prate of the anatomical arrangements,—the inscriptions,—and, above all, the concours." The editor then denounced the "levellers, or rather the annihilators" who "advocate the doctrines of unbounded freedom, free trade, free *grade*, free—every thing." Such reformers, he asserted, "may be distinguished and characterized by their choosing the French for their *beau ideal*," and he condemned their efforts to introduce "Gallican arrangements" into English medicine.[20] Radicals and reactionaries thus agreed that French medical polity, praised or vilified, had acquired an important place in English discourse about professional reform.

During precisely the decades when the Paris School grew so prominent, in England there was a widespread perception that the medical profession was degraded. A small elite, the "pure" physicians and surgeons (who in principle restricted their practice to either physic or surgery), enjoyed considerable social and financial success. They included the leaders of the Royal Colleges of Physicians and Surgeons and the medical officers of the metropolitan hospitals. The elite practitioner's prestige came not so much from medical knowledge as from social origins, family connections, and gentlemanly achievement, including for many a liberal Oxbridge education. The rank and file, on the other hand, occupied a subordinate and insecure position. Those known as apothecaries, surgeon-apothecaries, or, increasingly, general practitioners made up the vast

# MEDICAL EDUCATION,
## IN PARIS.

Dr. Caldwell, educated in the Medical Schools of London and Scotland, Graduate of the Literary and Medical Faculties of the French University, and established in Paris, receives a *limited* number of Medical Pupils.

The numerous advantages which the French Metropolis presents to Students of Medicine and Surgery, especially in the *commencement* of their studies, are so generally known as to require little explanation. But many young gentlemen who come to Paris, not knowing much of the language, and being strangers to the customs of the place, lose much valuable time for want of having their studies directed; and finding their situation while they remain in many respects irksome and unpleasant, relax their exertions, get connected with society injurious to their morals, and return to England without having fully availed themselves of the beneficial opportunities here presented to them.

In order to obviate these and other inconveniences, often experienced in a foreign country, young Gentlemen received by Dr. Caldwell, are provided with such society and domestic comforts as to render their situation advantageous and agreeable. They are directed in the various branches of Medical Science, connected with the Hospitals and University; receive Anatomical Demonstrations combined with Physiology, and enjoy regular Conferences on Medical and Surgical subjects, etc. — These Conferences, being conducted in French Medical Society, afford means of acquiring the Language without interruption to professional studies.

Dr. C., in thus imitating a plan long adopted in England by many Medical Professors and respectable Practitioners, has been kindly presented with the following testimonials, relative to this object in the French Capital.

" *We, the undersigned, Professors in the* Faculty of Medicine of Paris, *consider that the*
" *Establishment of* Dr. Caldwell *presents to* Young Gentlemen, *who come to study in* Paris,
" *the greatest advantages; and that, both with regard to* Instruction and Morality, Students
" *and their* Families *will find in* Dr. Caldwell *all the* Security *desirable.*

" December 14, 1827.

| | |
|---|---|
| Dr. CHOMEL, *Professeur de Clinique Médicale.* | Dr. DUPUYTREN (Bon), *Prof. de Clinique Chirurgicale* |
| BOYER (baron), *Profess. de Clinique Chirurgicale.* | ADELON, *Professeur de Médecine légale.* |
| ROUX, *Professeur de Pathologie Chirurgicale.* | ANDRAL, *Professeur d'Hygiène.* |
| RICHERAND, *Profess. d'Opérations et Appareils.* | ORFILA, *Professeur de Chimie Médicale.* |
| FOUQUIER, *Professeur de Pathologie Médicale.* | DESORMEAUX, *Professeur d'Accouchemens.* |

" Dr CONOLLY, *Professor of Physic in the London University.* "

For particulars apply to Dr. Caldwell, 15, *rue Saint-Germain-des-Prés,* or at the Faculty of Medicine, Paris. Applications may be also made to Mr. James Nisbet, bookseller, 21, Berners-Street, London; Rev. F. Monod, jun., Minister of the French Reformed Church, L'Oratoire, and to most of the other Protestant Ministers residing in Paris.

Fig. 6.1. Broadside advertising a supervised plan of medical study in Paris for British students. The plan, offered by the British Dr. Caldwell in 1827, promised to smooth the student's way into a foreign medical world and to circumvent the language barriers and moral risks of professional improvement abroad. (Courtesy of Historical Collections, New York Academy of Medicine Library, New York.)

# OUTLINE

## OF THE ADVANTAGES ENJOYED BY MEDICAL STUDENTS
### In Paris.

Admission to all the Lectures of the Faculty of Medicine; of the Faculty of Sciences; of the Faculty of Letters; to the Hospitals; to the situation of Dresser; and to the Medical Library, etc., free of expense.

Subjects for Dissection cost a few francs.

The Winter Courses begin in November. The Summer Courses begin in April, and continue until the end of August.

## INSTRUCTIONS
### TO GENTLEMEN WISHING TO GRADUATE.

The only Medical Degrees granted by the French University are, Dr. in Medicine, and Dr. in Surgery. They require four years' studies, and subject the Candidates to undergo the same Examinations for the one as for the other (*no apprenticeship is required*).—The following list of Examinations may give some idea of the System of Medical Education now pursued in France:—

I. *Examination.* Chemistry, Pharmacology, Botany, and Natural Philosophy.

II. *Exam.* ........ Anatomy, Physiology, and a Specimen of Dissection.

III. *Exam.* ...... *Pathologie interne et externe,* or, the Theory of Medicine and Surgery.

IV. *Exam.* ...... Materia Medica, Therapeutics, *Hygiène,* Legal Medicine, a Report to write on a given Case of Poisoning.

V. *Exam.* ........ *Clinique interne et externe,* or, The Practice of Medicine and Surgery, Midwifery, Three Questions on Medical and Surgical Subjects to be answered in writing; Six cases of different Diseases, methodically taken in the Hospitals.

VI. *Exam.* ...... *Thesis,* written and printed, either in French or Latin, and publicly defended during one hour before six Professors.—The other Examinations are also public.

The Expenses, including quarterly payments (called *Inscriptions,* and which are received by the Edinburgh University, etc.) together with the different *Examinations, Thesis,* and *Diploma.* are, in all, about FIFTY POUNDS.—He who thus obtains the Degree of Dr. in Medicine or Dr. in Surgery, *in France,* may also acquire the other Degree, by submitting a second time to the *Vth Examination,* and by defending a *Second* Thesis, which is an additional Expense of TWELVE POUNDS.

*N. B.* Gentlemen who have not taken the Degree of *Master of Arts* in their own Country. are, previous to being admitted to their first Medical Examination, required to produce the Diplomas of Bachelor of Letters, and Bachelor of Sciences, granted by the Parisian Academy;— these may be acquired during the period of Medical Studies.

The Paris Degree, like *that* of Edinburgh, authorises the individual possessing it, to practise in England, and in other parts of the British dominions, etc.

⁎⁎ *The above Statement is presented in order to avoid the trouble of writing on these subjects.*

Fig. 6.1 *Continued.*

majority of the regular profession but stood at its margins in status and legitimacy. Ordinarily the general practitioner took the license of the Society of Apothecaries and the diploma (the lowest grade of recognition) of the College of Surgeons; and, with the rise of gentility early in the century, this link with trade through the Apothecaries' Hall further debased their position.[21]

Because most practitioners could not aspire to the trappings of gentility and access to patronage that conferred status on the elite, their prospects for upward mobility were limited. Individually, the justification for claims to distinction they might make—medical knowledge and skill—was of scant utility. Collectively, their inability to raise licensing standards without support from the Colleges of Physicians and Surgeons and the Society of Apothecaries blocked efforts to improve the group's standing. As historian Irvine Loudon and others have shown, an emerging sense of corporate identity among general practitioners drove a reform movement that persisted throughout the first half of the century. The most vocal of these medical reformers complained that low educational requirements encouraged the overproduction of practitioners, divisive competition, and low fees; while the failure of the state to grant certified practitioners a legal monopoly left them vulnerable to competition from dispensing druggists and unorthodox healers. Only with passage of the Medical Act in 1858, with its inclusive register of all legally qualified practitioners, was the regular profession partly unified—a consolidation leading to the confident declaration by one editor that "medicine in this country has, both as regards Science and Polity, entered upon a new era."[22] Yet the aspirations of general practitioners went largely unfulfilled, for the Medical Act would reinforce their place at the bottom of a professional caste system.

It was in this context that reformers publicized a selective construction of French medical polity as a protest against the established order and a plan for change. In 1841, for example, printed under the familiar epigram "'They manage these things better in France.'—Sterne," an editorial in the *Medical Times* asserted that "in France, medical *polity* and medical legislation are brought to a degree of perfection, which, viewed as a whole, are not equalled in any other country." Pointing to the "decay" of the medical profession in England, the author asked, "Do we not see that giant curse of the country, exclusive and corrupt power, influence, interest, cemented in a bond of social and private despotism, as well as the hydra of quackery, in every chamelion-like form and shape? Do we not see all these vampyres and many more triumphing over the neglect, obscurity, discouragement and oppression of medical merit, talent, genius, and skill?"[23] To this degradation, the example of French polity offered a source of salvation. As the *Lancet* put the argument succinctly in 1847, "In medical legislation we are a century behind the French nation."[24]

Those English medical practitioners who most vigorously invoked the Paris School as a model were those most anxious for change, but they were not all cast in a single mold. Provincial surgeons and physicians (often holders of Scottish M.D. degrees) were inclined to use the French example to argue for meritocracy in the profession and for state suppression of quackery, but generally maintained a conciliatory posture toward the London corporations and opposed the centralization that France exemplified.[25] Metropolitan reformers were more intent on dismantling the corporate privileges of the Royal Colleges and Apothecaries' Hall and the monopolistic private control of London hospitals. But while various reform interests pressed the French model into service, those who used it most stridently saw themselves as champions for the general practitioners. English medical polity, they maintained, had to be altered fundamentally before knowledge and skill could function properly in determining the rank of the practitioner in the profession or of the profession in English society.

To trace the French impulse in English medical reform is beyond the scope of this book. A narrow focus on one key example, however, will illustrate wider patterns. One of the most aggressively pursued efforts to promote models of French medical polity in English professional reform turned upon the decline-of-science argument. This was the assertion that England was behind France in medical *science*—an invidious comparison of French vitality with English lethargy. Like the better-known claim, popularized by Charles Babbage in his *Reflections on the Decline of Science in England* (1830), that the physical sciences and mathematics in England were in decline, the decline-of-science argument in medicine did not suggest that England was slipping backward in science, but that it was slipping behind France.[26] A London medical editor writing in 1830 typically explicated the rapid strides of French science in order to "expose the truly humiliating, the almost degraded, and the unquestionably backward state of medical science in England." Taking pathology as his example, he noted that "in France, under a superior system, or one better calculated at least for the *promotion* of science, the disciples of Bichat, and Laennec, have made strides that distance all competitors." He asserted that "our continental neighbours have outstripped us beyond dispute—we follow, rather than lead, in the march of medicine."[27] As one practitioner charged, "France in medical science is nearly half a century in advance of England."[28] The exodus of English students to Paris, growing reliance on French literature, and prominent proselytism for Parisian ways by some converts made French ascendancy increasingly unmistakable.

The complaint about the *science* of France surpassing that of England was the cornerstone for a larger rhetorical convention used in deriding the prevailing order of English medicine and demanding change. "It is the science-killing tendencies of our old corporations that have awakened in us the whole severity of our opposition to them," one declinist asserted. Seconding the denunciation of the Colleges and Hall in 1845 by the National Association of General Practitioners, he charged, "All our statements resolve themselves ultimately into one grand accusation—they oppose the progress of science."[29] In declinist polemics, the elite's neglect of science and neglect of the general practitioner were often coupled. In 1836, George Webster made this point explicit in his address to the organizational meeting of the first British Medical Association, a society consecrated to the interests of general practitioners that included among its leaders such French-experienced reformers as Robert Grant, Marshall Hall, Robert Liston, Augustus Bozzi Granville, James Johnson, and William Farr. "Had the constituted authorities, the colleges, the corporations, and the halls done their duty (*cheers*), we should not have been obliged to meet this night, to take the matter into our own hands, and form an association," Webster told the assembly. "But instead of protecting the *profession*, I fear they have frequently oppressed it; in the place of advancing *science*, I fear they have rather acted as drags on the wheels of improvement."[30]

Statements about English backwardness usually were framed in the context of explanations for French achievements. And it was here that the link connecting the decline-of-science argument with programs for reform was welded. Claims about English inferiority in medical science, as voiced by reformers, pointed to the superior system of medical polity that nurtured science in France.

Declinist rhetoric used to promote change conformed to a strikingly regular pattern, which can be displayed by several representative instances. Especially through the early 1830s, one of the most touted restraints on English medical science was the dearth of corpses for anatomical teaching and investigation. The legal system compelled anatomists to rely on the illegal traffic of the resurrectionist, a risky way of procuring bodies that stigmatized all who anatomized and raised the cost of extensive study. "The obstacles which impede the study of anatomy in this country are such, and the facilities presented to the study in foreign countries are so great, that those English students who are desirous of obtaining a thorough knowledge of the science desert the schools at home, and repair to those abroad," reported the committee of the House of Commons appointed in 1828 to investigate anatomizing in England. "Their principal resort is to Paris, where 200 English students of anatomy are now pursuing their course of instruction."[31] Critics—in this case, radicals and conservatives alike—insisted that the shortage of cadavers depressed anatomical knowledge and hampered new contributions.[32]

The abundant, cheap, legal supply of bodies in Paris was a standing backdrop for denunciations of the English system. It went far toward explaining French achievements as well as the "hundreds of English students" abroad who, as one observer put it in 1832, were "seeking for those advantages which are denied them at home."[33] Noting that "the London hospitals were in a great degree deserted by students of medicine who found greater facilities for dissection at Dublin and Paris," in 1825 one medical practitioner told members of the Liverpool Literary and Philosophical Society that, as the secretary wrote in the minutes, "it was owing to this circumstance that France possessed a greater number of good anatomists than Britain, and that notwithstanding the great merit of a few eminent practitioners in this country, skilful surgeons were more abundant in France."[34] In testimony before the 1828 parliamentary committee, witnesses persistently urged legislation modeled after the French plan to provide anatomical material. "They dwell upon the practice of the schools of Paris," a writer in the *London Medical and Physical Journal* explained, "because it approaches most nearly to the plan recommended by most of the witnesses for adoption in this country."[35] The Anatomy Act passed in 1832 in the wake of several murders that were committed to procure cadavers for dissection— "the demand for *dead subjects*," as one Englishman wrote from Paris in that year, "which of late has elicited cupidity to crime & shocked the public mind to an unbearable degree"[36]—alleviated the problem. But its provisions fell far short of Parisian arrangements, and English students continued to travel to Paris to study anatomy and operate on the dead body while reformers continued to complain that at home "supply falls miserably short."[37]

A second source of the depressed condition of medical science was the way senior appointments were made at London's great hospitals. Critics charged that nepotism, social influence, and commercial connections, not skill or scientific ability, figured most prominently in the choosing of medical officers. "There is scarcely a physician or surgeon, attached to an hospital or dispensary in London, who has not obtained his appointment through interest, vote-making, or intrigue, and not one on the grounds of knowledge, experience, or eminence," one critic claimed in 1833.[38] Placing wards in the hands of socially elite physicians and surgeons who did not particularly care about scientific investigation, the declinist argument went, meant that England's richest resources for generating and disseminating medical knowledge were underexploited. The recourse to Parisian wards and autopsy rooms by English practitioners bent on scientific inquiry was held up as compelling testimony to the corruption of hospital government in London. "So little liberality is there in the British hospitals, that Englishmen are driven abroad to pursue investigations which they have no chance of prosecuting under the existing monopolies at home," Thomas Wakley, editor of the *Lancet* and a leading radical reformer, asserted in 1838.[39]

The example of the Paris School offered a solution: "Our hospitals ought to be placed under the control of the Government, and the medical officers chosen by concours," one reformer argued in 1842.[40] In Paris, critics of London hospital governance charged, a meritocratic system favored clinicians dedicated to scientific investigation who put the resources at their disposal to good use. By instituting *concours* in England, then, "we should have the great hospitals of the country purified from the present system of misgovernment and nepotism," substituting "the favouritism of science, talent, and industry" for a corrupt and degrading system.[41]

Reformers also inveighed against the direct financial stake London clinicians had in teaching, and its dire consequences for English education. The leading hospital physicians and surgeons, they maintained, regarded teaching more as a means of making money than as an obligation of office, and the stiff fees they charged for clinical instruction barred many students from the wards. Students themselves complained about the high cost of clinical experience; "I am completely sick of this system of extortion, of taxes upon knowledge," one pupil at St. Bartholomew's (who later sought experience in Paris) wrote in 1834 to his mother. "This plan is full of corruption."[42] As with the supply of dead bodies, access to living ones was stymied by a medical polity that enabled clinicians to "make merchandise of the sick poor."[43] Contrasting the openness of Paris to the student with "the cold reserve and neglect he is likely to meet in London," Wakley charged that "our hospitals are manors, and our museums are preserves; and every man who is not either an agent or a keeper, or who has failed to take out a 'certificate' for a year or six months' perambulation, is regarded by the functionaries as a trespasser on the property."[44] As Wakley summed up, "The dresser *buys* his office—the interne *wins* it by merit. This fact speaks volumes."[45]

The French example provided a model for change. Reviewing the "mercenary" plan of clinical teaching in London, one observer urged that emulation of Parisian arrangements placing clinical professors on a state salary and severing their income from student fees held out "some hope of redemption from this state of degradation."[46] Some reformers urged legislated reconstruction of hospital management, fashioned after the Paris mode of placing patient care, teaching, and research all under state control.[47]

The most fundamental cause reformers cited for English degradation was the low esteem accorded to science by the institutional leaders of the profession, those Wakley called "crafty, intriguing, corrupt, avaricious, cowardly, plundering, rapacious, soul-betraying, dirty-minded BATS."[48] Reformers assailed the Royal Colleges for devaluing science as a determinant of professional recognition and smothering incentive to scientific enterprise. "The old corporations," one practitioner noted, "are obsolete—effect—moribund. They form in their cadaverous aspect the vivid contrast to the life and freshness of science that is on the wing abroad."[49] "Our chiefs," another critic commented in 1843, "are recipients of so much per annum (their *private* property being the most valued item)—they are denizens of an aristocratic square—acquaintances of the noble—agreeable fellows in society—carriage-owners—gentlemen—bustling men of business; any thing, in short, but those patronized humble beings—*men of science.*"[50] The Apothecaries' Hall and the Surgeons' College were in a position to regulate standards in education. Yet records of the Society of Apothecaries make it clear that at least through the 1830s deficiency in Latin, not in natural science, was the most common reason some candidates for the license failed.[51] By keeping formal requirements and knowledge actually tested in examinations low, the established elites further depressed the scientific education of general practitioners.

This situation too was turned on its head in France, reformers maintained, where medical government made scientific achievement the cardinal claim to professional reward. Therefore giving scientific accomplishment a comparable importance in the assignment of professional rank in England and making requirements for qualifications more rigorous were pivotal in plans for invigorating English medical science and uplifting the profession. Instead of examinations held in secret—the practice at the College of Surgeons and Apothecaries' Hall—they should be conducted with the openness of French proceedings.[52] Radical reformers also called for legislative reorganization that would bring a "*representative government*" to the profession, making it "a republic of men of letters," and abolishing "the distinction of ranks in what ought to be the commonwealth of science."[53] Science, reformers argued, made no distinction between physic and surgery, and, since their unification after the French Revolution, neither did the Paris School. Reformers looked forward to a time when better-educated practitioners would occupy a place in society commensurate with their scientific attainments, uplifting the standards and respectability of the profession as a whole. Thus, in assailing the elite for neglecting science, one reformer typically affirmed that "the real distinction, the true respectability of our profession, is its science. It is to us what valour is to the soldier, piety to the priest, chastity to woman. . . . It is our only title to existence as a profession—our only claim to support."[54]

These examples could be multiplied and refined, but it is the general pattern that matters here. By the 1820s the decline-of-science argument had become part of a standardized rhetorical formula deployed in aid of a wide array of professional reforms. It was one part of a larger argument that conformed to a fixed pattern. Typically, the writer asserted that medical science in England was in decline, then identified a source of its low standing and explicated how it kept science down. He next turned to the comparable situation in France and showed how the French system better fostered science. Having established the need for change and pointed to the appropriate model (and usually having affirmed the importance of science to the profession), he then proposed how change after a French blueprint could elevate medical science in England. The argument was often closed by a codicil stating that ultimately the reforms that declinists sought required legislative intervention.

In using the decline argument, reformers were looking for more than institutional change alone. They also claimed for science a fundamentally new importance to the English medical profession, one they sought to sustain by pointing to the value system underlying Parisian medical polity. Certainly the elite physician or surgeon regarded natural science as one part of his domain, but that was not what principally set him apart from lower orders of practitioners. Declinists, on the contrary, reflecting the wider emergence of science as the value system of the English middle classes, placed science at the heart of professional identity. It was in part the chasm separating this image of science as the symbol of professional identity from the reality of professional definition derived from social position that gave the idea of science such promise as a tool in promoting professional change. Unable to advance the profession from within the established system, reformers went outside it to find the nucleus for a new ideology of professional identity in science and in the paradigm of meritocratic French polity, in which command of science established entitlement to preferment.

These reformers spoke about the decline of science and the French solution for several audiences. They saw themselves primarily addressing the masses of the profession, general practitioners whose collective position they hoped to elevate. Through the decline argument they explained to the rank and file the causes of their degradation and identified those to blame. Further, by showing general practitioners the possibility of upward mobility, reformers sought to transform them into an energetic and vocal body standing united under the banner of science. Reformers were speaking as well to a broader audience, especially those in a position to legislate change, and did so in language designed to tap into the power of English chauvinism to motivate action. They were self-consciously playing on what one French surgeon described as "the national pride of the English, which is greater, perhaps, than that of any other civilized nation."[55]

Above all, though, these reformers were speaking to each other and to themselves. Through their oratory they made professional degradation understandable and affirmed that they knew the solution. Their production of rhetoric was itself one form of action; aside from exhibiting their leadership and exercising sometimes deeply felt admiration for French medical ways, it may have provided the reassuring sense of doing something to promote professional redemption. It also gave reformers the satisfaction of denouncing high-placed sinners and exhorting them to repent while declaring as evidence of their own sanctity their allegiance to science.

Enthusiastic praise for French medical ways, not surprisingly, incited resentment from other English practitioners. The very artifacts that French-experienced practitioners held up as emblems of a new and better faith became targets for derision. "I do indeed wish some exposure could be made of the *use* which is made of the Stethoscope," one English critic wrote to a colleague in 1842. "It is the '*conjuring stick*' . . . of a superior order of quacks; and many *honest* men, I believe, attach a confidence to its revelations the truths of which I am quite sure *they* have not the power of ascertaining." He noted that a recent book on the physical signs of disease "speaks of persons 'too stupid, too lazy, or too old' to learn the value & use of the Stethoscope; perhaps I am one of these, but I am sure I am more *clever*; more *industrious*[;] & most young men make it of more value to *them selves* than their *patients*."[56]

So too laudatory representation of Parisian medical science and medical polity by radical reformers provoked a counterrepresentation from English conservatives, who both contested claims about French superiority and lambasted the enthusiasm of those voicing them. More often than not, the socially and institutionally entrenched elite elected not to dwell on the state of English *science* but instead sought to dispel criticism by concentrating on the excellencies of English *practice*. Protesting against "the attempt to excite a *French* feeling here," for example, the editor of the conservative *London Medical Gazette* asserted that in medical knowledge "not merely to be speculated about in the closet, but to be converted to useful practical purposes in the chambers of the sick, the English are immeasurably before their Continental neighbours."[57] A valuation of practice above all else, they asserted, informed the intellectual and institutional structure of English medicine. "It is one advantage arising from the peculiar constitution of the London medical schools, that, with few exceptions, the instructions, which you here receive, have, in a greater or lesser degree, a *tendency* to *practice*," Sir Benjamin C. Brodie, Bart., F.R.S.—a leading target for assaults from radical reformers such as Wakley—told his students at St. George's Hospital in 1838. "I have no doubt that the praises which are bestowed on some of the continental anatomists are well founded," Brodie acknowledged; "but nevertheless, I assert that ours is the better method with a view to the education of those who wish to become, *not mere philosophers, but skilful and useful practitioners.*"[58] So too, "although the medical men of the Continent receive a more elaborate scientific education than those of England, and have a more minute knowledge of morbid anatomy, that is, of disease, as an object of natural history," one conservative wrote in reply to criticisms of London hospital education, "as practitioners, they are mere children, compared with the physicians and surgeons of England."[59]

Conservatives also denounced radicals for recklessly sacrificing English honor by "appealing to French arrangements as the *beau ideal* of every thing that is excellent about medical affairs."[60] They dismissed what one called "the absurd Frenchified system now vigorously attempted to be palmed upon them" and what another stigmatized as the pathological behavior of "Gallomaniacs."[61] Conservative polemics were further animated by the politically resonant anxiety that what was being called for was not reform but revolution. "Some, who hope to gain, and, for obvious reasons, cannot lose by any change, are anxious to follow the example of the French at the period of their revolution," a conservative journal editor charged in 1832, "and would annihilate all existing colleges and corporations—all institutions—all grades—all educational regulations—all those means and appliances which fit men for the practice of a difficult art—all those distinctions which give a rank and a name to medicine as a profession."[62] Conservatives propagated their own, unflattering portrait of Parisian arrangements "to shew the actual working of this much-lauded machinery of the French School."[63] In depicting what was most noteworthy about the Paris School they, like their opponents, dwelled on such emblems of French polity as *concours* but did so to recount their failings and to pronounce them unsuitable to English society.[64]

There was of course a good deal of middle ground between radical reformers who proselytized for the French model as a blueprint for change and the ensconced elite suspicious of all things French as threats to their privileges. What those who sought to elevate the medical profession shared—radical and conservative reformers alike—was the premise that professional uplift chiefly depended on change in medical institutions and governance.[65] "It is no longer disputed that misgovernment, generated and cherished by defective medical laws, is at once the foul and odious source of all the grievances which vex, injure, and harass the profession," a *Lancet* editorial asserted in 1842.[66] The programs the *Lancet* endorsed were the sort that elite London physician Thomas King Chambers no doubt had in mind when, a year earlier, he complained in a private letter to recent Oxford graduate Henry Acland about the reform proposals "daily put forth by persons who are really totally ignorant of the subject however loud and long they may discourse upon it." And yet Chambers concurred with their underlying assumptions about where change had to come from, noting, "I am of [the] opinion that the only mode of reforming our Profession would be to apply the process of reform to all the old institutions."[67] Elevating the medical profession meant reforming professional polity: on that English observers tended to agree, however much they disagreed about what measure of change might be desirable. In such a context, French medical knowledge and technique, whatever their merits, were not so likely as models of French polity to propel professional reform. Reformers, accordingly, gave polity—not epistemology—the lion's share of their attention as they urged Parisian models on the English medical profession.

## AMERICANS AND FRENCH POLITY

The elements of French medical polity that were boldly prominent in English accounts were, by comparison, obscure in the model of French medicine depicted by Americans. While in Paris, American physicians did try to understand the workings of the French system, largely to sort out their own options for study. They in turn recounted what they learned for the benefit of compatriots, and in guidebooks and letters they sketched those features of French polity the foreign student needed to grasp. As medical tourists describing a foreign landscape—as they did when visiting Switzerland, Italy, Austria, or the Netherlands—they also reported on the structure and functioning of French medical institutions, the relationship between practitioners and the state, and the values that characterized the profession. Yet such elements of French polity attracted less of their attention than it did that of their English counterparts, and Americans were much less inclined than the English to tease out the implications for reordering things at home.[68]

Once Americans returned to portray an image of the Paris School with an eye to reform, their attention to French polity dwindled further. While easy to see when viewed in the context of English-American comparison, this relative dearth of attention is difficult to document. All of the major elements of French polity that appear in the English depiction of the Paris School can be found in the collective American depiction. Yet, taken as a whole, in the latter they were featured less prominently, cited less routinely, and urged much less insistently as models for change.

When Americans did assess—not merely describe—French polity, they tended to see it as an unpromising template for professional reform in the United States. This is not to say they did not admire the French system. Some aspects of it Americans envied but recognized as unrealistic examples for a young nation consecrated to democratic ideals. Others they found admirable but irrelevant to professional reform in America. And still others, even those that facilitated the opportunities for study they relished in Paris, Americans judged to be dangerous if not deplorable models for emulation. Even to the most devout American disciples of Parisian medical ways, much of the French system at best was fine for France but irrelevant to American needs and possibilities, and at worst represented oppressive Old World despotism and corruption they were proud the New World had escaped. Skeptical about the viability of Parisian models of medical polity in the sociopolitical climate of America, and ambivalent about their appropriateness to the problems that most disturbed regular physicians, antebellum Americans looked more to other aspects of French medicine in fashioning programs for professional reform.

Much of the explanation for American attitudes' diverging so markedly from those of the English rests in the fact that the specific problems plaguing physicians in each country—problems to which French models might conceivably promise solutions—were not the same. In the United States, even more than in England, the period between the 1810s and the 1850s was marked by a widespread perception of professional degradation. Complaints were legion, but regular physicians voiced particular themes with regularity and ardor. Overcrowding and a decline in educational standards were targeted as leading evils. The proliferation of for-profit medical schools, sometimes with dismal standards, greatly increased the production of regular physicians, leading to competition that further undercut professional solidarity. "Do send me anything you may write about our professional troubles," Alfred Stillé complained in 1844 to George Cheyne Shattuck, Jr., about the growing mob of ill-trained holders of M.D. degrees. "The grand source of them all is the humbug of the 19th century, *Science made easy*."[69] Medical professor Samuel Henry Dickson advised his nephew in 1846 to think well before studying medicine. There was no profession, he cautioned the young man (who chose law instead), "which holds out so little chance of 'success' or advancement and this which was always true is especially so at the present time."[70]

Apprehensions about professional decline were equally informed by changes outside the ranks of regular physicians, changes critical to an understanding of the sociopolitical context in which French models for reform were invoked. What most disturbed regular physicians was the growing prominence and power of organized groups of antiorthodox physicians such as the Thomsonians and, toward midcentury, homeopaths. These practitioners attacked the practices of regular physicians and competed with them for paying patients. Their vocal disparagement of the orthodox profession, and the receptive audiences they found among the American people, signaled the regular profession's degradation.

Starting in the 1820s and continuing through the Civil War, the medical profession came under aggressive popular attack. The challenge grew partly from the earlier republican critique of professional aristocracy that had its roots in the American Enlightenment, expressed in the programs of Thomas Jefferson and Benjamin Rush for the simplification and dissemination of medical knowledge. But criticism of the professions, including medicine, came to be infused with new political urgency. The rising democratic impulse was evident in the ascendancy of the Jacksonians and their campaign against special privilege and chartered corporations. Characterized by a romantic longing for the values of an earlier, simpler American way of life, the Jacksonians targeted privileged groups, aristocracy, paper money, and monopolies as signs of growing corruption in society. The skepticism of claims to special knowledge and authority conferred by formal education that Alexis de Tocqueville observed when he visited the United States in 1831 informed a growing popular indictment of what botanical physician Wooster Beach typically denounced as "King-craft, Priest-craft, Lawyer-craft, and Doctor-craft."[71]

The assault on orthodox medicine was expressed most forcefully, especially by adherents of the Thomsonian system of botanical healing, in the campaign against professional monopoly. "The medical monopoly deserves to be abolished," insisted one botanic practitioner in 1841. "The law which deprives one class of men of their rights and gives special privileges to another, is not just. It violates the first principles of democracy."[72] Echoing the theme of liberation that pervaded the rhetoric of democratic politicians, antiorthodox reformers called for emancipation of the American people from established medicine. "There is not a greater aristocratic monopoly in existence, than this of regular medicine—neither is there a greater humbug," one reformer charged. "False and dangerous must be that science which exists—not from any truth or utility in itself, but from legislative enactments, cunning, and deception, which strictly speaking *enslave the people* to it and its votaries."[73]

What has been too little emphasized about the rhetoric of the Thomsonians and like-minded radical medical critics such as hydropaths is the extent to which it was based upon a caricature of the regular profession.[74] Far from enjoying a monopoly, de facto or de jure, regular physicians functioned within a remarkably open medical marketplace. In representing the regular profession as a bastion of monopoly in American society, critics were using prevalent polemical conventions to construct a straw villain that was easy to attack rather than depicting social reality. Their assault on medical monopoly is best regarded as a symbolic crusade. It was an outlet for antiauthoritarian sentiment; but the authority being assailed derived not from a legal monopoly so much as from claims to the exclusive possession of special knowledge.

This assault was most dramatically expressed in the campaign against medical licensing. Starting in the 1830s, the Thomsonians and their Jacksonian allies led a drive in state legislatures for the repeal of licensing laws. Deploying the antimonopoly rhetoric of free trade and egalitarianism, they persuaded legislatures to virtually abolish legal regulation of medical practice. By midcentury only a few traces of a licensing system remained, and, as historian Matthew Ramsey has concluded on the basis of a transnational study, "the American medical field was the freest in the Western world."[75]

The licensing laws that existed before repeal provided chiefly an honorific distinction. Penalties for unlicensed practice, even when enforced, were often trivial—as in loss of the right to sue in court for uncollected fees. The highly successful battle against licensing could not do away with medical monopoly in America, for there was none to be abolished; instead, it helped undermine the idea that specialized professional knowledge should constitute a valid source of distinction in America society.[76]

The assault upon the regular profession was an attack on professional mystery, the possession of secret knowledge concealed from or unknowable to ordinary citizens, and on all claims to authority by merit of its possession. Samuel Thomson typically asserted, in the preface of his *New Guide to Health*, that while other realms of knowledge such as religion and politics "are brought where 'common people' can understand them; the knowledge and use of medicine, is in a great measure concealed in a dead language, and a sick man is often obliged to risk his life, where he would not risk a dollar."[77] Insisting that "the spirit of the medical profession must be revolutionized, to be in harmony with the spirit of the times," reformers called upon doctors to abandon "their Latin Diplomas and antique technicalities."[78] Physicians' use of Latin was assailed as a symbol of their attempt to keep the language of medicine inaccessible, a tendency expressed more profoundly in their needlessly intricate theorizing about the body in health and sickness. The mystification of medicine, like the claim that regular physicians had privileged access to knowledge of anatomy, physiology, and pathology, was illegitimate, and any prestige held by merit of it should be taken back by the people.

Such assaults grew from cultural and political commitments most boldly articulated in the radically democratic ideology of the Jacksonians, but resonated with convictions about the proper relationships among knowledge, authority, and deference that were widely held in American society. Within such a climate, the example of French medical polity as model for reform could hardly be seen as very promising. Calls for legislated change that would protect the regular profession in recognition of its possession of special knowledge, for example, or that would encourage privileged access to the education that defined a regularly trained physician, were not only unlikely to garner popular support but almost certain to act as lightning rods attracting condemnation. For regular physicians newly returned from study in Paris and impressed by what they had witnessed there, leading characteristics of French medical polity that seemed admirable and desirable also seemed patently unrealistic guides for reform in America.

Paris-returned Americans recognized that the vigor of medical science and the standing of the medical profession in France grew in large measure from state support, encouragement, and protection. "Medicine is not cultivated any where in the world so thoroughly as a science as in the great European capitals and the facilities of their immense hospitals afford the most extensive means of perfection in all departments of medicine and surgery," Cornelius Comegys, preparing to depart to Paris, explained in 1850 to a friend. "All this arises from the fostering care of their governments who not only richly endow their schools but numerate their distinguished teachers."[79]

Americans often returned from Paris convinced that the lack of government involvement in medical affairs of their own country was one source of professional degradation. "If the government of the United States were to pay the same attention to the encouragement of medical science as in France, where it has been placed under the particular direction and patronage of governments it would be immensely improved," a Philadelphia medical student, plainly mirroring the views of his teachers, wrote in his 1820 M.D. thesis.[80] State "encouragement of medical science" sometimes meant legal provisions for human dissection, or the modest financial support that some state legislatures did provide to medical schools, but often it was a euphemism for legal protection of regular physicians from alternative practitioners. "So long as the laws of the country suffer quacks and charlatans of every description to live in a state of piracy against the world," one physician wrote from Paris in 1847, "it cannot be expected, that American physicians will devote their energies to such an extent, as to rival the French in their attainments, who are not protected merely, but spurred on, and animated, by the 'powers that be.'"[81]

Regular physicians making the case for professional reform, however, generally were hesitant about pointing to the relationship between the medical profession and the state in France with any expectation that this example would be of much service in America. This was abundantly clear in the case of licensing. While calls for the reinstatement of licensing laws were heard from regular physicians after repeal,[82] the French model was remarkably little invoked in appeals for government protection of the profession.

Underlying this reticence was a recognition not only that such demands were unlikely to be met but also that they would incite popular ire. Licensing laws and calls for their reinstatement, one regular physician in Chicago noted, "put it in the power of quacks to raise a cry of persecution and represent the profession as greedy monopolists, and thus excite some feeling in their favor among weak and credulous people."[83] And such fears were well grounded. In 1847, for example, the editor of an antiorthodox medical journal depicted the founding of the American Medical Association as a reactionary move "designed to give the profession in America some portion of that power of which they have been stripped by the democratic spirit of the country" through such means as the annulment of "tyrannical medical laws." Decrying "the great Sanhedrim of the profession," he denounced its program as "relics of the corrupt and aristocratic organization of society in Europe." Making the opposition between European and American polity unmistakable, he went on to conclude that "the spirit of American liberty is at work in this country upon all the ancient notions and usages imported from Europe by our fathers, and moulding our national character—our social arrangements, opinions and sentiments, into more perfect accordance with the great principles of liberty and justice."[84]

To a remarkable extent, regular leaders accepted that restrictive statutes on medical practice were out of keeping with the prevailing tenor of American society. "Laws regulating medical education, & restraining the practice of medicine, never have been enforced, (except vexatiously upon a few individuals,) in our country," a New Haven physician wrote in 1846 to a colleague in Albany, "& they never can be enforced."[85] Indeed, two years earlier a committee of the Albany County Medical Society had cautioned that agitation for restrictive laws on medical practice was politically dangerous, noting further that it would be "utterly impossible to enforce them so long as they are not in accordance with public sentiment." The committee, headed by Thomas Hun, who had recently returned from six years in Paris, concluded that "quackery must be suppressed not by legislation, but by enlightening the public as to its dangers. The dignity and respectability of our profession is to be promoted not by asking for legal privileges, but by an increase of individual zeal and a more cordial coöperation."[86]

Much the same reserve characterized the use made of French models in calls for the state to elevate standards of American medical education. Orthodox reformers widely maintained that without legal discriminations between regularly educated physicians and their competitors, it was unrealistic to envision dramatic improvements in requirements for an M.D. degree. "As long as Legislatures declare every man a 'Doctor' who sets up a sign with his name on [it]," Robert Peter complained to Elisha Bartlett, "what chance is there for lengthening courses and rendering more stringent the regulations of Med. schools?"[87] However, many regulars believed that an open system accommodating wide variation in the educational acquirements of regular physicians—not a uniform and strictly regulated plan—was best suited to American society and geography alike.[88] American circumstances, one regular reformer asserted, made European models "wholly inoperative or impracticable, in relation to the profession in this country."[89] As Joseph Pancoast, a Philadelphia medical professor recently returned from Paris, told his students in 1856, "However excellent the European system of medical instruction may be for their own students and their own people, the general methods pursued by the best appointed medical institutions of this land are, under all the peculiar circumstances of the country, the best devised that we could adopt."[90]

Other means by which the French state supported medical study, such as laws for the provision of cadavers, were also little cited in American compared with English programs for reform. Like the English, Americans envied the supply of anatomical material that government policies lavished on Parisian teachers and students. The ease of anatomizing in Paris remained among the leading lures attracting American physicians to the French capital, while the pathoanatomical orientation of French medical knowledge and investigation made Americans who had returned home anxious to gain increasing access to bodies for dissection experience, surgical practice, and postmortem examinations. And the demand for cadavers for medical instruction certainly mounted over the antebellum decades.[91] Many regular physicians railed—as one visiting Paris did in 1850—against "the short-sightedness and ignorance of two-thirds of those composing our State legislatures, that no legal provisions, of a generous character, have been devised for aiding or facilitating practical anatomy."[92] Yet, unlike English reformers, who demanded change at home by self-righteously pointing to the French government's encouragement of anatomizing, Americans seemed reluctant to use the French model in making a strong case for legal reforms.

Popular prejudice against desecrating bodies of the dead was one check, as it was on English reformers. But it was also the democratic political sensibilities of the American public that made demands for the legal provision of cadavers for medical study odious. Calling for legislated provision of bodies to American medical schools would be asking the state to assure the privileged access of physicians to precisely the kind of exclusive, private knowledge that was used to set the orthodox brotherhood apart from other healers and to assure the preservation of professional mystery by encouraging the profession's cultivation of esoteric learning inaccessible to the common man and woman. To cite Old World precedent in demanding legislation placing cadavers in the hands of regular physicians would have flown in the face of the same popular sentiment that had demolished licensing laws.

Another reason why French arrangements were cited less often and less boldly by American than by English reformers is that invidious comparisons with French cultural achievement simply did not have the same polemical force in America as in England. English reformers could point to French superiority in anatomical science, and to the throngs of English students crossing the Channel for anatomical study, confident that such claims would be humiliating. In America, on the other hand, there was not the same expectation of cultural parity with France, much less superiority—only the pervading faith that in due course, the New World would outstrip the Old.

Similar patterns are evident in American and English readiness to invoke the value system that in France ordered institutional arrangements and professional rewards. French meritocracy, for example, embodied in the use of *concours* to determine professional appointments, was a persistent refrain in the demands of English reformers. Yet, again, it was a French medical model that American reformers only occasionally urged, and then almost always with ample qualification. American physicians admired what they, like the English, saw as a meritocratic ethos in the Paris School. Moreover, they saw it as being very much in harmony with the temperament of their own society. Yet they regarded it with ambivalence—as a model that promised little utility in their own programs for reform and that, indelicately used, could actually reinforce existing professional ills.

Nowhere was American admiration for French meritocracy and its workings in the Parisian medical world clearer than in the collective story they told about how certain leading figures in the Paris School had lifted themselves up from poverty to professional eminence. Most often Armand Velpeau or Guillaume Dupuytren were cited, but sometimes it was Jean Civiale, Jacques Lisfranc, or others, almost always surgeons. It was a narrative endlessly repeated in the diaries and letters of American physicians in Paris, in the accounts of the Paris School they composed for American periodicals, and in the guidebooks they wrote for Paris-bound students. The tale of their careers, as Americans told it, though drawing its elementary plot from real life, was so stylized in its recounting and so didactic in its moral lessons that it took on all the proportions of a professional fable about Paris medicine.

"Velpeau," John Young Bassett put the story line tersely in an 1836 letter from Paris to his wife, "from a poor boy without money, time, education, or friends, has by industry made himself one of the first surgeons of Europe."[93] Joynes, on the other hand, filled pages of his Paris diary in 1840 with a detailed narrative making the same point. The young Velpeau, Joynes related, crushed his forefinger while laboring with his father, a poor but respected blacksmith, and, while convalescing, "with great assiduosity spent his time reading all the works on medicine in the Tours public library" ("particularly all that had any relation to the subject of his disabled finger"). A physician to the local hospital recognized Velpeau's ardor for medicine and took up a collection from neighbors to enable the young man to travel to Paris, where he "worked incessantly at the profession" and, "with zeal & determination," thrived. To underscore the latter point, Joynes closed his diary entry by writing, "His income is about 30,000 francs."[94]

Velpeau's story resonated with deeply held American myths, showing how "one who, without family, without education, without means, and with nothing but his own native intellectual vigor and superiority to depend upon, can emerge from the cloud by which he is surrounded, and soar through regions of ineffable brightness, a shining mark, to guide and control his high-born, rich and college-bred brethren."[95] Though a French surgeon, his biography was that of an archetypal American hero, scripted like the life stories of contemporaries ranging from Andrew Jackson to Samuel Thomson. This was not the Horatio Alger story of postbellum America, in which good luck and charm drove the rise from rags to respectability, but an earlier American success myth in which industry, character, and self-discipline alone brought elevation.[96] "Twenty years ago, Velpeau came to Paris without a profession, without money, and without friends—a poor boy from one of the provinces," Moses Linton summed up in a letter from Paris in 1840. "A laudable ambition and untiring industry has made him what he is—a towering monument to the often repeated, but seldom appreciated adage, 'labor vincit omnia.'"[97]

No less than other fables, the Velpeau story was meant to teach a moral lesson, which Linton neatly encapsulated. Americans spelled out that lesson clearly and threaded the life stories of other Paris clinicians into essentially the same narrative. F. Campbell Stewart, for example, related how Velpeau, Dupuytren, and other eminent surgeons had "arisen from the lowest estates of life, and many from the uttermost depths of poverty," exemplars, he urged, "which go to prove that it is only necessary to use proper exertion and attention to ensure success, even under the most disadvantageous circumstances."[98] So too New York professor of surgery Valentine Mott, in his 1842 Paris memoirs, offered the surgeon Lisfranc as "another example of a self-made man, illustrative of what genius, and effort, and industry may accomplish when fostered by the liberal encouragement, free competition, and almost gratuitous instruction everywhere dispensed by the judicious arrangements of the schools of this capital."[99]

As Mott's remarks suggest, though, while this professional fable about self-made men bore a message that had powerful resonances in antebellum American culture, it equally taught a moral lesson about French medical polity, especially *concours*. It was *concours* and the meritocratic ethos that informed it that made these life histories possible. As Stewart stated it plainly, Velpeau and the others, "without friends or interest, would never but for the Concours, have been able to work their way to the high positions which they now occupy."[100]

Though not blind to its abuses, Americans admired *concours* as an institution that, as Gardner put it, "makes talent, not influence, the necessary requisite for promotion."[101] The French system of conferring professional rewards through *concours* embodied meritocratic ideals that were at the core of the American self-image, ideals largely shared by regular professional leaders and their Jacksonian critics alike.

Some Americans visiting Paris did urge *concours* as more fair than "our boasted republican system" in the making of hospital appointments.[102] Gardner, citing recent appointments at the New York Almshouse, complained that "a large proportion of the hospital medical officers of the United States are indebted for their situations to rich relations, or powerful friends, and not to their genius," and urged that "a far better system prevails in France, where situations of this description are open to the struggles of all."[103] And some institutions, such as the Medical College of the State of South Carolina, took up the language of *concours* in making faculty appointments.[104] Trying in 1839 to recruit Shattuck to a vacancy in pathological anatomy, a member of its faculty wrote that "in the new faculty we retain the old organization of an extended course of instruction, vacancies in the professors to be filled by concours & in fine the whole establishment [torn: to be placed on a] most liberal footing."[105]

Yet despite American admiration, and in sharp contrast to its vigorous deployment as a model in English programs for professional change, *concours* never became a very prominent feature in American calls for medical reform. The success of *concours* as it functioned in France depended upon government control of medical schools and hospitals and a putatively detached tribunal, operating by law in a public forum, to objectively gauge the merit of candidates for clinical or teaching posts. Many Americans would have had to agree with Chandler B. Chapman, who wrote from Paris in 1851 that "the system of concours, after all its real value here, would be by no means adapted to . . . the United States, from the fact that our institutions have received no government aid and care."[106]

More than this, regular physicians were uneasy with the image of placing medical appointments under the control of American government, ruled by public opinion. They endorsed the proposition that professional rewards and appointments should be made according to merit; the problem was just how and by whom would merit be appraised? Many of the regular profession's ills, after all, were attributed to a misguided public unable to distinguish between the virtues of true physicians and the false claims of quacks. Some regular leaders who admired *concours* even dismissed the French model by asserting that an analogous system was in place in American institutions. "We have already, virtually, such a system, more effective and satisfactory in its operation than would be a closer imitation of the method pursued in France," Austin Flint suggested in 1854.[107] In America, he went on, through healthy competition among medical schools for paying students, the market provided a natural *concours*. What he did not need to spell out was that in these regular medical schools, decisions about merit were firmly controlled by regular physicians. A system of *concours* modeled after the French plan meant placing such decisions ultimately in legislative hands, the very same legislatures that were repealing licensing acts and increasingly granting legal charters to homeopathic and Eclectic medical schools. In the eyes of regular reformers, while *concours* offered an appealing image of meritocracy, it presented a disturbing specter of the tyranny of American public opinion.

If observers generally were agreed in their admiration for the putative meritocracy of French medicine, however, they found other aspects of the value system that ordered the workings of the Paris School more troubling. This was especially true of prevailing attitudes toward hospital patients, and toward the expectations of patients themselves. Americans reveled in the free access to the body that clinicians and students enjoyed at the French bedside, but were disturbed by what they judged to be a pervasive objectification of the sick. Ambivalence toward the French system in this instance shifted uneasily between envy and disgust.

Americans in Paris never doubted that free access to the bodies of the sick grew not merely from formalized government polities but also from wider, distinctly French sensibilities. The assumption that the sick were hospitalized partly as a source of medical knowledge and instruction was fundamental to the organization of Parisian institutions. "Here in Paris every thing in the hospital line is new to an American," Montrose A. Pallen wrote home to St. Louis in 1857; "for the benefit of the student all are infinitely superior to those of the United States, but for the patients far otherwise."[108]

Pallen's last point, one other observers commonly made, troubled many American visitors, as did the extent to which patients were made objects for instruction, which Pallen professed left him "shocked."[109] Americans who compared hospital patients in France with those in the United States found satisfaction in "the difference in their respective sensibilities," proud that even the poorest Americans would not tolerate degradations they believed French patients endured as a matter of course.[110] Chapter 8 will explore the ways American physicians found the treatment of patients witnessed in Parisian wards both disturbing and threatening; as one American wrote from Paris, "Verily, there might be an 'Uncle Tom's Cabin' written on this and other conditions."[111] Given such attitudes, the value system that encouraged easy access to French bodies—despite its evident benefits for teaching and research—was plainly not an example reformers were likely to use in promoting change in the United States. Instead of embracing this model of French medical polity they in large measure shunned it, reaffirming their own instead.

Going abroad taught Americans about what they valued at home. They returned with admiration and sometimes gnawing envy for much of what they had witnessed in France. Equally, though, they often returned with a reinforced and newly clarified faith in the superiority of American polity (in more than medicine alone) to that of the Old World. Paradoxically, yet reflecting an experience travelers often share, their voyage left them both dissatisfied with the state of things at home and confident that American arrangements were vastly preferable to what they had seen abroad.

"In my opinion, there can be no better lesson of patriotism than a year's residence in Paris," Joynes wrote home in 1841. "The American of common sense & correct principles who observes with attention the character of the people (I say nothing of *politics*) *must* return loving his country more than ever, and blessing his stars that he was born an American."[112] Such nationalistic pride was a common theme in the writings of American physicians in France, as in an 1833 letter from William Crawford to his sister asserting that "the advocates of oppression who have sneered at the government of the U.S. as an ideal dream, a bubble about to burst, [will] see that it is a reality and be made to tremble for their own situation."[113] What they celebrated most was the promise of the new nation and its freedom from the restraints that ordered life in the Old World. "America is not cumbered with massive equipage," one American wrote in his Paris diary in 1838; "we are light."[114]

Most became more critical of American affairs—political and medical—after returning home. Perhaps the most pervasive complaint about American medical polity by physicians who had observed the French system was that it forestalled excellence. Like novelist James Fenimore Cooper, some few physicians returned to decry the tyranny of public opinion in America and the leveling effects of unrestrained democracy. Stillé was among those who over time fell prey to antiegalitarian bitterness. "A higher aim in professional culture," he wrote to Shattuck in 1857, "is improbable, perhaps impossible, under a political system which recognizes no virtue or worth in any knowledge beyond what every mechanic's or tradesman's son may obtain in the common schools." Deploring what he called "the democratizing tendencies of our political system," Stillé wrote that "I cannot find much ground of hope for a higher standard of professional education than we now have so long as popular sovereignty is recognized as the central doctrine of our political faith."[115]

Yet the measure of Stillé's gloom was unusual. Overwhelmingly, American physicians discovered in Europe a pride and faith in the fundamental tenets of the American system. "There was a time when I began to fear that we had too much republicanism in our own country," Robert Peter wrote to his wife from Europe in 1839. But "I am more and more satisfied with our country—our own institutions and our people.—We are outstripping the Europeans in every thing that we take in hand in earnest."[116] Even Jackson, Jr., ardent disciple of the Paris School that he was, came while in France to see the freedom of American life from government interference as cause for pride. The American in Europe "becomes necessarily interested in the different public questions wh. constantly arise, in the state of the society he sees about him, the happiness or misery of the people etc.," he told his father. "It is thus that I rejoice to reflect that I am born in a country where the word Government is hardly known and never felt in the sense wh. the inhabitants of this hemisphere are obliged to feel it." As Jackson concluded, "When I reflect upon all these things wh. I daily see around me, I rejoice, I say, that I am an American."[117]

English medical reformers, many of them at least, selectively used the example of French medical polity to call for radical reform, if not revolution, in the social order of English medicine. By and large, however, American physicians returned from France to embrace the structure of American society and the place accorded the professions within it. Most tended to be confident that despite its many evils, the American order of things was preferable to what they had seen in the Old World and should not be overturned. Throughout their careers, many continued to bemoan the shortfalls of their own medical system but championed programs of reform that were in keeping with the main currents of American society rather than at odds with them. French medical polity, however much Americans admired or envied certain of its elements, was as a model for professional reform judged to be unpromising, undesirable, and un-American.

### AMERICAN USE OF FRENCH INSTITUTIONAL MODELS

Despite the reluctance of the Americans, compared with the English, to call upon models of French medical polity in promoting professional reform, French patterns did enter in important ways into the reorganization of antebellum American medical institutions. Disciples of the Paris School often pointed explicitly to the French example in urging such changes. However, the avowed aim was not to directly alter the social structure of the profession or its place in society, but to reform medical knowledge and its cultivation. French models of medical polity, that is, were selectively used to reshape the American institutions in which French notions of medical teaching and investigation—and the empiricist ideals they served—could be pursued.

Sometimes the plan to transplant French institutions into American soil was direct, as in the endeavor of Pierre Louis's Boston pupils to re-create his Société Médicale d'Observation in 1835 as the Boston Society for Medical Observation.[118] Other societies, such as the Baltimore Pathological Society and the Pathological Society of Philadelphia, though less explicit in their Parisian provenance, were also institutional forums for cultivating the French program. They provided a platform for reporting clinical and pathological observations and a stimulus for members to keep records.[119] This is not to say that they were always a success. "The Pathological Soc. of which such grant [grand] things were hoped, is thoroughly defunct," Stillé complained from Philadelphia in 1844, noting that "it is very odd that with all the ability amongst the members of our profession here there should be so little of that feeling which shows itself in medical association for scientific progress."[120] Even county and state medical societies, which historians ordinarily have dismissed as mere political associations designed to advance the socioeconomic interests of their members, sometimes promoted serious investigations of the relationships among local environment, disease, and treatment that were animated at least in part by the Parisian imperative to reconstruct medical knowledge through the direct observation and analysis of nature.[121]

It was by changing American patterns of teaching medicine, though, that reformers used French organizational models to the greatest effect. As Paris-experienced Americans returned to become professors, they changed the content of what was taught at American medical schools more than the structure of those institutions. Given legislative and social realities, aspirations to reproduce the French educational system would have been patently unrealistic, and Americans were reticent in using the French example to call for legal changes that might nudge things in that direction. Still, emulation of a French program was evident when in 1836 the faculty of the Medical College of Louisiana created a Chair of Special Pathological Anatomy and Clinical Practice, "it being made the duty of this chair to institute autopsies of all cases that die under his charge during the course,"[122] and when in 1842 the faculty of the Medical College of Ohio asked trustees to "let a distinct Professorship be erected to be entitled the Chair of Physical Diagnosis and Pathological Anatomy" and to "let the incumbent of such chair attend every morning at 8 o'clock at the Hospital to teach a limited number of students not exceeding ten in number at any one time auscultation and Percussion."[123]

Structural changes were most dramatically expressed in efforts to shift the locus of instruction from the lecture hall to the clinic. The limited access to clinical experience throughout the antebellum period has been stressed in chapter 1, while the fitful emergence of organized clinical instruction and growing ties between medical schools and hospitals, especially in the decades after the Civil War, have been traced by several historians, especially Charles Rosenberg and Dale Smith.[124] What matters here is the extent to which the antebellum move to give medical students practical clinical training was self-consciously cast in a French tradition.

Some students were able to study in American hospitals long before the influence of the Paris School was strongly felt in the United States. Often that experience was informal and arrangements ad hoc. "I have paved the way to combine the speculations of authors with the experience of practitioners," a medical student in Philadelphia wrote in 1805 to his preceptor in Savannah, "by cultivating an acquaintance with the officers of the two great medical institutions of this city—viz—the Hospital & the Alms-House."[125] And at some medical schools such as Harvard, which drew on the Massachusetts General Hospital after that institution opened in 1821, "students attending the lectures are admitted gratuitously to the surgical operations & clinical practice of the Hospital," one physician advising a relative on how best to pursue medical study wrote in 1824.[126] Most physicians and pupils alike, however, assumed that students would acquire practical training in apprenticeship, at the domestic bedside of their preceptors' patients.

During the second quarter of the century, however, there was mounting insistence that much of medical education and investigation could be conducted properly only in a hospital. Two hallmarks of Parisian praxis—the stethoscope and postmortem examination—fueled this conviction. Americans encouraged the use of the new instrument in ways ranging from donating a manual on the stethoscope to a local medical society, as Abel L. Peirson did in Essex, Massachusetts, in 1829, to teaching by example in an effort to see its use "Americanized," as Jackson, Jr., put it in 1832.[127] Yet most agreed with Philadelphia professor Samuel Jackson, who noted in 1827 that use of the stethoscope "tis only to be learned in Hospital practice, for in private practice the cases are scattered & we have few opportunities for post mortem examinations."[128] The stethoscope made it difficult for ambitious students to rely on apprenticeship alone, for it became all but impossible in that context to fully acquire Parisian techniques of physical examination, much less clinical investigation.

Teaching students the meaning of signs elicited by physical examination at the bedside by displaying their underlying lesions was another essential element of the French plan of instruction. Many Americans returned eager to employ systematic autopsy as a research tool, and more than one began notebooks in Paris that they subsequently filled with observations made in American hospitals.[129] Paris-returned professors urged the need for postmortem examinations and students took up this lesson, as when a Charleston student wrote in his 1839 M.D. thesis that "the French, have arrived at greater precision in diagnosis and pathology than any other nation, and this is owing to attention to post mortem."[130] Sometimes autopsies were possible in private practice, perhaps more frequently in the South where the bodies of slaves were particularly vulnerable. But even there, it was seldom an easy matter. "I applied at Mr. Haxall Taylor, etc for help in an autopsy," Gooch wrote in his diary a few months after his return from Paris. "Dr. Rives very courageously agreed to help me and after much humbug to find Mr. Cagbill, who was the agent for Mr. Walker the master of the slave Henri and whom I found at the church. About noon, we began the autopsy and at 3 we had finished." Kentuckian Ludsford P. Yandell found his course easier when, in 1826, he was able to record in his diary the "Post-Mortem Examination of a servant Boy belonging to my Father."[131] William M. Boling wrote to Bartlett in 1847 that he was trying to make good use of postmortem examinations in his study of remittent fever in the vicinity of Montgomery, Alabama, and other physicians had promised, "should opportunities present, that I should have the examination of their subjects." Yet he recognized "the difference in the opportunities of private practitioners and Hospital physicians," and had to conclude that his cases were so few "that my notes as yet are of little value."[132]

Over the course of the antebellum period, medical teachers increasingly won the privilege of bringing students into hospitals for clinical teaching and, to a much lesser extent, to perform autopsies. This was a highly checkered process, however, and while faculty members traded on their symbiotic relationship to hospitals—in which their medical services were exchanged for a teaching forum—they seldom gained the full measure of access they wanted. Lay trustees often denied faculty requests to autopsy all bodies not claimed within a day or so after death, just as they routinely protected patients and their own authority by limiting student access to the wards. In 1857, for example, the Board of Guardians curtailed clinical teaching at the Pennsylvania Hospital in

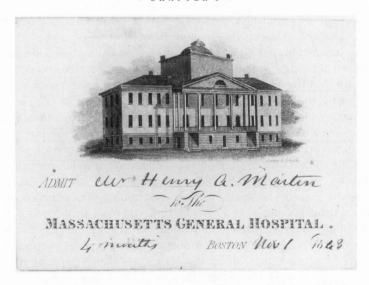

Fig. 6.2. Ticket admitting Henry Austin Martin to clinical study at the Massachusetts General Hospital in Boston in 1843, two years before Martin would receive his M.D. degree from Harvard. Although calls informed by the French example for student access to hospital experience grew increasingly strident, hospital instruction remained limited in antebellum America. (Courtesy of Francis A. Countway Library of Medicine, Boston.)

a kind of move that was repeated throughout the country. "The medical board, minus I suppose the chief resident, assumed and exercised the right of bringing what patients they saw fit before the class," an Ontario medical student in Philadelphia reported home, "which so shocked the Guardians, fearing that some dreadful exposures would be made improperly; and piqued them that their authority should thus be trampled upon, that at their last meeting they passed a resolution abolishing the clinic."[133]

Especially early on, then, Americans who returned from Paris eager to introduce elements of French clinical teaching found themselves up against formidable obstacles. American hospitals were tiny compared with their Parisian counterparts and were not under centralized government control. Trustees, often willing to admit small groups of students under the supervision of a medical officer-teacher, certainly would have balked at the idea of the crowds of sometimes two hundred pupils at a time who followed the great Parisian professors. Older faculty members often remained convinced that the practical experience most students needed could be adequately acquired in apprenticeship, and, given the growing competition among medical schools for pupils, were reluctant to increase formal work required for the M.D. degree. Even if hospital training might be desirable, requiring it might drive students into the lecture halls of less demanding competitors.

It was partly for these reasons that as Americans returned from Paris, the clinical instruction they offered tended to be in private courses and in non-degree-granting schools.[134] Such small, optional courses circumvented many of the forces that worked against adding requirements to the curriculum. In opting for this format, however, instructors were not merely conceding to the constraints of the American context. They were also following the model of clinical teaching that they themselves had most valued in Paris, namely, private courses taught outside the official curriculum to a small group of students for a fee.

After Gerhard returned to Philadelphia in 1833, for example, he began to offer private clinical courses that focused on diseases of the chest, stressing the use of the stethoscope in physical examination and the use of autopsy in disclosing internal lesions. Thus in 1837 Josiah Clark Nott, just returned from Paris, advised a medical student headed for Philadelphia to "follow Gerhard *unremittingly* in his Hospital, his clinique is good." Nott cautioned that, "you will see I think much to object to in Gerhard's practice—but he is a profound pathologist and you should not permit any '*mauvaise honte*' or false delicacy to prevent you from assisting in *every* post mortem examination that he makes."[135] Although Gerhard's stature increased over time and his hospital affiliations became more secure, he continued to offer such clinical instruction over the next couple of decades. "Gerhard who is the present attending Physician at the Hospital, gives good clinics," one student wrote home from Philadelphia in 1856. "He is very fluent and quite humorous," and "is allowed to be the best auscultator in Philadelphia," although the student added that the fee for the class on practical auscultation was "respectably large."[136] In many respects, the student could just as well have been writing from Paris rather than Philadelphia. The private clinical course was a French transplant well suited to the American voluntary system of medical education. Ambitious students typically combined such clinical courses with the regular course of lectures and other optional courses on fields such as practical anatomy.

By the 1840s, though, the faculties of many American medical schools recognized that just as clinical instruction was drawing a steady stream of students across the Atlantic to Paris, so it might give their schools a competitive edge within the American marketplace. The French origin of the educational model they took up—or at least the luster of the Parisian image—was unmistakable in their use of the term *clinique* as the most common way of denoting such programs of instruction. As one later observer commented, American medical schools had succumbed to a "clinique epidemic."[137]

The faculties of small-town schools, threatened by this movement, tried to refute the advantages claimed for clinical instruction that gave city schools the upper hand. In 1848 Robert Peter, having just mailed circulars advertising the medical department at Transylvania, told a colleague that they could be optimistic about the school's prospects in the coming year. Two years earlier he had observed that some clinical teaching had been instituted at the Lunatic

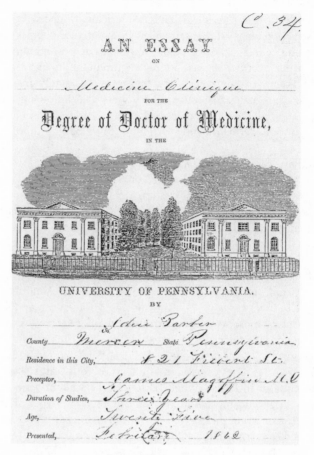

AN ESSAY

ON

*Medecine Clinique*

FOR THE

Degree of Doctor of Medicine,

IN THE

UNIVERSITY OF PENNSYLVANIA.

BY

*John Parker*

County *Mercer* State *Pennsylvania*

Residence in this City, *821 Filbert St.*

Preceptor, *James Magoffin M.D.*

Duration of Studies, *Three Years*

Age, *Twenty Five*

Presented, *February 1862*

Fig. 6.3. M.D. thesis submitted at the University of Pennsylvania in 1862. The student's choice of a title—"Medecine Clinique"—reflected the strong identification American physicians made between hospital instruction and the French medical tradition. (Courtesy of Department of Special Collections, Van Pelt–Dietrich Library Center, University of Pennsylvania, Philadelphia.)

Asylum, noting that "it is a better *clinique* than the Marine Hospital of Louis[ville]," Transylvania's leading rival.[138] Yet, well aware that his school, in the small town of Lexington, could boast no large hospital, Peter complained bitterly about the prevailing vogue of *cliniques*. "It is the fashion now," he wrote, "to *talk* much about *cliniques*, and many a farce is enacted in that relation, very interesting and *attractive* to the *young* students." He suggested that "it will be fashionable for a time with the mass of physicians in the great West to talk of Hospitals &c &c as the great desiderata to students, and to depreciate the good and wholesome clinical instruction of the private practitioner to his pupils." As he concluded derisively, "The one requires the centralization of a crowd from distant points around the beds of the pauper inmates of the infirmaries of the large cities—the other exhibits every day practice in the sphere of the future operations of the pupils."[139] Even at the time Peter wrote, however, such arguments coming from proprietors of small-town schools looked to many like special pleading and over time seemed increasingly disingenuous.

Yet while the *cliniques* boasted by American schools drew on the prestige the French model of clinical instruction was acquiring in America, they did not necessarily incorporate much of its substance. The actual experience designated by the term *clinique* varied enormously. Most often, a medical school *clinique* meant practical teaching at a dispensary set up for the treatment of poor outpatients and the instruction of students, not teaching in the wards of an inpatient hospital. The student's opportunities to trace the full history of a case, much less witness an autopsy, were quite restricted. Even when a hospital was the venue for a school's *clinique*, often the site of instruction was not the bedside but an amphitheater in which patients were exhibited.[140] "Within a few years the practice has been adopted by most of our medical schools of examining and prescribing before classes for such poor patients as may choose to present themselves for that purpose, the professor making such practical remarks as the circumstances of the cases may suggest," the editor of the *Buffalo Medical Journal and Monthly Review* observed in an 1847 article titled "Cliniques." "This, which is not strictly speaking clinical instruction, is commonly known by the term prefixed to this article, a gallicism which, as it also signifies bedside teaching, is equally incorrect. As the name has passed into general acceptation we will not object to it, although we should have preferred one philologically more correct, and supplied from our own vernacular. The more homely expression, *Dispensary instruction* would please us better." Noting that this system "has long been virtually in vogue," he observed critically that "some appear to regard it as an adequate substitute for true clinical or Hospital instruction," but concluded that "to render the system of practical instruction complete, it is obvious that *cliniques*, and hospital attendance, are both required."[141]

As this editor's remarks suggest, by the late 1840s widespread criticism was being leveled against attempts to capitalize on the image conjured up by the term *clinique* and, by renaming dispensary work, to draw upon the cultural bounty that French clinical training conferred. These American teachers were marketing the illusion of French clinical training with little of its content. Writing in 1855, a Tennessee physician cautioned students against being taken in by deceptive language in selecting a medical school. A proper school, he advised, "should possess the advantages of a well-arranged *Hospital*—not one in name only, but in truth, not a mere college clinique." He warned that "College Cliniques" did not fulfill the educational functions of "regularly established Hospitals"; "we have witnessed them," he asserted, "and we say to students, do not be entrapped by them."[142]

Calls for bedside clinical instruction intensified after the Civil War, but change remained gradual. When a committee of the Cincinnati General Hospital proposed a new plan of clinical teaching in 1872, it reported that "it is only lately that clinical teaching has been brought to its due application by the medical teachers of this Country." Calling for "systematic bedside training," they asserted that "this is now done in all European hospitals and the want of it is the Crucial defect in American Medical education." Two years later the case for reform in Cincinnati was still being argued, and a new proposal reiterated that "in carrying out this work it is not intended to interrupt the old plan of the daily lectures in the amphitheater of the hospital but to add thereto a practical course of bed side teaching which has given such renown to the hospitals of Europe."[143]

Much of the public rhetoric about clinical instruction was posturing by the faculties of profit-oriented schools eager to attract clients, but the movement for change was also driven by a deeply felt conviction that the French plan was a better way of educating physicians. It was with relish that in 1873 Lundsford P. Yandell, Jr., told students attending his course on clinical medicine in Louisville how, at a competing school in Cincinnati, a single patient was hired to appear before the class regardless of the topic: "he was lectured upon for Bright's disease of Kidneys, Chronic rheumatism, diarrhea &c as the occasion might arise." But it was with evident regret that, standing in the amphitheater, Yandell told the class how much better it would be if they were taught at the bedside, as was done in Paris and London, predicting that "eventually clinical medicine will almost entirely supercede theoretical."[144] By the time Yandell spoke, a reform impulse had been well established; but a fuller integration of bedside clinical instruction into the curricula of American medical schools would be realized only gradually over the next half century.

The campaign for clinical teaching was sustained by the underlying epistemological ideals Americans associated with the Paris School, an institutional expression of the program to cleanse medical knowledge of rationalistic embellishment and reground it in sensual experience. Seeing hospital training as an education of the senses was of course not peculiar to those who had studied in the Paris Clinic. "The student must see, and hear, and feel for himself," New York physician Samuel Bard had asserted in 1819. "The hue of the complexion, the feel of the skin, the lustre or langour of the eye, the throbbing of the pulse and the palpitations of the heart, the quickness and ease of respiration, and the tone and tremor of the voice. . . . Where can these be learned but at the bedside of the sick? and where shall a young man, who cannot be admitted into the privacies of families, or the chambers of women, acquire the necessary information, but in a public hospital[?]"[145] Yet the new valorization of the senses by the Paris School redoubled the importance attached to educating the senses through direct encounters with disease in hospitals. "We fear that the great advantages offered by the Hospital as a school for *practical medicine*, has not yet been fully appreciated by the Profession," the medical faculty of the University of Louisiana admitted in 1849. "But the time will come, and that soon, when both the teacher and student will not only talk of *clinical* medicine, but the one will hasten to teach, and the other to learn, medicine in the only way in which it can be safely taught. To make a good—a practical physician we must educate all the senses; the touch; the eye, &c."[146] Through such an education, a University of Pennsylvania student who wrote his M.D. thesis titled "Medicine Clinique" asserted in 1862, "vain delusive theories are fast sinking into merited oblivion."[147]

Clinical education, in other words, was depicted as a mainstay in the battle against the spirit of system and the false authority systems engendered. At the Medical College of Ohio, a faculty committee charged in 1831 with defining the objectives of the professor of clinical medicine argued that he must take nature as his only text; "he must not adopt a *method*, nor proceed with his instruction in any other order, than that of the class[es of disease] which chance may throw in his way, and which throughout the whole course of instruction are to constitute the texts or occasions of his lectures." Clinical instruction, they insisted, "does not, therefore, occupy itself on *Systems* of pathology or therapeutics."[148] The same animus against the authority of theory was evident at the Baltimore Almshouse. "What are the objects of a School of Practical Medicine?" an 1834 report began. "They ought to be of much higher order than those which commonly obtain: far above that of inculcating whatever truth or falsehood, science or superstition[,] hypothesis or empyricism may have obtained the sanction of the schools as legitimate medicine." Insisting that "no systems of practical rules, be it ever so ample, can furnish authority for every case," the report urged a plan of instruction "elevated far beyond the servile drudgery of enforcing dogmatic routine."[149]

This insistent call to hold established teachings in abeyance and observe afresh intersected with American cultural regionalism to promote western and southern medical separatism. "If *they* have descriptions and plates of disease," a southern medical professor wrote in 1844 of northern teachers, "we have here the *living tableaux*, the diseases themselves."[150] Clinical education, accordingly, was at the core of the antebellum movement for regional separatism in medicine, and especially for distinctly southern schools. In the 1850s, the New Orleans School of Medicine made regular instruction at the bedside of hospital patients more central to its curriculum than had any other medical school in America. At the Charity Hospital, the student was shown at the bedside how to use the stethoscope in physical diagnosis and encouraged to "follow the body to the *dead house*, with scalpel in hand, and there examine *for himself*, to see if the diagnosis was correct."[151] Students were given free access to the wards, where they examined patients themselves and then submitted their case reports for review by a faculty member—the "chef de clinique," as the clinical professor was called.[152] As Erasmus Darwin Fenner, founder of the school, stated his goal: "Why should not New Orleans become the Paris of America?"[153] At the same time, Fenner insisted that "this Institution is of special importance to the Southern Medical Student, on account of its presenting the very types and varieties of disease he will meet with when he goes into practice."[154]

French medical polity failed to offer thoroughgoing solutions that seemed either desirable or viable in the American context. American physicians—even the most ardent disciples of the Paris School—responded to it not with unguarded admiration but with an ambivalence informed by the values and sociopolitical realities of their own country. By and large, they made little use of such French models in their programs for professional reform. The modest institutional changes that partly followed a French blueprint failed to elevate the standing of the medical profession in antebellum society in any direct or dramatic way. Americans, like the English, found in French medicine what they believed were promising solutions to the degradation of their profession; but just as they faced somewhat different problems, so they found in the French model different solutions.

# "Against the Spirit
# of System": Epistemology
# and Reform

THE GAP between English and American uses of the French model in programs to elevate the medical profession, pronounced in the case of medical polity, was even wider in the case of medical epistemology. While English reformers who drew on the French example made relatively little reference to French epistemology, Americans made it central in their plan for reform. The most valuable lesson of the Paris School, as they depicted it, was its stand for empiricism and against rationalism, and in an allegiance to that example they saw the greatest promise of transforming not only medical knowledge and practice but also the place of the profession in American society.

American and English representations of the Paris School were constructed out of substantially the same materials: it is comparison that draws attention to the differing rules of selection used by their builders. Reading the selective stories the Americans and the English told about French medicine with the contingency of their construction in mind reveals fundamental and important differences between their expectations about professional uplift and their assumptions about professional identity. These differences, in turn, disclose an American approach to professional reform in medicine based on understandings of professional identity distinct from those that prevailed not only in England but in the rest of the Western world.

To understand why some American physicians so ardently deployed their version of the French empiricist ideal in programs for reform, one must comprehend the particular social status of this epistemological stance in the United States. Empiricism and antirationalism had powerful resonances in antebellum American society that gave the epistemological program of French medicine special meaning to its disciples and encouraged them to see in it the promise of intellectual and social salvation. The perceived inadequacy of changes in professional polity and the structural alterations they would bring to provide solutions to professional problems in the American context was part of what gave the ideal of empirical truth such force. To reformers, the empiricist ideal offered not only a promising vehicle for professional change but also a satisfying claim to certainty that they could cling to in a time of disorder and a haven of rigor and authenticity in a society they believed to be riddled with mediocrity and imposture.

## THE ENGLISH AND FRENCH EPISTEMOLOGY

"Our ultra reformers are ever appealing to French arrangements as the *beau ideal* of every thing that is excellent about medical affairs," the editor of the *London Medical Gazette* asserted in 1833; they "look across the straits of Dover whenever they want something to put in place of what displeases them at home."[1] No doubt he had some grounds for this conclusion, for during the decades between Waterloo and midcentury, models of French medical polity were prominent in demands for reform. Those who sought to change the governance and institutions of English medicine, as one reformer explained in the *Lancet*, tried "to stimulate the apathy of the members of our Legislature by frequently holding up before their eyes the example of other nations."[2] Yet reformers were reticent about invoking other French models—especially those of epistemology and patient care. English medical radicals and conservatives alike tended to deplore French patient care and, far from holding it up for emulation, frequently denounced it. The case was different with French epistemology, however. It is difficult to document that which is missing; but in the English depiction of the French medical model compared with its American counterpart, epistemology was scarcely visible.

This is not to say that English medical travelers to Paris took no notice of the prevailing commitment to sensual empiricism and revulsion against rationalism. They were enthusiastic about opportunities for eyes-, ears-, and hands-on access to the body that the Paris School encouraged. And even though earlier experience in the London hospitals typically left them less awed than Americans by the Paris Clinic, many nonetheless were impressed: "I am tormented wth more opportunities than I can embrace," John Green Crosse wrote from Paris in 1815.[3] Yet in depicting medical Paris while in its midst, English observers tended to pay much closer attention to the institutional policies and legal arrangements that facilitated access to experience than to underlying assumptions about the nature of knowledge. That selective attention persisted in their representations of the Paris School after their return.

In England, the decades when the Paris School grew prominent also witnessed intensifying denunciations of rationalistic system building in medicine and avowals of strict allegiance to empirical observation. "The pruriency of Descartes for hypothetical reasoning, or rather hypothetical quibbling, was a death blow to medicine," one English medical editor charged in 1823; "since then, physicians have only employed themselves in chimerical speculations and arbitrary explanations, believing it sublime to aspire to first causes." He went on to call for "our *system builders* and *theorizers* to repent"—to overturn their misplaced faith in "REASON."[4] Others equally deprecated system building but were convinced that the age of reason in medicine was drawing to a close. "The Pomp of System has long dazzled and misled the medical Student," Charles Fergusson Forbes told his London medical class in 1819. But "happily for Mankind, the Delusion is nearly at an End—The real Treasures of Medical

Science are now unfolding, & consist in permanent and universally acknowledged Truths, and not in the pomp of Theory, or the parade of System."[5] By 1844, another English practitioner could assert that "hypothesis has been discarded in the study of medical science," suggesting that "for it the scrutiny of facts has been substituted."[6]

The ideal of gaining knowledge through direct observation of nature was a pervasive theme. "There is but one way to obtain knowledge," John Abernethy urged anatomy pupils at St. Bartholomew's Hospital in 1819; "we must be companions with the dead."[7] Those who urged that teaching at the London hospitals should place greater emphasis on bedside instruction persistently stressed the importance of learning by seeing. Thomas Wakley counseled students that "the great immediate object of the student in visiting London is to consult the book of nature as laid open to his view in the Hospital, [and] in the dissecting room," though at least one pupil from Sheffield repeatedly complained in his diary that his teacher at Guy's Hospital, as he noted after one class, "as usual dwelt too much on Theory."[8] Rhetoric denouncing rationalism persisted despite the greater attention bedside instruction would receive over time. In 1849 Walter Hayle Walshe, for example, a physician with Paris experience who had translated Pierre Louis's treatise on phthisis, introduced his course on clinical medicine at University College Hospital by telling students that there were two categories of practitioner—"those who theorize prior to experience, and base treatment upon such theory—the so-called *Rationalists*; and those who, unbiassed by preconceived notions, record, analyze, count and interpret the results of observation of the action of remedies—the *Observers*." As Walshe asserted, "It is to Observers, and not to Rationalists, [that] all the real triumphs of our art are due."[9]

Those who encouraged medical research echoed the same call to base knowledge on direct sensual experience of nature. At the first meeting of the newly organized Pathological Society of London in 1846, its Paris-experienced president Charles J. B. Williams argued that medical knowledge had been held back "because it has hitherto been taught and treated too metaphysically,—too much by closet speculation,—too much by book description, mystified, or cramped. . . . Too little has been done by physical demonstration—too little by appeals to the senses—too little by direct observation and experiment—too little by habits of that careful and accurate investigation of phenomena, to which, alone, Nature discloses her truths." By contrast, "we do nothing without an appeal to the senses," Williams insisted, "and this is one distinguishing feature of the Society."[10]

The theme of sensory experience as a counterforce to rationalistic systems that appeared in English rhetoric, however, differed in several important ways from its expression in America. First, it was never so prominent or so central to programs for reform in England as in the United States. Second, when it was deployed in English programs, it was cast chiefly as a tool for improving the medical profession's knowledge and perhaps its practice—not its standing in

society. Finally, the antisystem impulse in England was not ordinarily presented in ways that identified it with the Paris School. Sometimes French participation in this intellectual current was made unmistakable, as when Paris-
experienced Edward Henry Sieveking, physician to Queen Victoria, copied
onto the cover of a volume in which he kept his reading notes, "Les systèmes
en médecine, sont des idoles auxquelles on sacrifie des victimes humaines."[11]
But the English movement against the evils of system was not portrayed as
being in any significant measure French in origin.

The Guy's Society for Clinical Reports, founded in 1835 and later renamed
Guy's Hospital Clinical Society, was the kind of context in which English celebration of sensual clinical experience and disparagement of speculation was
most confidently expressed. "The establishment of the Guy's Society for Clinical Reports will form the Commencement of a new era in the history of medical
schools in this country," Thomas Hodgkin, then president, urged at the close
of its first year. "The example must spread from us to others, and it is to see
how the attachment to sober realities, the habits of close observation, and the
massive experience, which such institutions are calculated to nurture, will
tend mightily to uproot the use of theory and groundless speculation, which
has for so long a time shed a withering influence on Medical Science."[12] Richard Bright told the members in 1840 that "every sense plays its part in the
successful prosecution of Medicine," and spelled out the importance of sight,
hearing, smell, taste, and touch.[13] The "observations" made at the bedside and
autopsy table and reported at the society's meetings, Samuel Ashwell claimed,
"are the surest protection against wild theories, and sweeping generalizations,
which still continue to retard Medical Science."[14]

Even in such programmatic statements of their stance, however, society members made little of its Frenchness and almost nothing of its potential for uplifting
the medical profession. Bright hoped that "a race of superior practitioners will be
spread abroad" as a consequence of the society's labor, while Benjamin Guy
Babington hoped "to see Medicine take a higher standing among the Sister-
sciences"; yet neither suggested that such improvements in knowledge and practice would bring any solution to the social degradation of the profession.[15]
Equally, despite the fact that the Paris School had significantly shaped the thinking of such leaders of the Clinical Society as Bright and Hodgkin, efforts to
situate the society's agenda in a French medical tradition were muted at best.
When Charles Aster Key cited approvingly "the simple method of enumeration
by Louis" in his 1837 presidential report, it was less to recognize French
influence on the work of the society than to applaud the Paris clinician for
marching in step with an enlightened body of English investigators.[16]

That the antisystem animus was little portrayed as French is underscored by
English depictions of Louis and his numerical method. As in America, Louis
had critics in England, those who snipped that "an undue value may be ascribed to this numerical method, and that the theory of not theorizing may
prove as delusive as any of its predecessors."[17] And some resented his bold

claims for the newness of his program, as did one reviewer of the first *Mémoires de la Société Médicale d'Observation, de Paris* who assailed its "arrogance of tone" and suggested that Louis "has gained a high place, but he has grown giddy."[18] The voices of Louis's English advocates, however, were even more strident. "If there be a name in the profession which we ought to revere, it is that of Louis," the editor of the *Lancet* asserted in 1846, praising Louis's writings for their "sternness of inflexible integrity and truth."[19] So too, speaking at a meeting of the Provincial Medical and Surgical Association in 1835, a Bristol practitioner proposed that a "revolution" had recently taken place through the "partial abandonment of theoretical systems." Citing Louis's work as a refutation to system-builders, he went on to urge that "statistical researches are likely to afford the most satisfactory solution of many difficult problems, which have been thought, heretofore, to lie within the region of speculation."[20]

Yet in praising Louis, English admirers often appropriated him for an English tradition, as Marshall Hall did by dubbing Louis "THE BACON OF MEDICINE."[21] Having summed up the message of Louis's *An Essay on Clinical Instruction*, newly translated in 1835, a reviewer wrote that "we anticipate the remark it will call forth: this is the 'Novum Organum' applied to medicine," and noted, "The remark is just, but at the same time the best eulogium for the system."[22] Speaking to his students at the University College Hospital in 1841, John Taylor lauded Louis's numerical method, suggesting "not that Louis is the inventor of the method, for it is no other than that of Bacon, so long in general use in the other physical sciences; but to him, far above any other man, is due the merit of insisting on the necessity of a systematic employment of it in medicine."[23] Offering a distinctly English compliment, one reviewer remarked, "It is, we say, the crowning and distinguishing glory of M. Louis, that he follows the only true path in physic, the Baconian path of rigid observation."[24]

Depicted as French or not, Louis's method and the broader empiricist movement played little part in the campaign to lift the English medical profession from its degradation. The reason for this was the underlying English assumption that however much the dismantling of systems and rigorous allegiance to empirical clinical observation might improve medical knowledge and practice, it would not significantly alter the medical profession's position in society. "The public," one reformer noted in 1838, "give station to practitioners rather in accordance with their birth, parentage, and education, than with any reference to their power of curing disorders. Indeed, it is worthy of observation that medical practitioners have rather fallen in the public respect, while their real knowledge has been increasing."[25] And what was true of the public, as reformers complained, was equally true of established institutions, such as the corporations and metropolitan hospitals.[26] Superior medical knowledge could hardly be depended upon as a professional leaven. It is not surprising, therefore, that the spirit of system was not a common element in English inventories of the evils responsible for the profession's social woes, even though it routinely appeared on American lists.[27]

AMERICANS AND FRENCH EPISTEMOLOGY

Americans brought with them to Paris different assumptions about the sources of professional degradation and returned with different expectations of how French medicine might be used to promote professional change. The privileging of empiricism and antirationalism in representations of the Paris School would become most forceful in programs for professional reform. Yet the American preoccupation with epistemology was already evident in depictions of medical Paris composed on the spot—in private records, such as personal diaries and letters, and in public writings, such as reports sent home for publication in medical journals. What emerges most prominently from these accounts is a stress on what was sensually experienced—what was seen or touched. In part, this expressed the enthusiasm of Americans for Parisian institutions and policies that provided access to the body on a scale new to them. Yet the chief object of their celebration was the education of the senses these facilities afforded. "While I remain in Paris," Anson Colman wrote in his first letter from France, "I must occupy nearly all my time in *seeing* and *hearing*; leaving it to memory to treasure up the impressions which the mind receives through these (*especially in Paris*) important organs."[28] Both the institutional arrangements of medical Paris and the undergirding philosophical tradition of the medical idéologues drew attention to sensual empiricism as one central feature of the Paris School.

Alden March pointed to another reason why so many Americans stressed what could be *seen* in Paris when he made his first diary entry after arriving in the city: "Great disadvantage in not being able to speak French."[29] Even those who knew the language often lamented that they could understand French lecturers only if they spoke slowly, and this barrier to grasping the theoretical content of Parisian instruction itself focused their attention on what they could actually see or otherwise directly experience. As R. A. Kinloch put it in a letter from Paris to a Charleston medical journal, "Though knowing little of the language upon my arrival, I was nevertheless determined to take in whatever information I could through my eyes, notwithstanding that but little could be forced through my ears."[30]

Yet deficient language skill was not the leading reason they so enthusiastically extolled access to knowledge gained experientially through sight and touch: the promise of learning from the bodies of French patients was what had principally drawn them to Paris in the first place. Describing a visit to Paris as a "tour of observation,"[31] as was so often done, affirmed the importance of actually being there, of seeing a lesion in the body's tissues at autopsy or discerning a lesion in the living patient by listening through a stethoscope. "These are things that cannot be done by proxy," David Yandell wrote to his father, "and the superiority of French hospitals over all others, consists in the facilities which they afford for these examinations in *propria persona*."[32]

An underlying message—and, for Americans, the critical one—was that what was most significant about Parisian medicine was a particular attitude toward gaining and assessing knowledge that transcended the Paris Clinic and the experiences it afforded. Moses Linton echoed Yandell by reporting that what mattered most about free access in Paris was that "every one can examine for himself the facts and truths." Equally important, though, was what Linton saw as the ascendancy of clinical empiricism over an earlier medical rationalism, an observation that enabled him to write from Paris in 1840 that "the time seems to have gone by when system-builders may expect the multitude to bow down to their idols, and yield a slavish credence to their dogmas and dreams."[33] Thus, typically, Thomas Stewardson told William Gerhard that he valued his time "collecting cases à la Louis at La Pitié, not so much on account of the absolute information gained and labour performed as for the influence which it has exerted upon my mind."[34] Experience in the Paris Clinic, such Americans maintained, instilled in them a sensibility that abhorred rationalism and embraced empiricism. The education of the senses Americans acquired in Paris and the ideal of sensual empiricism for which they made the Paris School stand took on their wider meaning by insuring that, as Linton put it, the "spirit of speculation be stayed."[35]

What was most worth relating about a complex medical world was not self-evident, and the stories Americans told about the Paris School varied widely. Yet in their reflections while still in Paris, one can see the beginnings of a process by which their experience was both simplified and symbolized. At its boldest, this was expressed in a proclaimed allegiance to *truth*, a very specific notion of medical truth that turned upon Parisian empiricism. Thus James Jackson, Jr., not only condensed Louis's program into an effort "to *learn* and not to *invent* truth" but seized upon this ideal as a standard for his own life.[36] For him as for other Americans in France, "truth" became a symbol of the battle against the errors of reason and a fitting emblem of Paris.

Selective perceptions Americans had of Paris while abroad, evident in the accounts they produced there, would be one basis for selective memory. After their return home, however, what physicians recalled and featured in their representations of medical Paris was informed more and more by the sociopolitical needs and expediencies of the American context. As they proselytized for French medicine in programs for reform, the polemical function of stories about Paris became even more pronounced.

At this juncture, what Americans publicly remembered about Paris also became increasingly selective. Their recollections were further streamlined and distilled into symbols that stood for both their own experience and the broader lessons of Paris, and the ideal of empirical truth emerged clearly as the sturdiest core of their depiction of the Paris School. Other aspects of French medicine that they had routinely noted while in Paris were trimmed out of their public pronouncements: with critics loudly assailing French medicine for its deplorable patient care and apathetic attitude toward healing, for example, its American disciples were decreasingly likely to voice such criticisms themselves, as chapter 8 will show. Selective memory involved more than just muting certain negative judgments, however. Often Americans writing in Paris talked about how Parisian ways could transform medical knowledge and practice; but it was only after returning home that they began to say much about how the French model could elevate their profession in American society. It was at this point that memories of Paris became strongly linked not just with the advancement of medicine but also with the betterment of the American medical profession.

In American reports from France there had been an underlying sense that something about Paris could not be fully conveyed by words: it was knowable only through the experience of actually being there. Many tried to re-create a sense of the Parisian clinicians by providing finely detailed descriptions of not just their ideas but also their appearance, gesticulations, mannerisms, and voice. Others used rhetorical forms designed to convey a facsimile of place. "Take my arm this morning, at 7 o'clock, and go with me to the Hotel Dieu," Elisha Bartlett began a letter to readers of the *Western Lancet* in 1846.[37] Augustus Gardner instructed readers of his guidebook that "you must follow me in imagination in my diurnal visit," and, like Bartlett, proceeded to walk them from his boardinghouse to the doors of the Hôtel Dieu and on into its wards.[38] Some wordless knowledge was held back; those who had experienced the Paris Clinic in person retained special, exclusive insight.

Yet the leading message of the Paris School as Americans depicted it—the ideal of empirical truth—could be offered to those who had not made the journey, and they could even make it their own. That, indeed, was one aim of returnees who urged this lesson on the profession at home and on its next generation in the classroom. When in 1841 Bartlett addressed the medical class at Transylvania on the epistemological lessons of the Paris School, for example, and a class committee requested that he publish his remarks, Bartlett replied by reconsecrating himself to the task of instilling in students the empiricist program in which he saw the profession's best hopes—of "inculcating sound philosophical and practical principles in Medecine, and in opposing the adoption and spread of those multiform and hypothetical systems of physiology and pathology and therapeutics, which have ever exerted, and which still continue to exert so disastrous an influence upon our Noble Science and our beneficent Art."[39] For their part, Bartlett's students took up his message and plagiarized his rhetoric in the process. When in 1848 a student at Transylvania wrote on "Young Physic" as his M.D. thesis, which he dedicated to Bartlett (and largely lifted from his publications), the student concisely stated the program that his teacher had embraced: "It is the alotted task of our age to remove the crumbling relics of a false philosophy," he asserted, "in order that our posterity may, upon the site of a grand but erroneous philosophy, build the Pyramid of Truth."[40] In ways such as these, Bartlett and other Paris-returned physicians not only proselytized for French medical epistemology but to a large extent Americanized it. The American profession, a student asserted in his 1852 M.D. thesis at the Medical College of the State of South Carolina, "has probably to struggle with no greater enemy" than "the spirit of system."[41]

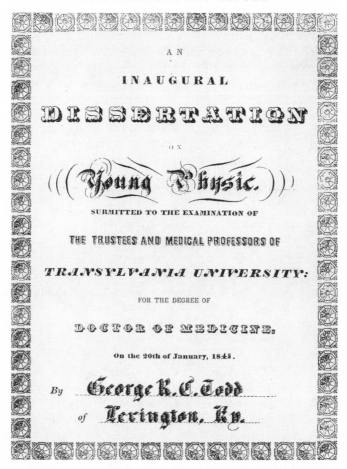

AN

INAUGURAL

DISSERTATION

ON

((( Young Physic. )))

SUBMITTED TO THE EXAMINATION OF

THE TRUSTEES AND MEDICAL PROFESSORS OF

TRANSYLVANIA UNIVERSITY:

FOR THE DEGREE OF

DOCTOR OF MEDICINE,

On the 20th of January, 1848.

By  George R.C.Todd

of  Lexington, Ky.

Fig. 7.1. M.D. thesis presented at Transylvania University in Lexington, Kentucky, in 1848, which the student dedicated to his professor, Elisha Bartlett. The rhetoric this and other midcentury American medical students deployed often emulated the animus against the spirit of system promulgated by their Paris-experienced teachers. (Courtesy of Special Collections, Library, Transylvania University, Lexington, Kentucky.)

## EPISTEMOLOGY AND AMERICAN PROGRAMS FOR REFORM

Just how were the epistemological ideals attached to the Paris School supposed to uplift the regular medical profession in the United States? This program for reform was far from monolithic. But while there was no single blueprint for change, three leading prongs to the design for reform can be identified. First, by escaping the reign of rationalistic systems, the regular profession would shed those features of its knowledge and practice that had come most under attack, depriving antiorthodox critics of their targets. Second, by cultivating empirical observation of nature, regular physicians would improve the character of their ideas and practices, with the expectation that such betterment would win public favor. And, third, having undermined the attack on orthodox medicine, regular reformers would go on to use the ideals of empiricism and antirationalism to discredit their irregular competitors, thereby affirming the superiority of regular medicine in ways consonant with American values.

The promise regular physicians saw in the reform program based upon epistemological change is best understood within the context of the ongoing assault by antiorthodox practitioners on the orthodox profession, and particularly on its mystification of medical knowledge. Accompanying their siege on professional mystery was the proclamation of an alternative—and assertively more democratic—medical epistemology. Common experience of nature, commanded by the ordinary man and woman, was a sufficient guide to health and healing and, moreover, the only source of truly authentic medical knowledge. "In the science of medicine, I assure you, there is no mystery," one botanic physician writing for the public urged in 1834. "There is nothing incomprehensible about it."[42] As another botanic put it, simple truths should replace the "unfathomable arcana of medicine."[43] What was beyond the ken of ordinary people could not constitute sound knowledge. "We wish to see the healing art brought home to our own firesides, and rendered so plain and simple, that it can be understood by all," one Thomsonian editor advised. "It is as easy to cure disease, as it is to make a pudding," he claimed, insisting that in medicine there should be "no mysticism—no bombast—no monopoly."[44] Contrasting the water-cure with orthodox medicine, a hydropathic physician echoed, "Our science is not buried in technicalities, nor our practice veiled in mystery."[45]

Critics underscored the evils of the putative mystification of medical knowledge by pointing to its dire effects on the people's health. Orthodox physicians kept a knowledge of healing and the laws of healthful living from the public. As one health reformer charged in 1856, orthodox doctors "do not aim to enlighten mankind in regard to their physical well being, but rather seek to envelop their processes of cure in deep and impenetrable mystery. This mystery possesses a magic charm for the uninitiated and ignorant. You have only to look about you to become aware of the credulity and superstition with which the Medical Profession is regarded." It was the health reformer's task, she continued, "to sow far and wide the seeds of truth that will eventually germinate and b[e] the means of redeeming the world from ignorance that so effectually blinds the mass of its inhabitants."[46]

More than simply making medical knowledge appear beyond the grasp of common Americans, though, the highly wrought, speculative systems of orthodox physicians, critics asserted, led to dangerous practice. "False theory and hypothesis," Samuel Thomson claimed, "constitute nearly the whole art of physic."[47] The target of critics' most violent denunciations was orthodox heroic therapy, aggressive depletion by bloodletting and mineral purgatives such as calomel and tartar emetic. Orthodox doctors, in their view, exemplified the corruption of established medicine by poisoning the American people. What led to this deluded practice in the first place was their purportedly blind reliance on rationalistic theories instead of on experience. Speculative systems of pathology and therapeutics represented not only the core of orthodox physicians' special knowledge but also the source of their murderous bleeding and purging. Accordingly, antiorthodox medical professors routinely illustrated their lectures by examples of cases "treated by the murderous systems," while their students wrote M.D. theses roundly denouncing orthodox physicians as "speculative theorists."[48] By placing their faith in complicated, rationalistic systems, regular physicians kept knowledge of healing from the public and misguided their own practice by obscuring from themselves nature's simple truths.

The persistent message was that medical knowledge should be simplified and access to it opened up. Once this happened, critics maintained, the authority of orthodox physicians would, properly, disintegrate. No longer would regular physicians be able to use artificially intricate medical knowledge to exploit and defraud the public. A better, simpler epistemology of common experience and common sense would improve health care, banish the evils of heroic drugging, and foster a healthier, more democratic, and more authentically American social order.

One impulse among regular physicians in the face of such popular attack was to turn inward in order to find in established tradition a stable core of professional definition and distinction. In the realm of practice, this influence encouraged regulars to proclaim more stridently than ever before their allegiance to the traditional therapies that had come under attack, transforming bloodletting and mineral drugs into symbols of orthodox identity.[49] A similar orthodox reaction was to loudly reaffirm the necessary complexity of established medical knowledge. Georgia physician Paul Eve told medical students gathered for an 1849 commencement ceremony that the source of "the unfavorable opinion entertained by the public for the medical profession is, that as a science it is the most difficult, obscure and complicated of all human learning. No other occupation in life involves such varied and minute knowledge."[50] The importance of initiation into the special knowledge that distinguished the regular profession was formalized in the new institutions set up to define and preserve orthodoxy. Emblemizing the conservative response to the attack on medical knowledge, in 1847 the newly created American Medical Association wrote into its Code of Ethics that "no one can be considered as a regular practitioner" unless he has been educated in regular medicine, mastering "the aids furnished by anatomy, physiology, pathology, and organic chemistry."[51] Assaults on the regular profession and the repeal of licensing laws drove regular physicians to underscore what defined their orthodox faith and distinguished them as healers.

The popular critique of professional mystery had a still more profound influence in molding regular physicians' attitudes toward established medical knowledge and expectations about how new knowledge should be gained. It created a socioeconomic and intellectual environment that fundamentally shaped epistemological change in American medicine, giving the turn from rationalism to empiricism special force. The assault on the profession intensified the symbolic meanings regular physicians attached to the ideal of empiricism they took up from the Paris School, enabled them to see it as a powerful agent for change, and helps explain why they so ardently embraced that ideal in the first place.

Instead of rejecting the popular critique of professional mystery, to a remarkable extent regular reformers sought to co-opt its epistemological message and thereby dissipate its political force. Empiricism adopted as a symbol of professional uplift was neatly suited to the sociopolitical tenor of American culture; and in embracing empiricism, regular reformers set themselves on a tack in some respects strikingly parallel to that of their critics. French empiricism could represent direct observation of fact open for all to see rather than shrouded as a professional mystery, and therefore offered a rallying point and symbol of professional advancement that promised to be resilient in the face of pervasive assaults against claims to privileged access to knowledge. It provided what could be framed as an epistemology of common experience, an epistemology well calculated to withstand attacks from monopoly-bashing exponents of Jacksonian democracy like the Thomsonians. The direct observation of nature of the Thomsonians was far from identical with the direct observation of nature of Paris-returned elite American physicians: the clinic and the autopsy table offered a context for observing nature quite different from the domestic bedside. Nevertheless, both versions of medical empiricism turned upon a vigorous insistence on the primacy of direct experience. Thus Samantha S. Nivison, in her 1855 M.D. thesis at the Female Medical College of Pennsylvania, urged that "as when the vail of the Temple was rent assunder in the hour of the great sacrifice, opening the sanctuary to all worshipers, so the penenetralia of each mind are opened, for the true physician."[52] Regular physicians took up an empiricist faith akin to that of their assailants and used it to launch a counterattack against them. "We go for *science*, in medical practice and in medical reform," one physician told readers of the *Boston Medical and Surgical Journal* in 1839, at once denouncing Thomsonians and proclaiming his orthodox faith. "And by science in medicine, we mean large experience, not theory."[53]

Regular reformers engaged in an energetic campaign of their own to demystify established medicine, with the intertwined aims of shedding the errors of rationalism and depriving assailants of a vulnerable target. Stripping medical knowledge of all needless embellishment, they argued, was a project in which the French had led the way. "They have served to extricate us from the mazes of hypothesis, in which we were before involved, [and] are daily unfolding to us new truths," a Philadelphia physician asserted in 1832, with the result that "the science of medicine has already become, in a great degree, freed from the paralyzing influence of mysticism, and the bewilderings of hypothesis."[54] Throughout the antebellum decades, reformers insisted that this cleansing of medical knowledge was an ongoing battle. Demonizing "subtle reasoning," "ingenious systems," and "the shackles of speculation," Stillé charged in 1848 that they had "contributed to discredit the profession, and to arrest the progress of knowledge." He called on regular physicians to abandon "the hypotheses which have more recently arisen and flourished" and urged that "Brownism and Rushism, Broussaisism and Hahnemannism, with all the other fruits of a luxuriant fancy and a poverty of facts, must descend the inevitable slope to oblivion."[55]

Bartlett's *Essay on the Philosophy of Medical Science* (1844) was a prominent example of calls to reform medical knowledge by demolishing rationalistic systems, what he called "the golden day-dreams and the fairy imaginations of a speculative optimism."[56] Paris-returned physicians believed they represented an enlightened core that had heeded this call, but they remained convinced that the masses of their profession languished unenlightened. As James Jackson, Sr., wrote to Bartlett after its publication, "I have no doubt that your book will be useful every where, but especially in the valley of the Mississippi, where some false systems of philosophizing have had too much vogue."[57] The objective reformers set for themselves, and for the regular profession, was to discard past errors and "avoid all useless speculation and vain embellishment."[58]

Just as dispelling the mystery of regular medical knowledge would do away with a leading target of attack by antiorthodox physicians, so too would reforming the excesses of heroic drugging. Irregulars pointed to aggressive bleeding and purging as the clearest emblems of orthodox evil and often blamed such practice on rationalistic orthodox systems—"the *doctrines of drugopathy*," as one hydropathist put it.[59] Regular critics, for their part, blamed "*heroic practitioners*" for "the sin of *having prepared the minds of men* for the reception of quackery in general, and particularly for that subtle, but most absurd species known as homoeopathy."[60] Historians have recognized that as the attack on orthodox ways led to a popular outcry against heroic drugging, regular physicians tailored their goods to the demands of the market, making their therapies increasingly milder to render them less vulnerable to ridicule and more palatable to paying patients.[61] The best way to oppose "homeopathy and its kindred delusions" was to give the public what it wanted by overturning "the reign of the drugging system."[62]

Yet regular protests against heroic drugging were fueled as well by the program for epistemological reform. "System-making" and "its spirit," a medical student at Transylvania urged in 1841, led unavoidably to therapeutic error— "an error, which sweeps a fearful number of yearly victims to an untimely grave." "Exclusive systems," he explained, "exert a secret but powerful influence over all our habits of thought and principles of reasoning; and, unknown to ourselves, perhaps, give their peculiar hue to every subject of investigation and reflection. Truth is no longer seen arrayed in simple, unadorned beauty, but disfigured and discolored."[63] It was reliance upon rationalistic systems that corrupted regular medical practice and stigmatized it as "a clouded mystery."[64]

Demystifying medicine and banishing all systems also promised to uplift the profession by promoting professional unity. Regular leaders routinely pointed to disagreements and rancorous arguments about medical theory and practice within orthodox ranks as a key source of professional degradation. The followers of a system became its creatures, intent on defending their creed. Such divisiveness undercut the profession's authority in the eyes of the public and provided a prime target for ridicule. Pointing to the diversity of opinion existing among orthodox doctors, a professor at the Cleveland Institute of Homoeopathy told his students in 1851, "Aleopathy is like a large army without tactics wandering in a glorious uncertainty."[65] Regular professional leaders rightly attributed such discord in part to an overcrowded marketplace and the competition for patients that ensued, problems that reformers sought to alleviate by the fee bills and codes of ethics of medical societies. Escaping the divisive influence of systems would enable regular physicians to stop squabbling among themselves and stand united in their opposition to their assailants. "When we reflect upon the difference of opinion which must necessarily exist in the profession, resulting from the stubborn and erroneous advocation of one or the other of these systems of medicine by its disciples," one student observed, "we can easily see that disease is not shorn of as many of its terrors as ought to be the case: nor should we any longer marvel at the fact, that the people have so little confidence."[66]

As reformers sought to liberate established medicine from its rationalistic past, they also called for positive improvement of knowledge and practice by the cultivation of empirical observation. "By means of it alone, can *medicine* be elevated to a rank amongst the 'Exact Sciences,'" a Kentucky physician argued in 1844, noting that Louis's studies on phthisis and typhoid fever had "given to our knowledge of those maladies certainty, where before were only chaos and confusion."[67] The overturning of rationalism would only half realize the program for epistemological reform. "The spirit of system is a propensity belonging to the human mind—and, even when the light of Philosophy is clearest, it will prompt, if not steadily repressed, to a departure from the onward path upon which that light falls," a South Carolina student asserted. Having escaped what he called "the spirit of system," though, next "the desideratum is, an acquaintance with all the *facts* within the sphere of our observation relating to disease—its symptoms—its causes—its remedies."[68]

The collapse of system meant the loss of a comforting illusion of certitude and direction. "In the present posture of affairs every medical man is compelled to build anew the foundations[,] to go to work as if the science existed in its original state of chaos and confusion, in order to fix for himself with exactness and certainty its elementary facts and principles," one medical student reflected in 1841.[69] "How shall we get out of this darkness?" Jackson, Jr., posed the question. "Can we do it by reading? The books contain more falsehoods than truths & of these last scarcely any that are proved. By theory à priori? The world has long enough suffered fr. this. But we can observe c̄[um] care the phenomena of Nature; we can collect our facts; & fr. these draw rigorous truths."[70] Praising Louis's application of the numerical method to bloodletting, another physician urged that the profession needed further studies "with the exactitude and in the philosophical spirit of the great French pathologist. Then, and not till then, will something like the same certainty, which distinguished the physical sciences, be introduced into medicine."[71] A repudiation of speculation coupled with an allegiance to empirical observation, Bartlett told his students, was "the first essential condition of the advancement of our Science, and especially of therapeutics—of its increased certainty, positiveness, completeness, and consequent usefulness."[72]

The same epistemological critique regular physicians made of their own knowledge and practice they turned against what they pejoratively labeled *sectarian* medicine, with the aim, though, not of reforming but of destroying it. They sought to discredit the principles and practices of antiorthodox practitioners by exposing their roots in speculative theory and to undercut their claims to epistemological purity. Homeopathy, Thomsonianism, and "all the systems of medical delusion" were consigned alike to "the morasses of false experience of vain hypothesis and delusive theory."[73] The crusade against the spirit of system thus became a crusade against alternative healers and outright quacks as well. The ideal of empiricism gave regular physicians a powerful weapon for assailing their rivals without offending the epistemological sensibilities of the American public.

Some orthodox reformers acknowledged that regular and irregular medicine shared an inclination to excessive theorizing; "there has ever been a veil of mystery thrown around the temple of medicine," one Alabama physician put it.[74] The combined result, they further acknowledged, was the degradation of medicine as a whole. Yet they denounced irregular practitioners as vastly more fanciful and indulgent theorizers than the worst offenders among their orthodox colleagues. "We find theories in the writings of the most celebrated physicians, even those who preface their work by declaiming against idle & visionary speculations in our science," one regular medical student acknowledged. But no "quack," he asserted, "ever gave a medicine without cherishing a theoretical indication of cure in his own mind."[75] "Sectarians" and "quacks," orthodox critics charged, were medical mystifiers par excellence: "our sage assuming friend, who with some false theory clothed in language as unintelligible to his patients as latin or greek to the unlettered urchin, assumes the dignity of a philosopher or benefactor and deals out a quantity of shrubbery or the roots thereof, the nature of which he is entirely ignorant."[76]

The language regular reformers used in condemning rationalistic orthodox systems was remarkably similar to the language they used in attacking antiorthodox systems such as Thomsonianism, homeopathy, and, as one Albany medical student put it, "all the systems and humbugs of the vast horde of quacks & impostures who, almost as numerous as the locusts of Egypt—'have overspread the whole land.'"[77] The test of empirical observation, regular reformers hoped, would disclose the errors of alternative medical systems and thereby undermine their appeal. As one regular medical student proposed, it would bring their hold on the American people to an end, and "in place of this monster shall reign order and benignity."[78] A Louisiana physician urged with equal bluster, *"Truth is might, and will prevail!"*[79]

Orthodox reformers maintained that epistemological change would also uplift the profession by enabling the American people—who they believed tarred all who claimed to be medical practitioners with the same brush—to distinguish between regularly bred physicians and quacks. "No department of science affords greater opportunity for deception," a Philadelphia medical student noted, urging that reformers could rectify this only "by stripping medicine as much as possible of its technical and useless ceremonies, and placing it upon a footing with all the other sciences that are intended for the benefit and convenience of mankind."[80] If medicine were laid open, patients would be better able to judge true merit. "The enlightened physician," an Albany medical student asserted, by basing all claims to public favor on ideas and actions "stripped of their mystery," would in the natural course of things win "the confidence of the community."[81]

By appealing to empiricism and antirationalism, regular reformers were seeking a sturdy basis for professional identity and authority that was in keeping with the prevailing values of antebellum society. They could not reasonably expect to elevate the standing of the profession by legislation or by dramatic changes in the education formally required of regular physicians. But they could hope to ground professional education and claims to authority in knowledge free from the encumbrances of speculation and validated by empirical observation. Thus one graduating medical student, urging that his fellow regulars avoid "the labyrinthian morass of speculation and hypothesis," asserted in 1840 that "as they elevate their standard of learning, . . . so will the worth of well educated physicians be appreciated, and their responsibility felt more suitably."[82] The public could not be relied upon to sanction legal distinctions that would discriminate between the regular physician and the quack; but reformers perceived more dependable criteria in an allegiance to empirical truth. "We should evidently be guided, in our practice, by those principles, founded on fact alone," asserted a Kentucky medical student in 1835. "It is this which should distinguish the physician from the empiric, & this alone should determine his superior claims upon an enlightened & liberal public."[83]

Many physicians perceived the French ideal of empirical truth as a singularly powerful resource in meeting the sociopolitical realities of antebellum America. Speculative medical systems corrupted by rationalism, on the one hand, and "sectarian" systems informed by rationalism and outright deception, on the other, were held responsible by regular reformers for the profession's low standing. Empiricism would rid American medicine of rationalistic systems, quell criticism, reduce professional divisiveness, and improve regular practice. It would temper the excessive bleeding and purging that were the main target of antiorthodox ridicule, and establish the folly of irregular therapeutics. All this would enhance the profession's standing and authority in the eyes of the public. To the intellectual elite who had studied in Paris, the ideal of empirical truth they had returned with from France offered a weapon for battling both the "brainless quack" and the "respectable humbug."[84]

## The Cultural Meaning of Empiricism

What remains puzzling about the program to use empiricism as a platform for uplifting the regular profession is its sheer durability in the face of a discouraging paucity of social change. The antebellum decades did witness a transformation in regular medical thought and practice, most especially the self-conscious move away from reliance on grand systems of pathology and therapeutics. But signs that the regular profession's status was significantly elevated as a consequence—the aim reformers confidently proclaimed—were few. Only the final third of the century saw the beginning of the extraordinary rise in public esteem for the medical profession that became pronounced in the twentieth century, and, perhaps ironically, when the dramatic change did come, it would be linked to both a new program for medical epistemology and a new relationship between epistemology and authority in American society. Yet antebellum reformers did not conclude that the problem was intractable or that its potential was exhausted, and continued with undiminished vigor to proselytize for sensualist empiricism and antirationalism as engines of social uplift. Indeed, the epistemological program that Paris-returned physicians had begun to urge in the 1810s and 1820s not only persisted but intensified during the 1830s, 1840s, and 1850s.

In part, as I have suggested, the particular appeal of empiricism to regular reformers must be ascribed to the social status of this epistemological position in America. The sociopolitical context of medical practice in the United States did not *cause* physicians to take up an empiricist ideal: during the first half of the nineteenth century a shift from rationalism toward empiricism was evident throughout Western medicine. But there is ample reason to say that the peculiar socioeconomic, political, and intellectual milieu of the antebellum United States redoubled the meaning this particular epistemological stance held for the American physicians who returned from Paris and for other regular medical reformers who embraced it. It made a commitment to empiricism matter more to them and let them see in it greater promise.

Yet the persistence of regular doctors in their campaign to bring professional uplift through epistemological reform cannot be fully understood in terms of a functionalist account of a reform agenda that went largely unfulfilled. Beyond its perceived utility as a tool in countering antiorthodox assaults on professional mystery, the ideal of empirical truth, as Paris-experienced reformers deployed it, promised to uplift the American medical profession by unmasking fraud and imposture both within the ranks of the orthodox profession and among its rivals. Truth, as they understood it, offered a weapon in their battle against the pervasive humbuggery that, in turn, they held chiefly responsible for the profession's protean social and intellectual ills.

Antebellum society was beset by a fear of deception, paranoid about being taken in and exploited. On the one hand, an American fascination with trickery and masquerade made possible the success of P. T. Barnum and his self-admitted cultivation of the art of humbug. On the other, anxiety about deception and its social consequences in daily life was deeply rooted in American culture. Historian Karen Halttunen has neatly captured these anxieties by pointing to the looming images of the painted woman and the confidence man as archetypal counterfeits, representations of imposture and hypocrisy that were seen as threats to American society and duly assailed. What these two imagined characters shared was a disregard for truth and the power to deceive through false appearances. The painted woman, more often a woman of fashion than a prostitute, seduced through the guises of extravagant embellishment and false etiquette, not the authentic charms of natural simplicity. So too the confidence man pretended honesty—a calculated forthrightness that was merely deceit—as the lure to draw in his victims. Dishonesty, artificial adornment, and calculated deception—all betrayals of republican virtue—were threatening to undermine American society.[85]

This preoccupation with deception and its social consequences, pervasive in American rhetoric ranging from advice manuals for boys and girls to political speeches, was a central theme in the oratory and writing of regular physicians. "Our age is one of imposture and unbounded credulity," a Kentucky medical student proposed in his 1850 M.D. thesis; "deception & craftiness is the order of the day, and public sentiment and belief very unsteady."[86] If quacks were dismissed as deceivers by their very nature, more disturbing were regular physicians suborned by the arts of deception. Orthodox leaders identified overcrowding as one source of the problem, for it compounded the inbuilt trickery of quacks with a resort to trickery by even well-educated, regular-bred physicians desperate to win a competitive edge. Orthodox medical schools, locked in competition, succumbed to this malaise. As Stillé wrote from Philadelphia to Shattuck in 1848, "The tricks, the falsehoods, the quibbles & equivocations, the downright frauds & moral felonies practiced by some of the medical schools of this city are enough to disgust an honest physician with his profession, and make him tear the diploma which confers upon him a title borne by so many whose proper place would be at the plough-soil or behind the counter."[87]

The lament about dishonesty and deception in medicine was for many regular physicians part of a wider lament about the condition of American society. Politics, in particular, offered a mirror to the ills that plagued medicine. Complaining in 1840 about a country "where commerce is synonymous with swindling," Stillé protested against "the contempt for virtue and uprightness" he believed pervaded popular politics.[88] Speaking before an entering class of Philadelphia medical students in 1854, Stillé denounced the quack, the medical system-builder, and the political pretender alike. "The shallow politician, the trickster of popular favor, the great man's familiar spirit, the creature of accident, may sometimes glide into place and power," he told the students, cautioning them that in medicine "the way is not smoother than in the political arena, nor the rivalry freer from shocks and strategems." Stillé warned that "the smooth and plausible deceiver, the crafty panderer to the sins and follies of patients, the cringing sycophant of doctors of renown, the oracular expounder of solemn nonsense,—or even the insolent denouncer of all science, the dealer in shameless imposture, the trader in nostrums, the brazen-browed quack, in fine,—may plate his sins with gold, and be worshipped by the people, as was the golden calf of ancient times."[89] As a Tennessee medical student echoed the point in 1857, "Most Physicians must have their hocus pocus upon which to ride into Practice as does the Politician into office."[90]

It was partly within this context that the ideal of empirical *truth* acquired such powerful symbolic significance in American medicine. The commitment to empiricism ascribed to French medicine represented a touchstone of authenticity in a world of counterfeit. Distilled to its essence, truth was what the American disciples of French medicine saw themselves bringing back from Paris and offering to their profession. As Stillé put it in his *Elements of General Pathology* (1848), a textbook he prefaced with an essay titled "Medical Truth," this ideal of truth was a bulwark against "metaphysical subtlety, the dreams of genius, or the frauds of charlatanism." Its lesson was "to abandon every hypothesis . . . [and] to lay aside the pride of reason."[91] His own aim was to avoid the false allurements of speculation and the false promises of reason, to avoid the temptation "to speculate on fanciful analogies, rather than to extract truth from facts."[92] Empirical observation "creates nothing, it does not even invent anything, it only *sees things as they are*, and discovers truth in what it sees," Stillé insisted. "Such was the genius of Hippocrates," he asserted; "such *is* that of Andral, of Chomel, of Louis."[93]

Epistemological issues were routinely expressed in an emotionally resonant idiom that spoke to anxieties deeply rooted in medical culture and the broader culture alike. In the rhetorical forms that became commonplace among regular physicians, epistemological positions became distinctly value laden, with empiricism and rationalism linked not only to divergent ways of knowing but more profoundly to integrity and dishonesty respectively. On the one hand, empirically determined medical fact was rhetorically identified with sincerity, honesty, authenticity, and, above all, simple, unadorned truth. On the other, rationalism was identified with deception, hypocrisy, and fraud, while its fruits were framed as captivating but ultimately false.

The assault by reformers on regular and irregular system-builders, like their adulation of the seeker of medical truth through empirical observation, gained force by being cast in the language of deception and honesty, imposture and forthrightness, guile and character. The mystification of rationalistic systems was depicted as a form of trickery dangerous to the people's health and the social standing of the profession. "Whether it stalks abroad bedecked with false advertisements, or lies more concealed and domesticated," a Philadelphia medical student urged, such deception "must be considered as highly reprehensible and injurious to the physical well being of the community."[94] Stripping away concealment was held up as an intrinsically noble professional pursuit. Thus, having just read Bartlett's newly published *Essay on the Philosophy of Medical Science* in 1844, Stillé wrote to Shattuck saying, "Dr. B. has done Science much good by showing her naked to the professed followers, many of whom venerate the Queen less than they admire her artificial trappings, her rich garments, & her glittering crown." Stillé lamented that "her unadorned perfections have little charm for them in whom the inventions of Art have taken precedence of Nature," but reaffirmed the commitment he shared with Bartlett and Shattuck to "consult Nature honestly."[95]

Much the same language was used to decry antiorthodox physicians as deceivers—as (in the words of one South Carolina medical student) "impostors and vain pretenders."[96] In the United States, an American physician in Paris reflected in 1847, "quacks and charlatans"—as he collectively denoted irregular practitioners—"live in a state of piracy against the world, robbing and killing all, who come in their way, or are allured by a false flag."[97] The success of Thomsonian and Eclectic physicians in competing with regular practitioners was likewise attributed to their dishonest cultivation of the arts of deception. A regular physician practicing in a rural Louisiana parish bemoaned this state of affairs: "Thomsonian Doctors," he wrote in his diary in 1837, "have totally infested the Country . . . & by decrying mineral medicines have cast doubts upon the regular medical faculty & have succeeded in fooling the people & killing thousands of the innocent dupes." The public, in his view, were beguiled by these "Root Doctors," taken in and duped by the Thomsonian practitioner just as they were taken in by other confidence men.[98]

Especially during the early years of homeopathy in America, when many of its practitioners were German immigrants, representing homeopathy as "nothing but German mysticism" was a maneuver regular physicians employed that redoubled its image as a speculative system by linking it to a widely held caricature of the German mind: homeopathy, as one critic described it, was the "result of habitual modes of thinking in Germany,—the result of a kind of unphilosophical dreaming among a people who often show themselves incapable of severe reasoning, as they are almost always transcendent in the observation of facts."[99] Thus the author of *The Anatomy of a Humbug, of the Genus Germanicus, Species Homeopathia* (1837) tellingly urged that "Germany is the land most congenial to ghosts, goblins and devils," and suggested that homeopathy—"baptized in the magic waters of that country"—was a throwback to "the reign of magic and witchcraft." He proceeded to represent homeopaths as foreign confidence men "duping and deceiving the credulous," as beguilers who "consider the Yankees fair game and an easy prey."[100]

By the 1830s, against the foil of the archetypal medical deceiver, a counter-archetype became prominent in regular medical rhetoric—what was denoted the "true physician" or, as often, the "honest physician." The attributes of the true physician were the antithesis of those of the deceiver: integrity, sincerity, allegiance to medical truth, and success won not by trickery but by honest dealings. Above all, true physicians were precisely what they seemed to be, and professed medical beliefs out of genuine conviction rather than artful calculation.

At the root of this transparent integrity was solid character. "A *good character*, is the only sure basis for a successful life," Hardy Vickers Wooten told the graduating class of the Memphis Medical College in 1853. He made it clear that outward appearances designed to win public approval were no substitute for inner virtue. "By character, we do not mean the mere reputation, or position which accidental or adventitious circumstances, or a course of conduct founded upon expediency, may give an individual; but the great aggregate of life, based upon fixed and conscientious principles, and made up of deliberate actions therefrom. A man may sometimes acquire a temporary reputation, as fair and bright as a summers morning, while the intrinsic character which shall mould his life, shall be as dark and forbidding as a winter's night."[101] Joseph P. Logan, speaking to the Atlanta Medical Society in 1855, denounced both "the fondness for *mystery* in the medical profession" and the pervasive imposition of *"humbug,"* and went on to suggest that professional degradation could be partly attributed to the public's failure to discriminate between "the unscrupulous pretender" who embraced these deceptions and "the true physician." "Notwithstanding the number of parasites and scullions who are hanging on the outskirts of our army, and have ever been a clog upon our march and a blot upon our escutcheon," he told the gathered members, "there is a noble array of determined and true men, who constitute an invincible phalanx pressing on under the banner of truth and philanthropy."[102]

In depicting *the true physician* as one marching "under the banner of truth and philanthropy," Logan invoked ideals so lofty and vast that they might be dismissed as having little relation to the often self-serving world of medical reform. But in fact, the assembled physicians who heard his words would have understood them to convey a specific message and charge. It was their philanthropic duty—an obligation of their calling—to disclose deception both outside and inside the ranks of the regular medical profession. "It becomes the duty of the honest and philanthropic physician, not only to adhere, *himself*, to the strictest principles of moral rectitude, in the prosecution of his professional duties, but also to use all honorable means in his power, to expose and suppress professional intrigue and dishonesty, under whatsoever garbs they may present themselves, and by whomsoever practiced," a student of Bartlett's at Transylvania wrote in his 1844 M.D. thesis, titled "The Moral Responsibilities and the Proper Qualifications of the Physician." "It is his duty, as a guardian to society, to expose popular humbugs that are often gotten up in the profession," he urged. "All such deceptions are, as I conceive, *dishonest*, and in the highest degree degrading to the medical profession; and lasting odium and disgrace should be branded upon the character of all who are guilty of such high handed imposture." Equally, he continued, the physician "should consider himself morally obligated to detect and expose that monster in the profession called *quackery*, in all its shapes and under all its clokes of disguise—whether found in *high places* or among the lower orders of those who style themselves *doctors of medicine*." All this, he insisted, was "the duty of the physician as a philanthropist."[103]

Viewed in this context, the language used by the American disciples of Louis in portraying their mentor, formulaic and repetitive as it was, appears unmis-

takably calculated to depict him as the epitome of an emergent American archetype: the honest or true physician. Louis, as Jackson, Jr., described him, was
"the most respectable and honest *truth-seekers* of the age."[104] Bartlett, on revisiting Louis in Paris in 1846, eulogized the French clinician as one who had
spent his life "not in barren speculation, but in . . . a love for truth, which no
temptation can alienate, which no passion or interest can corrupt, and which
no obstacle can turn aside." Louis, as Bartlett depicted him, was the antithesis
of the confidence man, an embodiment of those characteristics that best represented the true physician. "If honesty of purpose, straight-forward, unbending
integrity; simplicity of character, and the highest and purest combination of
personal and social qualities, can constitute legitimate titles to our veneration
and love," Bartlett asserted, "no claims can be stronger than those of Louis."[105]

The Louisian program pursued by his American disciples was couched in
similar terms. When Jackson, Jr., proclaimed his intention to emulate Louis's
labor "to *learn* and not to *invent truth*," he not only consecrated himself to
empirical observation and truth seeking but also denounced all who created
enticing but empty illusions.[106] Deploring Broussais and the misguided efforts
of all system-builders, Jackson told his father that "the vain attempt to *invent
truth* is to be fol$^d$ by an attempt, wh. I hope & believe will not be so unsuccess-
ful, to *discover it*."[107] Jackson praised his codisciples by singling out in them
those features he most revered in Louis: he wrote of Gerhard, Pennock, and
Ashbel Smith that "they are all honest and intelligent observers . . . [who] will
represent truth," and of Bowditch as one "whose mind & talents & eminent
*virtue* (I mean honesty), love of truth for its own sake together with a due
degree of rigour in pursuing it I prize daily more & more."[108] Jackson proudly
counted himself as an initiate of a congregation "all inspired with the holy
desire to discover truth," confident in the admonition of his master, Louis:
"'Seek & you shall find.'"[109]

In the American context, then, divergent epistemological positions took on
distinct moral valences. Those physicians who advocated the program for epistemological reform they had witnessed in France, and others in America who
took it up, framed it above all as a campaign to seek truth and expose falsehood. Moreover, by systematically associating empiricism with truth and rationalism with falsehood, they implicitly identified these polar epistemological
positions with good and evil, respectively. The mystification of medical knowledge was not merely misguided but morally wrong, not least of all because it
sacrificed the lives of patients and blocked the pursuit of empirical truth that
alone could guide medical advancement. Reformers regarded the crusade
against the spirit of system as a moral crusade, and the homiletic language they
so often used reflected the way they understood the task at hand. It was their
conviction that programs for epistemological change bore moral meaning that
endowed their proselytism with moral legitimacy, beneficence, and philanthropic selflessness, as well as an underlying sense of mission that was more
than merely metaphorical.

The rhetoric of empiricism was in part designed to impel action, to drive a
program of reform that would improve regular medicine and expose antiortho-

dox medicine as humbug. Yet it was designed to reassure as much as to convert or reform. It served an important symbolic function for reformers by affirming that they had identified a key source of the profession's ills and a remedy to meet them.

The language of honesty and deception, authenticity and imposture, truth and falsehood offered physicians a vocabulary and set of images for talking about rationalism and empiricism in ways at once gripping to their listeners and compelling to themselves. But their use of that language also points to the wider meaning they found in the program for epistemological change as a vehicle for articulating, understanding, and acting on anxieties pervasive in their culture. Regarding their enterprise this way helps clarify why the American physicians who traveled to France so ardently took up empiricism in the first place and why reformers so urgently proselytized for it in America. An ideal of empirical truth held out comfort and hope to orthodox physicians who saw their professional world being pulled apart at the seams. It offered to the American disciples of the Paris School and others who adopted its epistemological message a way not only to uplift their profession from its degraded position but also to bring order and meaning to their own lives.

## WHAT MADE REGULAR EMPIRICISM DIFFERENT?

The peculiar social and cultural standing of empiricism in antebellum America empowered it in multiple ways, making an allegiance to it seem a promising avenue to reform that was singularly resilient in the face of popular criticism. And yet everybody who practiced medicine in nineteenth-century America claimed experience as a sanction for their ideas and practices. Even those denounced as the rankest speculators by Paris-returned physicians—be they professionally eminent system-builders such as Benjamin Rush or pridefully unlettered antiprofessionals such as Samuel Thomson—confidently asserted that their medical explanations and therapies grew from experience and were validated by success in practice. As one New Hampshire physician wrote to Bartlett in 1847, "Sometimes I long for the appearance of a good strong-headed, fearless exposition of the medical twaddle which under the name of Experience, flows in such streams from the press."[110] How, then, did the American physicians who had studied in Paris make French empiricism—*their* empiricism—distinctive? How did they distinguish regular empiricism and their ideal of empirical truth from all the other medical empiricisms on the American market?

In part, as chapter 5 showed, while the American disciples of the Paris School celebrated the newness of French empiricism, they at the same time asserted its special legitimacy by linking it to a medical tradition extending back to the Hippocratics. This was important partly because it framed French empiricism as a learned, cultured empiricism, something to be scrupulously distinguished from the empiricism of the host of upstart medical "empirics" who claimed that experience was on their side. Indeed, the long-standing identification of the "empiric" with the charlatan and of empiricism with quackery placed regular physicians in a troubling semantic quandary. Orthodox physicians who proclaimed the empiricist faith, disturbed by the common use of the term *empiric* as a derisive epithet for the quack, sometimes explicitly urged their colleagues to call unqualified healers and mountebanks something else. Thus a medical student at the University of Pennsylvania wrote his M.D. thesis to assert "the importance of Empiricism to the Scientific Physician" and "to protest against the use of a word whose definition comprehends so much that is useful, and which defines the very foundation of true Medical Knowledge"— "that word is Empiric, and is used in this sense as synonymous with Quack, Charlatan, Imposter &c." He urged that *empiricism* be reserved for regular medicine, and, as for the irregular physician, "call him ignoramus, but not an Empiric."[111] Some regular practitioners resorted to terms such as "scientific empiricism" or "rational empiricism" in an effort to distinguish professionally respectable empiricism from its more sordid alternatives: the modifier *rational*, in this case, referred not to any epistemological position but was intended only to indicate that this empiricism was reliable, proper, not irrational. Even if "rational empiricism" seems an oxymoron, its use pointed to the concerted effort by regular physicians to lay claim to a professionally reputable empiricism methodologically and morally distinct from the mere experience of their competitors.[112]

The observation of nature that the American disciples of the Paris School claimed as the core of *their* empiricist program was to be direct, but not naive. "Observation is, to a considerable extent, a matter of method and training," Stillé insisted, demanding "a cultivation of the senses."[113] It required a trained eye, ear, and hand—in other words, an education of the senses. Beyond training the student how to observe, though, regular medical education was to inculcate revulsion for the seductive but false charms of rationalism and a resolute allegiance to honest, empirical observation. The experience of the regular-bred physician, accordingly, would have a character quite different from the experience of the untutored pretender, however much both claimed nature alone as their guide.

A regular education also gave the physician mastery of the technical and conceptual tools central to the French program for making and analyzing empirical observations, tools such as the stethoscope, the scalpel, and the numerical method. Their full exercise could not be limited to the domestic bedside, and therefore the empiricism regular physicians claimed was further distinguished by the locus of its exercise. Regular physicians, like all medical practitioners, said that their knowledge came from experience at the bedside of the sick; but they further claimed a knowledge of the natural history of disease that could be derived only from experience in a clinic. The wards and autopsy room of a hospital were physical spaces separate and distinct from the sites of domestic healing.

The adherents of regular empiricism also were expected to have a command of such sciences as physiology, pathology, and especially anatomy. Empirical study of normal and pathological anatomy was at the heart of the French program for medicine, and mastery of these sciences and their techniques was frequently invoked to distinguish the "true physician" from the "empiric." Anatomical dissection and the special access both to the body and to experiential knowledge it exemplified was a particularly powerful wellspring of the physician's identity. At a local medical society meeting in 1834, for example, the speaker began by acclaiming the turn away from rationalistic systems: "Truly medical men dream no longer over favourite & long standing theories—They are content to adopt the surer course, to read nature in her operations, & compel her to give up her secrets to the persevering inquiries of her votaries." He went on to defend anatomical dissection as an essential and distinguishing feature of the regular physician; "without it a physician is a disgrace to himself, a pest in society, & would maintain but a level with steam & red pepper quacks." Even here, though, the speaker took care to assert that the fruit of anatomical study—although special knowledge that required labor to master—was no mystery but knowledge laid open. That, indeed, was an argument against legal restrictions on human dissection. "Light is every day breaking forth upon the subject," he told the assembly of physicians. "Free discussion has got hold of it, & truth will appear. Truth loves light, it invites investigation."[114]

However confident the American followers of French medicine were that their empiricism was special, and however sturdy their faith that it was inaugurating a new era in medicine, throughout the antebellum period they anguished over the fact that its virtues lay more in future promise than in demonstrated results. This perduring anxiety was expressed in what bordered on an obsession with medical certainty. One comfort enjoyed by the dogmatic systematist, orthodox or antiorthodox, was a sense of certainty that, albeit false, was reassuring. "In quackery uncertainty is perhaps all that is doubted," one medical student quipped.[115] As empiricists tore down the edifices of rationalism, they were often left with a disconcerting sense of instability—an underlying suspicion of all medical knowledge that was a discouraging counterpoint to the exhilarating promise of disclosing truth through future labor. "Our poor Pathol$^y$ & yet worse Therapeutics," Jackson, Jr., wrote to his father; "shall we ever get to a solid bottom? shall we ever have fixed laws? shall we ever *know*, or must we be ever doomed to suspect & to presume? Is *perhaps* to be our qualifying word forever & foraye? Must we for ever be obliged to hang our heads when the Chemist & the Natur. Philosoph. ask us for our laws & principles? Must we ever blush to see the book of the Naturalist, his orders & his genera with their *characteristics invariable*, while we can point to no such equivalents?"[116]

Some boldly proclaimed that the French empiricist program was at last bringing certainty to medicine. "By a close attention to the disease during life, a careful record of the symptoms kept, and a *minute examination* of *the body after death*, the scientific physician was enabled to come to conclusions amounting to a certainty," an Albany student expressed a commonly held view in 1849.[117] It was doubtless with mixed reassurance that professors at the University of Nashville read in one student's M.D. thesis the confident assertion that medicine was attaining "almost mathematicle cirtainty."[118] Most regular physicians who addressed the issue did not claim that certainty was imminent, but argued that a commitment to empiricism would in time bring something authentic and lasting. What was singular about the empiricism Americans claimed for French medicine was that it would begin to establish empirically determined, certain truths in a medical world wherein all too often claims to experience were merely false fronts for alluring speculation, empty theorizing, or calculated imposture.

Bartlett's *Enquiry into the Degree of Certainty in Medicine* (1848) was the best-known assessment of the certitude vouchsafed by a thoroughgoing program of empiricism. In his empiricist brief of four years earlier, *An Essay on the Philosophy of Medical Science*, Bartlett was openly iconoclastic, applauding the leveling of systems. But in this treatise he was more at pains to identify what was emerging from the rubble.[119] After serving for years as mayor of the mill town Lowell, Massachusetts, Bartlett had become deeply disillusioned by political posturing. He shared the dismay of a friend who wrote in 1844 that with the downfall of Whiggery, "I never felt so sad in all my life," recognizing that "conservatism is at an end . . . & Rowdyism must rule."[120] While he had never stopped practicing medicine, after leaving the mayoralty Bartlett reimmersed himself in his profession, pursuing further study in New York and Boston, making a second tour of study to Paris in 1845, and increasingly devoting himself to medical teaching and writing. In writing his *Enquiry into the Degree of Certainty in Medicine*, Bartlett—no less than the French sensualist Cabanis had done on the eve of the French Revolution, in his 1788 essay later published as *Du degré de certitude de la médecine* (1798)—sought to reassert some measure of stability in a world in which medical, social, and political certainty all seemed to be slipping away.[121] At the same time, Bartlett's treatise was an assertion that French medical empiricism was more than merely an elite bludgeon for system bashing: it would lead to positive medical knowledge, to enduring truth.

Claims that the empiricist program would bring certainty to medicine carried the further assertion that regular empiricism, unlike the mere experience of other healers, was progressive. That was a key element in what regular reformers saw as its distinctiveness. Irregular experience was dismissed as unprogressive; as one physician writing to a lay friend about "botanics and eclectics" insisted, "Whatever may be said of the favourable treatment that is made by these irregulars in many cases,—there [sic] general tendency is the destruction of all enlightened progress in medicine."[122] The regular physician, on the contrary, was urged to recognize that (as a student at the University of Pennsylvania put it) "the science to which he has devoted himself is a progressive one."[123] Bartlett, addressing students in Lexington, proposed that "it seems to me that the chief cause and reason of slow progress and the want of certainty, positiveness and completeness, of medical science, in most of its departments, and especially in this of therapeutics, are to be found in the general prevalence, always, from the time of Hippocrates to our own day, of vicious and inadequate methods of investigation, growing out of a vicious and inadequate philosophy."[124] Empirical observation modeled after the French plan, he proposed, offered the pathway out of this situation.

To establish the promise of the empiricist ideal ultimately meant putting empiricism to work in programs of medical investigation. This was an aspiration shared by many of the Americans who had studied in Paris, eager to exercise the ideals they had taken up there. "I burn to do something," Jackson, Jr., wrote from Paris to a friend, "wh. will advance the science or that portion of it wh. I now love like life."[125] Jackson told his father, "I am bro't to think that the medical man's life may be *most usefully* spent in the collection of facts," and went on to explain that "it can be done, well done, scientifically done but in one way. Numerous histories of the lives of individuals fr. the uterus to the grave must be carefully collected. . . . This cannot be done by one man—there must be a society, a body of men, all impressed c̄[um] *the difficulty of observing well*, all impressed c̄[um] a sense of its importance, all feeling & knowing that without it we *cannot* reach truth." As he went on to describe his fantasy, he asked his father, "Suppose there were ten of us in Boston & its environs who shd. thus associate & observe carefully during ten years or twenty? We begin with the child" who are born under our care: each of us keeps a record of all thus belonging to him: these records are to be copied by a clerk into a book wh. is the property of the society. Each month we meet together: the subject of the ev'g is the additional material during the past month wh. appears upon the pages of our book." Over time, he continued, all of the illnesses of this population would be observed and recorded, collectively informing a morbid natural history "not painted by the imagination, but rigorously deduced fr. facts." The younger Jackson went on to imagine the expansion of the society, from Boston, to Philadelphia, New York, and thence to European cities. "Wld. there not be truth & useful truth there?—to set such a wheel in motion, wld. it not be to have been useful?"[126]

Jackson recognized that his plan was, as he termed it, "utopian," and two days later scrawled at the end of his grand scheme: "On read^g over these pages, I am almost tempted to burn them."[127] What his plan exemplified, though, was the longing felt by many of the Americans who traveled to France to validate its program by putting it into practice at home. More often than not their ambitions were blocked, even when their plan for investigation was on a scale vastly more modest than what Jackson envisioned. "I am collecting medical observations," Ashbel Smith wrote to Jackson in 1834, "but I have not time to digest and compare them for *my own* improvement—to appear as an author, I have no ambition. Last winter I dissected with great care 7 bodies. I neglected my patients and they grumbled; this winter my scalpel has not tasted dead flesh."[128] Bassett, having returned from Paris to Huntsville, lacked access to even a tiny clinic and so instead expressed the passion for empirical investigation he had acquired in Paris by keeping meticulous meteorological records and systematically correlating changes in climate with his empirical observations of the region's diseases.[129] What is most striking is not how little in the way of concrete results those who took up the empiricist banner produced so much as the dogged devotion they brought to what was often an arduous and discouraging endeavor.

Jackson had little opportunity to fulfill his aspirations, for he died soon after his return to Boston. His mantle fell partly to his friend Gerhard, as did their joint plan to translate Louis's treatise on phthisis. "I still consider myself as pledged to continue the translation of Dr Louis work," Gerhard wrote to Jackson, Sr., only a few weeks after returning from Paris, in his letter of condolence. "Both your son and myself had regarded that work as the first of a series of joint efforts to extend sound pathological views in America, this design is frustrated but it is still a consolation for me that our names will be associated with that of a teacher so much beloved by us both."[130] Gerhard did manage to win clinical posts in Philadelphia that gave him the kind of facilities for investigation— limited though they were—that few Americans enjoyed, as others relentlessly pointed out in reminding him of the responsibility he had to put them to good use.[131] "I continue my observations at our little hospital although I regret much the slender materials I possess and the difficulties wh seem inseparable from observation in this country," he wrote to Jackson, Sr., the following year, describing case reports he had submitted for publication. "These reports from our own hospitals will attract the attention of American physicians more than the observations collected at Paris against which there is an absurd feeling of distrust."[132] Gerhard's investigations would lead to important results, including confirmation of the distinction Louis had drawn between typhoid fever and typhus fever, prompting one New Orleans medical editor in 1846 to designate Gerhard "the Louis of America."[133]

The American physicians who took up the French ideal of empirical truth left little doubt that fundamental differences distinguished their medical empiricism from everyman's and everywoman's medical experience. They recognized, however, that ultimately the American program of empirical observation patterned after a French model would be judged by its fruits. This recognition, in turn, redoubled the significance they attached to what Stillé called "the sincere and honest investigator of nature"[134] and reinforced the underlying sense that research was a philanthropic activity. The realities of antebellum American society gave Paris-returned physicians only limited opportunities to devote themselves to a life of research. But that should not obscure the fact that many of them, no less than the more renowned Germany-returned American researchers of the final decades of the century, invested medical investigation with a distinct sense of mission. Even if pure research had little place as a career option in the medical world of antebellum America, it was with unreserved admiration that in 1834 Gerhard could write to Jackson, Sr., of Louis's consecration to what Gerhard called "pure science."[135]

## COMPARATIVE PERSPECTIVES ON IDENTITY AND REFORM

American and English reformers selectively lionized the features of the Paris School that they believed were most likely to elevate the profession in their own country while passing lightly over other aspects that were either undesirable or irrelevant to the possibilities and needs of their professional culture. What they did select out of French medicine points to broader national differences in expectations about professional reform and assumptions about professional identity. Viewed within its European context, one of the most arresting features of English medicine was its freedom from state regulation; yet viewed from the perspective of American comparison, English reformers' expectation that the state and its agents should to a considerable extent both define professional identity and effect change is unmistakable. English reformers looked more to legislated, structural solutions to the profession's problems. Americans, on the other hand, looked to France principally for cognitive and technical tools that would transform knowledge and most especially practice. They saw Parisian empiricism as a tool for improving performance in an open marketplace, with public approbation conferring prestige in a society that cherished the myth of egalitarianism. In approaching reform, they took for granted the notion that professional identity was not dependent on the state but turned above all on practice.

In studying professional reform in antebellum American medicine, historians have tended to focus on the institutional organization and formal structures of the profession—particularly medical schools, societies, and licensing. These are important; but this emphasis on institutions, professional organization, and the role of the state in attempts to understand antebellum reform is also somewhat Whiggish. It has been shaped by models of *professionalization* that have a strong teleological odor about them, and shaped by our knowledge of where dramatic professional elevation came from much later, especially during the Progressive Era. English-American comparisons draw attention to another reform tack at least as important to antebellum physicians but much less studied by historians. This was the distinctly American stress on uplifting the profession by transforming practice (and its epistemological underpinnings)—on changing not formal structures so much as individual thought and behavior.

This American approach to professional reform was empowered by a conception of professional identity also rooted in practice, and it too deserves closer scrutiny. Regular doctors obviously did not share the antiprofessional animus of their critics, nor were they willing to concede that all people were equally able to interpret the secrets of nature. They did agree with their assailants, however, that relying on direct experience of nature was the best guarantee of good practice. They also agreed that the theoretical edifices of rationalistic medicine were dangerous and must be torn down. Most of all, though—and to an extent that may have been singular to American medicine—they agreed that practice, not the possession of or access to special knowledge, was the most crucial source of a medical practitioner's authority and identity.

Historians have long stressed a tension between the democratic allegiances of antebellum society and the aspirations of the professions for distinction and special privilege, and to the extent that professional identity was enhanced by membership in an exclusive society, possession of an M.D. degree, or licensing, this is fitting. Yet from the perspective of English comparison, American medical reformers, living in a society in which the power of class was more covert, embraced a concept of their identity and authority as professionals that was in considerable harmony with egalitarian ideals. Using French empiricism as a vehicle for improving knowledge and practice, regular physicians believed, could bring uplift in a society prepared to honor natural merit but antagonistic to artificial distinctions in rank. For antebellum American physicians, in contrast to their English counterparts and American descendants, the definition and authority both of the profession and of each individual physician came not primarily from a place assigned by any formal structure or certification, but from practice.

This singular rooting of American professional identity in practice is largely why epistemology—the French ideal of empirical truth and disparagement of system—seemed so promising to those antebellum physicians who sought to reform and elevate the medical profession. Yet, as the next chapter will show, it also made certain other aspects of French medicine deeply threatening, and made sorting out the relationship between science and healing an especially freighted task for the American disciples of the Paris School.

# Science, Healing, and the Moral Order
# of Medicine

AMERICAN and English observers, however much they differed in assessing French models of medical polity and epistemology, were in remarkable agreement in their evaluation of another aspect of French medicine—the performance of the Paris clinicians as healers. Both the Americans and the English insisted that the French were inferior as healers and that their inferiority stemmed from a flawed value system. This French model was not to be emulated, even selectively, but to be denounced and shunned. Instead of promising professional uplift it threatened corruption, and even those who gave their hearts and minds to French ways took seriously the task of avoiding its taint.

What in 1824 one British practitioner in Paris characterized in his diary as "the feebleness of French practice" was a routine theme in English depictions of the performance of the French as healers.[1] In England, both critics of the Paris School and others who extolled its scientific achievements maintained that, as one English practitioner modestly put it, "we are indisputably the best practitioners in the world."[2] Often praise for French science was followed by cautions against its practice. "It is remarkable that, with all the light to be derived from morbid anatomy, the treatment of disease should be so deplorably bad in that country," one English practitioner charged.[3] French clinicians were stereotyped as ardent in their desire to understand disease but apathetic in their efforts to cure. "I thought the French students more curious to know precisely the situation of the disease than interested in its treatment," one practitioner visiting Paris in 1828 wrote home. "Indeed, they seem to think that the perfection of medicine consists not so much in keeping patients alive as in foretelling with precision the appearances which will be found after death."[4]

American physicians, the focus of this chapter, generally concurred that the English surpassed the French as healers, asserting all the while that Americans surpassed them both. Yet, far more than the English, Americans attached an element of danger to the model of healing witnessed in France. Nationalistic chauvinism informed both English and American appraisals, but Americans further projected onto their image of French patient care a broader wariness of Old World corruption. To the American practitioner—whose professional identity was rooted more in practice than in institutional or legal structures—falling too deeply under the sway of French values threatened to vitiate performance at the bedside and character as a physician. And to the American reformer—who sought to uplift the profession by improving the practice more than by altering polity—this French model threatened to undermine efforts at professional elevation.

Americans in Paris devoted considerable energy to depicting the evils to be avoided and gave more attention than did the English to denouncing the French clinicians' brutality, lack of interest in actively curing disease, objectification of the sick, and valuation of knowledge over healing. After their return, they were on guard against displaying French traits that might signify deeper corruption. In expressing their Parisian commitments as investigators and healers, they took pains to reassure others and themselves that they had avoided the double risk of being suborned by the French example—the risk, that is, of being converted from a true physician into a mere natural historian or into a therapeutically feeble skeptic. It was their arbitration between the ideals of the Paris School and the realities of American society that for the first time made the tension between the physician's identity as healer and identity as scientist salient in the American context. This was the moment when the trope of the heartless medical scientist became established in American culture, where it has occupied a prominent place ever since, and when concern over transforming patients from subjects of healing efforts into objects of scientific scrutiny started to become a central theme in anxieties over the conduct of American medicine.

## THE SPECTER OF FRENCH HEALING

The Americans who traveled to France made it clear that medical therapeutics had neither drawn them across the Atlantic nor become any part of what they wanted to take home. "I am far from being disappointed in the estimate I had formed of the capacity of the French physicians in discovering the exact seat of disease under the most complicated appearances; their skill is truly wonderful," James Cabell wrote from Paris in 1837; "but I have little confidence in their application of remedies."[5] Some aspects of French clinical practice, especially diagnosis and surgical technique, won American acclaim. But despite diversity and change over time in French practice, and notwithstanding occasional exceptions (American Broussaisists routinely praised topical bleeding by leeches, for example),[6] American observers generally repudiated the medical therapeutics of their French mentors. Over time their perception of French medical treatment became both stylized and routinized, informed as much by their expectations as by anything seen through their own eyes. Thus in 1855, a newly arrived American wrote home with an air of assurance that his compatriots could learn much in Paris about diagnosis, "but in the treatment we are much better physicians than the French, and have as a general rule little to learn from them which would not be better learned at home."[7]

Sustaining this perception was a central tenet of antebellum medical thought, namely, that treatment had to be specifically matched not to diseases but to patients and environments, individually fitted to age, gender, ethnicity, class, occupation, and moral status, as well as to climate, topography, and population density. Indeed, disease-specific treatment implied a routinism that was a sure sign of quackery. Diagnosis could suggest therapeutic plans, but the same disease might demand opposite treatments in different environments or in different individuals. This belief meant that native born and immigrant, African American and European American, private and hospital patient, Northerner and Southerner, American and European all had different therapeutic needs.[8]

Treatment appropriate for the inmates of French city hospitals, accordingly, would be inappropriate in managing the ills of most Americans. Just as American physicians assumed that therapeutic knowledge suitable for one part of the United States might be inapplicable in another, they had long held that the therapeutic requirements of North Americans differed from those of Europeans. Since the late eighteenth century, the belief that American constitutions and diseases were more robust than those of Europeans had been firmly entrenched in American thinking. Benjamin Smith Barton, for example, echoing the views of Benjamin Rush, his predecessor at the University of Pennsylvania, told his students in 1815 that the same disease that demanded depletion in Americans, to drain off excess energy, in enfeebled Europeans ordinarily required the opposite, stimulation.[9] Thus a medical student attending lectures in Lexington in 1828 copied into his class notebook his professor's direction that for treating inflammation, "In *Paris* we would stimulate by Porter, Bark &c— In Kentucky we would bleed & purge."[10]

More significant still was fact that Americans witnessed French practice only in large urban hospitals where both physical conditions and the socioeconomic class of patients bore little resemblance to the case of American patients attended in their own homes. The conviction that cities remolded constitutions and their diseases, though encouraged by antiurbanism, was solidly based upon principles that all American physicians—rural and urban—shared. They further argued that the treatment of American hospital patients—debilitated by poverty, inadequate diet, and degraded habits—was ill-suited to managing the ills of Americans seen in private practice.[11]

Even the sick poor who peopled hospitals in the United States, American physicians insisted, required treatment different from that given the patients who filled the Paris clinics. The therapeutic needs of Americans could not be extrapolated from hospitalized French men and women, those drawn, as Charles Caldwell, recently returned from Paris, told his medical class at Transylvania in 1841, "from the very dregs of society[,] a class whose constitutions have been depraved by intemperance and want, and modified by vice, habit and climate until they possess no analogy in constitution or disease to any class in our own country."[12] In voicing such a perception, Americans were making a point as much about the political and social order of their own country as about French practice. The Mississippi physician and racial theorist Samuel A. Cartwright carried this thinking one step further, drawing on observations he had made in France to assert in 1853 that southern slaves were hale and hardy compared with the poor of Paris. "The treatment best adapted to the diseases of the half-starved paupers of the European hospitals, is so little applicable to our full-fed negroes, as to drive their owners from all those doctors who pursue such a practice in the treatment of their people. Not because they dislike European learning, but because their negroes die under it."[13] Cartwright's political argument, reflecting his pro-slavery radicalism, was heterodox even within the South. But the medical point he was making was commonplace: French therapeutics could be harmful at the American bedside.

Surgery was a different matter, for antebellum Americans not only admired the skill of Parisian surgeons but also believed that unlike medical therapeutics, the mechanical aspects of surgical therapeutics studied in Paris could be transported and applied to American patients in American environments. Yet the broader treatment of patients by surgeons in the Paris hospitals left most American observers profoundly uneasy. "It is astonishing that the French who excell so much in the science of medicine should be so far behind in practice," Henry Bryant told his father in 1843, having seen two operations for femoral hernia shortly after reaching Paris. "I have no wonder that so many of the patients die[,] I only am astonished that any of them live."[14]

French medical therapeutics was far from monolithic, and Americans studying in Paris recognized diversity among the prescribing habits of French clinicians. Yet the overarching and enduring feature of French practice, as American observers depicted it, was skepticism about the value of interventionist medical treatment and a promotion of expectant method—*médecine expectative*—that gave primacy to the healing power of nature. "The *expectante* system is almost universally prevalent, in the management of cases of every description," F. Peyre Porcher wrote from Paris home to South Carolina in 1852, while George Suckley similarly wrote to New York on "the prevalence of the 'let alone treatment.'"[15]

In the appraisal of most American observers, however, the Paris clinicians were not just practicing in ways better suited to France than to America: they were inept as healers. Americans doubted that the mild expectant plan was sufficiently vigorous even for French patients, leading one to pronounce the practice he observed in Paris "more successless than that pursued in any other *cultivated* portion of the globe." But, as he asserted, while "French practice *may* cure French *men*; it *kills* Americans."[16] Having witnessed the French clinicians at work during his recent visit to Paris, Joshua Flint informed his students at the Louisville Medical Institute in 1838 that their practice was "inert, lame and inefficient, to a degree surprisingly in contrast with the show of science and research which appears in their writings." He insisted that "I am not an advocate for the heroic practice," but protested that French therapeutics represented "the other extreme, a reprehensible impotence of curative appliances, which is sometimes quite as mischievous. I defy any unprejudiced, sagacious, experienced physician to follow the medical clinic of the Parisian hospitals, and mark the prevailing inactivity of the treatment pursued, without being tempted to apply to it, over and over again, the sarcastic definition of the Roman empyric, 'a meditation on death.'"[17] Even the most ardent disciples of the Paris School maintained that in medical therapeutics the French were inferior: "impotent" and "useless" were among the adjectives Jackson, Jr., selected in writing privately to his father.[18] Thus the author of a book promoting the benefits of Parisian study qualified his admiration by stating in a footnote, "I do not allude to any advantages to be gained from a knowledge of French *practice*, for I believe that our own systems of treatment are, in most respects, far superior to those pursued by the majority of the French faculty."[19] As Levin Joynes summed up in a letter from Paris to his family, "It is believed very generally that the French doctors know how to discover and observe disease, but not how to cure it, and that the surgeons are a sort of butchers who are good only for cutting."[20]

Yet the Americans who studied in Paris did not merely dismiss the Parisian model of healing. Unlike certain aspects of French polity, for example, on which Americans commented but did not dwell, the behavior of the Paris clinicians as healers occupied a central position in American reports. And *this* French model they derided as offensive to American sensibilities. The moral judgment they passed on French healing grew not so much from the perception of Parisian therapeutic efforts as weak and ineffectual in themselves as from the suspicion that therapeutic ineptitude was an outward sign of a deeper perversion in values.

What is remarkable about the American depiction of the moral order of the Paris Clinic is its uniformity across a wide spectrum of American physicians and its durability over time. From the 1810s into the 1860s, both critics and champions of French medicine largely shared a vision of a Parisian clinical world in which the relationship between knowledge and healing was in some measure corrupt. Critics of the French presence in American medicine who had observed practice in the Paris hospitals for themselves sometimes portrayed publicly and gleefully what committed American disciples were likely to mention privately and perhaps ruefully; but the most prominent features in their portrait of encounters between doctor and patient in the Paris hospitals were strikingly consistent. For American critics, the perception that the Paris clinicians who were touted as the best medical scientists in the world were also among the worst healers was an effective vehicle for assailing the wider French impulse in American medicine. For the disciples of the Paris School, who drew different lessons from similar premises, it was a source of troubling questions about the nature of French medical science, the meaning of its cultivation in America, and their own identity as American physicians.

French clinicians, as Americans portrayed them, by and large placed little value on preventing suffering or preserving life. Americans criticized the French physicians they observed for the "barbarous indifference to pain and risque inflicted on his patients."[21] At the same time, they broadly shared the perception that "the French set, in the abstract, a lower estimation of life, and are therefore more regardless of saving it, than any other people," and that "hence the struggle of the practitioner to triumph over disease is neither eager nor obstinate."[22] Surgeons in particular were depicted as brutally indifferent to guarding their patients' lives. "Life is very little esteemed in this city," Robert

Peter wrote from Paris to his wife in 1839. "The great hospitals here—are no better than charnel houses and butcher shops—Thousands die and (and are dissected) from common surgical cases—One man operates on women, who never saves a case; and in the greatest hospitals, five out of a hundred of the cases of common amputations, only—are saved."[23] While the introduction of anesthesia in the 1840s in some ways transformed the image of surgery, it did not fundamentally alter American judgments on French surgical brutality. "Maisonneuve is a perfect rusher—a stunner—a butcher," William Williams Keen wrote from Paris to his parents in the mid-1860s. "If he killed a man I verily believe he wd think 'oh! well! its only 1 more Frenchman less. There are 35,000000 more left.'"[24]

Such attitudes, Americans widely maintained, enabled the French surgeons and physicians alike to regard patients as objects to be studied more than as subjects to be healed. Anson Colman, explaining the opportunities for study he was enthusiastically embracing, made this point in a private letter. "One circumstance which never occurred to me until I came to Paris, and one too which has an immense effect in multiplying the advantages which Physycians derive here," he explained to his wife, "is the great redundancy of population, and the consequent *cheapness*, or rather *the non importance of human life*!!—This gives every opportunity for investigating diseases; of experimenting; of operating; of examining them in their minute details every morbid condition to which life is incident; and finally when the poor devils make their final exit, [they] are, as a matter of course the property of the Hospitals in which they died for the purpose of dissections."[25] Caldwell, a critic of all things European, displayed a more vituperative polemical aim when, making much the same point, he sent home an open letter for publication in the *Western Journal of Medicine and Surgery*. In the Paris hospitals, Caldwell suggested, "true *disease-curing* and *life-preserving* medicine and surgery are but little known or regarded—most assuredly they are but little *practised*." There, "patients are received but to be *ausculted* and otherwise *diagnostically* treated, die and be *post-mortemized*, for the instruction of the *eleves*, *internes* and *externes*, and the improvement of the profession by furnishing the *material* for writers and printers—and there the process ends."[26]

Americans rhetorically underscored the doubtful propriety of this medical order by depicting treatment in the Paris Clinic as a theatrical event, as spectacle. Too often the aim of the doctor-patient encounter seemed to be extravagant display rather than healing. And just as Americans sometimes reported on the seedy character of French theater and its habitués (casting themselves in the detached role of outside observers), so too they expressed their uneasiness about the clinical scenes they witnessed partly by casting them in the language of theatrical production. Surgeons were portrayed as caring chiefly about flaunting dexterity and manual skill, not exercising their power to heal. "With finished tact and adroitness, and, with the utmost show of every thing but *feeling*, the instruments are flourished, and the operation performed," Caldwell wrote in 1841, describing what he had seen in Paris, "and the patient (all at least that remains of him) is promptly removed, that the table may be ready for the reception of another, who is similarly dealt with—and thus—until the drama of the morning is closed." As he insisted, "The surgeon is satisfied with a dextrous and showy operation, though the subject of it should die."[27]

Regarded as a medical tableau staged for the act of healing, such a surgical performance had something counterfeit about it, captivating but hollow. As historian Martin Pernick has shown, Americans accepted the infliction of pain in surgical operations as warranted by the potential good done for the patient, an ethically sound trade-off.[28] Parisian surgery, however, appeared all the more morally problematic and brutal precisely because the suffering of the patient went unredeemed by the aspiration to cure. "The operation, as a spectacle, seems barbarous," New York physician George Suckley wrote from Paris in 1858, describing an operation by Pierre-M.-E. Chassaignac he had attended.[29] Without healing as its leading objective, the drama played out in the surgical theater was at risk of being reduced to *mere* show.

Internal medicine was equally described in terms of theatrical display, but here the performances that seemed to be valued above healing were the physician's pronouncement of a diagnosis at the bedside and verification of it before an eager audience at the autopsy table. "It must strike every observer who walks in the hospitals of Paris, that the great ambition of her medical men seems too much absorbed with the desire to verify the justness of their *diagnosis* and *prognosis* by the *autopsies* and *post-mortem* examinations of their patients, rather than scrutinizing and seeking sedulously with unremitted vigilance for remedies for healing the maladies of the sick," Valentine Mott commented in 1842.[30] Describing the clinician Pierre-Aldolphe Piorry as "not simply an enthusiast on the subject of physical diagnosis, but a monomaniac," Edward Warren, who studied in Paris in the mid-1850s, noted that Piorry "seemed to think that the whole art of physic consisted in ascertaining the nature and the extent of lesions, and then in verifying the diagnoses by a *post mortem* examination. With the cure of disease he did not concern himself, leaving the result to nature alone." As Warren explained, "I have repeatedly seen him trace upon the surface [of the patient's body] the exact seat and the gradual extension of the malady, and then patiently await the conclusion, in order to demonstrate the correctness of his original diagram." Warren commented that "this system of *ante-mortem* delineation and *post-mortem* verification of pen-and-ink sketches upon the integuments of the *living* and scalpel demonstrations upon the organs of the *dead* always seemed to me the *ne plus ultra* of scientific infatuation, to say nothing of its cold-blooded cruelty"; Piorry, though, was rewarded by "the applause which was to greet the professor's final triumph as a diagnostician and a limner."[31]

The perception that French physicians tended to be satisfied with understanding disease made the French model of healing reprehensible in the eyes of most Americans. It was a conception of clinical duty that seemed premised on the disturbing assumption that the physician had no moral obligation to heal. The most devoted American acolytes of the Paris School perceived their mentors' scientific devotion and therapeutic apathy as a weakness in professional character. When Jackson, Jr., first witnessed Louis's practice, he was indignant at his preceptor's lack of interest in curing patients. In a letter from Paris that his father later published, the young Jackson praised highly Louis's clinical teaching and skill at arriving at a diagnosis. But before publishing the letter, the elder Jackson deleted his son's comment that after Louis made his diagnosis, "he finishes there—he is very weak at therapeut[ic]s, and is perfectly satisfied c̄[um] a correct diagn[osis]."[32]

Most troubling of all was the suspicion—articulated only by critics of the wider French impulse—that some French clinicians actively subverted healing to the interests of science. According to this view, the expectant method could represent purposeful avoidance of intervention with the aim of advancing the study of pathology. Thus Robley Dunglison, who had studied in Paris but was critical of the growing hegemony of French medicine in America, told his Philadelphia students in 1844 that among the French clinicians "regret was felt when the sick got well, as it disappointed them of opportunities for *post mortem* examination," and, further, "that the physician did not prescribe treatment in many cases, under the apprehension, that if he did, he might thereby disturb the *post mortem* appearances."[33] "In the Parisian hospitals," Henry H. Smith, just returned from Paris to his teaching post at another Philadelphia medical school, reported to his class in 1855, there was "often noticed such an intense devotion to mere scientific investigations, as causes the prescriber to forget the cure of the patient, in his anxiety to study the pathology of the complaint."[34]

Parisian surgeons were similarly criticized for trading the lives of patients for surgical knowledge and operative skill. "Their proportion of losses, in surgery particularly, is immense," Peter wrote from Paris in 1839. "Indeed, human life, is not esteemed of much value in the hospitals of Paris—an experiment is worth a dozen lives."[35] Philippe Ricord, for example, had contributed much to surgical knowledge, another American observed, but through "means of equivocal propriety" and "doubtful morality."[36] Echoing this view, M. M. Rodgers insisted that "although French instruments and manual dexterity stand unrivaled, . . . the end in this case does not sanctify the means." As he wrote from Paris in 1851, "The coolness with which fearful experiments are carried on for the purpose of establishing personal reputations and private theories is astonishing to anyone who is in the habit of placing any value upon human life, or feeling sympathy for suffering humanity."[37]

Americans, then, depicted a sinister image of clinicians whose enthusiasm as scientists suborned their identity as healers. If no single Paris clinician fully embodied the moral debasement they collectively projected onto this imagined heartless medical scientist, the French novelist and social reformer Eugène Sue came close in his portrayal of Dr. Griffon, physician to a large Paris hospital who appeared in Sue's novel *Les mystères de Paris* (1843). "The 'learned doctor,'" Sue narrates, "considered the wards as a kind of school of experiments . . . a human sacrifice made on the altar of science; but Dr. Griffon did

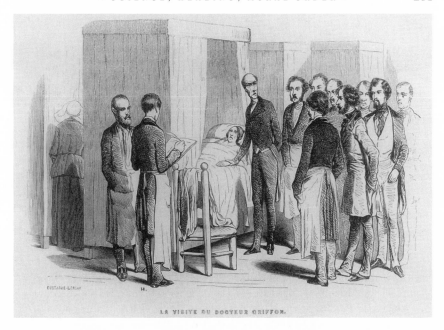

LA VISITE DU DOCTEUR GRIFFON.

Fig. 8.1. Dr. Griffon, a creation of the novelist Eugène Sue and shown here lecturing at the bedside in a Paris hospital, describes to students the postmortem appearances they will discover once the young woman patient dies. (From Eugène Sue, *Les mystères de Paris*, rev. ed. [1843; Paris: Charles Gosselin, 1844], 4 vols., vol. 3, between pp. 174 and 175.)

not think of that. In the eyes of this *prince of science*, as they say in our days, the hospital patients were only a matter of study and experiment." Followed by a band of students, he enters the ward with an acquaintance, the comte de Saint Rémey, who, distraught by the scene in front of him, is reproved by Dr. Griffon, "All these fine feelings must be left at the door. . . . Here we begin on the living those experiments and studies which we complete on the dead body in the amphitheatre." They proceed to the bed of an actress who has died overnight, where Dr. Griffon decides to "make a man happy" by allowing one of his students to dissect the woman's body rather than doing it himself. As the other patients look on, the delighted student uses a scalpel to incise his initials into the actress's arm, "to take possession," as Griffon puts it. As the ward rounds continue, the comte learns of a particularly murderous experiment Griffon proposes to conduct on one of his "subjects," a young girl. "If you were not a madman, you would be a monster!" the comte charges in despair. "'Confound the man! Why has he so much science?' said the count . . . 'Eh! It is simple enough,' said the doctor in a whisper. 'I have a great deal of science because I study, because I experimentalise, because I risk and practice a great deal on my *subjects*.'"[38]

Sue captured the imagination of American physicians who traveled to Paris after his immensely successful novel was published (and, soon, translated into English). "I have just finished the Mysteries of Paris by Eugene Sue and if the

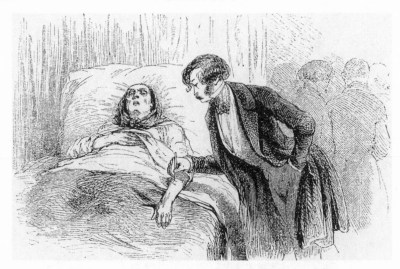

Fig. 8.2. In Eugène Sue's novel *Mysteries of Paris*, a medical student carves his initials into the arm of a dead actress, claiming her as his own for the dissecting table. (From Eugène Sue, *Mysteries of Paris*, 3 vols. [Paris, 1843; London: Chapman and Hall, 1846], 3:300.)

account which he gives of the state of morals in Paris is correct as he affirms it to be, the French must be the most utterly abandoned people on the face of the globe," Bryant, recently arrived in Paris, wrote in 1843 to his father. "I was almost frightened reading it for the scene is laid principally in the Cité and the Quartier Latin my future haunts. It is all the rage here[—]everything is mysteries de Paris, shawls and almanacks, hats and gingerbread."[39] Oliver Wendell Holmes, for his part, was incensed by the novel and its depiction of "heartless experiments" and "experimenting homicide." As revealing as his pique, though, was Holmes's belief that "Dr. Griffon may very probably stand for the founder of the numerical system," that is, his own mentor, Pierre Louis.[40] Whether or not Louis was Sue's model, many American physicians believed that the novelist's image of "the prince of science" devoid of the moral sensibilities they esteemed captured a disturbing reality. The image of the heartless medical scientist emblemized a corrupt value system in which the proper ranking of healing above knowledge was inverted.

## Brutalization and Character

To the American physicians who studied in Paris, this French model was not just deplorable but menacing—clearly to be left behind in Europe. Yet by the act of traveling to Paris for professional improvement, and even more by casting themselves as disciples of the Paris School, they were placing their character as healers at risk of being tainted. As much as they relished the opportunities Paris afforded them, a disturbing suspicion remained that through their relationship to the Paris clinicians they had placed themselves in the compromising role of collaborators. As Americans, they took comfort in the conviction that national traits distinguishing them from the French—especially practicality and sturdy morality—would preserve their integrity as healers intact. But they also realized that as students they were susceptible to the models set by their mentors and needed to be wary of falling under their sway. "A young man in Paris will need to be constantly on his guard, and be well fortified by sound general principles, to avoid the danger of *false science*," Rodgers warned in closing a letter from Paris to the *Buffalo Medical Journal* in 1851; "he must resist the allurements of show, and the eclat of '*cutting*,' or the community to whom he ministers the healing balm will have reason to regret his 'tour to Europe.'"[41]

To understand just how the specter of French healing threatened Americans studying in Paris, we must situate their apprehensions within the wider context of antebellum American assumptions about what made—and unmade—an effective healer. The link between scientific knowledge and the physician's professional identity was tenuous. Elite physicians valued their learning and often disparaged their ill-educated compatriots, those "who," as one critic put it, "know as much about Anatomy, Physiology, Pathology, Materia medica and Pharmacy, as a pet cat does about the battle of Waterloo."[42] But they recognized that scientific expertise was not a necessary criterion for membership in the regular profession. A respectable physician could remain ignorant of most natural science; thus in 1848 an eminent physician could tell those gathered for the first meeting of the Alabama State Medical Association that "we have no medical schools, no public libraries, nor large pathological collections or public infirmaries, to aid us in the cultivation of medical science," yet could go on without contradiction to say that "in all the practical branches of medicine at least, we have kept pace with our professional brethren in other parts of the country."[43] The knowledge required to sustain professional identity was knowledge about practice, what most physicians initially gained by apprenticeship and developed by experience at the bedside.

Conversely, as Daniel Drake admonished his medical class, "knowledge alone may make an able but cannot make a useful or acceptable physician";[44] it neither established identity as a regular physician nor guaranteed success as a healer. "The main purpose of the study of medicine," John Ware told his students at Harvard in 1850, "is to enable us to treat disease. This is the ultimate object, which is to be kept in view at every step." Warning against the pursuit of scientific knowledge for its own sake, he cautioned that a zealous student of anatomy, chemistry, or pathology might be an incompetent healer. "Of course it is desirable that he should be a perfect anatomist," Ware recognized; "but if he takes the time necessary to make himself a perfect anatomist, he may neglect what is necessary to make him a good practitioner."[45]

What was critical to the physician's image and performance was *character*. It was character that signified medical integrity and guaranteed correct behavior.

The American physician functioned within a medical marketplace in which, as one student astutely noted in his 1848 thesis, "his position is rather felt than defined."[46] Character earned patient confidence and gave the physician "the armor of *moral influence*, without which he is powerless to wield successfully the weapons of his art," as another student put it.[47] Elisha Bartlett, as a young practitioner freshly back from Paris to Lowell and scrambling to make ends meet, wrote optimistically to his father in 1828 that "a few years will place me above the fear of want.—I believe I can rely with confidence on the character I have gained and am gaining—and so long as *that* remains unimpaired I have little to fear."[48]

Medical education marked a critical period in the shaping of professional character, and, like education in general, was regarded as a morally transforming process. As a period of transition it was also seen as a time of danger— particularly subject to the influence of both fortifying and corrupting forces. "You are now upon that stage of life, where the formation of character is inevitable," Hardy Vickers Wooten advised students at the Memphis Medical College in 1853. "You have reached the forming point in your histories," he told them, and "whether the matter enlists your attention or not, your characters will nevertheless form, and your destinies be moulded, for good or evil."[49]

Brutalization was seen as an inbuilt danger of medical education. Professors warned their students to cultivate gentleness and a sympathizing spirit as counterbalances to the hardening influence of their professional studies, while records left by students themselves display sometimes acute reflection on the ongoing transformation in their own sensibilities. "The study of Medicine does have a manifest tendency to harden & corrupt the heart," Joseph Jones, studying in Philadelphia, wrote to his father in 1853. Spending every evening in the dissecting room, he reported, "renders our hearts liable to be corrupted and hardened," while it tended to "render the sensibilities Callous, [and] brutalize the feelings."[50] H.V.M. Miller, a professor of obstetrics in Tennessee, echoed this view when he cautioned students in 1847 that "anatomy, however indispensable it may be, tends certainly to freeze up the springs of human feeling, and destroy our sympathy for human suffering."[51] In the dissecting room students tended to forget that the body was more than an object, Ware warned Harvard students; yet "the influence exerted is so gradual, the change in our habits and feelings is so insensibly brought about, that we are not aware that it has taken place."[52]

The experience of human dissection was the most commonly cited example, but it was only one ingredient in a complex and subtle process. While a Charleston student agreed in his 1846 M.D. thesis, "The Effects of the Study and Practice of Medicine on the Mind and Character," that "the heart of the young student becomes tainted" by work at the dissecting table, he maintained that studying the sick poor in a charity hospital threatened a more profound "moral lethargy." "The frequent witnessing of diseases which are the result of libertinism, and hearing them spoken of by grey-headed men, without one word of moral remarks," left students "shocked and our senses disgusted, . . .

*blunted* and perverted." Reflecting on the consequences for the character of the future healer, he noted that "the medical student has to undergo trials which few or none pass through unscathed."[53]

Ultimately more brutalizing was the potential of an elite medical education to draw attention away from healing toward detached scrutiny of disease. Some students, Ware told his class, their character as true physicians still being molded, "become interested in the history of disease for itself alone." He cautioned that "there is danger of failing to keep constantly in mind its relation to practice; of regarding it too much as a mere scientific pursuit. This is a fault into which men of the highest education are perhaps most apt to fall. They acquire the habit of studying disease merely as an object of science."[54]

The threat of hardening often was cast as particularly dangerous for women, both by those who opposed women's medical education and by women physicians who based special claims to being *natural* healers in those putatively feminine characteristics held to be most imperiled by medical training. Both groups, historian Regina Morantz-Sanchez has argued, starting with similar premises about woman's nature, tended to embrace Victorian gender stereotypes that identified femininity with a refined moral sensibility and special capacities for caring, sympathy, and nurturing.[55] The conviction that there was some inbuilt danger of brutalization in medical education, a potential for blunting the moral senses and feelings of sympathy, threatened qualities of character that were a linchpin in the claim made by the first generation of women physicians to a special aptitude for healing. To opponents of the medical education of women—including physicians such as Ware, who earnestly warned his male medical students "to resist whatever may tend, in any degree, to diminish the tenderness, the delicacy, the purity of mind, which are so peculiarly required in the performance of our duties"—the hardening influence of medical education on women insured what in 1850 he called "defilement" of the "moral constitution."[56]

Ware's charge that women were peculiarly susceptible to the debasing influences of medical study was to be both extended and popularized in the second half of the century. Novelists who depicted women physicians and medical students seemed especially intrigued by their work in the dissecting room and keen to gauge the influence of that experience on delicate sensibilities. Thus the fictional medical heroine Ruth Bolton reacted with "nervous strain"; Atalanta Zay found that "the dissecting-room was a trial"; and Grace Breen judged parts of her medical training "almost insuperably repugnant."[57] Philadelphia author and humorist Charles Heber Clark took this a step further in *Out of the Hurly-Burly* (1874) by portraying Henrietta Magruder as a woman physician who, by successfully hardening herself, had been morally transformed. "Mrs. Dr. Magruder," as Clark presented her, is a professor at "the Woman's Medical College" in Philadelphia; "an enthusiast in the study and practice of medical science"; and "a woman of such force" that she effortlessly dominates her husband.[58] Mr. Magruder becomes suspicious when, repeatedly, he finds himself waking from his evening nap with "a peculiar feeling of heaviness in his head and a queer smell of drugs in the room." As the narrator puts it, "A horrible thought crossed his mind that Mrs. Magruder intended to poison him for his skeleton—to sacrifice him so that she could dangle his bones on a string before her class." He confides his suspicions to his brother, who hides in a closet as Mr. Magruder retires for his evening nap and his wife "pretended to have the 'sewing circle' from the church in the parlor."[59]

At nine, Dr. Magruder quietly climbs the stairs to the room where her husband lies sleeping, followed by the "sewing circle." Then,

> when the whole party had entered the room, Mrs. Magruder closed the door and applied chloroform to her husband's nose. As soon as he became completely insensible, the sewing in the hands of the ladies was quickly laid aside, and to Magruder's secreted brother was disclosed the alarming fact that this was a class of students from the college.[60]

The professor proceeds to lecture on her husband's nervous system, attaching a galvanic battery to him to demonstrate her points, and quizzes the students (who have spent their morning dissecting) about anatomy. Practice at therapy comes next: the pupils venesect his arm, cup his shoulder blades, and apply a mustard plaster to his back and leeches to his nose. The brother, watching from the closet all along, is especially apprehensive about the students' "hovering around Magruder's leg with a saw and a carving knife," but "the professor restrained these devotees of science," who, instead, merely "held out his tongue with pincers and examined it with a microscope." When the doctor begins to demonstrate the use of the stomach pump, Mr. Magruder suddenly revives and his brother bursts from the closet to tell all. The doctor and her "seekers after medical truth," the narrator ends the story, "said Mr. Magruder was a brute, and he had no love for science. But Mr. Magruder said that as for himself, 'hang science!' when a woman became so infatuated with it as to chop up her husband to help it along."[61]

Clark's story was one of burlesque, not the tragedy of, for example, Nathaniel Hawthorne's "The Birthmark" (1843), in which a man's compulsion to delve "into the heart of science" leads him to perform a fatal operation on his bride.[62] Yet his humor played on an invidious stereotype of the woman doctor hardened by medical study and bereft of the moral sensibility Victorian culture assigned to femininity, a stereotype reinforced by cartoon sketches published with Clark's text depicting Dr. Magruder with top hat and a full beard.[63]

The target of Clark's humor was a contested image, challenged particularly by women physicians who recognized the power of fictional representations to shape public expectation and perception.[64] Sophia Jex-Blake, for example, one of the first woman physicians in Britain and a leader of the movement there, later confronted this issue in her 1893 essay "Medical Women in Fiction," in which she concluded that "the *genus* medical woman" was ill-served by most of the novels she reviewed, whose heroines she thought unconvincing.[65] She found an appealing counterimage, however, in *Mona Maclean, Medical Student* (1892), a novel by Graham Travers (the pen name of Margaret Georgina Todd)

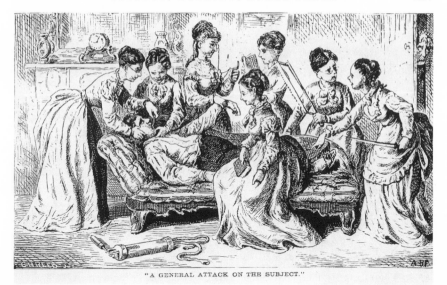

"A GENERAL ATTACK ON THE SUBJECT."

Fig. 8.3. Medical students from "the Women's Medical College" in Philadelphia perform experiments on the drugged husband of their professor, Dr. Henrietta Magruder. This satirical short story reflected deeper fears about the hardening, brutalizing potential of medical study, especially for women. (From Max Adler [Charles Heber Clark], *Out of the Hurly-Burly: or, Life in an Odd Corner* [Philadelphia: George Maclean and Co., 1874], chap. 5, pp. 68–84, on p. 77.)

she believed was "manifestly written *from the inside*."[66] To illustrate what earned her approval, Jex-Blake cited an exchange in which the twenty-five-year-old Maclean defends her pursuit of medicine to "an accomplished man of the world":

> "You must be becoming hard and blunted?" He looked at her as if demanding an answer. "I hope not," said Mona quickly, and her eyes met his. . . . "I don't think blunted is the word. It is extremely true, as some one says, that pity becomes transformed from a blind impulse into a motive." He seemed to be weighing this. "You dissect?" he said presently. "Yes." "Think of that alone! It is human butchery." "Of course you must know that I do not look upon it in that light. . . . It is difficult to discuss the question with one who is not a doctor" ("nor a scientist," she added inwardly).[67]

The perception that women students might be particularly susceptible to the hardening tendencies inherent in medical education gave women's medical educators special reason to insist that their graduates weathered the ordeal with moral character intact. As with other objections brought against women's medical education, they turned it around to show how anatomical dissection, properly regarded, fortified and refined the physician's moral sensibilities. At ceremonial gatherings held at women's medical colleges, orators routinely framed medical education as morally uplifting. "We know it has been objected

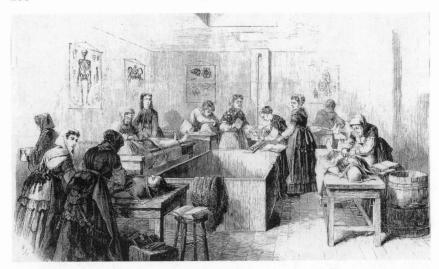

Fig. 8.4. Students dissecting at the New York Medical College for Women, as depicted in *Frank Leslie's Illustrated Newspaper*. This image of poised students in feminine dress, and the text that accompanied it, contested suspicions that a woman's character would be tarnished by medical study. (From "New York Medical College for Women," *Frank Leslie's Illustrated Newspaper*, vol. 30 [16 Apr. 1870], p. 73.)

that familiarity with such subjects as belong properly to the science of medicine, with anatomy and kindred studies, cannot fail to injure or destroy those feelings of delicacy and refinement which add peculiar lustre to the character of woman," Emeline H. Cleveland, professor of anatomy, told students assembled for her introductory lecture at the Female Medical College of Pennsylvania in 1858. The concern about the medical woman, which Cleveland stated in order to dispel, was "that her gentleness might give place to the characteristic boorishness of a *degraded* manhood."[68] As Cleveland elaborated her rejoinder, addressing students a decade later, "We feel sure that, on the contrary, you have found the study of Anatomy 'a hymn in honor of the creator,' . . . that the study of medicine has but strengthened your womanly feeling, your reverence for the Divine."[69]

When they published a defense of the New York Medical College for Women in 1870, accordingly, it was a deft choice on the part of editors at *Frank Leslie's Illustrated Newspaper* to feature three pages of drawings depicting women students at work in the dissecting room. Framed in a setting calculated to leave lay viewers squeamish, the confident, engaged, beneficent expressions on the dissectors' faces belied any suspicion that they had been morally debased. And lest some unobservant reader miss the point, the text recommended that studying these faces "will throw no little light upon the character of the persons engaged in following the course."[70]

Male physicians similarly argued that not all who studied medicine became hardened, and, sometimes using natural theological arguments, also drew attention to the potential of the dissecting table to uplift rather than degrade. "The heart is not hardened, nor the natural sympathies extinguished, by the exercise of a human art, although the hands may be bathed in blood," a Louisville professor encouraged his students.[71] Nevertheless, as a Philadelphia student wrote in his M.D. thesis, "The Formation of Medical Character," in 1840, the perception that "the study of medicine has a peculiar tendency to harden the disposition" made it particularly incumbent on students to cultivate an "affectionate sympathising spirit."[72] Most agreed that medical study did not *necessarily* harden the student; it did, though, have a potential for brutalization that in turn threatened to undercut the healer's character.

In Paris, antebellum Americans often were watchful for sources of danger and found much to write home about. Some of the hardening and brutalizing influences they confronted were ones they had already met while studying in America. But the scale and ease of access to the body in Paris intensified its assault on American sensibilities. Enraptured by the opportunities for anatomical dissection at the Clamart and the École Pratique, for example, Americans could also be troubled to find some denizens of those places "entirely hardened," devoid of reverence for the dead body. As Augustus Gardner described the "learned professor" at the dissecting table, "The blood and pieces of flesh upon the floor, he regards, as the sculptor does the fragments of marble lying round the unfinished statue."[73] Uneasy at seeing the body regarded as an object like any other, Henry Williams wrote from Paris in 1846 that "I saw among other operations a large tumor cut from the side of the neck of a most beautiful girl of twenty. After the operation was finished," he reported, "the Professor took the tumour, and instead of passing it gravely round the room for the examination of the students, as a Boston surgeon would have done, he cut it into five or six pieces, and tossed them round the room to so many different parts of the amphitheatre."[74] It was not without a sense of irony that Americans witnessed evidence of French *sang froid* in themselves, however. As Williams wrote to his sisters on his progress in dissecting, "C'est drole, n'est ce pas, qu'on peut être particulierement heureuse dans une salle ou il y a toujours vingt cinq cadavres?"[75]

Witnessing Parisian clinicians at the bedside could leave still deeper impressions. Observing Philibert-Joseph Roux at the Hôtel Dieu spit on his patient after a surgical operation led one observer in 1851 to write in his diary that the French surgeon's "unmanerly way of treating patients must be disgusting to every person of feeling."[76] Gardner, who witnessed the same behavior and accused Roux of "brutality," reported that "the outrage was observed by many who stood around, and the wanton violation of the feelings of a fellow-man, sunk deep into their hearts."[77] The worry for Americans was that instead of holding on to that sense of outrage and using it as a moral shield against such scenes, they would become inured to it—that if they repeatedly witnessed such displays, their character might be subtly transformed.

French treatment of women—in its perceived brutality, indifference to modesty, and insensitivity to suffering—particularly elicited American disgust.

Edward Warren recalled Antoine-Joseph Jobert de Lamballe at the Hôtel Dieu as "a surgeon of skill and dash, and his special infatuation was the cauterization of wombs. . . . He kept a supply of hot cauteries with which, through an ivory or horn speculum, he seared the cervix of every woman who entered his wards." In the mid-1850s, as Warren recounted, "twice each week he held his *grand clinics* in the amphitheater, at which he did this operation on so large a scale that the atmosphere of the room was rendered insufferable by the fumes and smoke of cauterized uterine tissues. . . . We called his *clinics* the 'barbecues' and his *daily cauterizations* the 'small fry,' while the surgeon himself was designated by the suggestive names of '*Le Chef*,' 'Old Griddle,' and 'Dr. Beelzebub.'"[78] Such practice Warren deemed "demoralizing," though he avowed that he had resisted its influence: "This was my first experience with gynoecologists, and it sowed the seeds of a prejudice against their specialty which time has only served to deepen and to intensify."[79]

The museological display of patients as pathological specimens in Parisian clinical teaching Americans found both singularly instructive and singularly troubling—an objectification of the sick, like the dead, that represented a clinical habit of mind to be actively resisted. "The French women," one American reported in 1857 on a touching course in midwifery, "resign themselves wholly into the hands of their physicians, and allow themselves to be stripped naked, and a diseased part examined, though the bed is surrounded by students. In labor the patient is wholly uncovered for the benefit of those around, and I have often seen more than fifty students watching this process of nature."[80] Describing Richard Liebreich's clinic on diseases of the eyes, a Connecticut physician wrote to his father that "two patients both women were selected from the *crowd* as illustrative of the subject of which he was to speak. They sat there, during the whole lecture, and finally were *passed* around the room, for us to examine." He added that "to an American," such a spectacle was "very repulsive."[81]

Americans also perceived a heart-hardening influence in the vivisectional demonstrations and experiments they witnessed in Paris. Just as Americans sometimes praised the clinicians as pathologists while denouncing their treatment of patients, so too they admired François Magendie as a physiologist while judging his vivisectional performances "cruel." Linton reported from Paris in 1840 that "his method is simply to pronounce his profession of faith, and then bring forward, or rather drag forward, as proofs, a parcel of poor dogs, that howlingly and unwillingly confirm it with their blood."[82] Writing home of a vivisectional demonstration on respiratory physiology he attended in 1836, Bassett described Magendie "as he stood, over a great big bitch, half flayed, & she kicking, while one of her puppies who had its chest laid opened & hashed & slayed in several places was walking about the table."[83]

Moreover, Americans sometimes identified vivisectional operations performed on animals with operations on hospital patients. Replying to a letter he had just received from Elias Samuel Cooper, an Illinois surgeon studying in Paris, one American commented in 1855 that "I suppose that there vivisections are not looked upon by the profession with that repugnance that they should look upon them or they would not be so cruel as to dissect these domestic animals alive and with every degree of cruelty as they seem to do. I suppose that you could witness operations of every class and grade upon the human subject almost daily and with the same inhumanity in degree as upon Animals &c &c."[84] Reflecting this perception of clinical inhumanity, a Connecticut physician, having just joined the crowd watching a woman give birth at the Hôpital des Cliniques, wrote home that the railed enclosure in which the woman was confined "seemed more like a *menagerie*, than anything else."[85]

French patients themselves appeared hardened, and the Americans who relished access to their bodies seemed taken aback by what they interpreted as resigned complicity in being clinically displayed and, in time, dissected. Indeed, the purportedly blunted sensibility of Parisian women patients was often cited as the moral precondition for *cliniques* on midwifery and the diseases of women.[86] Such open display of the female body, S. S. Satchwell wrote from Paris, "strikes a medical stranger from North Carolina, at least, with some surprise, however much it may comport with the vitiated taste and depraved morals of the French nation."[87]

Indeed, a persistent theme in American reports was that the demoralizing atmosphere of the Paris hospitals was typical of the broader hardening of the moral senses by Parisian life. "The whole scene of noisy and soulless caraussal made me sick," Bartlett wrote home in 1826, expressing "disgust" at a *grand fête* he had just witnessed. When he went on to say that "it was a most revolting and brute exhibition of the degradation of the dignity which ought to belong to human nature," his language could have referred equally to the streets or to the clinic.[88] "Beneath the appearance of elegance and refinement," William Walker wrote in 1850 to the New Orleans *Daily Crescent*, "there lurks in this Parisian world, an amount of depraved taste and sensual vulgarity which chokes up the aspirations of the higher Art, and degrades men who might otherwise soar beyond the depressing influences of the world they live in."[89] Replying to a college friend's concern about "the choking influence of a Parisian atmosphere," Jackson, Jr., wrote from Paris that he felt it essential to stay on guard, agreeing that "there seems to be as it were a miasm arising fr. its whole surface wh. not only does not favour but wh. actually deadens all religious feeling."[90]

Senior physicians and the families of Americans studying abroad particularly expressed worry about the French moral values and social mores that daily threatened to blunt the sensibilities of young physicians, concerned that the very experience of living in Paris could debase their character as healers. Breathing in the atmosphere of Paris day and night, no less than breathing the air of the hospital wards and dissecting rooms, posed risks of infection. Reports of students who returned morally ruined were not uncommon; "the temptations to profitless amusements, and vice, are very great, and it must require more than an ordinary stability of character, wholly removed as one is from the restraints of social and domestic influence, to resist the allurements by which he is surrounded," Austin Flint, then in his forties, wrote from Paris. "Observation shows that in not a few instances a residence here becomes attractive not so much for its scientific advantages, as for the abundant resources for dissipation."[91] Another physician wrote from Paris to St. Louis recounting in great detail "the immoral influences to which a young man is subjected," especially the temptations of "the common women." "When to these temptations, occurring *every day*, you add the entire removal of all the restraints of public sentiment, it will not be difficult to predict the course which most young men will pursue." Residence in Paris, he concluded, was "destructive of all the better habits" and "higher moral feelings."[92]

Yet while the concern that Americans might be corrupted by the vices of Parisian life was serious, the much greater concern was that their character as physicians would be tainted by the medical values of the Paris School—that excessive enthusiasm for science might undercut a commitment to healing. This latter danger was more subtle and more difficult to guard against. Thus, when in the summer of 1833, preparing to leave Paris, Jackson, Jr., told his father that he had come to see himself as one who would "make Science his sole mistress," the elder Jackson had reason for his apprehensions about his son's future.[93] Many worried that the American studying medicine in Paris might be seduced by French ways, but most especially seduced by science.

## THE NATURAL HISTORIAN AND THE TRUE PHYSICIAN

Looking back in 1861 at nearly three decades that had passed since his studies in "the wards of my Master the great Louis," Henry Ingersoll Bowditch, now professor of clinical medicine at Harvard, reflected in a lecture at the Massachusetts General Hospital on both the contributions the Paris School had made to American medicine and the dangers it had posed to his generation. He held up for the assembled students two images of the physician whose integrity as a healer had been undercut by excessive allegiance to the French model. The first was that of the *Natural Historian*, the physician who had come to "look at all disease with the non chalance of a Naturalist." With interests purely "scientific," the Naturalist saw human disease "as a great piece of Natural History." Healing was not the aim of this medical natural historian, who tended to "scoff at all puny attempts in therapeutics" or "hope of giving relief." Bowditch portrayed the Naturalist as "fiendish," "gloating over human suffering"; "heartlessness," he suggested, "seems to be the characteristic of this scientific student."[94]

Bowditch's second image was that of the *Skeptic*, a physician still committed to helping the sick but who had lost faith in the power of active therapeutic measures. "In some persons this scepticism culminates in a contempt for all treatment," Bowditch suggested. Skeptics "believe in Nature as a kind mother" while neglecting the therapeutic arsenal. The Natural Historian and the Skeptic, Bowditch insisted, were models the students listening to his words were to resist as they assumed the character of physicians. "You will judge from this," Bowditch told them, "that I deem the duty of the physician to be some thing more than 1$^d$ a Natural Historian or 2$^d$ a mere nurse."[95]

The specter of these two images—the Naturalist or mere "Natural Historian," the Skeptic or "mere nurse"—posed a troubling problem for the Americans who returned from Paris, especially for those who sought to make French ways central to their identity. As earlier chapters have shown, they optimistically looked to French medicine as a source of definition, distinction, and professional reforms. Yet the darker image embodied in these portraits meant that however much they allied themselves with the Paris School, they needed to distance themselves from some of its values. At the American bedside, the French model of healing threatened to discredit the practitioner rather than to bestow a competitive edge in the marketplace, just as it threatened to degrade rather than uplift the American medical profession.

This was especially a problem for those intent on pursuing medical science along French lines after their return. Reconciling their aspirations as scientists with their obligations as American healers was difficult, for it required distinguishing their own scientific cultivation from the image of the hardened natural historian indifferent to suffering. They confronted the pervasive reminder that "something more is necessary in order to cure diseases, than the mere knowledge of the pathological lesions in which they consist."[96] However eagerly some Paris-returned Americans sought to incorporate certain French tools and ideals into their research and patient care, they needed to make it clear that their character was that of not a French clinician but a true American physician.

While in Paris, Americans often reflected on what it would mean to "get frenchified," as one put it, or to contract what another called "*Francomania*."[97] They assumed this process would involve change in knowledge and values, and watched with curiosity as they found evidence of alterations—including hardening—in their own sensibilities. Gabriel Manigault, describing an operation performed by Armand Velpeau at the Hôtel Dieu in which, as Manigault hinted, the surgeon's eagerness to show students the beating of the exposed carotid artery hurried the patient to the "dead house," noted that "after a few of these I became so accustomed to them they produced no effect on me whatever."[98] As Gardner wrote, recounting vivisectional demonstrations he had witnessed, "one gets to bearing them without much sentimentality."[99] "You will think I am growing hard hearted," Williams wrote from Paris to his sisters in 1846, "but I must say it is very funny to see some of the children operated on. To say nothing of the noise they make, it requires about nine men to hold one of them still on the table, and then after it is finished to see them spin round like a top as they sometimes do."[100]

Nevertheless, many displayed a guarded vigilance against signs that transformations catalyzed by their Parisian experience were going too far. They were aware that by studying in the Paris hospitals they were collaborating in a system that served clinicians and medical students better than it did the sick.[101]

Even as they took full advantage of access to the body in Paris, they sometimes expressed revulsion at the values that made those opportunities possible. Young Jackson wrote enthusiastically to his father describing the "touching" course he had been following for two weeks and the knowledge about uterine disease he was gaining from it, and then paused—as if catching himself—to add that "altho' I am glad to avail myself of the opportunities here offered for acquiring it, I cannot but rejoice that the state of society is such in our own country that the same knowledge cannot be acquired there."[102]

So long as Americans remained in Paris, they were to a large extent free to indulge their scientific inclinations while reassuring themselves that their integrity remained sound. Their expressions of disapproval, scorn, and occasional outrage were a means of affirming those traits of character that made them different from the French and of assuring those at home (and themselves) that they had not succumbed. It was precisely such criticism that made it possible for them to present themselves as exposed and experienced, yet not tainted.

As they looked homeward, they often insisted that the journey had intensified their appreciation of American values. Permeating their letters and diaries is a contrast between American purity and authenticity and European corruption and artifice. "Coming to France has had an effect on me entirely different from what any one could suppose," Bassett told his wife in 1836. "Instead of strengthening me in infidel opinions, it has disgusted me with them." Reflecting on the moral tenor of American society that he had regarded with cynicism in Alabama, he wrote home that "if I were a citizen of *Paris*, . . . & if I had a son, I would send him there to avoid learning 'French morals,'" though he admitted that "I'd send him back again to learn 'French Science.'"[103] French sophistication and spectacle often figured as metaphors for moral decay and elicited longings for the simplicity and innocence of an imagined American Eden. "Surrounded by scenes of grandeur, where temples & towers, & castles & cathedrals meet the eye in every quarter, and statues of the first masters are almost as common as *stumps*," Bassett wrote home, "I long to be where they are not; where the rocks are unpoluted by the chizzel & the forest remains uncultivated & where I honestly believe the human heart is purer." As he continued, "If we have not the breathless monuments of art of this 'grand nation' neither have we its breathing monuments of misery."[104] On his return voyage, Bassett wrote in a private memoir that "I never knew I was so much of a patriot: I never knew how strong I was attached to home until I left it."[105]

Medical Americans leaned heavily on faith in American exceptionalism and a romantic image of New World purity for a guarantee that behavior at the American bedside would not be vitiated by the more odious of Parisian clinical values. Their endlessly repeated assertion that American society would never permit the brutalizing treatment endured by French patients offered reassurance that they would not transplant this French model to America because it *could not* be transplanted; the soil of America was different and would reject it. Describing the exhibition of women's bodies in a touching class in midwifery, one American in Paris reassured himself by asking rhetorically in the *New Hampshire Journal of Medicine*, "How many of our American women would be thus willingly exposed? I am proud to believe *not one!*"[106] Gardner similarly reported that "modesty is scarcely known among the women here," and wrote of Dubois's *clinique* at the Hôpital des Cliniques that "it is in this building, more than any other, that the great difference between the American and French woman is made apparent."[107] Another American, having described a "barbarous" new surgical method, concluded that it "will scarcely answer in our democratic country."[108]

Even as they established buffers between themselves and the French clinical ethos, the prospect of leaving Paris focused the attention of some Americans on their aspirations to proselytize for French medical science and to conduct investigations of their own. Thomas Stewardson, who had just spent eight months "collecting cases à la Louis at la Pitié," wrote in 1834 to William Gerhard that "I long to get home to pursue the same course there." To that end, he asked Gerhard's aid in promoting his application for the post of intern at the Pennsylvania Hospital. "I regard the spending [of] 2 years there in collecting cases as almost a necessary base work for my future success in the line which I prepare myself," he explained.[109] Most realized, though, that in the United States they would have to earn a living chiefly by treating private patients. "I remember I have yet to establish myself as a practitioner of medicine, & that I am advancing in years without having yet made any effort to gain the means of establishing myself respectably in the world," Charles Jackson, writing from Paris to his brother-in-law, admitted in 1832. "It is this that impresses upon me the importance of time & hastens my return home." Like other Americans, he was aware that some ambitions acquired in Paris would have to be shed. "Behold me then between two attractions my love of Science, & that of my friends & my home—Between these two forces I endeavor to maintain the *'juste milieu.'*"[110]

The institutional and economic realities of American medicine constrained scientific enthusiasm incited in Paris. Yet it was in order to avoid the suspicion that ardor as a scientist had vitiated character as a healer that some Americans were compelled to moderate their longing to pursue research, as the case of Jackson, Jr., exemplifies. Jackson's conversion into a disciple of Louis (traced in chapter 3) left him ready to consecrate his life to studying the natural history of disease. "The science of Pathology," Jackson wrote from Paris in 1832 to his boyhood friend William Henry Channing, "will require more than my whole life most actively spent. I burn to do something to write or to leave something 20 or 30 yr's hence which shall *last* . . . —something truly and essentially useful, wh. will advance the science or that portion of it wh. I now love like life." Looking five years ahead, he told Channing, "I tremble for my onward steady course, making truth and science my only pole-star."[111] Channing, bound for the ministry, wrote back chiding that "I do think you act too much on the principle, that scientific medicine est vitae summum bonum."[112]

As Jackson contemplated his return, he, like his compatriots in Paris, worried about the compromises ahead. The day after writing Channing, Jackson drafted a letter to his father suggesting very tentatively that perhaps his stay in Europe might be extended. "I must indeed work for my bread, but in working if you take fr. me the interest wh. search after pathological truth inspires, I can no longer work well."[113] He wrote again the next day, stating his case more boldly: "Remember my dear father, that I have a prospect of living 30 or 40 yr's—that for 10 or 20 I must prepare."[114] The elder Jackson preferred to let his son decide for himself, but urged "that you ought not to do so without some cogent reasons. After your return much time must be spent before you can get into business—and during that time you may be doing much to prepare yourself—and your opportunities for observation and study will be very favorable. The rooms occupied for our private school as well as the [Massachusetts General] Hospital will give you important facilities."[115]

James's experience in the coming months with cholera intensified his perception of himself as a disciple of Louis, and after half a year in Britain he returned to Paris more committed than ever to pathological investigation. Louis wrote to the elder Jackson in October 1832 urging that the young man devote four years exclusively to pathological study, and James, while he had no expectation that his father would approve, nonetheless wrote to him in November imagining how "4 years thus spent in Path^l research wld. give me a vast advantage over my confrères."[116] The prospect of returning to practice preyed upon his mind: "In very truth I look forward with fear & trembling to the day when I *must* employ my time to earn money instead of to learn truth," he told his father. As he lamented, "What a pity it is that our's is a mixture of Science & Trade."[117]

By February 1833, James had grown more assertive about the new image he was embracing of his identity and his future. Before he came to Paris, his vision was "almost bounded to becoming a good physician," he told his father; "now my much more ardent desire is to do my part in clearing away some of the clouds wh. hide the truth in our difficult medical sciences. I am beginning to regard myself as one whose education has been such that it is in his power & whose disposition is such that it wld. be his delight to seek & find *truth*, pathological & therapeutic." He intended to spend six more months collecting cases in Louis's wards, then sail for Boston.[118]

A month later, though, Louis proposed a different plan. Writing late in March directly to the elder Jackson, Louis said he had never intended to suggest that James spend four or five more years in *France*. Rather, "my only wish was that you should allow your son to devote himself exclusively to observation, for several years in *Boston*." Louis urged that "you ought to consecrate him for a few years to science," adding, "in my opinion it is a duty."[119] The very same day James wrote his father seconding Louis's proposal; "each m'g as I rise & each n't as I lie down it is c̄[um] a renewed hope that it will be my happy lot to spend a few y'rs in this manner." As he insisted, echoing his French father: "It is my *duty*."[120]

The elder Jackson judged the plan unrealistic and told his son so, but suggested they defer the final decision until James was back in Boston. Knowing the realities of American society, he was confident he could prevail over the young man's naive ambitions, but tried to soften the blow by proposing they spend some months together making observations at the Massachusetts General. "As to carrying science forward,—making discoveries,—that you must do as well as you can at home—you have nature before you here as well as in Paris—not so conveniently—but sufficiently," Jackson, Sr., wrote in April.[121] He wrote again in June, "I feel as if it were not quite fair to allow you to indulge too fondly expectations which cannot I think be realized in the manner you propose to yourself. To a certain extent your plan may be accomplished—but I think it may be done as well if you engage in business as if you do not—or nearly [as] well—so nearly that for the difference it can scarcely be wise to forgo the advantages of engaging in practice."[122] Distressed by his son's obsession, a week later he wrote yet again, "There are more difficulties than you see in doing the thing *a la Louis*. Boston is not Paris nor N. Eng. France."[123]

The father's will prevailed. In mid-July 1833 James left Paris to return to Boston and the following year received his M.D. from Harvard. While father and son did make clinical observations together at the Massachusetts General, the younger man also made plans to start a private medical practice.

Later, in 1835, the elder Jackson felt constrained to clarify why his son, as an American physician, could not follow Louis's plan and devote himself exclusively to scientific investigation. It had been impossible "because," as he explained,

> in this country his course would have been so singular, as in a measure to separate him from other men. We are a business doing people. We are new. We have, as it were, but just landed on these uncultivated shores; there is a vast deal to be done; and he who will not be doing, must be set down as a drone. If he is a drone in appearance only and not in fact, it will require a long time to prove it so, when his *character* has once been fixed in the public mind.[124]

As one of the most eminent physicians in the United States, the elder Jackson did not lightly dismiss his son's intellectual aspirations. But he understood something his son had not learned: even the appearance of excessive devotion to science threatened to taint his *character*, and thereby to undercut his integrity and identity as a healer. Justifying the plan he had imposed upon his son of starting in medical "business," Jackson continued:

> Among us, where the hands are yet few in proportion to the work to be done, every young man engages as soon as he can in the business of life. The public estimation of his character is decided early in life; earlier than in Europe. . . . But, if an individual were to go very far in the other extreme, his reputation would be fixed, as one, who perhaps loved knowledge and knew how to acquire it; but who was not disposed to use it, and who perhaps did not know how to apply it. . . . Such at least were my fears.[125]

As it happened, James never had to come to terms with all the difficulties that freighted his aspirations. Within a month after his graduation and just before his medical practice was to open, at the age of twenty-four he grew ill with what he diagnosed as typhoid fever, and died.

The elder Jackson had a good grasp of the realities of his profession and his nation. One had only to read the pages of the *Boston Medical and Surgical Journal* the year James died to find testimony to the kind of attitude that animated the father's concern. Denouncing practitioners who identified with French medicine as riding a "hobby," the writer of an anonymous letter asserted that "physicians should never resemble those philosophers who pursue science or literature in the abstract, either for its own sake, or to furnish materials for others to employ. All the pursuits of practising physicians should have a practical tendency."[126] Pursued in the United States, Louis's plan would have transformed the young Jackson's identity from that of a true American physician into what Bowditch had styled the mere "Natural Historian."

Paris-returned Americans faced resentment, notwithstanding the éclat their experience abroad brought them. "We have rarely seen a man go to Paris, but it made a fool of him," the editor of the *Georgia Blister and Critic* snidely expressed a widely shared attitude in 1854.[127] But those who returned with aspirations to scientific investigation faced not merely resentment but also suspicion. In the eyes of many American physicians, the French zeal for science and neglect of healing made the science itself look suspect.

Criticism of Louis was one vehicle for casting doubt on his American proselytes. He was, as one American described him in 1840, "doubtless one of the first pathologists of the age," but his achievement was tarnished by the fact that "therapeutics do not advance side by side with pathology; or the power to cure with the knowledge of what is to be cured."[128] So too a Philadelphia medical professor told his class in 1844 that it was "lamentable to witness the almost exclusive attention, which has been paid by many, of late years, to diagnosis," which he deemed the only practical yield of Louis's numerical method. "As a matter of scientific research it might be interesting to understand disease, even if we did not attempt to cure it; but as practising physicians and philanthropists, the alleviation and cure of disease must be the grand desideratum."[129]

To allay suspicion, Americans who returned from France with ambitions of pursuing empirical investigations needed to represent their allegiance to science in ways that made it seem subordinate—indeed, subservient—to their obligations as healers. Wariness about what would happen if a physician became too ardently devoted to science was not just the anti-intellectual grumbling of the medical masses but a concern of even the best-educated physicians. Though an elite practitioner like Bostonian John Collins Warren could privately contrast "practical" contributions with what he called "recherché," this was an invidious distinction not to be drawn in public.[130] An ardent American Parisian might argue defensively, as Stillé did in 1857, that "the physician's duty is two fold, he is at once a philosopher and a healer of the sick," but most sought to recast the American medical philosopher as a devout utilitarian.[131]

One way of subduing the chorus of American criticism against French models of healing was for the disciples of the Paris School to stop voicing such

criticism themselves, at least in public forums. Even in Paris, Americans sometimes were guarded lest their reports on patient care impugn French medicine
at home. Williams, having vividly depicted scenes of clinical brutality in letters
to his sisters, pleaded with them not to recount those segments of his letters
even to other family members. "If you must read *any* thing, at least be careful
not to read . . . [the] bad passages, or the Hospital anecdotes to anyone."[132]
Jackson, Jr., having written to Channing that periods spent studying internal
lesions by auscultation in Louis's wards "are the most delicious of my Parisian
hours," broke away from his enthusiasm to write that "such a term is only for
medical ears or if others hear it, the word 'delicious' has reference to the hopes
wh. this employment excites of being able to alleviate human suffer[in]g at
some future period."[133] After returning to the United States, the American Parisians became even more guarded in expressing their own negative judgments
on this French model of healing.

At the same time, they took pains to publicly celebrate the practical utility
of French medical science in general and of the researches they conducted in
America in particular. "Dr Louis is still as much as ever interested in the 'pure
science,'" Gerhard told Jackson, Sr., in 1834.[134] In presenting Louis's work
(and his own) to the wider American medical profession, however, Gerhard
recast it as not "pure science" but a foundation for practical therapeutics. In
collaborating on a translation of Louis's study of phthisis, for example, Gerhard and Jackson, Jr., recognized that to make the work palatable to Americans
they would have to do more than simply convert the French text into English.
To appeal to practical American physicians, Gerhard told Jackson that "we
must say something upon the treatment much more important than all the
negative results" and suggested they point to the benefits of hygienic measures
and the palliative value of opiates. Gerhard wrote that "you will probably agree
with me that Louis['s] book[,] excellent as it is, is still a collection of materials
which are of utility only to the limited number of individuals who are sufficiently interested to work them up and incorporate them in their own collections of facts—this is true in France, perhaps still more so in America." To
make the text "of immediate practical use," Gerhard proposed concentrating
on conventional methods of diagnosing phthisis rather than use of the stethoscope, despite its centrality in Louis's approach. Having made the book seem
appealingly practical, then and only then could they "urge upon the physicians
every where the necessity of statistics upon this important question impressing
it upon them in such a way that they may feel its utility," spelling out the
importance of counting in a new introduction on "la Methode."[135] Emphasiz-
ing the practical relevance of studies on the natural history of disease further
affirmed that their commitments to science and to healing were not in conflict,
and that their identity remained unsullied.

These Americans were insistent that they could use the tools of the Paris
School to simultaneously serve truth and improve practical healing. The promise of Parisian epistemology to uplift American medicine and the medical profession, after all, hinged in significant measure on its promise to improve ther-

apeutic practice. The belief that therapeutics had to be individuated to person and place provided one foundation for their confidence, for it suggested that the only sure way to produce therapeutic knowledge suited to the American habitat and peoples was direct observation of the operation of therapies on American patients in American environments. If therapeutic conclusions drawn from Paris hospital patients had doubtful applicability to Americans, that in no way belied the conviction that the technical and conceptual tools of the Paris School employed at the *American* bedside would transform American therapeutic practice.[136]

The broader problem was how to reconcile their own aspirations with the manifest failure of investigations in the Paris Clinic to make the French better healers. If, that is, the French held the key to uplifting practice, why had they not used it already? And what made the Americans so confident that they could do better? The answer to both questions centered on the basic problem that the French clinicians were *French*—that they lacked sound American values, especially practicality, morality, and a primary commitment to healing. Americans took courage from the conviction that New World purity, virtue, and practicality assured that medical knowledge would serve its proper end, that is, healing. In the final analysis, the American disciples of the Paris School believed that if anyone could use the lessons of French medical science to transform practice, they were the ones to do it.

Practical utility, then, was framed as a leading aim of natural historical investigations into disease, whatever intellectual passions may have animated them. It was this that ultimately made Louis, cast by his disciples as avatar of the true physician by merit of his allegiance to truth, a less than ideal model of the true *American* physician, committed above all to healing. The memorialization of Jackson, Jr., by American Parisians as a model physician was possible in part precisely because he died so young—died *before* he made all the compromises that an American physician had to make to avoid endangering his professional character. "What would he not have done in time!" Louis wrote to Jackson's father in his letter of condolence.[137] Though James acceded to his father's demands, his early death meant that his character never was tarnished by his holding fast to the pursuit of what he called "pure science" once the duties and responsibilities of practice as a healer commenced. Therefore Bowditch, far from denigrating Jackson, Jr., as a mere natural historian, was able to present his example in clinical lectures in the 1860s as "what I deem a Model Student." Jackson was "one the foundations of whose character was planted deeply and strongly on the ground," Bowditch told the Harvard class, "and this with a keen sense of the demands of Truth was the beacon light of his life."[138]

For most Paris-returned physicians, American realities obviated making a choice between science and healing: that was a dilemma only later generations would fully confront. In antebellum society there was virtually no place for the full-time medical scientist, no pathway by which the medical "Natural Historian" could consecrate a career exclusively to "pure science." A small number of the American physicians who studied in Paris—Charles Jackson (who gave up medical practice within four years of returning home), Jeffries Wyman, and Gabriel Manigault, among others—opted out of medicine entirely after their return to the United States in order to follow careers in natural history, devoting their time to fields like mineralogy, botany, and comparative anatomy. But those who remained in medicine did not have the option of sacrificing their identity as healers in favor of the single-minded pursuit of morbid natural history. If the American disciples of the Paris School did not strike a Faustian bargain, it was not least of all because no one made them the offer.

## THE SKEPTIC AND THE TRUE PHYSICIAN

Of the two extreme representatives of the French model of healing Bowditch cautioned his students to shun—the *Naturalist* and the *Skeptic*—the latter ultimately appeared more threatening to the regular medical profession in the United States. There was little risk that droves of physicians would neglect patients and assume the French mantle of the heartless medical scientist. However, any one of them might fall prey to skepticism, losing faith in active remedies and trusting their patients to the healing power of nature. The singular rooting of the American physician's identity in practice made therapeutic skepticism doubly threatening, for an erosion of confidence in the power to battle disease held the wider potential to enfeeble and degrade the entire orthodox profession.

The American skeptic who abandoned the orthodox therapeutic arsenal, like the medical natural historian interested only in "pure science," was in fact an imaginary creature. Records of actual practice show that throughout the antebellum period, the regular physicians most vocal in their allegiance to the healing power of nature, including some who openly professed their therapeutic skepticism, still prescribed active treatments, including most of the mainstays of the orthodox materia medica.[139] The skepticism they urged was a critical French attitude they believed should inform empirical observation and reassessment of therapies at the American bedside. They took from France not a mode of practice that eschewed drugs but a conceptual tool that they, as American healers, could apply in determining what was best for their patients. By the time Bowditch spoke in 1861, he like some other elite physicians feared that while the skeptical French influence had done good service, extremists were heading too far, leading toward the virtual abandonment of once-overused but potentially valuable therapies such as bloodletting.[140] During the preceding four decades, however, the assault on skepticism had been more sweeping in its denunciation of what many called the "do nothing practice."[141] Critics projected onto the skeptic a host of deeply felt anxieties, suspicions, fears, and resentments, vilifying this straw figure as a dangerous professional evil and the antithesis of the true physician.

At midcentury, physicians who reviewed the changes the French impulse had wrought in American medicine—disciples and detractors of the Paris

School alike—commonly concluded that while the preceding decades had witnessed imposing progress in knowledge about disease, there had been few new contributions to the therapeutic armamentarium. Yet therapeutic thought and practice had changed fundamentally. The severity of heroic depletive treatment declined dramatically as physicians came to use therapies like bloodletting and mineral cathartics less frequently and less aggressively. By the Civil War, physicians still used virtually all the remedies associated with heroic depletive practice but increasingly relied on stimulating and palliative treatments. To many physicians, the move toward therapeutic moderation itself represented improvement; as one summed up in 1850, "Our physicians have commenced a long-called-for revolution, in impressing upon their patients that medicine should never be taken if it is possible to do without it."[142]

This change had been a leading aim of the crusade against the spirit of system. By mounting an empiricist program that would unmask the deception and fraud of rationalistic systems, reformers sought to put an end to the excesses of heroic practice. The remedies that made up the established materia medica should not be arbitrarily abandoned, reformers argued, but their worth had to be freshly appraised by direct empirical observation. Regarded as part of the broader campaign against system, "'scepticism,'" as a Transylvania medical student urged in his 1841 thesis, "so far from being an unpardonable sin, 'becomes a cardinal virtue.'"[143]

Empirically reassessing the limits of art also meant reappraising the power of nature. It was the archsystematist Benjamin Rush who had declared, "As to nature, I would treat it in a sick chamber as I would a squalling cat—open the door and drive it out."[144] Reformers insisted that Rush's attitude was sustained by the hubris of rationalism and that, with the demolition of his own bankrupt system, nature should be given a chance to prove its worth. Empirical study of the natural course of diseases—and the recognition that some are self-limited—would provide a stable foundation for judging what credit particular interventions deserved and what was owed to nature. The empiricist program the French example impelled was only one of many engines of therapeutic change (others included antiorthodox criticism, the example of homeopathic success, and public attitudes that both of these encouraged), but its aim of moderating heroic excesses was attained with remarkable success.

By the time the hegira to Paris began, American physicians already associated a mild therapeutic plan with the French. In 1815, a medical student at Harvard attending the elder James Jackson's lectures on therapeutics copied into his class notebook, "There are two modes of healing diseases—(1.) active treatment—& (2) by wait$^g$ for ye efforts of nature—the French call this latter Medicine Expectante."[145] A decade later, another student attending what must have been much the same lecture recorded that there were in therapeutics "two methods—Active and Watching—or *a la francaise*—Expectante."[146] In the first method, Jackson told his students, the physician tried "to break disease"; whereas "in the second he watches the operations of nature—guarding against accidents."[147] Both the expectant plan and the idea of the healing power of nature had histories extending back to the Hippocratics. Yet by the 1820s, a mild, expectant therapeutic plan that relied on the healing power of nature, contrasted with an active, aggressive one that sought to break the disease, was clearly linked in the American mind to the Paris School.

Proponents and critics alike made this link. The pronouncements advocating therapeutic skepticism and the expectant plan that drew the most attention—by Jacob Bigelow in the 1830s, Elisha Bartlett in the 1840s, and by Holmes at the start of the 1860s—all expressed a therapeutic philosophy widely perceived as in some significant measure derived from French medicine.[148] The harshest critics of the expectant plan made it equally clear that they saw it as French-informed, speaking as they did of "the 'Expectant' plan of treatment, first systematized amongst the French"; "Expectantism—the system of medication pursued by some French physicians, and practiced to some extent in this country"; and "la medicine expectante."[149]

This identification of faith in the healing power of nature with the lessons of the Paris School gave American physicians their most concrete example of how the French impulse was altering their work as healers. In practice, the expectant plan was far from passive: when in 1832 visiting physician Walter Channing directed that the prescription "Medicine expectante" be written into patient records at the Massachusetts General Hospital, for example, Holmes, then his young house officer, proceeded to administer ipecac, opium, and calomel and to bleed by cupping and leeches.[150] At the same time, this identification provided a clear target for resentment against the French presence in American medicine, albeit one drawn in caricature.

The English novelist George Eliot lucidly portrayed this pattern in the reactions of *Middlemarch* villagers to her medical protagonist Tertius Lydgate. When he arrived in Middlemarch in the 1830s, Lydgate was fresh from study in the Paris hospitals. He longed to have charge of a small hospital where he could pursue clinical research for "he had known Louis in Paris, and had followed many anatomical demonstrations in order to ascertain the specific differences of typhus and typhoid." As one Middlemarcher introduced Lydgate, "He is likely to be first-rate—has studied in Paris, knew Broussais, has ideas, you know—wants to raise the profession."[151]

Lydgate soon became renowned for seeking to reform his profession's knowledge and social structure in accordance with his commitments to Parisian medicine, making the town's established physicians sense that "whatever was not problematical and suspected about this young man—for example, a certain showiness as to foreign ideas, and a disposition to unsettle what had been settled and forgotten by his elders—was positively unwelcome." His research aspirations fueled suspicion "that Doctor Lydgate meant to let the people die in the Hospital, if not to poison them, for the sake of cutting them up." It was when Lydgate criticized another practitioner for heroic drugging and inattention to the healing power of nature that resentment already mounted against him fueled the false rumor that he was a therapeutic nihilist. Resentful of his Parisian pretensions and suspicious of his reformism, the other medical men of Middlemarch found in Lydgate's advocacy of the healing power of nature and criticism of heroic practice an effective platform on which to "show him up."[152]

Such resentments and diffuse animosities against Paris-experienced physicians clearly were at work in the United States. What made therapeutic skepticism and *médecine expectante* professionally dangerous was the American understanding of how the physician's identity was established and maintained. From the 1820s, the rising strength of antiorthodox medical movements was the critical element in transforming regular physicians' confidence in their heritage into a conservative ideology of orthodoxy. The principal symbols of tradition to which regular physicians turned were heroic depletive therapies, especially bloodletting and calomel, the most conspicuous targets of antiorthodox assaults. The identification of these treatments with regular physicians and their function as emblems of the profession were by no means new; but between the 1820s and the 1850s their standing as symbols of orthodox medicine became stronger and more uncompromising. Yet it was to the value of these therapies in *principle*, not so much in *practice*, that orthodox physicians pledged their faith. Indeed, proclaimed faith in these therapies became loudest at midcentury, when the eclipse of heroic depletive therapy appeared a real possibility.[153]

It was within this reactionary context that in the 1820s, just as the influence of the Paris School was growing prominent, *heresy* (not just ignorance) first became a prominent issue in American medical culture. Advocates of the healing power of nature made up the most distinguishable group of regular physicians in antebellum America to challenge the power of the orthodox armamentarium, and therefore also the group of regular physicians held most suspect by conservative physicians looking for ways of not only setting themselves apart from alternative healers but also purifying orthodox ranks. This skepticism seemed all the more undermining because it was voiced by an elite, including many committed disciples of the Paris School. Although it was the skeptic Holmes who in 1860 coined the phrase "nature-trusting heresy" to describe the therapeutic movement in which he was participating, the term *heresy* used without his jocularity was frequently employed to stigmatize the position he defended.[154] Skeptics were branded with "infidelity to the healing art."[155] In the eyes of assailants, moreover, the skeptic's loss of confidence would dissipate that of the public. Whether or not the emphasis some regular physicians placed on the healing power of nature was actually impelled by the homeopathic example and propaganda—and a common perception held that it was— many practitioners rightly believed that it would be taken by antiorthodox physicians as an endorsement of their systems.[156] Reviewing in 1847 the argument by a regular practitioner that the apparent success of homeopathic treatment testified to nature's healing powers, an orthodox physician concluded in disgust that "absurdity and heresy can go no farther."[157]

Critics' portrayals of the American nature-truster bore a remarkable resemblance to depictions of the passive, indifferent, and doubtfully moral Paris

clinician. Asserting that effective intervention was "paralyzed by medical skepticism," one rural Ohio practitioner charged in 1858 that some regular physicians "have embraced dark and cheerless expectancy, and are seeking to convert the active and hope-inspiring practice of medicine, into a sad and gloomy
'meditation on death.'"[158] It was imperative that the practitioner at least make
an effort to interrupt the course of disease; as another physician asserted, "I do
not believe it is our duty to stand by and do nothing: we ought to study every
disease, and interfere."[159] The image of the heartless medical scientist was also
invoked to stigmatize nature-trusting. In a paper on puerperal fever delivered
at the Cincinnati Academy of Medicine, for example, a physician who linked
the "expectative method" with "worship [of] Indifferentism or Nihilism" proclaimed that "he who, keeping in view the diagnosis of the puerperal processes
alone, leaves the poor patients to their fate, appearing perfectly satisfied in
demonstrating at the post-mortem examination the by him presaged pathological alterations, has fulfilled his duty as physician but half."[160]

The darkest images of French healing were appropriated for the American
discourse on the healing power of nature, used to denounce the expectant
method. It was not so much to criticize French clinicians as to discredit the
character of any American who might pursue *médecine expectante* that in 1842
the editor of the *Western Lancet* declared that "the temporizing course pursued
by the French renders their therapeutics often inefficient. In anatomy, physiology, and pathology, they stand unrivalled; but beyond this they seem scarcely
to look. Having made a *diagnosis*, the next most important matter is to prove
its correctness; and, as this can only be verified in the *dead body*, more enthusiasm is manifested in a post mortem examination than in the administration of
medicine to cure the disease. *The triumph of these physicians is in the dead
room*."[161]

Invoking the French model, then, was a way of associating nature-trusting
with a flawed value system. "Some one has said that a fatal termination of
disease is considered by the French practitioners to be an element of success in
the management of cases, because the physician is then enabled, by an autopsy,
to verify the correctness of his diagnosis!" a Louisville medical professor told
his class in 1854. He acknowledged this to be an "exaggeration"; but having
placed this image in the mind of his listeners, he went on to say that "the
French physician is oftener satisfied to watch the progress of disease, and,
relying on the recuperative power of nature, content himself with the regulation of diet and hygienic measures."[162] The message to the students was that
should they cast their lot with the American nature-trusters, they too would
begin to resemble the French whose behavior and morals they had just been
invited to deplore.

Pervading the assault on nature-trusting was the underlying sense that it
disrupted proper power relationships at the bedside—not the relationship between doctor and patient so much as between physicians and the therapeutic
arsenal. For heroic practitioners of Rush's mold, nature was to be subjugated
to the physician's will through bold wielding of art. Medical submission to the

sovereignty of nature seemed to recast the physician in a meek, dependent, subordinate role. In 1860 a Georgia physician who blamed nature-trusting for the fall of bloodletting, addressing physicians gathered for the annual meeting of his state's medical association, sneeringly quoted an example of the kind of celebration of medical submissiveness he held responsible: "'How tenderly and patiently has Medicine, once so bold, aggressive and alert, learned to wait on Nature, following her hints, assisting her efforts, and relying chiefly on her own healing and recuperative powers.'"[163] So too Samuel Jackson told the College of Physicians of Philadelphia in 1845 that the notion "that *the physician is the mere servant of nature, which cures nearly all diseases*" was "the prevailing and most injurious error of the present time," one he believed "calculated to derogate from the honor and utility of medicine." Instead, he proposed, the dictum should be reversed, to say "that *nature is the servant of the physician*. She is to be carefully observed, and, like a servant, she is to be encouraged in all her laudable determinations; nay, further, like a servant, she must sometimes be tolerated, even in her errors."[164]

The language of gender provided critics with an effective medium for representing nature-trusting in ways that simultaneously devalued it. Traditional practice—sometimes called heroic by its adherents, but over time more often not—was almost uniformly framed as *active*. It was, as Drake told his students in 1830, contrasting it with the "expectant" plan, characteristically "energetic & bold."[165] The active practitioner, confident in his mastery of the orthodox armamentarium, vigorously took charge of the disease by using forceful, "decisive measures." A student listening to medical lectures at the University of Michigan in 1865 recorded in his class notes that sometimes the practitioner had to employ "Thunder and Leightning" drugging, while another student attending lectures in Charleston wrote in his class notebook in 1851, "Dr. Dickson says he is he is [sic] not afraid of any article of the materia medica[;] says he want to & would use a thunder bolt if would come under his power."[166] Metaphors to describe this therapeutic approach were more commonly drawn from warfare and the battlefield than from nurturing and domesticity.

By contrast, the expectant plan was routinely described as "a *passive* course,"[167] with its treatment characterized as mild rather than bold, its attitude watchful rather than interventionist, and its practitioner a handmaiden to nature rather than a commander of medical art. Samuel Chapman told University of Pennsylvania students in 1830 that this therapeutic approach was "highly dangerous; in as much as it has a tendency to dictate a feeble and inert practice, and to make us irresolute and timid."[168] The gendering of active (heroic) medicine and expectant medicine as masculine and feminine respectively not only conferred a particular character on the mode of practice associated with nature-trusting but also served to marginalize, devalue, and dismiss it.

These rhetorical strategies did not, obviously, identify the expectant method of practice solely with women: most of its adherents were men, many of them eminent in the regular medical brotherhood. But the language used to polarize active practice and expectant practice, and to attach to these polar positions

gender dualisms that in Victorian culture were both established and easily recognizable, also fostered gendered representations of the physicians who chose
between what were styled as active and passive roles. Disgusted by Holmes's
widely publicized 1860 proclamation of the nature-trusting faith, Samuel
Gross—the Philadelphia surgeon immortalized as the manly and heroic presence in Thomas Eakins's painting *The Gross Clinic* (1875)—wrote to a lay
friend that "as to Dr. Oliver Wendell Holmes he belongs to a class of nampy
pampy men who, if they are not a positive disgrace to medicine, are certainly
a great hindrance to it."[169] If medical men followed the course of the skeptic
Bigelow and his ilk "to abandon the use of active agents" and embrace the
expectant method, a New Orleans physician charged in 1859, "it is time to
abandon the practice of medicine to homoeopaths and old women."[170] The
president of the Medical Society of Virginia would even scoff that if the physician's task was merely to stand at the patient's side while nature did the work,
then women would be qualified to practice as physicians. He maintained, in
fact, that faith in the healing power of nature had "embolded" women to enter
the profession:

> She would blunder in physic no worse than the rest,
> She could leave things to nature as well as the best,
> She could feel at your wrist, she could finger your fee,
> Then why should a woman not get a degree?[171]

The young men gathered for Bowditch's clinical lecture at the Massachusetts
General Hospital in 1861 were being encouraged to see more than a weak
model of healing in his depiction of those physicians who took up the expectant plan—those who, in his words, "believe in Nature as a kind mother" and
who assist her by "gently . . . helping Natures laws." Becoming a "Skeptic" was
to be seen as a threat to their identity, not least of all for the potential it bore
to transform them, as Bowditch warned, from a true physician into "a mere
nurse."[172]

Those who defended their allegiance to the healing power of nature argued,
with reason, that their assailants were deploying a crude and misdrawn caricature: their convictions in no way rendered the physician subservient or passive.
"Nature should be our chief reliance," one physician commented in an address
before the Massachusetts Medical Society, "and when the processes she institutes are going on regularly, the less we interfere the better. The province of the
physician is to become satisfied of that fact." As he explained, "He is to decide
when to act and when not to act. He is to remove obstacles from her path; to
incite her when she flags; to sustain her when she seems on the point of discouragement; to check her impetuosity; to interrogate her, and supply those
cravings which are generally the indications of her necessities; and, whenever
possible, to concur with her in her efforts."[173]

The American nature-trusters insisted that they were not mimicking French
clinicians or succumbing to the extremes of Parisian inactivity and indifference
but that, influenced by a French way of seeing, they were empirically observing

disease and treatment afresh and employing orthodox therapeutics with judicious moderation. Expectant medicine as it was promulgated in America— what toward midcentury increasingly was called conservative medicine— sought to strike a balance between the extremes of heroic aggression and French passivity. "The conservative physician," Flint remarked, "is by no means a timid practitioner. He does not repudiate any of the potent measures embraced in the materia medica, but he does seek to employ them with a nice discrimination."[174] Keeping close watch over the operations of nature, no less than drugging, was doing something. "Typhoid Fever is a disease that requires no active treatment," a Nashville medical student wrote in his 1859 M.D. thesis, "yet it must be watched closely, . . . demanding the especial supervision, and untiring watchfulness of a Physician."[175] What was emerging by midcentury was the beginning of a new model of the physician's therapeutic duty that would vie for dominance in the final quarter of the nineteenth century, one that eschewed gratuitous interventionism and, like other realms of American culture, privileged watchfulness, supervision, and vigilance.

The most committed American disciples of French medicine who led the nature-trusting reform asserted that skepticism was their duty. In his *Essay on the Philosophy of Medical Science* (1844), Bartlett lamented the victims of "*rational* physic" and denounced "the abominable atrocities of wholesale and indiscriminate drugging." Unconvinced by the value claimed for traditional heroic practices in, for example, the system of Rush, Bartlett proudly affirmed that "there is probably no man more entirely skeptical in regard to their alleged properties and virtues, than I am."[176] Skepticism, as Bartlett and like-minded physicians understood it, was the only honest therapeutic posture a true student of the Paris School could adopt—a necessary tool for disclosing therapeutic delusions and clearing the way for reconstructing therapeutics on a reliable empiricist foundation. The expectant plan, in turn, was the practice of a physician who had escaped the sway of the spirit of system.

This was a harder course to follow, nature-trusters asserted. They were not deluding the public by administering medicines by rote, even when theirs was an unpopular course. It was a truism, which a Philadelphia student spelled out, that physicians "often employ medicines contrary to their own judgments, either, to have the appearance of doing something, or to silence the clamours of the friends of the patient."[177] While some patients resisted heroic treatments, regular physicians frequently complained that public insistence on traditional therapies was a leading impediment to change, and in hospital case record books from the antebellum decades, instances of patients' requests for heroic therapies outnumbered instances of resistance to them.[178] Keeping to the expectant plan meant holding firm against the temptation to pander to public taste by the easy imposture of drugging. Thus in 1850, John Young Bassett wrote in the *Southern Medical Reports* with obvious pride that, unconvinced any treatment was suited to the typhoid fever he observed in Alabama, "I boldly determined *to do nothing.*"[179]

Equally, physicians like Bartlett were shunning the worse fraud of deluding patients into believing that the physician cured by art when in fact nature did the work—precisely the deception they identified with homeopathic practice. Homeopaths, nature-trusters such as Bartlett and Holmes maintained, had recognized the central truth that nature often healed the sick; homeopathic practice, in their view, was tantamount to letting nature take its course unimpeded.[180] But instead of admitting this, homeopaths cloaked their practice in mystery, that is, Hahnemann's rationalistic system—beguiling to some of the public but fundamentally dishonest. A young physician in San Antonio, Texas, wrote in 1855 to his brother of the dilemma that by midcentury faced many American physicians: homeopathy, with its "infinitesimal delusions and arrant nonsense," he saw as a "swindle"; yet he was persuaded that the cure of disease came from "the forces of nature rather than the effects of poisons," and therefore judged orthodox drugging to be "the practice of a cheat."[181] In the effort to win paying patients, he concluded, hypocrisy was unavoidable: he *had* to be an imposter. The nature-trusters, however, were suggesting an alternative, more honest, and in their view more arduous course, namely, exercising the "moral courage" to follow the expectant plan.[182]

The nature-trusting impulse and the broader transformation of medical therapeutics that accompanied it constituted the clearest fulfillment of the campaign for epistemological reform at the antebellum American bedside. Better practice, reformers hoped, would both improve the standing of the regular medical profession in the eyes of the public and undercut the antiorthodox challenge. At the same time, establishing the role nature played in healing was part of the plan to demystify medicine, for it would expose the true worth of the therapeutic agents celebrated in medical systems. The massive doses of the heroic practitioner and the tiny pills of the homeopath both would be stripped of their rationalistic embellishment, seen for what they really were, and judged empirically on their merits. As with the broader empiricist program for reform, skepticism was presented by its adherents as a campaign to seek truth and expose falsehood. Yet it was persistently assailed by conservative, orthodox physicians for its damning association with French therapeutic indifference and its heretical complicity with "sectarians." It was only insofar as the American skeptics were able to distance themselves from these derogatory connotations, an arduous and never entirely successful endeavor, that they managed to reframe nature-trusting and the expectant method as parts of a professionally responsible program for reforming American medicine.

For the disciples of the Paris School who took up this program, therapeutic skepticism did not represent a concerted attempt to transplant French models of healing to the United States: in such an enterprise they saw more danger than promise. They did, though, see it as one important exercise of their commitment to an ideal of empirical truth, an exemplification of sound character rather than a threat to it. As they understood it, it was a duty of the true physician—the American archetype they took care to distinguish in turn from the apathetic Parisian healer, the heartless French medical scientist, the system-bound orthodox traditionalist, and the sectarian trickster. Americans who pursued the expectant plan, they maintained, exemplified character sturdy enough to not give in to the seductiveness of system (Rushian or Hahnemannian) or to the tyranny of public opinion, but to stand steady in their allegiance to truth.

# Americans and Paris in an Age of German Ascendancy

BY THE middle of the nineteenth century, Erwin Ackerknecht asserted, "*French medicine had maneuvered itself into a dead end*, as all empiricisms had done so far in medical history." He argued that "by 1848, Paris 'hospital medicine' had come to a dead end, its momentum spent," while the dust jacket of his book declared that the Paris School was "swept away by the Revolution of 1848." Ackerknecht went on to invoke the massive shift toward German cities in the stream of foreign medical students that once flowed to Paris as the most powerful testimony to the exhaustion of the French program. The influx of foreign practitioners after the peace of 1815, according to this interpretation, affirms the intellectual vitality of the Paris School. Equally, the redirection of students after midcentury is a clear indication that the vigor of the Parisian medical model had been exhausted. "French medicine paid for its practicalism, clinicism, and conservatism by losing its superiority to Germany," Ackerknecht insisted, that is, to both the states that later would form a unified Germany and other German-speaking centers in Austria-Hungary such as Vienna. With the creative promise of the Parisian empiricist program lost, those abroad in search of medical science at its forefront abandoned Paris in favor of the next-ascendant German centers, where the laboratory sciences purportedly ostracized by the Paris clinicians were vigorously cultivated.[1]

Historians of French medicine have begun to question this understanding of the Paris School. The emerging image of the Parisian medical world of the first half of the nineteenth century is more complex than Ackerknecht's portrait, while the notion that by the Second Empire the exhaustion of the empiricist program brought the whole thing to a halt has come to appear simplistic.[2] Yet the same fundamental assumptions that informed Ackerknecht's account continue to structure the standard narrative of nineteenth-century American medicine. Indeed, the premise for explaining patterns of American medical migration to Europe that Richard Shryock took for granted over a half century ago— that is, that a mid-nineteenth-century shift from Paris to Vienna and Berlin should be attributed to an underlying shift in "scientific supremacy"—has been surprisingly little qualified over time.[3] The most authoritative recent history of American medical education, for example, characterizes this shift as "testimony to the unchallenged superiority of nineteenth-century German medical science."[4]

The shift in destination that commenced in the 1850s was real enough, though American traffic to Paris remained remarkably brisk even after the Civil War. The interpretation of this shift, however, is more problematic. The experiences and expectations of American physicians in Europe during the third quarter of the nineteenth century suggest patterns of change that do not mesh well with the intellectualist assumption that what chiefly attracted students to one center rather than another was the prospect of studying at the cutting edge of Western medical science. I have argued in earlier chapters that the reasons for Americans' journeys to Paris cannot be equated with the stories they later told about its significance or the meaning they came to attach to their studies there, and the same is true of the reasons for Americans' increasingly making their way across the Rhine. If—as I want to suggest here—it was not chiefly the stagnancy of empirically rooted French medical science and the contrapuntal vibrancy of new German modes of scientific medicine that initiated the redirection in migration, we must begin to reconsider the shifting French and German presence in American medicine as well as the origins and meaning of late-nineteenth-century battles over how *scientific medicine* should be defined.

## "OVER THE BEATEN TRACK"

If the Paris School reached a dead end in 1848, there was no indication of it either in American reports or in patterns of migration by American doctors. The revolution of February 1848 temporarily converted lecture halls into what one American described as "theatres of political discussions," while at the hospitals students took advantage of the opportunity to study wounds inflicted at the barricades, but the workaday routine was soon restored.[5] Some American doctors in the French capital applauded the revolution, just as others detected in it "a strong smell of sulphur" and welcomed the coup d'état of Louis-Napoléon Bonaparte and his installation at the end of 1852 as Emperor Napoléon III.[6] But political turmoil did not dissuade Americans from embarking for Paris, and during the 1850s the number annually making the journey grew markedly—by one historian's estimate, doubling what it had been the preceding decade.[7] "Scarcely a day passes without the arrival of new members of the medical profession from America," one observer in Paris noted in 1853, "and probably every steamer carries home some who have just completed their tour of observation and study here."[8] So large was the influx that by 1853 the American Medical Society in Paris, founded two years earlier, was reported to be larger than its older British and German counterparts, the Anglo-Parisian Medical Society (founded 1837) and the Verein deutscher Aerzte in Paris (founded 1844).[9]

In Paris, Americans continued to follow much the same eclectic routine of medical studies that their predecessors had pursued for nearly two generations, with access to the body—facilitated by paid private instruction—paramount in what they valued. But there were shifts in the kinds of courses most prominent in American reports, particularly a greater emphasis on specialties. In early-nineteenth-century America, medical specialism had been distinctly illegitimate—a hallmark of the charlatan.[10] In Paris, however, the practice that

Americans observed was conducted in hospitals that often were explicitly devoted to one or another class of malady, and therefore their experience was of a system in which de facto specialization was vastly more pronounced than in the larger medical world of Paris encompassing private practice. Many of their private clinical courses focused on midwifery, for example, or on diseases of the skin or of children, and were conducted in "special" rather than general hospitals. One American, contemptuous of "specialists as they are called," wrote from Paris in 1844 protesting signs of the subdivision of the profession "into eye doctor ear doctor nose doctor and belly doctor."[11] Nevertheless, even from the early decades of the century Americans felt comfortable concentrating on one or a few "branches," so long as they did not declare any intention of becoming a specialist. Americans generally spoke of studying diseases of the skin or of the eye—not dermatology or ophthalmology—but the specialized focus of their work was nonetheless apparent.

From the late 1840s onward, Americans displayed a more self-conscious awareness that medical specialties were central to what Paris offered them, an awareness underscored by their growing use of the term "specialties" rather than special "branches," as had been the convention. The cultivation of "specialties," one American physician suggested in 1856, "seems to be a French peculiarity."[12] Augustus Gardner, who wrote in 1848 that "my great object in visiting Paris" was to study midwifery, betrayed a common defensiveness when he insisted that "the study of a specialty" was more demanding than preparation for general practice, for before turning to "his own specialty" the aspirant had to master the full compass of medical knowledge. "Whether the new world will give encouragement to such a procedure, time will determine," Gardner noted. But he contrasted "the poor man in America, at the same time, physician, surgeon, accoucheur, attempting to be skilful in operations on the eyes and ears, percussion and auscultation, [and] the diseases of women and infants," with the French clinicians who "have each taken one branch and pursued it, aiming at perfection and attaining an approximation to it."[13]

By the 1850s, Americans were following specialty courses confident that they would find esteem at home for the kinds of knowledge they were acquiring in Paris. Courses taken with Julius Sichel at the private eye clinic he established in 1832 or with his pupil Louis-Auguste Desmarres proved in the late 1840s and 1850s to be among the most popular. "Not one in twenty of those who graduate at Boston knows anything about eye diseases, and though after some experience he can learn to distinguish them yet it is nothing to the certainty he can acquire here," Henry Williams wrote back to Massachusetts in 1846 after completing three months with Sichel.[14] Although it was in Prussia that Hermann von Helmholtz had invented the ophthalmoscope in 1851, it was in France that a significant number of Americans first learned how to use it. Thus an Atlanta medical professor studying at Desmarres's eye clinic in 1857 reported enthusiastically that the ophthalmoscope "has done as much and perhaps will do more for diseases of the internal eye, than the great discovery of Laennec and Avenbrugger has done for diseases of the chest."[15] Even though many specialties were recognized by chairs in the official Paris curriculum only in the 1870s, instruction was widely available much earlier through private courses—and these, after all, were the pivot upon which the studies of Americans turned.[16] The students who took such private specialty courses in Paris were the first large cohort of Americans to embrace and proselytize for specialism as an appropriate professional model for medicine in the United States.

Americans in the 1850s vigorously took advantage of instruction in experimental physiology and microscopy—"collateral sciences," as they tended to be known—still hard to come by at home. As recent historical work has shown, such laboratory sciences were much better integrated into the Parisian medical world than earlier depictions of stark antagonism between the ward and the bench had suggested.[17] Moreover, Americans claimed that in both fields they were more ardent students than the French. Many Americans frequented Claude Bernard's physiological lectures and demonstrations; "in the class which attended the Spring Course of Lectures on Physiology by Bernard," George H. Doane asserted in 1853, "and which was quite a numerous one, there were only two who were not Americans."[18] Austin Flint, in Paris the following year, noted that "the name of Claude Bernard is well known in the United States, not from his works, for I am not aware that any of the few publications that have as yet emanated from his pen have been translated, but mainly through the letters of American physicians who have attended his lectures or followed his demonstrations in the laboratory."[19]

In microscopy, Charles Robin's courses won a devoted American following. "He gives two courses, one theoretical, in which he gives description of the histological tissues; the second one is practical in which he shows them all under the micro[sco]pe in addition to all morbid and malignant growths," Cincinnati medical professor John A. Murphy wrote from Paris in 1854. Predicting the coming importance of the microscope, Murphy asserted that "the results of investigations now going on with it, joined to the physiological researches of M. Bernard, will produce a great change ere long, in the treatment of disease, as well as in pathological anatomy."[20] In the same year, another American wrote from Paris that Robin's class "is generally confined to a small number of American students. Nachet, one of the principal manufacturers of microscopes, told me that his best customers were from America, and that nearly all his most expensive instruments were sent there."[21]

The significance Americans attached to a trip to Paris also began to change at midcentury, for it had become an expected step in the career building of any American physician with ambition and means. In 1845, Daniel Slade, who had just graduated from Harvard College, included study in Paris as an assumed stage in professional training as he sketched a plan for his future. "My way is clear for at least 6 years if my health and prosperity continue," he told a friend. "3 years and a degree of M.D.—and then two years in Paris and Europe—After that I may begin to look after a wife."[22] As more and more Americans journeyed to Paris, the power of that experience in setting the traveler apart from the masses of an overcrowded profession was diluted. Parisian study gradually became less a source of distinction and special identity and more an expected rite of passage into competitive professional life.

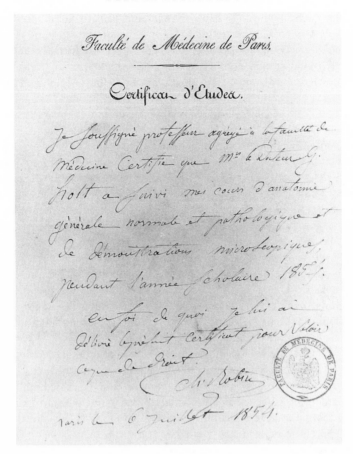

Fig. 9.1. Certificate signed by Charles Robin, affirming that William J. Holt had taken his 1854 course in Paris on normal and pathological anatomy, which centered on microscopical examinations. Starting in the 1850s, microscopy, along with experimental physiology, powerfully attracted the attention of Americans studying in Paris. (William Joseph Holt Papers, courtesy of Manuscripts Division, South Caroliniana Library, University of South Carolina, Columbia.)

Part of what was lost was the heady sense of discovery that had permeated reports by the first generation of American travelers. "I do not flatter myself that I shall be able to speak of anything here, that is really new to the well-informed medical men in America," one physician wrote from Paris to a New Jersey medical journal in 1853.[23] Another told the editor of a Cincinnati medical journal in 1868 that he hesitated "to go over the beaten track," for, as he explained, "every one has read or heard a great deal about this gay capital, if he has not visited it."[24]

Over time, accounts of Paris and guides for medical visitors had become increasingly standardized. The reports of early visitors structured the perception of those who came later and helped establish conventions for describing the Parisian medical world. By 1855, for example, Robert Harris could write to the *American Medical Gazette* giving his judgments on the most and least interesting hospitals, offering his opinion that bedside lessons were the most useful instruction available, and comparing the relative standing of American and French clinicians in diagnosis and treatment—all after only one week in the city and prefaced by his admission that while he could read French "pretty well," he could understand the spoken language only with great difficulty.[25]

The complaint grew common that many medical Americans, taking their visit for granted, were less than diligent in their studies. "There are at present a number of American Students here," Edward Jenkins wrote from Paris to his brother in 1853, "but not very many who really deserve the name of Student."[26] In the same year, another American complained that fewer of his compatriots really made the effort to learn French. "You will meet those who have been here but two or three months, who knew not a word of French when they arrived, who say they understand all the professors say, and get along very well," he told readers of the *Western Lancet*; "I do not believe a word of it. I know it is false."[27] "About the time he is to go home," Harris claimed, the typical American "begins to understand what the lecturers say and to profit by their teaching; but his money is all gone, and he cannot stay any longer; so, buying a box of the newest medical publications and some instruments, he takes passage for home, and says very little about this the dark side of the picture."[28] Underlying such criticisms was the suspicion that some physicians were chiefly after the ornamental value of the journey, not knowledge or experience. A Charleston observer in Paris commented in 1854 that while "many are very hard and regular students, others [are] amateurs, who stroll in a morning or so, look at a great gun, find hospitals, before breakfast, not the things they are reported to be, and that is the last you see of them *here*."[29]

The very fact of having studied in Paris *did* continue to confer some measure of distinction and professional advantage. In 1857 John Kane had been in Paris several months when a downward turn in his family's finances led him to propose returning home to Philadelphia immediately; he reassured his father that "I have now, the credit at least of having studied abroad."[30] Just as some physicians worried when plans were being made to create the American Medical Association that it would be the instrument of "some clique desirous of ascendancy,"[31] so too four years later, when the American Medical Society in Paris was organized in 1851, a Boston physician—who, in a revealing slip, called it the American Medical *Association* in Paris—worried that it might "become the tool of some domineering clique." As he noted critically, "It is an accomplishment to have been a student, if but for a single week, in the hospitals of Paris—and many a one who has the reputation of having completed his medical studies in foreign institutions, has hardly achieved more than to enter at one door and pass out at another."[32] His characterization was unduly harsh. Compared with the first generation of American "Parisians," however, as a group those who traveled to Paris in the 1850s embarked for France with less sense of mission, passed their time in Paris without the same experience of conversion, and returned with much less invested in their identity as disciples of the Paris School.

Many Americans nevertheless regarded their journey with a spirit of awe and celebration. Even if the French medical world had become familiar to every physician who read a medical journal, to the individual practitioner who made the trip, their experience of Europe remained fresh. And they still reveled in access to the body beyond anything they could enjoy at home. Into the 1850s, those Americans consecrated to the Paris School continued to depict the ideal of empiricism as what was most important about the French medical model. Yet experience at the bedside and dissecting table was what most attracted American doctors to Paris and what seemed to assure that their migration there would continue.

## PARADIGM LOST OR PARADISE DECLINING?

During the decades when Paris stood unrivaled as a magnet for American doctors abroad, many of them included on their itineraries not only British but also German and Italian cities. Through the 1850s, those who visited German-speaking centers often did so as tourists, but ordinarily did incorporate medical institutions and figures into their sightseeing. After a year and a half studying in Paris, Charles Jackson explained that "I resolved to lay aside the scalpel & stethoscope for a while & take a tour through the most interesting portions of Europe." When he visited Vienna in 1831 it was as part of a leisurely grand tour, and only when cholera appeared just after his arrival did he decide to take advantage of the epidemic to study at the Allgemeine Krankenhaus, the massive civic hospital.[33] Elisha Bartlett interrupted his study in France for a sightseeing tour in 1846, returning to Paris to write that "in medicine, except physiologists and microscopists, I do not think the Germans are doing much and the Italians are doing less. At Heidelberg I saw Naegaile the famous obstetrician, and at Berlin Muller the great physiologist."[34] Alfred Stillé visited central Europe in 1851, but not for study; "during the two months, nearly, that I have spent in Vienna, very little of my time has been given to medical affairs," he wrote home, though he did observe the pathologist Carl von Rokitansky and the clinician Joseph Skoda at work (and judged the latter "a thorough bred pig").[35]

Throughout the first half of the century, Vienna and Berlin were second only to Paris, London, Edinburgh, and Dublin in the medical curiosity of Americans. James Jackson, Jr., from the outset hounded his father for permission to study in Germany after his time in France and Britain. "I am daily more and more firmly persuaded of one thing viz: that I shall regret all my life not having become acquainted with German medicine," he wrote in 1832 to his father, who doubted that there was much in German medicine worth learning. "Let us for a moment look forward 20 yr's my dear father, and suppose, what is certainly supposable, that I have a son to educate in Medicine and that by that time there shd. have been some g$^t$ discovery or advancement in the German school wh. like the discovery of Laennec has added a new luminary to our art and changes the face of some imp$^t$ branch of our science," James wrote the next day. "Of what vast importance will it be that I am familiar with the history and labours of that school."[36] The father finally consented, but only after the young man's intense devotion to Pierre Louis had made any plan that would take him away from Paris unwelcome.[37] James still considered "making a rapid run," though Louis said it would be a waste of time; but by the start of 1833, his work in the Paris Clinic led him to write that "my conscience *asks me very seriously* whether I have a right to go to Germany. Louis & my conscience say 'No.'"[38]

Many who did visit, even chiefly for tourism, found much to admire in German-speaking medical centers. Like most who passed through Vienna, William Horner, a recent Philadelphia medical graduate abroad in 1848 for studying in Paris and "travelling" and "sight seeing" in central Europe, found the size of Vienna's Allgemeine Krankenhaus overwhelming; "it would be difficult to conceive of a school more exactly suited for the study of disease," Horner wrote to a former professor.[39] Valentine Mott, who in 1840 visited Berlin and Vienna, reported on the work of the ophthalmic surgeon Friedrich Jaeger at the Allgemeine Krankenhaus and suggested that "in no part of Europe is this branch of surgery cultivated and practised with more success"; and Harris, visiting a decade later, reported that "the best Obstetric clinique [in Europe], is that of the great General Hospital of Vienna."[40] American physicians like E. Williams, who in 1854 spent five months in Vienna "in attendance at the great general hospital with its vast materials and celebrated professors," plainly took pleasure in writing home that they had seen in action the Viennese clinicians whose names were becoming well known in the United States, such as Rokitansky, Skoda, Johann R. von Oppolzer, and Joseph Hyrtl.[41]

Reports by Americans who included Austria and Prussia in their European tours, combined with translations and summaries of German works in the American medical press, meant that the medical community in the United States was generally aware of facilities and activities in Vienna and Berlin. Until the 1860s and 1870s, however, most elected to study in Paris instead. "I do not think I shall meddle with Germany as a residence," Henry Williams wrote his sister from Paris in 1846. "I can learn everything in Medicine here that I could in Germany, and if I should go there, I should lose all the time (some months at least) from Medical study, which would be required for learning the language."[42] Levin Joynes wanted to spend six months exploring German medicine in 1841 before returning home from France. "But to one who does not know the language, it would be folly to go to Germany to study, unless he has at least four months to throw away in acquiring it," he told his father, explaining that he had resolved to visit England instead; "I abandoned all ideas of going to Germany, and why should I regret it after all?—for there is no *Paris* in Germany. To exchange one for the other would be 'paying dearly for a whistle.'"[43]

Yet by the early 1850s, as American attention increasingly focused on clinical specialties and fields like microscopy and experimental physiology, some older physicians could be heard complaining that the Paris School was slipping precisely because it was departing from a strict focus on their kind of clinical medicine. Stillé told George Cheyne Shattuck, Jr., in 1851 that New York physician John Appleton Swett, a contemporary who had judged things declining when he recently revisited Paris, might have a point. "I do not wonder Swett should have felt that there was a falling off in the scientific status of the present generation of physicians in Paris," Stillé admitted. "Yet," he continued perceptively, "the change is perhaps less in them than in himself. When a man has devoted himself as he, and you, and many of our associates did, in Paris, to a certain field of investigation, it is not easy to enter upon a new one with the same interest, or estimate so highly those who cultivate it." Stillé reflected that "I begin to find it no longer a matter of wonder that men who have become accustomed to practice with a certain degree of knowledge should have so much difficulty in being persuaded that there is still more to learn."[44]

Grumblings that Paris was not what it had been were generally muted and tentative. Nevertheless, early in the 1850s some Americans did begin to suggest that the kinds of instruction they valued in Paris might be equally obtainable in Vienna. "Nothing can be conceived more admirable than the arrangements at Vienna for instruction," Doane, comparing the advantages of Paris, Berlin, and Vienna for studying diseases of the eye, wrote in 1853, after his return to Vermont. "Having for a short time experienced them, I regard it almost as a duty to call to them the attention of those who have in view a visit to Europe, after the completion of their studies here. There were only five Americans in Vienna last winter, while Paris could boast of between three and four hundred.* These latter crowded every private lecture-room, and clinique of the 'Quartier Latin' to their own discomfort, and that of the teachers; while in Vienna the same, and in many cases, greater facilities exist, unknown and un-improved."[45] Flint, addressing medical students in Louisville the following year, typically told them that "Paris has been generally considered to possess greater facilities for pursuits connected with medical science, than any other city in the world." He went on to note that "of late there has been some diversion in favor of other places, such as Berlin, Vienna, Giessen, and Dublin," but concluded that "the supremacy of Paris is still maintained."[46]

Some Americans did begin to assert that the Paris faculty was not being kept up to its earlier standards. In part, the clinicians Americans had most identified with the Paris School seemed, as David Yandell put it in 1847, "to belong to the by gone generation."[47] More than this, some observers suggested that the changing political climate had lowered scientific standards for making medical appointments, which sometimes hinged upon imperial favor rather than *concours*. Although the revolution of 1848 did not profoundly interfere with the studies of Americans in Paris at the time, some believed its aftermath was more intrusive. Stillé, writing to Shattuck after revisiting Paris in 1851, noted that "the political state of the French capital is unfavorable to scientific progress, & the peers of our old masters do not at present exist there."[48] Another Philadelphia physician reported in 1854 that "to the stranger who was familiar with the Institutions in 1840, it does not appear, on a return at present, that much progress has been made," noting that "in the Faculty, the gain scarcely compensates for the loss, and if the reputation of the School of Paris depended upon that alone, it might well be supposed to be upon the decline." Yet he dismissed the notion of decline by pointing out that what Americans most valued—not teaching by the faculty but private instruction by more junior clinical officers—remained intact.[49]

In 1855, however, this changed dramatically. On the first of January, Americans then in Paris reported, an edict by the dean of the faculty suppressed all teaching by *internes* of private clinical courses. "This is greatly to be regretted," Robert A. Kinloch wrote from Paris two weeks later to the *Charleston Medical Journal and Review*, "since most of our young men have derived what practical knowledge they obtained in Paris, by the freedom they have heretofore enjoyed of entering the hospitals, and examining the patients more closely with the intelligent '*internes*', than they could possibly do when following the physician or surgeon in his daily visit."[50]

Kinloch went on to say that "many explanations have been offered, but I believe none of them sufficient to account for the procedure." He noted that "amongst other reasons, the '*internes*' sometimes tell Americans that they believe our country-woman, Mrs. Clarke, . . . to have been the cause of the change, from her *close scrutiny* of the male patients." Kinloch dismissed the rumor about Nancy Talbot Clark—whom he had earlier encountered in the clinics—as "only a '*funny*' explanation, and no doubt a scandal upon the good lady."[51] Another American who reported that the cause of the dean's action "did not seem to be well understood" nonetheless noted that "it was said to be owing to an abuse of the privilege formerly allowed to the *internes*, and which it was thought had resulted in injury to the patient."[52]

Other observers agreed that this new move boded ill for Parisian medical study by Americans. In spring 1855, Henry H. Smith, a professor of surgery who had studied in Paris sixteen years earlier, revisited the city to collect pathological specimens for the University of Pennsylvania and concluded that "in comparing the present position of Paris, as a residence for the young American student, with that which it held in 1839, I am sorry to say that its advantages appeared to me to have diminished." He lamented that "its private clinical courses have been much impaired by a decision of the Dean, which has forbidden the formation of private classes under the charge of the hospital *internes*." Such private instruction in Paris, he explained to Philadelphia medical students after his return, had "caused hundreds to seek its hospitals after the completion of their preliminary courses elsewhere; but now it is forbidden, and the student is limited to the public visit of each morning in connection with the crowds who follow the rounds of each surgeon." Smith predicted that just as Paris had superseded Edinburgh as the favored destination for Americans, Vienna might well supplant Paris as "the great centre of medical attraction."[53]

The edict was not unprecedented, and earlier proscriptions on private courses seem always to have been temporary. In 1845, for example, extolling the extensive opportunities for private clinical instruction that he had taken advantage of in Paris, Alexander Wilcox had declared, "Unfortunately all this is at an end. Last January, [Mathieu] Orfila, the Dean of the Faculty, and the managers of the hospitals, put a stop to these private courses. The reason assigned for this was, that such repeated examination was injurious and cruel to the patients. But those internes who were engaged in the business said that the real opposition was on the part of their fellow internes, and arose from their jealousy."[54] Wilcox warned that "if this privilege be not again granted, Paris has in my opinion lost its great charm for the American student."[55] Yet private arrangements continued. As Yandell had explained in 1848, "Some years ago private clinical instruction in the hospitals was sanctioned by the administration, but being carried by the *internes* to too great an extent, the patients made such loud complaint that it became necessary to prohibit it." He noted, however, that "under the present system private clinical teaching is conducted *sub rosa*," and suggested that "the laws of a hundred faculties and administrations would be little heeded by the *internes*, when pecuniary reward was in question."[56]

Even if the dean's action of 1855 was temporary as well, its timing assured serious, far-reaching consequences for Americans. In 1845 the Paris School had reigned as unquestionably the leading place for professional improvement. It was secure not only in its status as the center of medical science but also (and more important for Americans) in its reputation as a clinical school unparalleled in the access students could gain to the bedside for modest fees. In 1855, however, the singularity of Paris seemed less self-evident. Some observers had been voicing qualified concern that the standards of the Paris School were slipping. At the same time, occasional reports from Americans were newly enthusiastic about the potential of German-speaking clinics as places for study. In Vienna, *Privatdozenten* had long offered private courses for fees, but the reorganization of medical teaching in the wake of the 1848 upheavals for the first time officially recognized and encouraged this practice. The University Law of 1849 sanctioning such private instruction stated that "private lecturers are not employed by the state, but are merely men to whom the state gives its permission to teach. By virtue of this permission they have the right to announce their lectures publicly and to deliver them in the rooms of the university."[57] Also at midcentury, American society as a whole was paying increased attention to German culture. Thus one American student in Paris wrote home in 1854 that he wanted to spend time in either Berlin or Vienna before returning, partly to study medicine but mainly to master German, for, as he explained, "fortune may bring me in contact with the German emigrants of whom such vast numbers pour into our country every year," and others echoed his conviction that learning German was good strategy in winning practice.[58] By 1855, then, there was a growing awareness that if anything threatened to impede access to private clinical instruction in Paris, there might be equally attractive opportunities on the other side of the Rhine.

During the second half of the 1850s, remarkably abruptly, invidious comparisons of Paris with Vienna began to proliferate in the American medical literature. No single bellwether led the flock across the Rhine, but reports from young physicians such as Henry K. Oliver, Jr., one of the earliest American disciples of the Vienna School, were critical in redirecting American attention. Writing from Vienna in 1857 to the *Boston Medical and Surgical Journal*, Oliver, who would later establish himself in Boston as an otolaryngologist, enthusiastically described the arrangements he found for clinical instruction. "The clinics are distributed throughout the entire day," he reported,

> so that one may go from the medical wards into the midwifery wards, and from there into the surgical, &c. Not to speak of other advantages, this single arrangement enables one to pick up as much medical knowledge in Vienna in six months, as a year or more at Paris, where all the clinics take place at the same hour of the morning. Each student who wishes, is charged with the care of a patient, whom he visits at least twice a day. On the first day of the patient's entrance, the student examines him and writes out the result and the history of the case generally. In this he is guided by the *chef de clinique*, who points out the main features of the case, teaches him to percuss, auscult, &c. The following day, the student reads the account of the case, as written off, to the professor at the bedside, who then examines the patient himself, and afterward questions the student, laying especial stress upon the means of arriving at the diagnosis. The advantage of this mode of lecturing, instead of just examining the patient and retiring to the lecture-room to enlarge upon the case, as in Paris and with us, can hardly be questioned.

The editor, Jonathan Mason Warren, who had studied in Paris a quarter century earlier, prefaced Oliver's letter by noting that "the superior advantages of the Vienna hospitals, for students, over those of Paris, have of late years attracted much attention. The great facilities afforded for both medical and surgical study and observation, have quite turned the tide in favor of the German institutions."[59]

As in Paris, what Americans most often celebrated about Vienna and other German-speaking cities was access, for a fee, to practical clinical instruction. This was a central feature in the comparisons of Paris with Vienna that became commonplace in the 1860s. "Little can be done . . . in Paris, except by comparatively few, because of so little being done in private classes," H. Z. Gill wrote to the *Cincinnati Lancet and Observer* in 1868, "while at the German cities every facility is afforded to strangers, at very low fees." Having just returned from two years of study in Austria, Prussia, France, and England, he was convinced that "private instruction in the general branches can be obtained in Germany more thoroughly and at less expense, perhaps, than in any other country," urging, for example, that "in Vienna, Prague and Berlin are offered the greatest advantages for personal examination of patients by members of the class." Praising the attention "given to teaching practical diagnosis, as well from physical signs as from chemical and microscopical means," he added that particularly in "the special subjects . . . Vienna affords the greatest facilities for the foreign students."[60] Thus in 1868 an Ohio physician wrote from Vienna to his mother, "There are some thirty American Students here and I think if the others in Europe only knew of the *advantages* here they would not waste their time in Paris."[61] Noting the abundance of clinical "material" available to the "*Privat-docent*" at the Allgemeine Krankenhaus, a Boston physician wrote from Vienna, "At any given time, one may find here a dozen or twenty series of interesting special courses going on, and never need wait long for a new course to commence, for the usual length of the great number of courses is from three to eight weeks." Such special courses offered for a fee, he concluded, "are what the foreigner wants; the teachers are ambitious, and the classes are small."[62]

Instruction in the clinical specialties loomed especially large in American appraisals. By the second half of the 1850s some Americans were proposing that among the chief reasons to visit Berlin was the Augenklinik of Albrecht von Graefe, who had himself studied diseases of the eyes in Paris with Desmarres, served as his *chef de clinique*, then returned to Prussia to establish a clinic of his own.[63] So too in 1860, prefacing a letter from an American in Vienna about courses on eye diseases offered by Jaeger and Ferdinand Arlt, a Boston medical editor noted, "It certainly well illustrates . . . the advantages claimed for that over other European cities, as the place for American students to complete their studies."[64] Similar comparisons in other specialties such as obstetrics and in fields like microscopy abounded. As Bostonian David F. Lincoln, writing from Vienna in 1871, summed up, "For us foreigners, Vienna is a school for *specialties*."[65]

In all their discussions about the advantages of Vienna over Paris, though, Americans made it clear that what they valued *most* was precisely what they had valued in Paris—not teaching by the great professors so much as ready access to practical instruction at the bedside. Patrick O'Connell, in a letter published by an American medical journal in 1872, wrote bluntly from Vienna that the assistants offering special courses to small groups in the clinic, not the professors, were the principal attraction: "Those who are the most prominent before the medical profession at large, those who have acquired a world-wide reputation already, perhaps, and who might be supposed to be the real foundation of Vienna's popularity, have practically little to do with it."[66] As Lincoln reported from Vienna, "The idea may still linger in the minds of some, that a student comes to Vienna to hear Rokitansky, Skoda and Oppolzer—or their respective successors. This can hardly be said to be the case." Instead, "the real glory of the school at present consists in the fact that one can learn anything, quickly and thoroughly."[67]

Certainly the appeal of Vienna and Berlin had nothing to do with any notion that their clinicians were better at therapeutics or at patient care in general than their Parisian counterparts. Just as Americans had long insisted that they were more effective healers than the French, those who traveled to Vienna and Berlin were equally confident in asserting superiority to the Germans. "In the Hospitals they study to know what is the matter; then they stop," Ohio physician Joseph Webb wrote from Berlin to his mother in 1866. "In 'Diagnosis,' they excel; but in *Treatment* we excel."[68] The Vienna School was notorious for having taken skepticism about drugging to the extreme of therapeutic nihilism.[69] And just as critics deplored the apostasy of Americans seduced by a French valuation of science over healing, they questioned the integrity of practitioners suborned by German clinical values. Commenting on physicians of "Teutonic proclivities," one American charged that "the day of triumph for such pathologists is not in that of the cure, but while by the side of the cadaver, scalpel in hand, holding up the diseased organs with 'I told you so' beaming joyfully from all the lineaments of the face."[70]

The conversion of sick people into objects of science, a model Americans made such a display of resisting in Paris, appeared to observers even more complete in the Viennese wards. This attitude toward patients seemed neatly embodied in the common practice of referring to them as *material*, a term Americans in Vienna more often than not self-consciously placed in quotation marks. "The 'material', as they call it here, is most abundant," one American studying in Vienna in 1865 wrote in a private letter to Lincoln in Boston, and Lincoln, visiting Vienna six years later, would report back that both professors and their assistants "have certain rights in regard to the use of 'material.'"[71] At the Allgemeine Krankenhaus—"a town in itself," as another Boston student wrote to his father—each professor was provided with a lecture room near his wards. "At the time of lecture this room is filled in with 'specimens' in the shape of men and women who are transferred from the other wards for the occasion. These patients are looked upon and spoken of as 'material' for the medical instruction and as such are submitted to examination by the students without much reference to any feelings which they as men and women may have on the subject."[72] Americans had long spoken of human cadavers as "material," but it was with the shift in migration from France to Germany that they fell into the habit of using this term to refer to living patients as well, with all the subtle alterations in clinical perception that accompany such a change in language.[73]

Americans protested that the treatment they witnessed in Vienna was perhaps even less suited to American patients than were the models that had left them ebullient but uneasy in France. "I thought that in Paris the patients were made subservient enough to the instruction & Enlightenment of the Students but here they are nothing but animals trotted out for the gaping crowds," William Williams Keen wrote in 1865 from Vienna. Like most observers he insisted proudly that American public opinion would never allow the kind of use of patients he saw in the Allgemeine Krankenhaus; "but it's certainly jolly for the Students. It's a magnificent place to learn & in many respects is far superior to Paris."[74] It was partly for this reason that Webb, visiting France after his studies in Germany, remarked in 1867 that "there are many reasons, why one should give Vienna the preference for studying medicine, over all other cities." As he wrote from Paris, "There is much to learn here; but I am satisfied that Vienna, is all things considered the *best*—you get more *at* the patient in Vienna, than here."[75]

In a shift growing from concerns in the 1850s that access to experiential knowledge in Paris was diminishing, Americans abroad increasingly concluded that Vienna and Berlin afforded greater advantages. What most of them

sought in German-speaking lands was neither any new epistemological departure nor the scientific brilliance of the German teachers. Some found the extent
to which the Vienna School cultivated specialism particularly appealing, as
they did its stress on newer microscopical and chemical diagnostic techniques
their compatriots had been studying in Paris. And some—a minuscule minority, upon whom the lion's share of historical attention has been lavished—set
off to Germany for scientific study in the experimental laboratory. But what
most American physicians wanted from Germany was the same kind of ready
access to bodies and practical clinical instruction (for which they expected to
pay) that for so long had drawn them to Paris.

## German Domains of Science

In the stories Americans told during the years when the shift in migration
began and in the accounts they left of their own deliberations, there was no
indication in the 1850s and early 1860s that the clinical empiricism of the Paris
School had become outmoded. Nor was there any sense that new ways of doing
medicine—the ascendancy of laboratory medicine in Germany—was what first
redirected American students. As most Americans told the story at the time,
the French model of medical science was little dimmed; what had declined was
the nature of the clinical experience they could acquire in Paris as compared
with Vienna and Berlin.

As the shift proceeded, however, a generation of American physicians would
come to see themselves as disciples of German medicine in much the same way
their predecessors had seem themselves as disciples of the Paris School. As
with Americans who had studied in Paris, what first directed their travels was
not necessarily the same thing as the meaning that they came to attach to their
journey; and that meaning would be altered yet again once they returned to the
United States and established their identity as German-experienced American
doctors. *Their* experience abroad was rooted in German rather than French
soil, and they were inclined to attribute everything unfamiliar that they found
in the European medical world to a distinctive German ethos. Departing from
the conventions of nearly half a century by pursuing professional improvement
chiefly in German-speaking cities, they were particularly susceptible to seeing
themselves as true disciples of German medicine.

Just how was it that the Americans who studied in Germany saw themselves
transformed by that experience? What did study in such varied cities as Berlin,
Vienna, Leipzig, and Breslau mean to American physicians of diverse backgrounds, expectations, and activities as students, and how did they capture and
convey that meaning by constructing an image of German medicine in the
stories they told about it? And how did they make the Germanness of their
experiences part of the way they understood their place in American medicine
and represented themselves? A full study answering such questions, though
much needed, must be left beyond the scope of this book.[76] But to understand

the legacy of the Paris School and its contested meaning in postbellum America (explored in chapter 10), we must begin to recognize how a new group of Americans during the years just after the Civil War were able to shape a special identity for themselves on the basis of their German experience and how that identity conferred upon them an opportunity and obligation to apply Germanic lessons to reforming American medicine.

The ways Americans became disciples to German medicine have been most fully explored in the case of those few who went to Europe with the principal aim of studying experimental laboratory science, not clinical medicine. Indeed, in the existing historiography, the experience of Henry Pickering Bowditch, who would become the first full-time professor of physiology in the United States, has often been taken as a canonical expression of the wider shift from France to Germany.[77] Bowditch, son of an affluent Boston merchant and graduate of Harvard College who served from 1862 to 1865 in the Union cavalry, began his scientific studies with Jeffries Wyman at Harvard's Lawrence Scientific School after the Civil War, then attended medical school at Harvard, where in 1868 he received his M.D. That same year he set off for Paris, as had his uncle, Henry Ingersoll Bowditch, in 1832, and his mentor, Wyman, in 1841. Like Wyman, from the outset the younger Bowditch was more interested in pursuing natural science in the laboratory than in garnering experience in the clinic, and before his departure Wyman advised the young man to devote himself, as Bowditch put it in a letter from Paris, "to physiology pure & simple."[78]

Bowditch arrived a decade after American migration had begun to shift to Germany, but at a time when Paris remained for many American physicians the first destination on an open-ended itinerary. He spent the first several months taking French lessons, attending *cliniques* at various hospitals, and trying unsuccessfully to arrange laboratory study with the physiologist Charles-Édouard Brown-Séquard. He then settled into what he looked forward to as "a very profitable Winter" studying microscopy and physiology in the laboratory of Louis-Antoine Ranvier, an assistant to Bernard.[79] By January he was, as he informed his uncle, "giving nearly my whole time to physiology," attending Bernard's lectures, seeing him "in the laboratory doing experiments & talking physiology," and working in the laboratory himself. "I seem to be drifting farther & farther away from practical medicine," he told his uncle. "I wish I could see my way clear to devoting myself entirely to the science of the profession," by which he meant experimental physiology; "a life devoted to studies of this sort affords a pleasanter prospect to me than any other I can think of."[80] He was disappointed to find that Bernard's laboratory, "where I work nearly every day, is dark, badly provided with apparatus & with no proper arrangements for pupils."[81] Yet he resolved, as he told Wyman, to "devote myself entirely to the *science* of medicine," and in April he asked a German physiologist visiting the laboratory for advice on how he might best "get a systematic course of physiology." As Bowditch reported to Wyman, "He advised me to go to Bonn for a few months this Spring to learn the language & to follow Max Schultze's course on Histology, then in the Autumn to go to Leipzig & study for a year with Ludwig

& after that to spend what time I have left with Virchow & perhaps with Helmholz." Writing from Bonn the following month, Bowditch told Wyman, "I have already begun to carry out this program."[82]

During the next two years, Bowditch reveled in the laboratory facilities he found in Germany and in the attention he received from German mentors, especially Carl Ludwig at the Physiological Institute in Leipzig.[83] He complained for months that learning German was "no joke," telling his uncle that "there is no use in trying to make believe that it is not a terribly hard language";[84] but, in time, he found great satisfaction in his mastery of both the German language and German ways of life. Above all, Bowditch consecrated himself to what he saw as German ideals of medical science, particularly the belief that the pursuit of scientific truth in the laboratory exemplified by his German teachers was the most promising direction for American medicine. He set aside any notion of clinical study and resolved to spend his time in Leipzig, Berlin, and Heidelberg but not in the clinics of Vienna.[85] In 1871 he returned to Boston and to the newly created full-time post in physiology at the Harvard Medical School, where he set up a laboratory of his own and proselytized for the German program.

Bowditch's European journey and his sense of discovering in Germany a new departure in medicine and a map to the biomedical future provided later medical reformers and historians alike with a powerful emblem of a course American medicine followed in the late nineteenth and early twentieth centuries. He was a harbinger of William Henry Welch, T. Mitchell Prudden, Franklin Paine Mall, Victor C. Vaughan, and John Jacob Abel, who believed that their studies in German laboratories in the late 1870s and 1880s had unfolded a blueprint for modern medicine, and returned to become leading architects of a new kind of scientific medicine in America. Nevertheless, Bowditch has attracted so much historical attention not because he was typical of American physicians in Europe but precisely because his experience was unprecedented. His aspirations were unconventional, the course of study he pursued in Europe was exceptional, his vision of the medical future was still unusual, and the career he was able to follow after his return to the United States was, for the time, positively unique.

The vast majority of medical Americans who traveled to Germany went chiefly for clinical experience, many for only a few months but some for several years. Opportunities for practical education in hospitals and dispensaries increased in postbellum America but failed to keep pace with rising expectations of the clinical experience essential to a prominent career. The Civil War slowed but by no means halted the stream of medical students heading for Europe; many young graduates, indeed, looked upon the war itself as a vast school of experience that gave them the kind of intensive seasoning associated with study in France.[86] After the war, for medical students who could afford it, a trip to Europe was part of an expected routine. As an established physician in Marianna, Florida, surveying his profession in 1868, wrote to his cousin in North Carolina, "For a young man to take rank at once above the ignorant herd that has thronged and disgraced our profession of late, he must take 2 years to graduate, 2 more in Hospital and 2 more in Europe making 6 years and 6 or 8,000 dollars."[87]

In Germany, many of the Americans abroad for instruction in the clinic spent some time studying histology, microscopic pathology, or chemical diagnosis in the laboratory. And some were enticed by the studies they sampled.[88] But it was in the clinic that many of them fashioned an image of distinctive German medicine that defined their sense of special identity and special mission. Bowditch had embraced an image of "the science" of medicine—distinguished from "the practice"—that he located firmly in the laboratory. But most American doctors who sought to link their identity and the future of American medicine to their experiences in Germany had something else in mind. They too embraced what they framed as medical science—and what is more, as *German* medical science—but theirs was a science rooted largely in the clinic.

One such physician was Clarence John Blake, who set off for study in Vienna just after the Civil War. Like Bowditch, a fellow Bostonian and his senior by three years, Blake had studied both at Harvard's Lawrence Scientific School and at its medical school. In 1864 he gained experience through a junior appointment to the newly opened Boston City Hospital, then as a surgical assistant during the final year of the war, and in 1865 received his M.D. degree. Though Blake was uncommonly reflective about the calculations that informed his choices in Europe and meticulous in writing about them to his parents and sister, his course displays patterns that were widely shared among the Americans studying abroad who took German medicine as their reference point in constructing a sense of mission and of self.[89]

During the first several months after he arrived in Vienna in October 1865, Blake sampled widely from what was on offer. He immediately arranged lessons in German (and fencing) and bought tickets to courses by Ferdinand R. von Hebra, "the head of all specialists in skin diseases," and Oppolzer, "the greatest diagnosticator in the world."[90] But what elicited his enthusiasm was less the famous professors than the Allgemeine Krankenhaus itself—"the largest in the world having accommodations for 3200 patients"[91]—and his access to the bodies of patients brought in "as specimens are used, and examined freely by us as illustrations of the lectures."[92] Along with another American and two English students he engaged a young assistant, Karl Myerhofer, for a paid private course in "*practical* diagnostic and operative midwifery" that took full advantage of these "living specimens": "that's what you cannot get in America," he told his father.[93] The women in the wards, he suggested, put up "but little objection to being used as living illustrations," adding that if they did, it was "quickly overcome by the sharp command [of the instructor] . . . or by the manual interference of the nurse." As Blake stated it, "The fact of being able to look at the patient in the light of 'material' is a great advantage."[94] He soon discovered that his German was inadequate to enable him to follow Hebra's lectures, which he dropped, and it was partly because Myerhofer spoke fluent English that Blake gave more and more attention to midwifery, justifying that

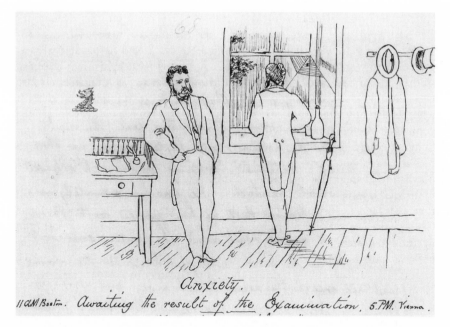

Fig. 9.2. Clarence John Blake's sketch in a letter to his sister of himself and a friend
waiting to learn the results of his examination in Vienna for a degree in midwifery.
(Clare to Dear Poppet [Agnes Blake], Vienna, 25 Apr. 1866, Clarence John Blake
Papers, courtesy of Francis A. Countway Library of Medicine, Boston.)

choice to his father by pointing out how much that branch did "to make or mar
the reputation of a general practitioner."[95]

Returning to Vienna in January after a two-week vacation, Blake outlined
plans that included courses on microscopic pathology, the diseases of the ear
and of children, and chemical pathology, as well as more German lessons. But
he resolved to make midwifery "the principle object of my Vienna pupilage,"
avowedly "without any idea of making a speciality of this branch." In no other
field, he told his father, had practical instruction been so deficient in his Harvard education.[96] In February he revealed his plan to take examinations for the
degree of "Magister in Midwifery," and, as preparation, for a month to "pay all
my attention to practice in the Lying in & womens wards, by this means I shall
get a chance to operate by turning the forceps &c on the living subject." The
degree, he told his father, "may prove useful at some future time in getting
some position from which to start a practice," adding that "every little helps
and a Vienna degree is worth much more than any to be got at home."[97] Late
in April he could write home proud not only that he had stood the examination
and been told "Sie werden Ihre Diplom mit Bene haben," but that his examiners had needed to translate only two of their questions into English.[98]

What Blake had seen of Viennese medicine convinced him by this point that
his future should lie in specialty practice. American cities like Boston, he was
persuaded, had populations sufficient to support "specialists," and Vienna was

"undoubtedly the place to study a speciality."[99] The question was, which one? He considered obstetrics as well as his father's "hints" that nervous disease was bound to be a growing field in the United States.[100] And he particularly explored the possibility of chemical pathology, partly because his own chemical studies at Harvard made "an inclination to this particular branch of science very natural," and largely to satisfy his father, a successful industrial chemist who persistently urged him to study in Justus Liebig's laboratory.[101] Yet the younger Blake remained convinced that "in the United States, a Chemist, although he may be an M.D., is a Chemist and not an physician," and although he pursued laboratory work while in Vienna, he told his father bluntly, "I have no wish to abandon the profession of medicine."[102]

Instead, once his midwifery certificate was in hand, Blake turned to a plan that had been in his mind for months and began private classes with Ignaz Gruber and Adam Politzer on diseases of the ear. "There is a fine opportunity to study that branch here as there are these two professors who attend to nothing else and who have large clinics," he told his father, underscoring again the importance of "speciality" training to making a career in Boston; "otherwise a young man might wait 10 or 12 years before getting anything like a remunerative practice."[103] Forgoing a long-contemplated course of study in Berlin, he decided to remain in Vienna "to get up the Ear thoroughly."[104] He took as well a course on microscopy and a separate microscopical class "on parasites," but it was clinical lessons on diseases of the ear that most intrigued him. "As yet I cant say how much there is to be learned or done in such a speciality as the Ear but certainly there is much more than I had supposed," he wrote home early in June. "Dr Gruber gives us opportunity to practice on his patients and I can now handle the tools pretty well." He also wrote to Edward H. Clarke, his former medical professor at Harvard, asking about "the chance for an Ear practice in B[oston]."[105] As Blake enthusiastically told his father a month later, "It is a speciality which here abroad is growing much as that of the Eye did and I think now is the time for a young man to step in and grow with it."[106]

When Blake first arrived in Vienna, he had assumed that study in Paris would be part of his European tour, and his letters home were filled with the conflicting advice he received from a network of American doctors at home and abroad about the relative advantages of Paris, Berlin, Prague, Heidelberg, Edinburgh, and other cities. From the outset his father encouraged him to keep up his French, but Blake complained that he had to put all his effort into German, "a difficult language to acquire."[107] The longer he spent in Vienna, the less disposed he was to leave it for Paris. "I have been thinking over the matter of studying in Paris and from all I've learned both from Americans and Englishmen who have been there am very much inclined to stay there only long enough to go thro' the hospitals & see the celebrities and the City," he finally told his father after half a year in Vienna. "Paris from all I have heard of it is hardly a city to study medicine in and I've been having here all the advantages of immense material and teaching which leads the medical world. It w'd hardly be worthwhile to live in so expensive and expose oneself to the temptations of

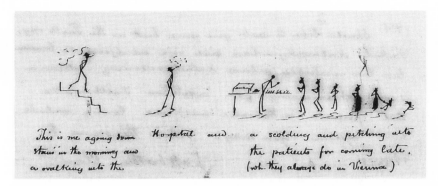

Fig. 9.3. Clarence John Blake's sketch in an 1869 letter to his sister of his routine at the Allgemeine Krankenhaus in Vienna, including his "scolding and pitching into the patients for coming late (wh. they always do in Vienna)." (Clare to Sister Agnes, Vienna, 29 Mar. 1869, Clarence John Blake Papers, courtesy of Francis A. Countway Library of Medicine, Boston.)

so loose a city as Paris."[108] Yet his decision, while partly based on reports about Paris, was informed as much by the intense satisfaction he felt having mastered the ins and outs of daily life in Vienna, its medical world, and the German language. Even the advantages of Berlin—formidable in pathology, he acknowledged—were "hardly an offset to the fact that I should have to learn how to live anew in Berlin & that much time would be lost in making the change."[109] Having paid his entry fee in Vienna, Blake wanted a full return on that investment, and when in summer 1866 he told his father about the guidebook he was writing for American doctors visiting Vienna, it was with obvious pride.[110]

Blake's conversion to German medical ways intensified over the next three years, as did his resolve to specialize in otology. By this choice, Blake saw himself "stepping into a domain of science where there is much as yet unexplored."[111] During his final months in Vienna, his letters were infused with an explicit language of science that had not been there during his first year abroad, and he confidently presented himself as a young American specialist who had donned the mantle of German medical science. Ophthalmology, he believed, offered a model for establishing otology as a specialty; "after a careful study of the ground and calculation of probabilities it seems to me that the domain of Aural Surgery will grow into a speciality much as the eye has done," he wrote to his father in April 1869. "The men taking it up now must be the builders up of it and be not merely givers of other mens prescriptions but above that, be observers and experimenters."[112] As Blake told his mother, he was "going into Otology head over heels in the hopes of being one of those who shall build it up to its proper rank as a branch of the Great Science. Since it is thrown in my way could I hit upon a better life work, do you think?"[113] In the clinics of Politzer and Gruber he studied the "science of Aural Surgery," assisted in performing "experiments," and took charge of examining new patients and performing operations. He also designed an instrument for removing polyps from the ear, which he hoped would help make his reputation in America.[114] As he told his mother, "I am sure I can busy myself with ears all the rest of my life and not have spare time for anything else."[115]

Despite his enthusiasm for German clinical models, Blake remained uneasy about the values governing patient care in the Vienna hospitals. Students, he told his father, were taught to value diagnosis more than therapeutics. "The great Vienna Hospital is in fact quite as much if not more a school for scientific investigation than an institution for the relief of the sick," he observed.[116] A mawkish short story Blake wrote while in Vienna particularly displayed his self-perception as an American who managed to stand apart from the moral order of the Vienna clinic. Set in a women's ward of "the great Vienna Hospital," where assistants busy themselves arranging instruments for the clinical lectures seemingly indifferent to the patients suffering "hopeless, alone," the protagonist, a young doctor from Boston, gives a young girl with an incurable disease comfort and a bunch of violets, which he takes from his buttonhole. Returning the following morning, he finds the girl has died. But, even as her cadaver is being carried away to be autopsied in front of the class, "there is a smile on her face and still clasped in her hands and pressed tightly to her lips is the bunch of withered violets."[117]

As Blake looked homeward, though, he could not but bemoan the "material" he was leaving behind. "The advantages for following up any train of reasoning or proving any theory by experiment on the living subject, are very great in Germany and I almost regret returning to America," he told his father. Yet he held out hope "of having eventually some material to work upon at home" and asked his father to pull strings that might win him an appointment at the Boston Eye and Ear Infirmary, explaining that "such a position will give material for study and be the best possible opening to practice as an Aural Surgeon."[118]

By the time he was preparing to return to Boston, planning to stop on the way for only a few days in Paris and London, Blake was eager to proselytize for German models and for his belief that "a radical change is needed in the American system of medical education and practice."[119] At the center of this program was the conviction that specialism and scientific medicine went hand in hand. "The general feeling among the men studying abroad is that a revolution in medical practice which has already commenced is to be extended to America viz. the splitting up of the profession into specialities," Blake told his mother; it was a reform necessitated by "the rapid advance of Med. Science."[120] There was no conflict, in his mind, between seeing specialism as an expedient pathway to a lucrative career and seeing it as the most congenial choice for "any one who loves Science for itself."[121] Blake's studies abroad had given him a new identity, and just as Stillé had come to see himself as one among a group of American "Parisians," so Blake imagined himself and compatriots who shared his education forming "a small circle of Vienna specialists."[122] Soon after his return Blake was appointed aural surgeon to the Massachusetts Charitable Eye

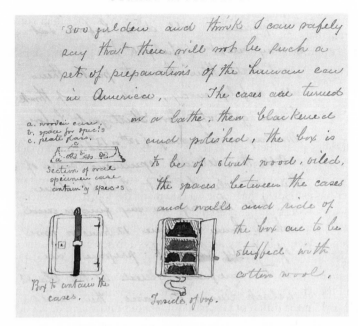

Fig. 9.4. Sketch by Clarence John Blake in a letter to his family of specimen cases he had commissioned to be made in Munich for shipping delicate preparations of the human ear back to Boston. (Clare to Dear Pater and Mater and Agnes, Munich, 7 July 1869, Clarence John Blake Papers, courtesy of Francis A. Countway Library of Medicine, Boston.)

and Ear Infirmary; was elected, in 1876, president of the American Otological Society; and, three years later, began editing the *American Journal of Otology*.

Blake and Bowditch shared neither identical visions of the medical future, nor aspirations for their careers, nor conceptions of what constituted "the science" of medicine. What they did share was the identification of their transforming experiences abroad with a *German* medical world, as well as the realization that transmitting the lessons of that world to the United States was at the core of their distinctive professional identity and defining professional mission. In German clinics and laboratories they—and other Americans—enjoyed a sense of discovery that was fading from the reports of their contemporaries who chose to travel "over the beaten track" to Paris instead. The German medical world was still vastly less familiar to Americans, and for that among other reasons it was easier to see in it a fresh departure. The power of that new German departure was all the stronger for its dual rooting in the laboratory and in the clinic. At home, the notions of medical science articulated by Bowditch and by Blake tended to be merged into a broader image of what German medicine represented, an image in which such social and technical hallmarks as specialism, diagnostic instruments, and reliance on the experimental laboratory often were conflated. What came to be deployed in the American context, more often than not, was a reified *German medicine* succored by patterns of reciprocal appropriation between laboratory and clinic that historians are only beginning to sort out.

## "ALL AMERICANS GO TO PARIS"

In the decades after the Civil War, the number of American physicians who visited Paris and toured its hospitals, far from trickling off, increased. As the tally of American doctors traveling to German cities soared—historian Thomas N. Bonner has estimated that some 15,000 made the journey between 1870 and 1914[123]—a growing number passed through Paris as well. But instead of engaging in prolonged study, increasingly they paused briefly to see the sights before heading on to Vienna or Berlin and getting down to serious work. By 1883, the author of a guidebook for the American physician abroad advised that "the study of medicine in Paris is so much less satisfactory than in Germany that almost all the American students who go to Europe do the greater part of their medical work in the different German universities and spend only a few weeks in Paris."[124] He was offering advice that had become commonplace; but his expectation that nearly all Americans in Europe for medical study would spend "a few weeks in Paris" is also striking. Thus a young Baltimore physician, abroad in 1877 to study medicine in Berlin, Vienna, and Strassburg, told his father with only a little hyperbole that passing through the French capital on his way home, he might run into a family acquaintance who was abroad, "because all Americans go to Paris."[125]

Even if we do not accept at face value the declensionist rhetoric that came to permeate French scientific and medical culture, French medical science and institutions were slipping behind their German counterparts. Nevertheless, the visibility of French medicine in late-nineteenth-century America, as historian John Burnham has displayed by an analysis of citations in American medical journals, was far more pronounced than most historians, preoccupied with tracing the rise of German medicine, have noticed.[126] More than this, being *less* impressive than German cities as a place for medical study did not make Paris *unimpressive* to Americans. "I have already seen enough to justify me in expressing the belief that the medical advantages of Paris, are greater than those of any city in the world," one recently arrived North Carolina physician wrote early in the 1860s. "Paris has, at no former time, been so justly entitled to this distinction as now."[127] His enthusiasm might have been tempered had Vienna or Berlin preceded Paris on his European itinerary, but echoes of his appraisal could be heard over the next several decades. Viewed through New World eyes that took as their benchmark Philadelphia, New York, or Boston, Paris remained imposing and surpassed anything easily available at home.

The official course of study in the hospital wards and lecture theaters continued to elicit the kinds of praise and complaint they had for decades. Americans still marveled that as foreigners they could enjoy the official instruction of the Paris School at no cost, a stark contrast to their remarkably uniform protest against German greed.[128] At the same time, the impediments to learning from the morning rounds of the famous clinicians persisted. As Keen wrote from Paris in the mid-1860s, "I tried the bedside Cliniques but gave them up because I could neither see (being but 5′ 4½″) nor hear (being crowded off by numbers) nor understand (being an Am. & not able to catch the then rapid conversational Fr[ench])."[129] Some decided the Paris hospitals deserved a portion of their time, even if German clinics merited more. Just before sailing from New York in 1866, Webb wrote to his sister that "I have made up my mind to spend eight or ten months, in the Hospitals of Paris or Berlin"; once in Europe, he was persuaded that Vienna was the best place for clinical study, but still decided to spend three or four months in Paris "after doing up Vienna."[130]

Other postbellum Americans arrived in Paris eager to pursue medical studies not so much in the clinic as in the laboratory, though sometimes they were disappointed by the arrangements they found. Bowditch's indictment of teaching in Bernard's laboratory is well known: "The want of a good laboratory for practical instruction in physiology is seriously felt in Paris," he told Wyman in 1869. "The Frenchmen acknowledge the great advantage that the Germans have over them in this respect."[131] His judgment echoed the rhetoric of French critics, part of a wider cultural jeremiad that confirmed and shaped the young American's perceptions. "I have just been reading a pamphlet entitled 'De la réforme des études médicales par les laboratoires' by a Dr Lorain in which the writer compares the advantages for studying medical science in Germany & in France much to the disadvantage of the latter country," he told his uncle a few weeks after writing to Wyman. "I hear the same story all round. The government lavishes millions on the army but leaves science to starve & freeze."[132] Nevertheless, Bowditch's growing enchantment with German science makes it easy to forget that when he first left for Europe, it was with high expectations for physiological study in the French capital. And the same letters in which he expressed the criticisms cited above also related his enthusiastic satisfaction with other aspects of scientific instruction he found in Paris.[133]

For American physicians who traveled to Paris in the 1860s to study natural science, however, learning once in Europe that opportunities might be better in German laboratories did not necessarily mean moving across the Rhine. That Bowditch's decision was by no means inevitable is clear in the choices made by his contemporary Stephen Henry Bronson. After receiving his M.D. from Yale in 1866, Bronson spent a year with Wyman studying comparative anatomy at Harvard, where Bowditch was among his classmates. Bronson's father, a New Haven physician, had visited Paris a quarter century earlier, leaving a record in his diary of his rounds of the city's hospitals, dissecting rooms, and museums, and in 1867 gave his son permission to go abroad, without, apparently, dictating the course of study he should follow.[134] "My object in going to Europe is not to travel, but to obtain facilities for the study of Comparative Anatomy and Medicine," the twenty-three-year-old Bronson told

Wyman. "Considering my limited knowledge of French and German, I do not know, in which of the foreign cities it would be best for me to locate."[135] In October 1867 Bronson boarded a steamship for Europe, pausing only briefly in London, where the naturalist Richard Owen seconded Wyman's recommendation that the Jardin des Plantes in Paris was the best place to study comparative anatomy, and gave him a letter of introduction to Georges Pouchet. Bronson's initial enthusiasm differed little from the reports Americans had been sending home for decades. "The unequalled opportunities, which one finds for study in Paris, impresses me more and more every day and I look about me with a feeling of awe," he told Wyman. "It is not strange, then, that this Mecca attracts from every quarter of the globe, pilgrims, who searching after truths, regard distance and separation as nothing."[136]

Like his medical forebears, Bronson began attending morning *cliniques* at a number of hospitals—La Charité, Hôtel Dieu, Hôpital des Cliniques, Hôpital des Enfants Malades, and St. Louis, writing in his diary of the latter hospital for the diseases of the skin that "here, one has the best opportunity to study those affections of any institution in the world."[137] And, again like his predecessors, he noted with some disapproval the way patients were used as objects for clinical instruction. Bronson seemed even more indignant, though, when at Jean-Baptiste Bouillaud's *clinique* at La Charité, he encountered a woman—unnamed, but probably Mary Putnam—among the crowd of medical students. "I noticed a *lady* there, apparently studying medicine, she had a note book in her hand and followed the *fellows* about the bed side," he wrote in his diary. "Imagine my disgust when informed that she was an 'American doctor' from N.Y. She follows all the Hospitals and seems to be an ardent follower of Gail Hamilton," the American feminist writer.[138]

Bronson followed clinical rounds with resignation more than enthusiasm, for, as he confessed to Wyman, his real aim was comparative anatomy, and after a few months he largely set aside hospital study.[139] He delivered his letter of introduction from Owen to Georges Pouchet, who arranged permission for Bronson to work in the comparative anatomy laboratory at the Jardin des Plantes, became his steady companion, and found him a French tutor.[140] With Pouchet he walked to the central market to buy live frogs for physiological experiments, to the place where stray dogs were taken to purchase "a very mild and benevolent looking animal" for the same end, and, as he wrote in his diary, "to the school of Clamart in order to get some ears for dissection."[141] He also took advantage of the official program of lectures and demonstrations on natural science, attending classes by Étienne-R.-A. Serres, Robin, Pouchet, Emile Blanchard, Henri Milne-Edwards, Paul Gervais, Armand de Quatrefages, and Bernard—discovering at the second lecture of Bernard's course that seated just behind him was his coworker from Wyman's laboratory in Cambridge, Henry Pickering Bowditch.[142] Most of Bronson's time, though, was spent in the laboratory, where he dissected the auditory apparatus of a deer, owl, iguana, kangaroo, and armadillo, among other creatures from the menagerie of the Jardin.[143]

Bronson heard all around him complaints about inadequate support for laboratory sciences in Paris, writing home, for example, that "Pouchet says, 'Everything is very dirty, we are beggars', meaning that they had little money"; yet at first Bronson was so overwhelmed by the wealth of facilities that he dismissed such griping as idle.[144] More and more, though, he began to echo the charge that the Second Empire was willing to lavish wealth on cutting grand new boulevards through the heart of Paris but little interested in supporting natural science. Nine months after dismissing Pouchet's complaints, Bronson was ready himself to assert that the Jardin was "in the stage of its decline."[145] The effect on laboratory work was demoralizing. "The teacher has no interest, whatever in instructing his pupils and the student is left alone to follow his own course where his fancy or inexperience inclines him," he told his parents. "The dearth of pupils in the Laboratory and the absence of seriousness in those who attend, are the legitimate results."[146] Bronson became convinced that opportunities for laboratory instruction were decidedly superior in Germany, and that if he wanted the best Europe had to offer, he would have to leave France.[147]

The deciding factor was language. For Bronson, as for many Americans, learning French had been a struggle, and he found so much satisfaction in his headway that within a year of arriving in Paris he had started making all his diary entries in simple French.[148] Having invested in learning one foreign language—and, perhaps equally, in negotiating the French scientific and medical world—Bronson was loath to give it all up and start over. "I am quite undecided to know what to do about Germany," he told his parents after a year and a half in Paris. "Germany is the most advanced now of all countries in science, the schools better and the facilities greater, but there is the language to be learned," he observed, adding gloomily, "I know about as much German as I knew French when I came here."[149] Returning to this theme several months later, he told them that "I think even if I was to remain another year abroad, I should prefer to remain in France, rather than to go into Germany. I find it takes so long to learn enough of the language to make it really serviceable."[150] In the event, Bronson did visit Germany before leaving the Continent and in Berlin even briefly engaged a German tutor, but he inspected hospitals and natural history museums as a medical tourist, not as a serious student.[151] Instead, he devoted his remaining time abroad to studying in England and Scotland, revisiting London where, as Bronson wrote in his diary (still kept in French), he went "à l'hopital St. Bartholomew—j'ai dit adieu au père Owen—il m'a donné un mémoire."[152] Returning to Connecticut in the summer of 1871, Bronson practiced medicine at the office he opened in New Haven and at the New Haven Dispensary until, at the age of thirty-six, he died in 1880.

During the 1860s, Paris also began to attract a newly emerging group of medical Americans, namely, women physicians. Both Bowditch and Bronson had traveled to France to study branches of natural science they believed could be better pursued in Paris than in the United States, and even though one emphasized experimentation while the other stressed morphology, what their work shared was its locus in the laboratory, not the hospital. But it was clinical access—what had drawn medical men to France for half a century—that women physicians would most seek in the French capital.

During the 1850s, a few American women who held M.D. degrees had studied in Paris, including Elizabeth Blackwell, Nancy Clark, and Emily Blackwell. But in the 1860s, as the numbers of women's medical schools and graduates rose, more and more women began to pursue professional improvement in France, as well as in Britain and German-speaking countries. "Nearly all of the pioneer women doctors in the first quarter-century after Elizabeth Blackwell's graduation went abroad," Bonner has asserted, and the advocates of women's medical education openly proclaimed the necessity of such migration at the time.[153] "It is almost impossible," Blackwell affirmed early in the 1860s, "for a lady doctor to get a *good* medical education without going to Europe."[154]

The American women who earned a medical degree abroad, few numerically but important culturally, established new precedents and a source of inspiration for medical women at home. When in 1871 Susan Dimock and Mary Corinna Putnam graduated at Zurich and Paris, respectively, they were among the first women from *any* country to earn European medical degrees, encouraging and enabling others to follow their example.[155] In the United States, at introductory and commencement addresses at women's medical schools that commemorated achievements and rallied the faithful for the struggles ahead, orators held up such examples as a cause for optimism. "In Paris women are now admitted to all the privileges of the medical schools and hospitals, and to the examinations for medical degrees," the 1869 annual announcement of the New England Female Medical College overzealously proclaimed, generalizing from the permission Putnam had recently won to take examinations leading to the degree. It went on to cite the case of Sarah Parker Remond, an African-American woman who had been studying in Florence, Italy, where she had just received her medical diploma.[156] Yet the women's medical schools founded in Boston, Philadelphia, and New York in the 1850s and 1860s, and others that followed, meant that an American woman *could* receive an M.D. degree in her own country, even if most American medical schools remained closed to her.

Like other American doctors who studied abroad, however, most women physicians who set off for study in Paris had no expectation of returning with a foreign degree. Gaining clinical experience in the United States—increasingly regarded as a key ingredient in any "*good* medical education"—was especially difficult for women students and recent graduates, blocked from most large hospitals. A common motif in addresses and catalogs of women's medical colleges was a self-congratulatory review of progress in educating women physicians, followed by lamentations over persistent obstacles to clinical training. Emeline H. Cleveland, professor at the Female Medical College of Pennsylvania, having recounted such a story of "progress" in 1866, cautioned that "in giving this brief history, we would not conceal the fact that it has been impossible in this early stage of the movement to secure to ladies all the educational advantages which are accessible to men." Access to "clinical facilities" remained the leading problem. In Cleveland's own city, "professional opposition, taking at last an organized form, has hitherto prevented the general hospitals and dispensaries of Philadelphia, from being available, to any considerable extent, to our students and graduates."[157]

Efforts to address this deficiency were three pronged. One approach was the creation of separate women's medical institutions—dispensaries and hospitals attached to the women's medical colleges. Crucial here was the work of such physicians with European experience as Elizabeth and Emily Blackwell in establishing the New York Infirmary for Women and Children (1857), Marie Zakrzewska in founding the New England Hospital for Women and Children in Boston (1862), Ann Preston in opening the Woman's Hospital of Philadelphia (1862), and Annette Buckel in setting up the San Francisco Hospital for Women and Children (1875).[158] Such facilities, Preston told her students at the Female Medical College of Pennsylvania in 1859, were critical to providing women with "*practical* instruction in medicine."[159]

A second strategy was lobbying for admission of women students to existing hospitals and dispensaries. In Boston, Samuel Gregory, the ever-optimistic proprietor of the New England Female Medical College, saw the founding of the Boston City Hospital in 1864 as an opportunity to stake his school's claim to municipal clinical resources. He proposed building new quarters for the school near the City Hospital "as the Harvard Medical College is located near the Massachusetts General Hospital," reasoning "that the City Hospital would afford the students greater advantages for clinical instruction than any private establishment."[160] Successes were significant, albeit piecemeal, providing limited access for some women students but virtually no positions of clinical authority for more advanced graduates.[161]

The third channel to clinical access was going abroad. The voyages American women physicians made to Paris were calculated investments in building successful medical careers. Simultaneously, their journeys during the 1860s were also self-consciously framed as contributions to the wider cause of women's medical education. Women's medical colleges pointed with pride to recent graduates in Europe, and most especially to faculty members abroad to improve their teaching and their institution's prestige. The New England Female Medical College boasted in 1865 that its professor of obstetrics and diseases of women and children, Minerva C. Meriam, planned "to go to Paris at the close of our next term to increase her practical experience in the great hospitals of that city, and return with additional qualifications the following term."[162] While Meriam was still away, her colleagues made use of her absence in Paris "to increase her knowledge and practical experience in the hospitals of that city" and her anticipated return to teaching in advertising their 1867–1868 session.[163] Sometimes faculty members were sent to France as an investment in a school's future. In 1860, Quaker women making plans to establish a teaching hospital in conjunction with the Female Medical College of Pennsylvania sent Cleveland to Paris to study obstetrics, just as they later sent Anna Broomall and Frances Emily White. Cleveland returned, having studied chiefly at the Hôpital de la Maternité, to become professor of obstetrics and diseases of women and children and resident physician at the school's newly founded Woman's Hospital.[164] Like professors from other medical schools, faculty members often went with commissions from their institutions. Thus Elizabeth Blackwell, revisiting Paris in 1866, arrived with a list prepared by her sister Emily of supplies needed for their school in New York; "I feel an immense responsibility in spending the hard earned money," she wrote from Paris.[165]

Through the first half of the 1860s, no institution in Paris was as central to the medical studies of American women as the Hôpital de la Maternité. Entering the doorway of the former convent led the woman physician from America into a kind of experience quite different from that enjoyed by her countrymen in the other Paris hospitals. She traded her status as a physician for what Blackwell had characterized as the disciplined and demeaning routine of a midwifery pupil; but in return she won obstetric experience perhaps unmatched anywhere. "You are very much mistaken if you think Vienna or Berlin better than the Paris Maternite for real knowledge," Marie Zakrzewska wrote from Boston in 1863 to her former student at the New England Female Medical College, Lucy Sewall, who after graduating had promptly set off for Europe. "For instance, in Berlin, no student, not even a male, is permitted to perform 'version' or do anything in the way of an operation. In Paris, every midwife gets her case of 'version.'" Sewall took her mentor's advice and continued her studies in Paris. In both Vienna and Berlin, Zakrzewska had counseled her, "the men take the places close to the beds and the women have to stand on the outskirts; while in Paris no man stands in the woman's way."[166]

The experience to be gained at the Maternité was widely recognized in America, and women's medical colleges boasted about graduates and faculty members who studied in its wards. At the Woman's Hospital of Philadelphia, Cleveland proudly informed prospective students that their instructor was one "who, to her available clinical advantages at home, had added the experience of a year's residence in La Maternite, Paris."[167] Helen Morton, a classmate of Sewall's in Boston, probably spent longer at the Maternité than any of her compatriots, and in 1864, after two years, she won a first-prize medal for her performance as a student from its École d'Accouchement. Morton then spent another two years there as an assistant instructor before returning to Boston, where later she became a successor to Zakrzewska at the dispensary of her alma mater.[168] Some American women—from the Blackwells and Clark onward—obtained permission to follow clinical instruction at other Paris hospitals as well; but such admission remained a matter of individual favor, not the official policy of entitlement enjoyed by men. As Cleveland, delivering her valedictory address at the Female Medical College of Pennsylvania in 1863, cautioned the graduating students, "In Paris, L'Ecole de Médecine is religiously closed, and general hospitals are entered only by personal favor."[169]

The centrality of the Maternité to the experience of American women doctors in Paris began to fade in the mid-1860s as gradually, individually, women gained access to the official instruction at the city's other hospitals. The cir-

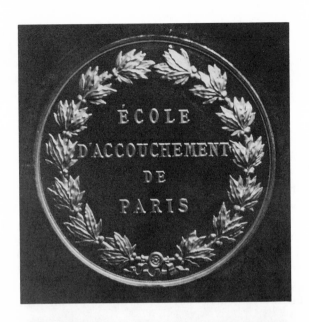

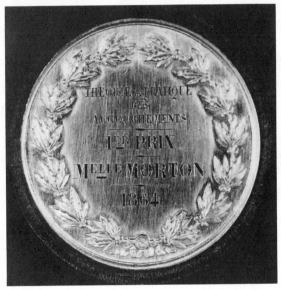

Fig. 9.5. First prize medal awarded to Helen Morton by the École d'Accouchement de Paris in 1864 for her performance as a midwifery student at the Hôpital de la Maternité, an institution central to the Parisian studies of the first generation of American women physicians. (Courtesy of Archives and Special Collections on Women in Medicine of Allegheny University of the Health Sciences, Philadelphia.)

cumstances of Morton's departure from the Maternité may have compelled them to look hard elsewhere. "I am excessively sorry to find that Miss Morton had a regular row with M^me Alliot [who directed the training of midwives], just two months before the close of the last session, & left the Institution with the other aide sage femme who sided with her," Elizabeth Blackwell wrote from Paris in 1866 to her sister Emily. "I tried to see M^me A, having a very good introduction, and she has avoided my visit with extreme rudeness. I fear in consequence of this, certain difficulties seem to be made to the admission of Mrs Merriam & Miss Putnam neither of whom has yet succeeded in gaining entrance."[170]

Perhaps Blackwell was right. But it is not clear that Mary Putnam ever *wanted* admittance to the Maternité. "You know when I first came to Paris," Putnam wrote to her mother from France late in 1866, "different advices that I did receive inclined me for a time to think of entering the Maternity. In fact I went to that gloomy establishment to make inquiries, but found myself confronted by several difficulties, among which my ignorance of French was pointed out to me as prominent, by the *directeur*." That, Putnam explained, came as a relief, for "I was in no hurry to seal my fate by entering that detestable place."[171]

The Parisian experience of Putnam (later Putnam Jacobi) can be used to illustrate both the ways American women were able to negotiate access to medical experience in France and the kind of rich opportunities American doctors in general could find in Paris in the late 1860s. The eldest daughter of Victorine Haven Putnam and the New York publisher George Palmer Putnam, in 1863 Mary Putnam graduated from the New York College of Pharmacy. Enrolling next at the Female Medical College of Pennsylvania, Putnam petitioned to be examined for the M.D. degree after one year and in 1864 graduated third out of a class of eight.[172] Putnam then gave several months to clinical study with Zakrzewska and Sewall at the New England Hospital for Women and Children; at the end of the summer of 1866, she boarded a steamer for Europe.

Like hundreds of American doctors before her, Putnam—pleased en route that she was "very little sea sick"—debarked in Le Havre, made her way to Rouen, wrote to her father of seeing the place where Joan of Arc was burned, and proceeded to Paris, writing home that she was "perfectly astonished and delighted by it."[173] She went first to a hotel across from the Tuileries Palace, then with the help of Elizabeth Blackwell, in Paris at the time, found more modest lodging in the Latin Quarter. Putnam began French lessons at once with a tutor to whom she had brought a letter of introduction from Austin Flint, and decided to defer medical study for a month, until she was better accustomed to the language and the city. "You have no idea of the overwhelming effect of Paris upon a person coming for the first time," she wrote to her sister Edith. "For the first few days I was as one intoxicated."[174] She saw Blackwell, twenty-one years her senior, many times during that month—later recalling that it was from her that she learned that in Paris, it was safe for a woman to walk alone in the evening.[175] Putnam told her mother that when the older physician left Paris, "she actually kissed me for the first time during the period of our long and friendly acquaintance! I was quite astonished, but very much delighted."[176]

Putnam had not arrived entirely committed to a life practicing medicine and, like Henry Pickering Bowditch, was still considering a career in laboratory science. Resolving "to devote half the time to clinical, and half to scientific study," she had left open "whether I would study medicine as subordinate to chemistry, or chemistry as subordinate to medicine." Like Blake, who in the same year was in Vienna and felt himself compelled to choose between being a chemist and being a physician, Putnam believed medical practice promised a more secure future. As one of eleven children she could not lean too heavily on financial support from her parents and wrote to her mother, explaining her decision, that "I see more chance of satisfying you if I am a practical physician than if, without fortune, I try to become a scientific chemist."[177]

It was not clear to Putnam, though, just what her options were for study. The guidebooks that celebrated the free and effortless access to the city's hospitals, dissecting rooms, and lecture halls applied to men only. She was "on the point of presenting myself again at the Maternity," as she told her mother, when letters from Sewall and a new acquaintance with the English physician Benjamin Ball redirected her plans "out of the compulsory channel in which they had been running."[178] Sewall, while visiting Europe several years earlier, had been greatly encouraged by the hospital access she enjoyed in London before crossing the Channel. Invited on ward rounds by individual physicians at the Middlesex and London Hospitals, she also reported to the Boston feminist Caroline Dall of "the Medical men" of London that "many of them call me Dr Sewall, treat me as if I were one of them, talk with me freely on all Medical matters and often take a good deal of trouble to show me their interesting cases."[179] Her London experiences helped encourage Sewall by the time she reached Paris, and she was later able to give Putnam an introduction to Jacques-Joseph Moreau de Tours, a clinician at the Salpêtrière, that was to prove crucial.[180] Ball, for his part, tried to gain permission for Putnam to attend lectures at the École de Médecine; though he "naturally failed," as she put it, he did secure her admission to clinical instruction at some of the hospitals.[181]

By the close of 1866, Putnam reported that she was "in full tide of hospital visiting."[182] Like her male counterparts, she favored hospitals distant from the École de Médecine and crowds of French students. Both the Salpêtrière and the Lariboisière, she explained, were "so far away from the schools, that, although both of them are very large hospitals, the medical students do not visit them, which is a great convenience for me." Moreau's *clinique* at the Salpêtrière, therefore, was "quite like taking private lessons."[183] And like her male compatriots, while she relished the access to practical experience in the wards, she was disturbed by the moral order of the Paris Clinic and told her sister that the French were "a people whose intellect has entirely consumed their conscience and feeling."[184] Later in life, she would urge Americans to emulate the strengths of the model of clinical instruction she had witnessed in France "without necessarily introducing into clinical practice the brutalities that so often disfigure the European treatment of hospital patients."[185]

But even though Putnam was now attending *cliniques* with American men (as Bronson noted in his diary with "disgust"), her experience of the official course of instruction was not identical to theirs. Once she was in the wards, in some respects gender figured to her advantage. Though regarded as an "anomaly," she also received "special treatment" from the professors, what she described as "the deference and politeness due to a woman, and the consideration accorded to a rather small person in a very large place."[186] When she joined the throng of students attending Léon-Athanase Gosselin's surgical *clinique* at La Charité, she judged the experience "magnificent," noting that "it is much crowded, but there is no difficulty in keeping near the professor, as the students yield me place."[187]

Putnam disdained the American medical tourists who made a fleeting appearance in the wards without seeming to appreciate the opportunities in front of them. In one of the first of a long series of reports on medical Paris that she sent to the New York *Medical Record*—published under the inverted initials P.C.M. and written, like articles sent to several newspapers and popular periodicals, to supplement her income—she noted how little was learned by Americans untutored in French who made but a "flying visit to Paris."[188] By contrast, "I cannot do a thing half way," she told her father. "When I was in Boston, Lucy Sewall considered me stupid, because I could not do things without having studied them, and could not accept her methods without question. In Paris, I am considered one of the most successful students, because I have been able to 'go the whole horse.'"[189]

Putnam had not entirely relinquished her commitment to chemistry, and even as she entered a routine of clinical study she sought to use another letter from Flint as entrée to a course in physiological chemistry. Expressing herself in words that could have come from Bowditch, she recognized that "a purely scientific life would suit me better than any other." Yet she realized that "many practical difficulties intervene. It costs more, pays less (pecuniarily) and, strange to say, I find much less facility for it here than for the medicine."[190] Discouraged by "the difficulties I have encountered in finding a laboratory where I can pursue certain chemico-medical analyses," by February 1867 she decided to put the plan aside and "concentrate my attention exclusively upon clinical medicine."[191]

Putnam nevertheless soon added work at the dissecting table and microscopy bench to her hospital studies. She began a class in anatomy, and her instructor obtained permission for her to attend a class of operative surgery at the École Pratique, a source of particular satisfaction because, as she told her mother, this was "one of the institutions that Dr. Blackwell prophesied that I could not enter."[192] Louis-Antoine Ranvier, who with André-Victor Cornil directed the microscopy laboratory where Putnam spent a couple of hours daily, also obtained permission for her to use the library of the École de Médecine.[193] While Putnam clearly saw her work at the École Pratique and in the microscopy laboratory as ends in themselves—significant elements in a plan of study cobbled together by special favor—she also saw them as "stepping stones" to further instruction. Realizing that she was now "in *two* courses of young men, one for anatomy, the other for the microscope," as well as attending clinical courses with male students, late in the spring of 1867 she began to think that this precedent might be put to strategic use were she to petition for admittance to the full range of lectures at the École de Médecine. It was a notion, she told her sister, that left her "in a whirl of the most intense excitement."[194] Her aim was permission to audit the lectures, as so many of her medical countrymen did; but over the next few months she extended her goal to registering for a medical degree. She revealed this plan to her father in November, writing that "my entrance to the École is a settled fact." She saw the prospect of being "the first woman ever admitted to the famous Paris École" as a good investment in her career and "a great thing for the medical education of all women."[195] But her confidence was premature, and a month later she had to write again to say her application had been rejected.[196]

In January 1868, however, Putnam was able to tell her mother that "day before yesterday, for the first time since its foundation several centuries ago, a petticoat might be seen in the august amphitheatre of the *École de Médecine*": she had been granted permission to attend Robin's lectures on histology, though not to take examinations for a degree.[197] As she later told her sister, "It is grand to be in the great amphitheatre of the famous *École*, after having been refused admission so decidedly!"[198] The train of events leading to this success had in part been put into play at a reception Putnam attended in October, given for Emily Blackwell by her sister Anna, a longtime resident of Paris.[199] Emily had good reason to use personal connections to aid Putnam, for only a month earlier Elizabeth had confided to her in a letter marked "Private" that she could think of only three women who might help the Blackwells realize aspirations for their medical college in New York, and one was Putnam.[200] Emily Blackwell introduced Putnam to an acquaintance who in turn introduced her to a woman of influence who pressed her case for admission, and by early summer 1868 Putnam had become the first woman inscribed for a medical degree, which she would receive three years later.[201]

It was around this time that her own democratic commitments, her growing friendship with a family of French socialists, and the violent course of political events that culminated in the suppression of the Paris Commune combined to radicalize Putnam in ways that, as historian Joy Harvey has argued, stayed with her throughout her life. In 1868, even as she was deriving satisfaction from her new presence in the amphitheater of the École de Médecine, she began to speak of her "deliberate and unqualified hatred" of Louis-Napoléon and all he stood for, sentiments shared by her new acquaintances the Réclus family—"radical republicans and socialists," as she described them.[202] By the end of the year she wrote to her father declaring her conviction that "the single saving element in France at this moment lies in the direction of Socialism."[203] By late 1869 she moved into the household of Elie Réclus, his wife Noémi, and brother Elisée, and in this politically committed milieu watched the approaching downfall of Napoléon III, civil war, and the start of the Franco-Prussian War.[204]

Putnam celebrated the proclamation of the Republic on 4 September 1870 and declined to leave the city with other foreigners before the gates were closed against the Prussians, writing of the Republic to her mother that "I feel really quite ready to die in its defense."[205] In the coming months, amidst the Siege of Paris she continued studying in the hospitals and finished her thesis, though the closing of the school meant she could not complete formalities for her degree. Thus toward the end of the siege, in the same letter in which she recounted finding shelter for a night in the vaults of the Panthéon with several hundred other refugees from the bombing outside—"the tombs of Voltaire and Rousseau sheltering the victims of the Prussian barbarians"—she told her father that she had finished her thesis. She wanted him to know, moreover, that she stayed not "for the empty bravado of playing at heroics" but as a witness who stood in solidarity with the ideals of the Paris Commune.[206] Before the war, Putnam had also fallen in love with a French medical student and the two were engaged just before he set off for the front; but when he returned, the relationship came apart.[207] The siege having ended, Putnam left for a visit to London, partly to await the reopening of the École so that she could take the last of the long series of required examinations and defend her thesis, and partly, it seems, to recover from her sorrow over the defeat of the Communards and the disintegration of her love affair.[208] She returned to Paris as soon as the École reopened, and, in July 1871, wrote home that she had passed her last examination and her thesis and was now "*docteur en médecine de la Faculté de Paris.*"[209]

Throughout her years in Paris, a medical women's network had been crucial to Putnam. Introductions from the Blackwells and Sewall had been key in initiating the chain of personal associations and favors that won her access to the Paris medical world. Putnam also spent a good deal of time in Paris with the Englishwoman Elizabeth Garrett, who was admitted to the École partly on the basis of the precedent Putnam had set and who received her degree before Putnam did, just before the Franco-Prussian War. Indeed, late in 1869 Garrett moved into the Réclus household with Putnam.[210] Other American women physicians also associated with Putnam in Paris, including Augusta and Emily Pope, twins who, after graduating from the New England Female Medical College, headed for Paris in April 1870 "to continue their education in the great hospitals of that city," as the school's next annual report put it.[211] Putnam became a guide and friend to the Popes, whose studies included work at the Hôpital des Enfants Malades. They remained until virtually the last moment before the city was sealed off for the siege, but left in mid-September 1870 for London. There they studied in a small hospital for women Garrett had established, and later returned to positions in Zakrzewska's Boston hospital.[212]

A medical women's network was also critical to Putnam's expectations about her career in the United States. Her hopes centered on a chair at the Blackwells' medical college, possibly in medical chemistry, and when she saw Elizabeth

Blackwell in Paris late in 1869, the older physician seemed encouraging.[213] Blackwell also helped arrange a loan for Putnam but privately was suspicious and a little disapproving. On the one hand, Elizabeth wrote to her sister Emily that "Miss Putnam, will certainly be of use," and noted that "I think it would be wise to help her to a certain extent, for she is wanted in the New York work." On the other hand, Elizabeth Blackwell was convinced that when Putman joined them in New York, "her object of course will be to make use of the Infirmary to push her private practice." Blackwell also found Putnam's dogged commitment to giving a "brilliant" performance in her examinations and thesis extravagant and a bit pretentious. "Dont build upon Miss Putnam," Elizabeth wrote again to her sister after some reflection. "I do not think she has stable character enough to make it desirable she should be any thing but an out-sider. Mind I've nothing new to say of her—only she is what she is—brilliant in intellect rather than solid in character."[214] For her part, as Putnam prepared to leave Paris she looked ahead with apprehension to "the unscientific *'milieu'* in which I shall be partially plunged." Indeed, implicit in Putnam's hope that she could catalyze in America what she described to her mother as "the creation of a scientific spirit, (which at present does not exist), among women medical students" was a judgment on Blackwell's generation and its understanding of scientific medicine that warranted the older physician's suspicions.[215]

In September 1871 Putnam returned to New York, where she became a member of the Medical Society of New York; joined the faculty of Blackwell's Women's Medical College of the New York Infirmary; married, two years later, the eminent German-Jewish immigrant physician Abraham Jacobi; in time became a member of the New York Academy of Medicine; and became established as one of the most prominent women physicians and teachers in America. Of her many professional achievements, though, singled out at her death in 1906 in the *New York Tribune* and virtually all other obituaries was "her successful entry into the Ecole de Médecine, encouraging scores of other women."[216]

Putnam's story, albeit singular, is suggestive of wider shifts in the place Paris occupied in American medical culture at a moment all too easy to label as one of French decline and German ascendence. To begin with, it underscores the newly emerging significance of Europe in the medical education of American women, who traveled abroad chiefly for clinical experience but, as in Putnam's case, often for laboratory experience, didactic instruction, and medical degrees as well.[217] In the 1860s, study in Paris—among other Continental centers— began to be seen as one of the most promising avenues an American woman could take in fashioning a medical career, a perception that in the 1870s and 1880s would grow commonplace. Women physicians in late-nineteenth-century American fiction often were portrayed as having European experience; and study abroad came to be represented not as the exceptional prerogative of an elite but as an unremarkable step. In Harriet Beecher Stowe's 1871 novel *My Wife and I*, Caroline Simmons, a young New Englander of modest means, has been studying with a local country doctor. When her father becomes ill, she is tied to home caring for him and her studies cease, but his death leaves her both "free of the world" and in need of supporting herself. "My desire is, if I could in any way earn the means, to go to France and perfect myself in medical studies," Simmons writes to her cousin. "I am told that a medical education can be obtained there by women cheaper than anywhere else." Later in the novel Ida Van Arsdel, daughter of a once-affluent New York family fallen on difficult times, also settles on medicine as her career. She has saved up some money "to make her studies with in Paris," and as the novel closes the two women make plans to sail for France where both will study medicine and Simmons, much like Putnam, will support herself as foreign correspondent for an American periodical.[218] What is striking is that Stowe presented the choice of Paris as the place for medical study by each of these characters entirely without fanfare. In a later novel, by William D. Howells, when the male Dr. Mulbridge first meets Dr. Grace Breen and tries to figure out her medical background—asking whether she has studied in Paris—he is taken aback to learn that she has not been to Europe:

> "I have never been abroad," said Grace.
> "No?" he exclaimed. "I thought all American [medical] ladies had been abroad."[219]

Increasingly, American women also pursued their European studies on the eastern bank of the Rhine. Novelists associated their women medical protagonists with work in Vienna, Berlin, and Zurich, while, according to Bonner, between 1870 and 1914 some six to eight hundred women from the United States studied medicine in German-speaking centers.[220] Still, the perception that American women could find in Paris medical instruction and experience difficult to obtain at home was remarkably durable. Not just the supporters of women's education but critics as well drew the special connection between women students and medical Paris. It was to disparage Paris medicine rather than to praise it that an American male physician naively wrote from France in 1880, "It would seem that Paris is the only place where female students are admitted to the same rights with the male."[221]

Putnam's story also points to some of the profound differences that distinguished Americans' experience of the Parisian medical world in the late 1860s from that of their predecessors. It is quite possible that Putnam, during her time abroad, wrote more on Paris than any other nineteenth-century American physician—in private letters, in professional journals, in popular periodicals, and in newspapers. From her writings, like those of her forebears, comes the heady sense of being at the center of things. What is missing, however, is the ardent celebration of empiricism that had so marked American reports from the 1810s through the 1850s—the sense that Paris particularly mattered because it was there that the medical barricades had been mounted against the spirit of system. In this respect, Putnam *was* typical of a postbellum American doctor in Paris. She was sensitive to the passage of generations and the medical ways they represented, something clear in her account of Bouillaud, who had once been among the most formidable of the Parisian medical lions. "Bouillaud has been a very distinguished man, but now his ideas are entirely out of date and the struggle he makes to *les faire prévaloir encore*, is really pathetic," she told her mother in 1867. "He is a man who bleeds for everything. His clinics are almost deserted but the heroic old fellow fights on, and revives the recollections of his youth. He has been *très gentil* to me, and I have fancied has an odd sort of fellow feeling for me, as if I, too, were fighting in an unpopular cause and deserved encouragement."[222] Putnam captured the change over time tersely when, in her first letter from Paris to the *Medical Record*, she suggested that recent French microscopical research on the pathology of tuberculosis "completely upsets the old descriptions given by Laennec and Louis."[223]

American doctors continued to visit Paris in the decades after the Civil War, but the ethos of Paris medicine, as well as the way its messages were discerned through American eyes, had changed. By the 1870s, in American medical journals, in professional addresses, and in private correspondence, assessments of the advantages for study offered by different European centers were less likely to compare Vienna with Paris than Vienna with Berlin. By 1880, an American physician in Vienna could write to a Cincinnati journal reflecting that "medical centres have their day like the states and empires of which they are so often the capitals, and if Vienna now holds out attractions, which at one time Paris possessed in the first degree, what is more conceivable than that Berlin in its turn may assume first rank?"[224] More and more, American doctors visited Paris as medical tourists or as tourists pure and simple. "I hope to be in Paris to-morrow evening," a young Baltimore physician, J. W. Humrichouse, who had been studying medicine in Vienna and Berlin, wrote home to his father in 1877. "How long I will stay in Paris will depend upon the collections in the Louvre which I have never seen, upon Versailles and many other things."[225]

# Remembering Paris

As migration to Germany continued, the stature of Paris medicine within the United States was increasingly eroded. Even if access to clinical experience had largely initiated the shift, once the redirection across the Rhine had become pronounced the reasons animating it were open to multiple interpretations. After returning home, young American physicians who spent their time chiefly in Germany and rooted their claims to special identity in that experience were inclined to proclaim the superiority of the German medical ethos and to denigrate the Paris School. "American Physicians [have been] held too long by the brilliant but illusory French writers," one observer asserted in 1870; "now they are turning to the more solid Germans with corresponding advantage."[1] Critics charged that whatever merit Parisian medicine once had was now a thing of the past.

The American disciples of the Paris School had not vanished from the professional arena, and many had become established leaders of the postbellum profession. Even if they conceded that younger physicians abroad were making the right choice by favoring Vienna or Berlin, many nevertheless resented what they perceived as an increasingly cavalier dismissal of the ideals of the Paris School of their era. The promotion of the experimental laboratory as a new foundation for scientific medicine, for example, often was accompanied by a disparagement of clinical empiricism that to older physicians threatened to undermine the profession's knowledge, practice, authority, and integrity. Far from resisting scientific medicine, physicians faithful to Parisian medical ways saw themselves defending it. Fully tracing the contested meanings of scientific medicine during the final third of the nineteenth century and delineating the role the German program played in reconfiguring American medicine are tasks beyond the scope of this book. Yet any real understanding of how American medicine was transformed during this period must take seriously the continuing French impulse as a key ingredient in the process of change.

Although the vigor and commitment that propelled the French impulse faded in the 1850s, after the Civil War the American disciples of the Paris School found a renewed sense of mission. By midcentury, they could no longer sustain an aggressive campaign for empirical truth and against the spirit of system by pointing to the dangers of rationalistic systems of the kind common in earlier decades, for such systems no longer loomed large in American medicine. But as the proponents of German medicine confidently proclaimed the promise of their program, aging American Parisians found new reason to guard the primacy of empirically determined clinical truth against forces they believed endangered it. What they were defending was not contemporary medical Paris but rather the Paris of their memory. That remembered Paris gained fresh meaning as they looked backward, assessing their lives, and forward toward the dissolution of the medical order they had labored so hard to establish.

## PROMOTING A NEW ORDER

"There was a time," Harvard medical professor James Clark White reflected in his commencement address of 1866, "when the French capital was looked upon by the medical profession throughout the world as the one and only seat of science, where alone the grand truths of our art could be discovered and taught. Students from every country went thither to complete their studies and to see the men whose names had been upon the lips of their teachers all through their early instruction at home as demigods in science, and whose opinions they had been taught to receive unchallenged as fixed principles." He noted that "Paris had then no rival as a school of medicine; she was the acknowledged front and centre of science." But that time, White proclaimed, was gone. "What position does she now hold?" he asked the assembled audience. "The earnest students of other countries no longer visit her exclusively, or even first or second, to complete their general studies, or to perfect themselves in any special branch of our art, nor is French now the universal or most important language of science, as it once was. The very names which then commanded such world-wide respect are now almost memories associated with the past, and are no more the representatives of the medicine of today."[2]

"What is the cause of this decadence?" White asked his listeners. "Why is it that the Wiener Schule holds at this moment the place then occupied by the Ecole de Medécine?" As he went on to propose, "Gradually the philosophic German mind, so sceptical and irreverent as to accept no dogmas unchallenged, and so patient and industrious in following the suggestions of nature to their very source, began to make itself heard." White concluded by asserting that "Paris has been living chiefly on the reputation of her past greatness, and the slight progress she has made has seemed complete stagnation by the side of the vast advance of her indefatigable Saxon neighbors."[3]

By the time that White spoke, just after the Civil War, his account of the decline of Paris and rise of Germany was one that most of his compatriots shared. However, his explanation for that shift—rooted in the "decadence" of French medicine and ascendancy of the "German mind"—was more idiosyncratic. Through his narrative White was trying to establish a new benchmark for American medicine, a new wellspring of professional distinction, and a new identity for his generation of physicians.

White was not a disinterested observer. Born in 1833—a year his fellow Bostonian James Jackson, Jr., had spent studying in Paris—White, in 1856–1857, was perhaps the first American physician of his cohort to spend a full year studying in Vienna. He was among the first professionally respectable American physicians to declare himself a specialist, in dermatology, and was among the earliest and most vigorous American proselytizers for the Vienna School.[4] White shared the expectation Clarence John Blake spelled out in a letter from Vienna that they would have "to fight tooth and nail against the narrow prejudices of many people." There was to be "a circle among the young men who have studied in Vienna," Blake wrote optimistically to his family. "Among us we have the nucleus of a Vienna club wh. shall meet in Boston and I hope in the character of moderate but radical reformers, inculcate some of the wise lessons wh. we have learned abroad."[5] Indeed, in 1865, the year before his Harvard address, White and five other Harvard medical graduates who had studied in Vienna during the second half of the 1850s founded the Wiener Club in Boston. At first the group met for dinners and the presentation of medical papers. Over time, though, as White would recall in a club scrapbook he put together in 1908, it became a dining club at which a nostalgic group of aging physicians savored Austrian wines "familiar to members during their residence in Vienna," acted out in costume "reminiscent sketches of our charming old life in Vienna," and joined together in singing such songs as "O Carry Me Back to Old Vienna."[6] The club, like the wider network of German-returned American doctors that began to take shape in the 1860s, was a fraternity that affirmed and preserved the special identity forged by their shared Viennese experience—what they themselves thought and spoke about as *German* experience.

The professional identity White and his cohort were crafting hinged upon a representation of German medicine as special and distinct. Stressing continuities between Parisian and Viennese medicine, or between the reasons why Americans elected to study at one or the other place, would have undercut such aims. The story White told to the 1866 assembly at Harvard instead celebrated the singularity of the German mind and its ascendancy as the mark of a new era in Western medicine. Just as an earlier generation returned from France to depict the Paris School as a turning point, so White was beginning the process of recasting the narrative of medical history in ways that would clarify the special mission of his generation. Still novel in the mid-1860s, the dominant theme of White's version of history—German ascendancy over French decadence—grew increasingly commonplace in America during the postbellum decades.

White, like many other young German-experienced physicians of his generation, succeeded in translating his self-perception as a representative of new German medical ways into a cogent public identity. Two years before White gave his commencement address, titled "The Past and Present of the School of Paris," his colleague on the Harvard medical faculty, Henry Ingersoll Bowditch, told the entering class that White "is peculiarly adapted to lead you to exact knowledge of what is now known by German science."[7] As White pushed successfully for changes in the Harvard curriculum modeled partly after a German plan, one observer reported to a Cincinnati medical journal that "Prof. White is decidedly Germanic in ideas, and he advocates a *higher* and *more scientific* course."[8]

Yet German medical science, as it was represented and understood in the United States, was far from monolithic. And the comment that White—or any other American doctor—was "decidedly Germanic in ideas" implied much but spelled out little about particular conceptions of scientific medicine. At the time of White's address, American physicians harbored widely divergent notions of what constituted scientific medicine, and even those who saw themselves as committed disciples of German medicine held sometimes disparate perceptions of what warranted special claims for its scientific character.

This variation can be displayed if we revisit the perceptions articulated by two other young Bostonians, Blake and Henry Pickering Bowditch, and compare the ways they depicted *science* in their reports on German medicine. Bowditch clearly embraced a distinction between the scientific foundations of medicine, pursued in the laboratory, and the practice of medicine, conducted in the clinic.[9] Like other Americans, he was impressed from the outset by German facilities in the laboratory sciences, writing in 1869 from Bonn that "it is wonderful to see the magnificence with which Science is treated here."[10] Later that year, he suggested that a fuller account of Carl Ludwig's "model institution" should appear in an American medical journal "in order that the medical profession may understand how science is valued here."[11] For Bowditch, such laboratories were the crucial site for both learning and advancing medical science. "I dont expect to spend any time in Vienna," he wrote a month later to his father, explaining that "I gave up the idea of going there when I concluded to devote myself to the science & not to the practice of medicine for clinical instruction is the great attraction of the Vienna School."[12]

The cultivation of science in laboratories, as Bowditch understood it, was at the heart of a German model in which the future of scientific medicine was rooted. "The patient, methodical & faithful way in which the phenomena of life are investigated by the German physiologists," he wrote from Leipzig, "not only inspires great confidence in their results but encourages one in the hope that the day is not far distant when Physiology will take its proper place as *the only* true foundation of Medical Science."[13]

Blake, too, was enthusiastic about the opportunities he found abroad for laboratory study, particularly in chemistry, and saw such work as a constitutive part of the new German ethos. Unlike Bowditch, however, he did not speak of the laboratory as if it were the sole defining locus of German medical science. For him, indeed, the clearest embodiment of German scientific medicine was clinical specialism. In part, specialties based their claim to *science* on their reliance on other sciences; thus, as Blake told his mother in 1869, "to be an otologist of any standing and not merely an 'Ear doctor'" required "scientific knowledge" of microscopical anatomy, physiology, acoustics, and so on.[14] Equally, though, the link Blake made between specialism and scientific medicine was welded by the meticulous cultivation of natural knowledge he witnessed in the Vienna clinic. "The thoroughness with which these Germans go into any one subject and stick to it is rather astonishing to the more grasping and superficial (in one sense) American mind," he wrote home, echoing a theme common in reports by American doctors. "There are Americans here and in Berlin who have been studying 'Eye' for two years or more and do not yet feel themselves fitted to practice and as for getting a sufficient knowledge of the Ear in six months it's mere nonsense."[15] Blake urged that what necessitated the splitting of medicine into specialties in the first place was "the rapid advance of Med. Science," and that "the study and practice of a specialty" was particularly well suited to "any one who loves Science for itself."[16] In the Viennese clinic he relished his daily communion with "the scientific men here" as well as their influence on him, writing home aphoristically: "the Vienna school breeds American specialists."[17] Blake, in other words, maintained that to be a medical specialist after the German model was to be scientific, and that his pursuits in the clinic were as authentically scientific and faithful to the German ethos as was the cultivation of scientific medicine in the laboratory.

In the United States, those who proselytized for a German model tended to elide distinctions between the activities of the laboratory and those of the clinic, incorporating both in a wider image of scientific medicine in which the kinds of knowledge produced and employed in these two sites, far from being in competition with one another, were mutually reinforcing. What was identified with Germany and German ways was a broader ethos characterized by a valuation of precision, exactness, thoroughness, and rigor that drew together rather than polarized the cultures of the laboratory and the clinic. This broader depiction of German medical science often conflated clinical specialism and laboratory experimentalism. The *exact method* that was the distinctive hallmark of the German experimental laboratory, for example, corresponded to the self-conscious quest for exactness in clinical science. The instruments of precision of the laboratory—including the most recognizable emblem of the physiology laboratory, the kymograph—were tacitly identified with what were styled as new instruments of precision employed at the bedside, such as the ophthalmoscope, laryngoscope, and otoscope. Moreover, the ideal of mechanical objectivity that came to characterize representations of knowledge produced in the laboratory had a clinical counterpart in the epistemological and aesthetic preference for standardization, precision, and visual representation in the depiction of knowledge about disease elicited at the bedside.[18] The German program for scientific medicine was multifaceted, but in America it tended to be depicted in ways that emphasized its unity and thereby enhanced its cultural power.

Part of what gave this image of German medicine coherence was the way it was contrasted with the past, and particularly with the Paris School. The utility of this polemical opposition in the establishment of a special identity for the Americans who proselytized for German medicine further depended upon a depiction of French medicine as exhausted. The postbellum Americans who championed the new order, in stressing its newness and Germanness, tended to gloss over the fact that many of its leading characteristics were neither entirely new nor entirely German. As chapter 9 recounted, by the 1850s and 1860s both specialism and such laboratory-based sciences as microscopy, chemistry, and physiology had become increasingly central components of French medicine and significant ingredients in the Parisian experience of physicians like Mary Putnam. The most lucid programmatic statement of a plan for regrounding medicine in the laboratory sciences—a polemic that in glorifying the "experimental physicians" of the future pointedly deprecated the "observing physicians" of the Paris Clinical School—had come from the French physiologist Claude Bernard in his 1865 *Introduction to the Study of Experimental Medicine.*[19] In the mid-1860s Boston medical students were told of "the importance of physiological pursuits, as opening to the medical profession the true way to the only accurate knowledge of disease and its treatment," and their counterparts in New Orleans were instructed that "all knowledge of medicine, thus gained renders it a Science, [while] all otherwise obtained is empirical," by professors whose consecration to physiology came from study in France, not Germany.[20] Yet the first generation of medical Americans to study in Germany, conscious of their departure from half a century of convention, wanted to see their experience as fundamentally fresh and different.

The success of the French impulse in American medicine and its status by midcentury as established tradition made French medicine an exceedingly usable foil. As an embodiment of the medical Establishment, it and its proselytes were the natural targets for ambitious young physicians eager to move beyond the medicine of their elders and to embrace a new crusade that would define their own careers. The Paris-returned enthusiast was sufficiently recognizable to be depicted as a comic stereotype. Thus medical satirist Edward H. Dixon published in 1866 the story of an American physician of three decades earlier "just arrived from Paris, dressed in the latest extreme, filled with all the knowledge of the French capital, and puffing and blowing like a speckled frog." Bursting into the library of a New York doctor, he enthused,

"Oh! my dear Doctor F——! mon cher Paris! Dupuytren! Lisfranc! Boyer! Roux! Larrey! and all the glorious constellation of worthies! Dear Doctor F——, I will tell you all, only give me time. You know nothing—you can know nothing. They know everything. Old things are done away, and all things are become new. Oh! mon cher Paris!" Thus the little man continued raving, alternately extending his arms toward "mon cher Paris," and looking round upon the Urse Major's elegant library with infinite contempt, assuring him in the most amiable manner it was all trash, and advising him at once to sell out, and go to Paris.[21]

Nostalgia for Paris remained an easy mark; by the postbellum decades, however, the target in ridicule of American Parisians was more likely to be the dotage of age than the exuberance of youth.

The clearest emblem of the French impulse that critics defined themselves against was empiricism. In making a case for the German program, they deprecatingly identified empiricism with *mere* experience, a necessary source of medical knowledge but an expression of clinical art rather than a sturdy foundation for medical science. Establishing the German program in America meant undermining the status of empiricism as a foundation for scientific medicine. *Exactness* was a watchword of this new program, which held out the hope that the "exact method"—the leading hallmark of experimental laboratory science—would bring precise rules to the bedside, would, in fact, begin to make clinical medicine an exact science.

Empiricism was most often disparaged in polemics that sought to establish new ways of knowing as the undergirding of a reconfigured scientific medicine. One of the most distinctive features of this plan was research on nonhuman animals, and an argument persistently used to promote vivisectional work was that physiological experimentation would yield medical knowledge more solid and exact than what mere clinical observation could glean. In the mid-1860s, Harvard medical professor Edward H. Clarke, an early proponent of what (in contrast to "the empirical method") he called "the physiological method," urged that without a knowledge of the physiological action of remedies, "therapeutics in the future will be what they have been in the past—empiricism." The physiological method, Clarke insisted, represented "the sure and only possible foundation of scientific medicine."[22] As another physician urging vivisectional work asserted in 1868, "all else is empirical and uncertain." As a guide to medical practice, "experimental physiology" promised once and for all time to supplant "superstitions" that, as he put it, "rule our art with a pure empiricism, and reduce the practice of medicine to a nurse's dogma, or an old woman's remedy."[23]

American physicians who sought to apply this program made it clear that they were in revolt against clinical empiricism. Empiricism, the Philadelphia physician and exponent of experimental therapeutics Horatio C. Wood noted sardonically, had sanctioned the therapeutic use of camel dung and dried frogs.[24] Wood and the other advocates of what they called physiological therapeutics further claimed that there were universal laws in therapeutics just as there were in the basic science, physiology, on which they sought to base it. Looking back in 1884, Wood asserted confidently that "the great therapeutic departure of the last decade is the general abandonment of the statistical method of therapeutic research, and the substitution therefor of the so-called physiological method."[25] Philadelphia medical professor Roberts Bartholow, another leading proselytizer for physiological therapeutics as "applied medical science," put it plainly in 1876: "The special advantage of the physiological method is its exactness."[26] The basis of therapeutics should not be empiricism and individualism but rationalism and universalism.

The laboratory was not to be the only site for acquiring *exact* medical knowledge, however; the instruments of precision that specialists saw as an emblem of their participation in the new scientific ethos expressed the ideal of exactness at the bedside. "These are the stethoscope, microscope, otoscope, laryngoscope, ophthalmoscope, electrical instruments, thermometer, sphygmograph, speculum, sound, and many other instruments of precision," one enthusiast explained to his students at the Medical College of Ohio in 1879. "They are instruments of precision, because they give us reliable and accurate information in the survey of the body—facts which can be determined in no other way."[27] In the image of scientific medicine acquired by postbellum medical students, work at the bench and use of instruments of precision at the bedside were increasingly conflated. "Mother, you dont know how perfect a science medicine is," one New Orleans student wrote home, describing the tools commanded by the modern physician. "The Microscope the Stethoscope," he told her, "the Speculum and ten thousand other instruments are in use to inform him as to the Conditions of the internal parts of the Body that he can describe it to you as if he saw through it like glass." As he wrote longingly, "How I wish I was rich, to have a complete Laboratory of my own."[28] Americans in Paris, of course, had voiced enthusiasm for the stethoscope in the 1830s and the microscope in the 1850s, but in postbellum America even these instruments were increasingly appropriated for a new German scientific tradition.

The point at which the new program most desecrated the empiricist ideals of the old was in its call for using the new sciences in constructing *rationalistic systems* in medicine. By the 1870s advocates of the physiological method such as Wood and Bartholow not only claimed a legitimate place for rationalism in medical practice—for reasoning from the laboratory to the bedside—but reinstated the language of *system* as a positive aim that had been all but banished from American medical discourse.[29] Physiology, as one physician put it in 1879, "leads the way to a rational system of therapeutics."[30] Faith in empiricism, according to this view, was precisely what the profession had to escape in order to bring clinical practice under the reign of scientific medicine. Held up as an ideal, "a system of rational therapeutics" would fulfill the goal "to develope a system in the treatment of disease which shall be founded on something more rational than tradition or empiricism."[31]

Such a fundamental transformation in American programs for creating and organizing socially relevant knowledge did not grow entirely from European models. Just as the plan to establish an ideal of empirical truth and demystify medical knowledge during the first half of the century came partly from France and partly from sociopolitical forces within American culture, so the new program for scientific medicine derived partly from German models and partly from wider changes in American cultural values.

What permitted a new kind of discourse about laboratory medicine and clinical specialization to emerge when it did was a broader shift in attitudes toward the place of specialized knowledge in American society that started to become pronounced in the 1870s and 1880s. The sociopolitical forces that had given empiricism its special meaning in antebellum America diminished, as did the symbolic power of empiricism itself. "Americans after 1870," Burton Bledstein long ago noted, "committed themselves to a culture of professionalism," and one attribute of the new professional ideal that began to take shape was the command of specialized knowledge unfathomable to the public at large.[32] Bureaucratic organization and specialized compartmentalization of work became increasingly prominent. In fields ranging from engineering to forestry, professional associations proliferated, giving members a distinctive badge of their special knowledge. The multiplication of institutions for higher education was but one sign of the elevated valuation of specialized knowledge and advanced learning. With what historian Samuel Haber has called "the reestablishment of the professions," such knowledge—its inner workings, its production, and its assessment—might remain mysterious to most Americans, but it won both esteem and authority for those who showed evidence of mastery over it.[33]

This gradual change in American culture enabled some American physicians to engage in a new kind of discourse about the relationship between epistemology and authority. A growing valuation of special knowledge gave both the experimental laboratory and clinical specialism heightened cultural legitimacy.[34] It was within this context that some physicians began to celebrate the promise of the laboratory for bringing about a cognitive and social transformation of their profession. What broader cultural changes offered to the American disciples of German medicine was not just a society newly receptive to claims to authority based on special knowledge but also a framework within which to define a new kind of professional meaning for the laboratory, the instruments of precision employed at the bedside, and the knowledge they produced.

During the final third of the century, physicians who sought to ground professional authority in German models of medical science had to come to terms with the underlying shift in professional identity it implied, from a primary rooting in practice to one in specialized knowledge. And this involved fundamental alterations in their understanding of the relationships among science, professional identity, and professional integrity. Those who looked to German models pinned their hopes on an image of the physician as an expert in natural science and claimed an accountability to science as the chief sanction for their actions. Like their critics committed to clinical empiricism, they maintained that the physician was more than a natural scientist, but they accorded to science a different place in the fulfillment of that further role. They partly shed the notion that the regular physician's identity and integrity were best guaranteed by interactions with patients and other practitioners in accordance with shared traditional values. Instead, they claimed an allegiance to the new sciences and their power to guide effective intervention as the ethical sanction for their program and the foundation for their definition as physicians, with the assurance that from good science—as they defined it—good practice would follow.[35]

An altered conception of the social role of science in medicine accompanied this new configuration of the relationship of science to medical practice, identity, and integrity. The shifting and contested allegiances of physicians can be seen in wider debates waged during the 1870s and 1880s over professional responsibility and propriety. One revealing example was the controversy over the section of the *Code of Ethics of the American Medical Association* that prohibited regular physicians from consulting with unorthodox practitioners on the grounds that the latter were medically and morally unfit. Those who had drafted the 1847 code, which was widely taken up by state and local medical societies, held that consultation with homeopaths sanctioned heterodoxy and degraded the regular profession.[36]

In the 1870s and 1880s this Code of Ethics came to be challenged from within orthodox ranks. Targeting the consultation clause in particular, some physicians began to insist in their local and state medical societies that they should be free to decide with whom they would consult, and called for annulment of the code or at least of the consultation clause. It would be much too simple to see all physicians with French experience lined up on one side of this issue, faced off against all those with German experience. What is intriguing, however, is that those American physicians who most vigorously proselytized for the new German program—physicians committed to the experimental laboratory sciences, and particularly elite specialists—were the ones who most actively opposed the Code of Ethics and its use to maintain professional standards. They believed that the advancement of the new sciences had rendered the code obsolete, and looked to science for more reliable criteria for professional integrity.[37]

One prominent argument against the consultation clause was that an allegiance to science rendered distinctions between competing medical belief systems made on any other grounds meaningless. Because "regular physicians claim to be scientific men," one activist in the movement to reject the code explained in 1883, they should be blind to arbitrary distinctions between orthodox and unorthodox medicine and free to accept any belief, "provided it stand the test of scientific work. As far as is known," he continued, "no scientific body places prohibitory rules upon scientific men in matters of ethics."[38] It was for this reason that Abraham Jacobi, as president of the New York Academy of Medicine, could reassure its members in 1886 that "the absence of ethical codes" from the organization was testimony to "its scientific spirit."[39]

Wood and Bartholow, who both wrote textbooks on practice that belittled clinical empiricism in favor of what Wood called a "rational system"—"the modern physiological school of therapeutics"—both thought the Code of Ethics was outdated.[40] What is more, both used the example of physiological therapeutics to sustain their argument that physicians who trusted in the natural laws revealed by experimental science no longer needed the artificial laws embodied in codes of professional ethics. "Homeopathy and allopathy are dreams of a by-gone time," Bartholow had asserted in 1872. "Modern science is indifferent to Hippocrates and Hahnemann. The therapeutics of to-day rejects dogmas, and the therapeutics of the future will accept nothing that can not be demonstrated by the tests of science." Wood shared this conviction, and he used his contribution to a textbook on therapeutics as an opportunity to assail the Code of Ethics and to affirm the liberty of scientific physicians to meet in consultation with whomever they pleased.[41]

The move to overturn the code was led by urban specialists. In New York State, where the battle was especially fierce, the most active opponents included New York City specialists such as Cornelius R. Agnew (an ophthalmologist), Fordyce Barker (a gynecologist), Abraham Jacobi (a pediatrician),

Henry Piffard (a dermatologist), and Daniel B. St. John Roosa (an ophthalmologist). These specialists stood to gain the most financially from abolition of the consultation clause, for not only did they practice in the urban centers where there were the greatest concentrations of homeopaths, but their claims to special expertise meant that they were the physicians most likely to be called in by a homeopath confronted with a perplexing case. At the same time, for physicians such as these who saw themselves as highly trained experts and masters of the new experimental sciences, personal liberty warranted by scientific competence provided a compelling sanction for doing away with the consultation clause. They saw their opposition to the code not as a sanction for homeopathy but as a denial that the distinction between homeopathic and allopathic creeds was any longer helpful. "Only one course can be open to those who value professional integrity, liberty, and advance," one like-minded physician wrote to Agnew, "and such a course, will contemplate the association in a common fellowship of all those who believe it time, to cast off the marks of ignorant exclusiveness."[42] It was a necessary step in the creation of a "pure, *scientific* democracy."[43]

More was at stake than freedom to consult with homeopaths, which even at the time was regarded as a partly symbolic issue. What mattered more was the underlying proposition that scientific expertise not only warranted what another physician described to Agnew as "liberty of opinion and of action" but also could be relied upon to guarantee correct clinical behavior.[44] Confidence in this power of the new sciences depended in the first instance on scientific advancement, something Jacobi chose to illustrate by pointing to the success of experimental therapeutics and by quoting Wood on the rise of therapeutics "from the position of an empirical art to the dignity of an approved science."[45] Opponents of the code looked forward to a profession made up of doctors educated as experts in experimental science and, as important, educated to accord that scientific expertise a new place in their identity as professionals. "While there is no hope at present of causing the state association to deviate from its old code stand," one physician explained to George F. Shrady, a New York medical editor and opponent of the code, "a sentiment can slowly be created among the younger men."[46]

Medical students, who were particularly susceptible to the vision of a medical ethos promoted in the name of new German scientific ideals, tended to be receptive to a depiction of empiricism as an emblem of stultifying tradition that hindered scientific medicine and the wider reordering of professional identity, morality, and social relations. "The claims of medicine to a position among the exact sciences no longer rests upon the dogmatic assertions of its too zealous supporters but has now for some years been conceded to have been proven beyond cavil or controversy," Joseph Davis Craig, an Albany medical student, opened his 1884 M.D. thesis, echoing the dicta of his professors but expressing a confidence that was his own. "Medicine," he asserted flatly, "has grown from the empirical into the scientific." He and his classmates, Craig noted with pride, had been educated in methods of a scientific medicine fundamentally distinct "from what they were in the old days when Empiricism was King." The mission of his generation, as he understood it, was to complete the task of bringing the exact method of the physiology laboratory to the clinic. "While the principles of physiology have come to rest on as firm a foundation as the laws of gravitation," he proposed, "it is now from clinical medicine that the profession has most to hope for in the lives of the next two generations."[47]

Viewing matters from "a student's standpoint," Craig looked ahead with assurance toward a wider cognitive and social reconstruction of the professional world he was entering. "While medicine was in great measure empirical in its practices a Code of Ethics of arbitrary law was necessary to hold coherently together its various members," he acknowledged. "But the laborers in the field of scientific medicine have, with the intellectual progress, grown tired of the restraint upon their full and free action and have dared to say that the law and conscience alone bind a doctor." As the practice of medicine became an exact science, Craig continued, the Code of Ethics became outmoded. "To-day the discussion is a heated one and full of perplexity," he noted, writing in the year that the state medical society of New York split over the code issue. "Ten years from now the interests of humanity will influence and guide the profession and a code of ethics will be only known as a matter of history."[48]

## "ON THE SIDE OF TRUTH"

What did this new program for American medicine look like viewed through the eyes of physicians consecrated to the ideals of French medicine? What meaning did German medical ways hold for Americans whose own studies in France had conferred upon them an identity as disciples of the Paris School, and for the larger community of American physicians who had taken up its teachings? What were the intellectual, social, and moral concerns that informed their judgments? More often than not, recountings of the history of American medicine have glossed over such questions and concentrated instead on how institutions and practices came to be transformed by those who emulated German models. In such accounts, the physicians who preserved their allegiance to the ideals of Paris medicine after midcentury—as a group increasingly likely to be elderly—have tended to be relegated to the background, and it is from that marginalized place that we occasionally hear their disgruntled protests against the brash dismissal of the old and the overconfident embrace of the new.

Yet as my focus has largely been their story, it is fitting that in my final chapter I call upon them once again to speak from center stage. Any depiction that tends to reduce them to aged reactionaries opposing the rise of scientific medicine profoundly misleads our efforts to understand the shifting course of scientific medicine in America. Too often, historians have treated the emergence of medicine cast in a late-nineteenth-century German mold, and especially laboratory medicine, as the emergence of scientific medicine. Yet in the appraisal of the American disciples of the Paris School, their medicine already was scientific: in voicing their apprehensions and challenges to some of the newer approaches they were not resisting scientific medicine but defending it.[49] Thus in 1857 Alfred Stillé, having just read the draft of a cautionary lecture given by George Cheyne Shattuck, Jr., to medical students in Boston, wrote to his fellow Parisian, "It is such lessons that must do more than most else to keep our younger professional brethren from straying away into the bypaths which at every step, almost, lead away from the direct road of true science and professional honor."[50] The physicians who drew attention to the dangers of the emerging program tended to be those committed to an ideal of science rooted in the empiricist crusade against the spirit of system. In postbellum America, what was most at issue in exchanges between leading proponents of the French and German schools was not the advocacy of or opposition to scientific medicine, but rather the terms in which an authentic, socially relevant scientific medicine was to be defined.

Some of the rifts that divided American physicians were generational, though at few points can a particular physician's position be simply reduced to age any more than it can be defined solely by French or German training. Debates in the United States over the medical utility of the microscope, for example, tended to be configured by age more than by German or French experience, however strongly the two variables were linked. In 1855, American observers were riveted by the battle in the French Academy of Medicine over the utility of microscopy in the diagnosis of cancer, and nearly all concurred that the clash represented what a year earlier one American called "the difference between the older and younger part of the profession."[51] Americans in Paris at the time reported that while younger French physicians and surgeons studied the microscope attentively, older practitioners, such as Velpeau, sought to "restrain the rashness and eagerness of youth" and chasten "the young school of Medical Philosophers."[52] Mirroring this alignment, many older physicians *in* America took the occasion to ridicule the scientific enthusiasms of the young "microscopical gentry."[53] Asserting early in 1856 that those skeptical of "the *microscopic* additions to science" were "nowadays called Old Fogies," one St. Louis practitioner proudly proclaimed: "I am an old Fogy. I believe that our ancestors, our fathers, knew something. I believe that a great deal of what is called progress is nothing but gyration."[54] Charging that "old men *know* what fools young men are, whilst these latter *think* old men fools," he was inclined to dismiss young diagnosticians preoccupied with this "philosophical toy" as "closet-dreamers" and "system-makers."[55] Nevertheless, although such generational divisions were real, they were hardly neat: Oliver Wendell Holmes, who neglected the microscope when he studied in Paris during the 1830s, later not only rued that neglect but became a leading proselytizer for medical microscopy.[56]

Most older American disciples of the Paris School neither inflexibly opposed these newer approaches to knowledge, nor unyieldingly defended the Parisian allegiances forged in their youth, nor yet again anguished over the wider med-

ical ascendancy of Germany over France. Indeed, some of the most stalwart of
the first generation in later years reflected critically on the naïveté of their
youth. By the early 1860s, Henry Ingersoll Bowditch worried that an overreac-
tion had set in against therapeutic intervention in general and bloodletting
in particular, and rightly identified the therapeutic skepticism he and his cohort had acquired several decades earlier in Paris as one impetus to this ex-
tremism. "On my return from Europe," he recalled before a Harvard class in
1860, "I took quite a delight in all the failures of my elders in their use of
drugs."[57] This skepticism, Bowditch elaborated a decade later, was part of the
lesson imparted by Louis. "He had moulded my medical mind into such a
rigid belief in the necessity of strict deductions from facts actually studied out
with the utmost care at the bedside that, for a time, I flippantly talked of all that
had preceded us as if their influence was to be deemed of no importance,"
Bowditch reflected; "I have had gradually to unlearn this grave error."[58]
Holmes, also a student of Louis in the 1830s, echoed Bowditch. "I had devoted
myself too exclusively," he reminisced late in life, "to the teachings of Louis";
"how strange it is," he noted "to look down on one's venerated teachers, after
climbing with the world's progress half a century above the level where we left
them."[59]

Revisits to Paris particularly provided an occasion for reflecting on changes
there. Elisha Bartlett, who returned twenty years after his first studies in Paris,
reported to an American journal on his walking tour of its medical precincts
and noted in detail concrete emblems of the place he recalled, such as the doors
of the Hôtel Dieu; yet he said little about what went on behind those doors. He
did visit Louis at his house, though, and used the report of his pilgrimage to
underscore what Louis (now fifty-nine) stood for, a life spent "not in barren
speculation, but . . . a love for the truth."[60] Henry Smith reported in 1855 that
the crossing to Paris "again settled me in the old and familiar wards of the
Parisian hospitals, in which I had formerly spent fifteen months." He revisited
the clinics he had known sixteen years earlier, but recognized that the advantages they offered the student had greatly diminished. "My old preceptors,
Lisfranc, Roux, Marjolin, and Breschet, were numbered with the dead," he
noted; "Velpeau and Civiale alone remained." Instead, "Malgaigne, Nélaton,
Chassaignac, Robert, Maisonneuve, Barth, &c., the young teachers of that period, are now the prominent clinical instructors of the present day." Still, the
physical sites of memory remained, and Smith noted that "the hospitals, with
one or two trifling exceptions, seemed to have remained stationary; even the
physiognomy of the incumbents of certain well-remembered beds were un-
changed, and it was difficult at first to think that No. 21 of the Ward St. Martha
was not the patient of a former period."[61]

Stillé observed after revisiting Paris at midcentury, "I found that 'tempora
mutantur et nos mutamur cum illis.'" As he told Shattuck, "I did not visit any of
the Hospitals, but was told that very little was doing in medicine," and he too
met with "our noble master" Louis.[62] Nevertheless, writing from Vienna on the
same tour, Stillé confessed that "from a slight observation here of some re-

cently educated men, hard students and diligent observers, I am sensible of being quite behind the age in several matters, and especially in all that relates to the application of chemistry to morbid processes; and at the same time I feel something of that want of appreciation of the methods of diagnosis at present employed which I blamed in my Seniors when I was studying auscultation & percussion." He concluded that "every day I lament . . . that I am at present in such a state of health as to be unable to learn even what I am anxious to know," adding that "my ignorance too of German is a very serious obstacle in my way; yet were I strong enough to bear fatigue and study at the bed-side I think I have still ardour enough in the pursuit of knowledge, and consciousness enough of my own short-comings to make me an attentive student."[63] For Stillé as for other committed American disciples of French medicine, however, while the medical Paris they revisited was dulled, the Paris that mattered more was the city of their memories, and it was little tarnished. *Paris* had come to recall not only a particular place but also a particular time and experience.

If aging physicians were ambivalent toward the confident enthusiasm of their heirs, and if few shared Stillé's unrealized longing to turn pupil again, many supported the aspirations of the upcoming generation. This strained co-existence between an attachment to an earlier medical Paris and its enduring lessons, on the one hand, and, on the other, a nurturing posture toward a younger generation eager to explore new pathways to medical advancement can be seen clearly in the case of Henry Ingersoll Bowditch. Historians have usually read the correspondence between Bowditch and his nephew, Henry Pickering Bowditch, written after the latter had set off for Europe, as a story about the rise of experimental laboratory physiology in America—have read it, that is, in the context of the trajectory that the younger Bowditch's career would later follow and (as I have used it in chapter 9) to exemplify the coming of the German program. Yet the resonances conveyed by this exchange of letters sound rather different if one tries to listen to the words through the ears of the uncle, attending to the meaning they held for his understanding of the past rather than the younger man's aspirations for the future.

Well before his nephew's departure for Europe, the elder Bowditch had come to terms with the shift from French to German ascendancy in medical science. "Germany now rises above France & justly I think," he candidly told students attending his 1861 clinical course at the Massachusetts General Hospital. But he went on to remind the class what should be retained from an earlier Paris; "to Louis," he noted, "we owe the strong tendency to accurate and minute observation of disease." Reflecting on the relationship between young and old, Bowditch suggested that "we all wish to be on the side of Truth."[64]

When in 1868 the young Bowditch first arrived in Paris, his uncle delighted in giving advice about how he should make his way, advice that drew on the elder physician's experiences there in the 1830s and stirred his nostalgia for that formative period in his life. "On arrival in Paris take a cab and drive to Hotel Beranger or to Peabodys rooms—and get into lodgings in the 'quartier Latin' forthwith until you can look about," he instructed his nephew. Once settled, he suggested, the young man should stroll to a café on the Place de l'Odéon. "Walk in, as if you knew every body. Look out for a paper, take it & sit down as if you had been there all your life and knew all about it—and begin to read 'Galignani,' . . . or still better one of the liberal papers—'Le National' as I remember." Then, "having settled yourself wait & read. Soon the garcon will ask your order—'Que voulez vous, Monsieur'? 'Café et pain, s'il vous plait'— you will answer in your blandest manner—& if you want to *blast the French-man* & convince him that certainly you know a little more than 'a thing or two' add et 'des oeufs cuits'. No *extra* words & sit down to read again as if you were perfectly cool & not sweating, *as I did at least at every pore* for fear you will not make out to get through in decent order your first meal." In this manner, Bowditch proceeded to relive a day in Paris by walking his nephew through it step by step, adding that "I feel like an old war horse that hears the bugle notes and I really long to go again." Asking his nephew to write letters frequently—to "make me your medical journal"—he pledged that "I will keep all & you shall have them at least when I pass to the land of shadows."[65] The younger Bow-ditch wrote regularly, reporting in his first letter from Paris that "on my first arrival here I went to your little hôtel Beranger where . . . the landlady said she remembered you."[66]

The uncle offered counsel on negotiating the medical world of Paris as well as its cafés, though his professional advice was rather more dated. When young Bowditch's plan to work in Charles-Édouard Brown-Séquard's laboratory col-lapsed, for example, his uncle wrote, "I advise you to learn from B. S., or if not from him from Monsieur Louis, who is the *best of the young hard-working, simple, practical experimental physiologists.*—Go to him. He is destined to be the *rising man* in France, and is one whose friendship in *future* you will enjoy."[67] The essence of the uncle's advice, that his nephew should find a men-tor of the sort he had found in Louis, was sound, but the assumption that the eighty-one-year-old Louis would be au courant with the laboratory life and promising young physiologists of Paris was naive. In the event, Louis, whom the nephew dutifully tried to seek out, was away from Paris for the season.[68] Nevertheless, the young man, describing his laboratory studies with Louis-Antoine Ranvier, reported that "Ranvier is just the sort of man you advise me to apply to; a young, hard working, enterprising man. His particular strong point is Histology but, as he says, Physiology, Pathology & Histology are so intimately united that it is impossible to study one without the others."[69]

The elder Bowditch wrote yet again urging that "I hope before long you will be able to see and to give my best love to the dear old master Louis,"[70] and this time his letter crossed in the post his nephew's report that he had "called on Dr Louis the other night & presented your letter. He seemed quite glad to see me, & talked a good deal about Boston people. He is rather feeble, but in pretty good condition for a man of his age[.] He wanted to be remembered to you & spoke of you with great affection."[71] The young Bowditch may have felt that this finally put paid to a pressing family obligation, for on the same day that he wrote his uncle he also wrote his parents of his visit to Louis, adding that "I am getting deeper and deeper into physiology."[72] From the elder Bowditch, though, the report of his nephew's meeting with Louis elicited musings on the passage of time. In his next letter he was as always supportive of his nephew's endeavors, writing, "I hope you are flourishing as a *Physiologiste enragé*." But he went on to reflect, "How the years roll on! It seems but yesterday when I was where you are now at Paris, with all its brightness & earnestness lifting me above myself —Now I have nearly finished my *active* life, though I hope to jog merrily on till I die."[73]

The nephew's growing insistence that experimental physiology represented the only true foundation for medical science, combined with his desire to pursue it exclusively and eschew medical practice, could not help but have been a little troubling to an uncle whose life in medicine had been consecrated to the epistemological ideals of the Paris School he remembered. Yet the elder Bowditch avoided disapproval, partly by resorting to self-deprecation whenever he dissented from his nephew's scientific passions: "I know I am an Old Fogy," he wrote in one letter, blunting any sharpness.[74] He asked to know all the details of his nephew's scientific studies but did so in ways resembling the affection of a doting parent more than the intellectual engagement of a peer. "Tell me all the curious things you see & all the odd things you do in your laboratory," he wrote late in 1868, "feeling assured that by so doing you will give me nothing but pleasure."[75] The nephew obliged but believed that what would interest his uncle were the doings of the clinic, not of the laboratory. "Since I wrote to you last I have kept at work pretty steadily at Microscopy & Physiology & have not been to many hospitals so that I have not much of interest to report," he opened another letter at the end of 1868.[76]

Nevertheless, the elder Bowditch could scarcely have been more nurturing, even if he did not entirely comprehend the medical world his nephew sought to enter. "I am afraid you think the idea rather a wild one," the young man wrote after broaching the notion of devoting himself entirely to the "science" of the profession, as he understood it, and avoiding "practical medicine."[77] He may have been right; yet the elder Bowditch supported his nephew's aspirations unstintingly. He put in a good word for the plan with the young man's father, telling him, "I think you are doing exactly right for Henry. . . . He has a sincere reverence for exact scientific truth—and a clear head to hunt it out."[78] And he wrote directly to the young physiologist encouraging him to "continue to devote yourself to pure Science," adding that "your course my dear Henry is I am sure upward & onward."[79] Still, the elder Bowditch, regarding experimental physiology as something akin to the emerging host of medical specialties, did press the young man to consider setting up practice in Boston as a physiological consultant—just as several years earlier Blake's father had encouraged him to consider a laboratory-based specialty in chemical pathology; as Bowditch put the question, "Why should not some physician want from time to time, to consult a physiologist proper, if Physiology be the groundwork of all Medical Practice?" He recognized that both the laboratory and specialism were parts of an emerging order, but was a little uncertain of the relationship be-

tween them. Concerned about his nephew's prospects, he hoped this plan offered "a somewhat practical as well as a scientific career as Physiologist."[80]

By the late 1850s, much of the crusading fervor that had once characterized
the proselytism of first-generation American Parisians such as Bowditch had
faded. Their campaign against the spirit of system had lost momentum—not
because it had failed but because it had been too successful. Rationalistic systems of a Rushian or Broussaisist cast were no longer menacing, and it had
become difficult to rally the troops against an enemy long since put to rout.
"One of the most efficient causes of the recent improvement in medical science
seems to me to be the virtual abandonment of all *exclusive systems*," a professor
at the Medical College of Georgia could tell his students by midcentury; "rejoice," he urged them, "you who start upon the career of medicine, that the day
of exclusive systems has, practically speaking, passed by."[81] Some M.D. theses
written in the 1850s and early 1860s continued to laud empiricism and rue the
evils of rationalistic systems, but by the Civil War their number had dwindled
almost to none.[82] Thus as the professional distinction brought by Parisian
study waned and as the shift in migration to Germany commenced, the power
of the empiricist crusade within American culture faded: it became not only
mainstream but somewhat redundant. The American disciples of the Paris
School, in turn, representing a program no longer defined and sharpened by
controversy, lost much of their binding, missionary sense of special identity.

The aggression of orthodox assaults against homeopathy (and to a lesser
extent other nonorthodox systems) should be understood partly in this context, for many regular physicians believed that they saw in homeopathy—
which, revealingly, they often called Hahnemannism—a rationalistic system
flourishing in the present that embodied the worst evils of the past. Indeed,
some of the wider animus against the spirit of system was displaced onto homeopathy, and in the 1850s and 1860s the demonization of homeopathy as an
"exclusive system" intensified.[83] At midcentury, denunciations of rationalistic
systems and their destructive consequences still were common, as in Stillé's
1848 call for his brethren to abandon "Brownism and Rushism, Broussaisism
and Hahnemannism, with all the other fruits of a luxuriant fancy and a poverty
of facts."[84] But even as Stillé wrote, no prominent orthodox physician any
longer publicly professed faith in Brownism, Rushism, Broussaisism, or any
other regular *system* of practice: homeopathy was singular, a real and present
danger. Thus in 1857, James Jackson, Sr., insisting that "I object to every *system*," explicitly compared homeopathy with the "Brunonian system" of his
youth.[85] As regular empiricists found it more difficult to find a clear target to
define themselves against, demonizing homeopathy as an enduring embodiment of the spirit of system helped sustain the momentum of the empiricist's
good fight.

With the rise of the German program, however, and especially as some proclaimed it the only true foundation for scientific medicine, the now-aging
American disciples of the Paris School discovered an invigorated sense of purpose and renewed sense of mission. Strident rhetoric about the stagnancy of

Paris and the vitality of Germany profoundly disturbed physicians who had made their commitment to French medicine part of their identity, and starting in the 1860s and 1870s the American Parisians grew defensive. At issue was the Paris of their medical youth, the remembered Paris that stood for the ideals around which they had structured their careers.

Their discomfort stemmed from much more than the shift of medical migrants abroad away from the site of their memory. In extolling the promise of experimental medicine, younger Americans who looked to Germany often derided clinical observation as inadequate and stultifying. They also zealously asserted the promise of the laboratory in terms so intemperate that some older physicians feared they were witnessing the revival of evils they had believed the empiricist campaign to have finally vanquished. By the mid-1870s, for example, Stillé found himself being assailed for relying on clinical empiricism (instead of laboratory experimentation) in his textbook on therapeutics.[86]

By and large, the American Parisians objected not so much to the knowledge and methods being imported from Germany as to promotions of this new ethos that seemed to brush aside all lessons of the past. In aggressively privileging new ways, they believed, some younger physicians were not only depriviliging but trivializing the empiricist program, including its valuation of clinical observation, as when in 1875 one admirer of Wood's plan for experimental therapeutics asserted that "physiological investigation has certainly achieved more exact progress than clinical experience."[87] Such proclamations, disparaging clinical empiricism, radicalized some of the American disciples of the Paris School. It was not the laboratory itself but overly sanguine claims made for its authority over medical practice that were seen as threatening. Bartlett, in his empiricist manifesto, had dismissed the laboratory as a source of knowledge about practice but had not explicitly denounced it. There was no reason to: when he wrote in the 1840s, the laboratory was making no pressing claims to dominance in American medicine. Vehement assaults appeared only when an upcoming cohort of postbellum physicians started to cavalierly dismiss the programs of their elders in the process of claiming that knowledge produced in the laboratory was the proper platform for uplifting medicine.

The goal proclaimed by proselytizers for the new German program to create a *rational system* of medical practice was an unmistakable rally calling old campaigners back to the barricades against the spirit of system. The language employed by those who denounced claims made on the laboratory's behalf is revealing. Typically, in 1876 one medical editor assailed a new book on materia medica by Bartholow for his reliance on the dictates of experimental physiology rather than on empiricism and the test of experience. "The practitioner, at the bedside of his patient," he insisted, "does not care to indulge in medical metaphysics. . . . No! He leaves that all to the speculative medical experimentalist." He went on to charge that "in his attempts to solve mysteries, known only to the Infinite, the modern speculator makes bold assertions, not guaranteed by a single fact, and[,] with an audacity unparalleled, will no doubt shortly give the medicinal effects of religion on the human soul, describing the

essence of the vital spark, its chemical constituents, and number of newly discovered elements contained therein."[88] He concluded that in a textbook designed for healers, "the space devoted to rabbits, guinea pigs and frogs might
have been utilized to a better purpose."[89]

In stigmatizing the physician who relied on the experimental laboratory as
"the modern speculator," this critic clearly identified the new rationalists with
earlier generations of systematists. "The speculative medical experimentalist,"
like the speculative system-builder, sought to ground medical knowledge upon
an unsound foundation. Even if these new systems were constructed from materials different from those constituting their predecessors, critics feared that
they shared many underlying epistemological flaws and threatened many of
the same medical and social consequences. Like the speculative medical systems of the late eighteenth and early nineteenth centuries, they held out the
kind of alluring but delusive promise of certainty that the faithful of the Paris
School had battled to unmask through their empiricist revolution.

The optimistic faith that experimental science would rapidly transform clinical practice therefore was a target for ridicule by disciples of the Paris School.
Stillé, about to turn seventy, condescendingly characterized that faith as the
search for a medical "Cloudland."[90] Conventional wisdom held that young
physicians tended to have greater confidence in the power of drugs than did
practitioners sobered by years of hard experience, and the belief that physiology would transform practice seemed to fit this pattern neatly. As one physician asserted, "It is only our younger, less-experienced and over-sanguine
members who feel such zealous and unhesitant confidence in their own skill
and in the definite and mathematically estimable potency of remedies."[91] Critics further charged that it was presumptuous and wrong to think that practice
could be derived from the basic sciences; this was not to deny the medical value
of physiology, but unless it could be shown to guide action, not just explain
how remedies worked after the fact, then physiology must remain an accessory
to medicine. "It behooves us to remember," Stillé insisted, "that medicine is,
above all else, humane as well as human, that its beginning, middle, and end
is to relieve suffering, and that whatever is outside of this may indeed be science of some sort, but certainly is not medicine."[92]

As critics such as Stillé viewed it, the goal of a rational system of practice
grounded in experimental laboratory science was to set up precise, universal
rules in a realm where such rules were inappropriate. Charles Stockton, an
upstate New York practitioner, charged that in their enthusiasm for physiology
its advocates sought "to try all cases before her tribunal, with recourse only to
established physiological laws." But such a plan ignored the individual peculiarities of the sick, which could be grasped only through empirical clinical observation. "This exact medicine," he continued, "can never traverse certain
unascertained limits; beyond those limits we come upon the province of indi-
viduality."[93] Sanguine claims made for experimental physiology threatened to
sidetrack the slow but persistent progress of practical medicine through empirical observation. "Unless we constantly hold therapeutics before our eyes," one

practitioner cautioned against the seductions of the laboratory, "our profession will become nothing but one of scientific amusement."[94]

The distinctive methods of the new program—and none more so than vivisection—were also seen as portents of epistemological and moral danger. Animal experimentation and its products represented needless and deceptive embellishment of clinical knowledge and the potential for brutalization that Americans had taken care to distance themselves from in Paris. The well-known protests by Harvard professor of surgery Henry Jacob Bigelow against the use of vivisection in teaching medical students expressed a long-standing nineteenth-century apprehension that visual impression held the power to transform the viewer into someone cruel and heartless, that exposure could demoralize the future physician and vitiate his or her character as a healer. Bigelow, who had studied in Paris three decades earlier, remonstrated in 1871 against "the cold-blooded cruelties now more and more practised under the authority of Science!" Disturbed in particular by moves to make vivisectional demonstration a significant feature in training Harvard medical students, Bigelow asserted: "I say it is needless. Nobody should do it. Watch the students at a vivisection. It is the blood and suffering, not the science, that rivets their breathless attention." Bigelow warned that "if hospital service makes young students less tender of suffering, vivisection deadens their humanity and begets indifference to it."[95]

Vivisection became a foil for those who would reassert the primacy the Paris School accorded to empirically determined clinical truth. Alfred G. Tebault, a medical professor at the University of Virginia, urged his students that action at the bedside should be informed by clinical observation, "not by recondite researches into the physiological action of medicines on the brute." Dismissing the latter as "the recreations of science," Tebault praised clinical empiricism by telling them that "there is no groping in darkness in this path."[96] Underlying denunciations of the place of vivisection in the moral order of scientific medicine was the conviction that its benefits did not warrant the costs: human dissection, physical examination, and clinical teaching might also hold brutalizing tendencies, but these practices were warranted by the clinically useful knowledge they provided that could be acquired in no other way.

Like proponents of the German program, those who remained faithful to Parisian ideals rightly recognized that a new epistemological order involved not only reconstructing medical ways of knowing but also establishing new canons of professional practice, identity, and integrity. Their wider apprehensions, like the aspirations of those who pinned their hopes to the German program, can be partly displayed by the stand many of them took during the 1870s and 1880s in the debate over the consultation clause of the AMA Code of Ethics. Physicians rallied in defense of the code for a variety of reasons, and the grassroots support it enjoyed can be attributed only in part to the way the French impulse had entered the American medical mainstream. Moreover, not all American Parisians favored preserving the code.[97] Yet it is striking that many of the surviving disciples of the Paris School energetically defended the code, and that they did so partly by contesting new claims made for the clinical and social authority of experimental science and by reaffirming their allegiance to a French-informed ideal of medical truth.

Those who defended the code were disturbed by claims that experimental science could be relied upon as an arbiter of professional conduct. In their view it was because science could *not* provide exact and invariant rules for practice that the physician needed the kind of guide to behavior the Code of Ethics offered. Austin Flint (known for his writings on stethoscopy, and soon to be elected AMA president), who led the move in New York to preserve the code, made this point plainly by linking his stance to a dismissal of the therapeutic certainty promised by experimental science. "The practice of medicine, when contrasted with other pursuits, is peculiar," he asserted in *Medical Ethics and Etiquette* (1883), written to defend the code. "The medical practitioner does not deal with facts and laws having the exactness of those pertaining to physics. In employing means for certain ends, he can not calculate results with mathematical precision. The problems of disease embrace many and varying elements, which can not always be estimated with absolute certainty. They offer a wide scope for the exercise of judgment in the practical applications of medical knowledge."[98] This inbuilt uncertainty was the reason further guides to behavior were required. Thus after listening to criticisms of the code at a county medical society meeting in Ohio, one member declared that "what he had heard here in this discussion reminded him of the absurd cry of certain self-styled moral and social reformers, who claimed that the advanced civilization of the nineteenth century had outgrown the Bible."[99]

Just as proponents, such as Bartholow and Wood, of the program for re-grounding practice on experimental physiology were leading opponents of the code, so too physicians such as Flint and Stillé, who unabashedly presented their textbooks on practice as bastions of clinical empiricism, were among its most strident defenders.[100] And just as Wood used an essay on his philosophy of therapeutics as an occasion to lash out against the code, so Stillé used an 1884 address professing his very different therapeutic faith as an occasion to defend it. Stillé accused the advocates of experimental medicine of seeking to impose their scientific laws like "a new delivery of the decalogue"; several paragraphs later he prefaced his defense of the AMA Code of Ethics by placing it in a tradition he traced back to "that most ancient of moral codes, the Decalogue."[101]

The language of those who defended the code typically was imbued with the moral indignation of people who saw the issue as "the survival of right over wrong" and who regarded moves to abolish the consultation clause as "a fire-brand of Nihilism in the profession."[102] But this broader protest was sustained by more specific charges against those who sought change, particularly the accusation that the assault on the code was the self-interested work of "a horde of New York specialists."[103] Those who opposed the code, according to this appraisal, had placed socioeconomic interests above professional integrity. Echoing this refrain, the members of a newly formed medical society (organized with Stillé's support) passed a resolution in 1883 reaffirming their allegiance to the code and stating that "we members of the West Philada. Medical Society look with regret and abhorrence on the attempt of certain mercenary men to destroy those principles which for forty-five years have been cherished and protected by the noblest and most honorable men of the medical profession."[104]

In an angry letter written in 1882 to Agnew, a practitioner in Canandaigua, New York, charged that by tacitly sanctioning homeopathy, Agnew and the other city specialists were flying in the face of true science. "If there were a particle, even of the 30th dilution of anything that, could be called *science* about this worse than midsummer madness, one could have a little patience," he snipped, "but there is not; it is a whim, a trick, a *trade* pure and simple." Calling homeopathy "the dream of a crazy-brained, dissatisfied German," he insisted that "whatever else may rise or fall in regard to this subject, that School, whose foundations were laid by Hippocrates and his followers, will stand—As in Christianity so in this, there is 'One faith—one baptism'—we of the Country are amazed by this action of the Roosas, Jacobis and Agnews and others and will not permit ourselves to be led by them for a moment—we do not and *will not trust them*." He told the New York City ophthalmologist, "I make no apology for this letter," concluding, "it is well you should hear from the *woods*."[105]

The presumption of urban specialists that their claims to expert knowledge placed them above the established professional order also drew from defenders of the code assaults against symbols of medical specialism and of experimental science in clinical medicine such as instruments. In his 1884 presidential address to the first annual meeting of the New York State Medical Association, which had broken away from the existing state medical society in order to preserve the code, Henry D. Didama, a physician from Onondaga County and leading defender of the code, urged "conservative progress" in practice and suspicion of promises of rapid progress or certainty. Didama particularly warned against "the innumerable instruments of precision, which promise to substitute mathematical accuracy for vague guesses and which are too often used, not to supplement but to supplant other and valuable methods of investigation." There was real danger, he went on, in "all the 'scopes,' all the 'graphs,' and all the 'meters'" for which clinical authority increasingly was being claimed, particularly by specialists. "These rightfully challenge recognition and study, while with unappeasable appetite they devour our substance if we attempt to add them all to our *armamentarium*."[106] It was perhaps fitting that Flint's last address, published posthumously in 1886 as *Medicine of the Future*, not only cautioned that "the only solid basis of therapeutics is clinical experience," but ended by warning against medical specialization as "a dangerous tendency."[107]

Intermeshed into the animus on both sides were conflicting ideals of science and its place in medicine that had far-reaching intellectual, social, professional, and moral implications. Indeed, some of the leading participants in the Code of Ethics controversy recognized that no amount of discussion, even among people of good will, could resolve the underlying incommensurability in their outlooks. "A division of the profession seems inevitable," Flint wrote to Agnew on the eve of the split of New York's state medical society in 1883, in a letter that he asked be kept private. "I would appeal to you to use your influence to prevent this, were it not that I must suppose you to be as firm in your conceptions of right and duty, as I am in mine."[108]

In this light, it is not surprising that stalwart disciples of the Paris School tended to meet the program for a new medical order with hostility, not diffidence. They perceived the promises of clinical power made on behalf of experimental science as the outer shell of a Trojan horse that endangered medicine intellectually, professionally, and morally. Thus in 1885, in one of the last addresses of his career, Stillé again railed before a gathering of medical students against both the dangers of experimental therapeutics ("the medicine that calls itself scientific") and the evil of those who rejected the Code of Ethics and met with irregulars in consultation, "as if there could be any fellowship between light & darkness, truth & falsehood."[109]

## THE ENDURANCE OF MEMORY

"Paris exists to me now only in the memory," Augustus Gardner wrote as he began his voyage back to America in 1847. "That city," he went on, "has vanished, for aught I know, into some such stuff as dreams, or the bodiless spirits of the air, are made of." Yet he was confident that his memories would endure. "The acquisitions I have made, and the pleasures I have enjoyed, I cannot be deprived of—they are yet mine." He did not expect to see again the Paris hospitals or the acquaintances he had made there, yet felt sure that "in a world of perpetual change, absence, like death, will embalm these summer friendships, and preserve them forevermore the same."[110] But in fact, as we have seen, memories of Paris were altered by both transplantation and time.

Parisian memories, however, reified as they became, played a powerful role in the cognitive and emotional lives of the American disciples of French medicine, and what Bowditch called "memory's fairy fingers" tightened their grip on these physicians as they entered old age.[111] It was their commitment to the lessons of a remembered Paris that, after midcentury, called some of them back to the fray to defend the ideal of empirical medical truth against forces that threatened to depose it. To this extent, aging American Parisians were concerned about the future of medicine, and concerned that the gains they had made not be swept away in the ardor of new enthusiasms. But as they approached the end of their lives, the first generation of American disciples of the Paris School also were increasingly preoccupied with the past, and in particular with how they and the French impulse would be remembered. Asserting the right to tell their own story and say what it meant was a final act in the definition of self, the writing of their own history and their own epitaph.

Physicians who revisited Paris decades after they had studied there often were surprised to discover a world unlike the one they remembered. Yet in no case did this seem to endanger the integrity of their memories. A persistent sense in their reflections on this new Paris was that *it* somehow lacked authenticity, and instead of sorting out a new medical world, often they set about seeking familiar emblems of an earlier time. Bowditch, who in 1867 traveled abroad to recover his health, visited Louis a few days after arriving in Paris and dined at his house opposite the Bois de Boulogne. "Louis was benign, and as beautiful in his old age as you can imagine a man to be," Bowditch wrote in his journal, particularly pleased by the autographed lithograph of Louis his former mentor gave him at their parting.[112] What most drew Bowditch's attention during his brief stay, though, were physical sites that conjured up the recollection of earlier days: "memories floated before me," he wrote fondly in his journal.[113] He visited the wards of La Pitié, "the scenes of my youth"; walked down the Rue de l'École de Médecine, "the scenes of my student life"; and "slowly retraced my steps over the hallowed ground of the Rue d'Orléans (now Rue d'Aubenton)" to touch the gate handle of the boardinghouse where he had first met Olivia Yardley, the young Englishwoman who became his wife.[114] Other memories came unbidden: walking past the doorway of a prison, for example, triggered recollections of the time thirty years earlier when he had concealed a human lung from the dissection room underneath his hat to examine it at leisure in the room of his pension, only to panic when he realized, passing the guard stationed at that doorway, that blood had begun to trickle down his cheek.[115]

Post-Haussmann Paris was physically transformed, however, with old structures torn down by order of Napoléon III to give way to wide, straight, tree-lined avenues, and even the sites of memory from the first half of the century could not be relied upon to have remained intact. Thus Holmes aptly referred to his return visit in 1886 as "a Rip Van Winkle experiment." He found in Paris that "my old master's name, Louis, is but a dim legend in the wards where he used to teach his faithful and almost worshipping students," reflecting that "*nous avons changé tout cela* is true of every generation in medicine."[116]

Increasingly, Americans tended to link the broader meaning of the Paris School and their experiences there to the clinicians they had followed—concrete emblems that stood for the whole; yet they too were impermanent. Writing in 1885, Edward Warren, who had studied in France three decades earlier, noted that of the great men he had heard in Paris—Trousseau, Velpeau, Piorry, Robin, Nélaton, Jobert de Lamball, Ricord, Maisonneuve, Andral, and Dubois—only Ricord survived. As Warren commented, "With a single exception all of them have paid the debt of nature, and their places have been filled and the busy world has forgotten them; but they still live in the memory of those who listened to their words of wisdom and eloquence as well as upon the proudest pages in the history of medicine."[117] In recollections of the Paris School, the mundane realities of practical clinical experience, a central preoccupation in the stories they had told during their student days in France, all but vanished from their narratives. Yet the essence of that experience endured, distilled into symbols—above all, the ideal of empirical truth—that stood both for the Paris of their youth and for its lasting meaning.

During the years when the image of French medicine was being eroded, the passage of time and of people were themes that took increasingly firmer hold on the first generation of American Parisians, and reflections on their lives often turned to disappointment and loss. Stillé cut short a revisit to Paris in 1851 when he learned that his youngest son and his mentor's namesake, Louis Stillé, was ill. On returning to Philadelphia, moreover, he discovered that his wife Caroline's mental illness had grown acute during his absence, and within a few days he committed her to Thomas Kirkbride's asylum for the insane. "You may easily suppose that such an event is not likely to leave me much of the profit I may have reaped abroad," Stillé wrote to his old friend Shattuck; "I feel more as if I should soon become an inmate of the same institution where C. is for the present. I try to keep myself as busy as possible but I feel more like one walking in a dream, than like a man who acts from routine & towards a settled purpose."[118] The bitterest disappointment for Bowditch came in 1863, when, like many American fathers, he lost his eldest son, Nathaniel, in the Civil War—the young man was fatally wounded in a cavalry charge. "His vanishing has caused a blank never to be filled in all my relations in this life," he replied to a letter of condolence. "It has taken from me much of the zest of my professional success; because I have been for years always moulding my life with reference to his future. Now that future is gone."[119] Nat had been studying medicine when war broke out, and his father had proudly looked to him as his medical heir. As Bowditch wrote in his journal on the first anniversary of his son's death, "How much has all the beauty of life gone from me. I seem to have nobody to look forward to as my successor, and the sweet hopes I formed of him are all vanished."[120]

Disappointments such as these were no more than individual variations on the toll extracted by a lived life; but what is striking is how recurrently loss turned the attention of these aging physicians to the legacy they would leave behind. Stillé expressed this at the death of Pierre Louis's only son, writing in 1857 to Shattuck, then in Italy and bound for Paris, "Of course, you will see L. before long in Paris, & I dare say will find him changed, as a man only can be by the irremediable wreck of all his hopes of leaving his name to an only heir." Stillé then turned to the trials and discouragements of his own life, to "expectations, sparkling hopes, which glittered in the young fancy, all ground away by the gnawing of care!" "Hope," he wrote, an "angel" that once "walked beside me, has winged his way [to] heaven. The dreams of usefulness & greatness," he reflected, "have dissolved away; &, instead of happiness . . . I have come to use as an incentive to li[ve] the desire to leave behind me a name—not for greatness, for that is not in me,—but for usefulness." Yet he could not help but "shudder at the thought" that those of the next generation "are to go through the same round of disappointment & despair. We flatter ourselves, perhaps, that they will shun the dangers we have encountered and hope for them as we once hoped for ourselves. Alas! the way of life is the same to all. It begins indeed, as [a] garden-path where all sweet perfumes & delicate hues [de]light the soul: but soon, this path extends beyond the [gar]den of childhood, and it is then plain that it was never finished as it was intended to be; 'thorns also & thistles' does i[t] bring forth, & we go struggling along it torn & weary [un]til at last we lie down in the house appointed to all."[121]

The much-heralded rise of German medicine and disparagement of the lessons of the Paris School played upon this pervasive sense of loss. The aging American pupils of French medicine realized that their professional colleagues were decreasingly interested in hearing their opinions—that, as Stillé lamented in 1871, theirs was "as the 'voice of one crying in the wilderness,'"—and that apprehensions they expressed about the coming medical order, as another physician put it, "will be set down to old fogyism."[122] This in turn altered the meaning of both private and public rememberings of Paris. As a primary allegiance to empirical truth came to be dismissed as outmoded and backward, the significance of memories of an earlier Paris was discounted; and there can be little doubt that the American disciples of the Paris School felt that denigration of their memory as a degradation of their identity.

Such a situation urged American Parisians to recall in new ways the Paris of their youth and to spell out its significance for their lives and profession. Nostalgia was one impetus to recollection. Yet remembering medical Paris and bearing witness to its meaning was also a moral act. As a new generation of physicians, such as White, began to rewrite history in ways that trivialized both the individual memories of older physicians and the wider legacy of the French impulse in American medicine, they reacted by telling a counterhistory drawn in part from their own lived experience, placing memory at the center of a moral discourse. If they were to keep the French impulse alive, it would be by making symbols of it, by distilling its lessons into what Kate Campbell Hurd-Mead, reminiscing about her own medical studies in Paris, would call a "memory picture."[123]

Various events offered older physicians an occasion to bring forward their memories for the benefit of the young, and of themselves. Some of these were private: a chance meeting at the 1876 International Medical Congress in Philadelphia between Bowditch and Ashbel Smith, who was "full of former Parisian memories"; Bowditch's confession to his son, as the latter departed for medical study abroad, that "I often think I have done more good to some poor weary patients by sitting down and telling them of a delightful European experience than by all the drugs I have ever poured down their throats"; or a visit paid in London to Sir James Paget by Hurd-Mead, freshly graduated and on her way to Paris, which the elderly Paget spent "chatting about his old friend, Dr. H. I. Bowditch" and, as Hurd-Mead recounted it, telling her "anecdotes of his student days in Paris."[124]

Other occasions, such as teaching, were more public. "When I was in Paris . . . " was a phrase that peppered the lectures delivered by French-experienced professors.[125] More and more after midcentury it was the memory of an earlier Paris that was deployed, not a model taken from contemporary France. Bowditch opened a course of clinical lectures at the Massachusetts General Hospital in the 1860s by presenting James Jackson, Jr. (whom he had known in Paris when both were young) as the model medical student. Bowditch told his class of Jackson's life, his character, and their tutelage under Louis, to which, Bowditch noted, "I owe most of my subsequent satisfaction in my Medical career." He used the lecture to remind his students what should be retained from that earlier Paris, and employed Jackson as a vehicle for displaying the values of the Paris they had shared together decades earlier.[126]

Death provided another occasion for remembering, a time for those still living to validate the meaning of their careers and the work of their confrères who could no longer speak for themselves. Writing an obituary of Bartlett in 1855, for example, Holmes emphasized Bartlett's commitment to "severe truth." Bartlett's treatise on medical philosophy had been "the abstract expression of that phase of truth practically illustrated in the admirable works of Louis and his disciples."[127] The memorializations of individual physicians who had studied in France became occasions to commemorate the larger congregation of American disciples of the Paris School. Thus in delivering the 1880 eulogy of the South Carolina–born physician James Berney, who had studied in Paris in the mid-1830s, the speaker recited to the assembled members of the Medical and Surgical Society of Montgomery, Alabama, a roll call of other South Carolina natives who, after medical study in Paris, had gone on to "become men of rank in the profession of medicine."[128]

The death of Pierre Louis in 1872 particularly prompted American remembrances, private and public. "Another real pang of sorrow shot through my heart this afternoon while reading in the 'Medical Times and Gazette' of August 31, 1872, the fact that my dear friend and most honored master in medicine, Louis, died at Paris, after a very short illness, at the age of eighty-six," Bowditch wrote in his journal. "It reminded me of many most precious hours spent in his society when I was young and just entering professional life. Is it possible that I shall never see him again? Can it be that the good God ('le bon Dieu,' as Louis called him at our last meeting) will not gratify these longings after a future, when the pure friendships we have made here shall be sanctified?" He proceeded to fill pages of his journal reviewing "the sweet and all-powerful influences exerted by Louis as a leader in medicine and as a dear friend upon my whole life," recalling in detail the time he passed as Louis's pupil in the wards and dissecting rooms of La Pitié forty years earlier. "And now he has gone and left me," Bowditch reflected; "another friend and guide of my youth, helper of my mind, dear to my heart, gone away." To his journal Bowditch confessed, "I feel that Louis's death has seemed to carry me nearer to the grave."[129]

One month later Bowditch spoke publicly about Louis's life to the members of the Society for Medical Observation of Boston. He reviewed Louis's scientific work, which he characterized as "the stalwart protest of a truth-loving man against all the theories then raging." He recalled the time he had spent in Paris as a youth and contrasted the Société Médicale d'Observation at Paris, where he had presented his first "observation," with the "emasculated," "lack-luster gatherings" of its Boston descendant. "In these microscopic, spectroscopic, thermometric, and chemical times," Bowditch noted, the work of those earlier days had to be seen as imperfect, and the skepticism he had acquired in Paris, naive. But seeing things not just with "*calmo currente*" but also "*con amore*," Bowditch did not belittle the message Paris held. He recalled his last meeting in Paris with Louis five years earlier (when Bowditch was fifty-nine and Louis eighty) and the inscribed lithograph Louis had given him. Louis, he remembered, "slowly read over the words, as if they were his parting gifts to me, his pupil." As Bowditch translated for the assembly, "'There is something rarer than the spirit of discernment: it is the need of truth.'"[130]

Such memorializations provided an occasion for those who remembered Paris and their youthful ideal of *la vérité* to recall the bonds they shared privately and publicly. When Bowditch published his eulogy as *Brief Memories of Louis*, he sent a copy to Louis's widow, who, in turn, sent copies of a French eulogy of her husband to both Bowditch and Shattuck. "La guerre, la famine, les désastres de pays; La commune, le bouleversement social, presque la ruine, et enfin la mort de mon cher mari que j'ai perdu le 22 aout 1872!" she wrote to Shattuck's daughter Eleanor Shattuck (who had visited her in Paris), recounting the misfortunes that the family had endured; "voilà pour faire couler des larmes! ce qui surprend c'est de survivre à de tels bouleversements: mais courage toutes les séparations de ce monde ne sont qu'un rendez-vous pour l'Eternité."[131] Bowditch also gave copies of his *Brief Memories of Louis* to fellow Parisians such as Stillé, who replied to the eulogy of "our Master" by telling Bowditch, "You are, of course, quite right about his influence on the medical *esprit* of our generation. All of the minute investigations of disease, the laborious & systematic analyses of thorough medical records, must be traced to him. They are in common use now by those who affect to sneer at the numerical method, not understanding that of which they speak. The labours of the German 'Association' for Scientific investigation is of this sort."[132] Bowditch sent a copy as well to the widow of Philadelphia physician Caspar Wistar Pennock, whom he had known as a student in Paris in the 1830s. "With this, I send my 'Brief Memories of Louis,'" he wrote to her. "Please take them as a token of my remembrance and love for the memory of your excellent husband."[133] It was a double act of remembrance.

The public display of Parisian memories was especially clear in the addresses Paris-experienced Americans gave on leaving their professional duties. This may have seemed the last chance to convey the lessons of one's own medical life to students, who all too often seemed headed in the wrong direction. The tendency on such occasions to dwell on the Paris of a half century earlier should not be regarded as a sign that the orator was living in the past or inattentive to the present. Often it hinted at a sadness at no longer being one of the Young Turks, but perhaps it is best seen as what recent literature on aging has identified as "part of a normal life review process brought about by a realization of approaching dissolution."[134] Not only were the speakers individually relinquishing their positions, but with the rise of German medicine they realized that Parisian supremacy could no longer be maintained. Marking a formal end to their careers, a presentation such as a retirement address was an occasion to affirm one final time that their memories mattered, and that their experience, toil, and devotion counted for something that would endure after they left the stage. Reminiscences on such an occasion could be part of the process of putting one's life in order.

In November 1882, for example, when Holmes delivered his farewell address to students and colleagues at the Harvard Medical School, he devoted most of it to recollecting the time he had spent as a student in Paris nearly a half century earlier. "I can hardly believe my own memory when I recall the old practitioners and Professors who were still going round the hospitals when I mingled with the train of students that attended the morning visits," Holmes reminisced. He had come to terms with the changes brought by the intervening decades, noting that "old theories, and old men who cling to them, must take themselves out of the way as the new generation with its fresh thoughts and altered habits of mind comes forward to take the place of that which is dying out." But then, "You young men who are following the hospitals hardly know how much you are indebted to Louis[,] . . . I say, as I look back on the long hours of the many days I spent in the wards and in the autopsy room of La Pitié, where Louis was one of the attending physicians." The names of Louis and the other Paris clinicians "are but empty sounds for the most part in the ears of the men of not more than middle age," but their message still mattered: "Louis taught us who followed him the love of truth."[135] Holmes was speaking of his own Harvard class, but in words he might equally have applied to his Parisian compatriots, when he wrote that "we know not who among us will be the last survivor, but whoever he is, he will be the heir of a great wealth of memories."[136]

Six months later Stillé addressed the medical class at the University of Pennsylvania on retiring from his chair of the theory and practice of medicine. Unlike Holmes, Stillé did not speak of his time in Paris, yet pervading his remarks was a plea that the banner he had taken up there and carried throughout his career not be trampled down by those eager to champion new ways. More medically engaged than Holmes, who had increasingly turned his energies to literary pursuits, Stillé was also more anxious to use this last opportunity to pass on his legacy to students. When he spoke in 1883, Stillé was deeply concerned that experimental medicine was seducing his students, drawing them away from empirical clinical observation. "I find the theses I have to examine are, some of them, full of chemical and physiological speculations instead of clinical facts," he had lamented to Bowditch the previous year. "Hippocratic-Louisian medicine is at a discount—for the present. But the earth turns!"[137] Seeing the lessons of Paris that he stood for being subverted, Stillé sought in his parting address the chance "of being held in remembrance as one who did not labor altogether in vain."[138]

Fig. 10.1. Lithograph of Pierre Louis, presented by the French clinician to his former Boston pupil Henry Ingersoll Bowditch when the latter revisited Paris in 1867. Five years later Bowditch read the accompanying signed inscription as part of his eulogy of Louis delivered at a meeting of the Society of Medical Observation of Boston. (Henry I. Bowditch, Collection of Autograph Letters and Portraits, courtesy of Francis A. Countway Library of Medicine, Boston.)

"The one principle that has shaped and governed my instruction was to oppose fact to theory," Stillé began, "to defend you against the intrusion of hypothesis and unsubstantial theories, the most dangerous of all your enemies, because the most seductive to the young and ardent mind." Stillé contrasted "empirical facts" with the "laws formulated by experiment" and warned his students not to give in to the "egotistical materialism" that threatened "the established order of things that links the present to the past and to the future." He wished there were time to give a detailed account of the history of medicine. As he explained,

My plea for medical history is to induce you to examine it for yourselves, being persuaded that you will learn from it that the unity and continuity of medical art have been maintained, not by theories of disease and of medicinal action, that have chased one another like jack-o'-lanterns along the road of time, but by the facts of observation honestly and laboriously accumulated from the beginning until now. This was the theme of a lecture that I delivered nearly forty years ago, and all these years of experience and study have so confirmed me in its truth that now, in this, my last public utterance, I cannot refrain from handing it over to you

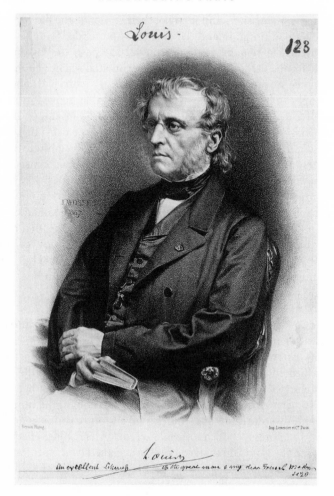

Fig. 10.1 *Continued*

as the sum and substance of my teaching and the best legacy I can bequeath to all my pupils.

Marking the close of his career with words that harkened back to the creed he had taken up in Paris half a century earlier, Stillé ended, "To you, to all who hear me, I offer my most earnest wishes for your success in life, bidding you to love mankind, to love your profession, and, above all, to LOVE TRUTH."[139]

As it happened, the following year Stillé had another chance to speak to students, this time to a medical student society in Philadelphia. Clearly reflecting the broader meaning his professional ideals had taken on in his own life, Stillé chose as the title for his lecture "Truth in Medicine and Truth in Life Inseparable."[140]

To the American Parisians and many of their students, the bid for hegemony by the new German program and the dangers it portended were to be resisted above all by calls to remember the lessons of the past, the lessons of Paris. Claims made for the medical authority of experimental science could represent the reemergence of rationalism and speculation, the very evils their generations had fought so hard to put down and had fought, moreover, in a battle that had helped give definition and meaning to their lives. Some among the younger generation, those who seemed to their elders intoxicated by the promise of German medicine, were *forgetting*, taking for granted the animus against the spirit of system to which those who had studied in Paris had consecrated their careers. *Remembering* the Paris of their youth and the battles they had waged under its banner—and conveying these memories to those too young to have shared their experiences—was the best way older physicians had of trying to ensure that never again would rationalism dominate medicine, that never again would speculation subvert medical truth. The preoccupation of physicians such as Stillé with history is telling, for to them it was not banal but imperative to warn younger members of their profession that if they could not remember the past, they would be condemned to repeat it. They had taken on a duty as custodians of memory, and, as they understood it, of truth.

Stillé lived to give voice to his memories and disappointments into the twentieth century. Writing to William Osler in 1900, he recalled the essay Elisha Bartlett had written half a century earlier on Hippocrates-as-sensual-empiricist, and reaffirmed the ideal it had championed. That essay, Stillé told Osler, "I read and enjoyed, as I do whatever helps to strip Truth of her gauds and present her in her native simplicity." He lamented, though, the inbuilt urge to embellishment, mystification, and "human invention" that his generation had failed fully to suppress.[141] In another letter to Osler, Stillé reflected that "I never supposed the Louis methods would be accepted by the profession generally. They were too laborious, and they gratified too little the thirst for popular applause and personal exaltation that contaminates so many, even men of merit." Despairing that Louis's lessons were being lost, Stillé told Osler that "not even their adoption and illustration by a certain number of physicians who drew their inspiration from the Parisian fount has sufficed to prevent their being overwhelmed by the deluge of German speculation on pathology and therapeutics."[142]

When Stillé died in 1900, there was no one left from his generation of American pupils of the Paris School to deliver his eulogy. It was instead Osler, born a decade after Stillé had completed his Parisian studies, who read his obituary at a meeting of the College of Physicians of Philadelphia. "I feel it a special privilege to be allowed to act as the mouthpiece of my colleagues in expressing our sense of the value of his work and the lessons of his life," Osler said, introducing his remarks. But the story he told the assembled physicians was history compiled by a descendant rather than remembrance voiced by a surviving peer, for he admitted that he had not known the man himself until Stillé was over seventy. Instead, what Osler memorialized was the place Stillé and his fellow disciples of the Paris School had occupied in the history of American medicine. "Coming out of the wilderness in which we had wandered for two thousand years, he entered the promised land," Osler told the Philadelphia gathering, and "saw the heathen dispossessed and the profession at last enter upon a heritage of scientific medicine."[143]

Indeed, during the 1890s, just after the remaining few members of Stillé's generation of American Parisians had lost the chance to tell their own story, Osler took up the task of commemorating the French impulse in American medicine, writing essays on Holmes, Bassett, and Bartlett, as well as a collective portrait of the American disciples of Louis. His historical essays were homage to his teachers and to his teachers' teachers. And in an age of experimental laboratory medicine, they were reminders of what Osler deemed an important tradition of clinical science—an assertion, in fact, of the clinical origins of scientific medicine. The clinician-teachers of the Paris School, Osler believed, figures such as Velpeau, Andral, and Broussais, had been all but forgotten; "scarcely one," he noted, "touches us with any firmness from the past," adding that "of a majority of them it may be said, they are as though they had not been." Yet "modern scientific medicine," he insisted, "had its rise in France in the early days of this century." He singled out the pupils of Louis because "they more than any others gave impetus, which it still feels today, to the scientific study of medicine in the United States." Their achievement, as he appraised it, had been "in substituting finally in the study of medicine, for speculation and theory, observation and method."[144] Osler saw himself as retrieving both lost voices and the vanishing memory of a tradition. Thus "An Alabama Student," his essay on Bassett based largely on letters Bassett had written home from Paris in 1836, letters Osler obtained from Bassett's daughter, was the most poignant precisely because Bassett was so obscure and uncelebrated. As Osler wrote in 1906 to Laura Bassett, who seventy years earlier had been the eldest of the toddlers Bassett was afraid might forget him while he was away in Paris, "I do not think that anything I have ever written is so frequently referred to by my correspondents as the sketch of your good father."[145]

Some Americans continued to travel to Paris for medical study, as they do today, but by the final decades of the nineteenth century such a journey had lost the sense of mission it possessed during the first half of the century. Medical visitors who sought out evidence of Laennec, Velpeau, or Louis did so more in the spirit that in 1865 had led William Williams Keen to report home on his "professional pilgrimage" to Padua to see the site where Vesalius dissected.[146] It was in this sense of professional pilgrimage—an act of veneration rather than of professional improvement—that in 1905, while attending an international medical congress in Paris, Osler organized an "American pilgrimage" to Louis's mausoleum. There Osler placed a wreath at the steps of Louis's tomb, then turned to pose with fifteen other Americans as the event was commemorated by a photographer. As Arnold Carl Klebs, one of those assembled, reported Osler's words, Louis's "special claims to remembrance" rested not so much on his contribution to medical knowledge and practice as on the judg-

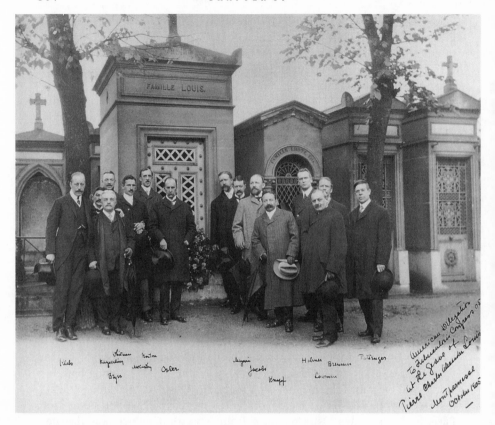

Fig. 10.2. Photograph of the pilgrimage of American physicians to the tomb of Pierre Louis in Montparnasse in 1905. William Osler stands at the center of the doors to the mausoleum of the "Famille Louis," and Arnold Carl Klebs stands at the viewer's far left. (Courtesy of Historical Library, Harvey Cushing/John Hay Whitney Medical Library, Yale University, New Haven.)

ment that "through his students he may be said to have created the American school of clinical medicine."[147] The ritual at Montparnasse was at once an act of filial piety that identified these pilgrims with a particular professional tradition and a memorialization of the legacy to American medicine of the campaign against the spirit of system.

# A B B R E V I A T I O N S
## A N D
## L I S T   O F   A R C H I V E S

| | |
|---|---|
| MA—Peabody Essex | Phillips Library, Peabody Essex Museum, Salem |
| MA—Schlesinger | Schlesinger Library, Radcliffe College, Cambridge |
| MD—MD Hist. Soc. | Manuscripts Division, Maryland Historical Society Library, Baltimore |
| MD—NLM | Modern Manuscripts, History of Medicine Division, National Library of Medicine, Bethesda |
| ME—ME Hist. Soc. | Maine Historical Society, Portland |
| MI—Bentley, U. MI | Bentley Historical Library, The University of Michigan, Ann Arbor |
| MI—Clements, U. MI | Manuscript Division, William L. Clements Library, The University of Michigan, Ann Arbor |
| MO—MO Hist. Soc. | Missouri Historical Society, St. Louis |
| NC—Duke | Special Collections Library, Duke University, Durham |
| NC—Duke Med. | Duke University Medical Center Library, History of Medicine Collections, Durham |
| NC—NC State Arch. | North Carolina State Archives, Raleigh |
| NC—SHC | Manuscripts Department, Southern Historical Collection, Library of the University of North Carolina at Chapel Hill |
| NH—NH Hist. Soc. | New Hampshire Historical Society Collections, Concord |
| NY—Albany Med. | Archives, Albany Medical Center |
| NY—Columbia | Rare Book and Manuscript Library, Butler Library, Columbia University, New York |
| NY—Columbia Med. | Archives and Special Collections, Augustus C. Long Health Sciences Library, Columbia University, New York |
| NY—Cornell | Division of Rare and Manuscript Collections, Cornell University Library, Cornell University, Ithaca |
| NY—NY Acad. Med. | Historical Collections, New York Academy of Medicine, New York |
| NY—NY Gen. & Biogr. Soc. | Library, New York Genealogical and Biographical Society, New York |
| NY—NY Hist. Soc. | The New-York Historical Society, New York |
| NY—NY Pub. Lib. | Rare Books and Manuscripts Division, The New York Public Library, Astor, Lenox, and Tilden Foundations, New York |
| NY—NY State Lib. | Manuscripts and Special Collections, The New York State Library, Albany |
| NY—U. Rochester | Department of Rare Books and Special Collections, Rush Rhees Library, University of Rochester |
| OH—Cincinnati Museum | Collections Division, Cincinnati Museum Center for Natural and Cultural History, Cincinnati |
| OH—Dittrick | Archives, Dittrick Museum of Medical History, The Cleveland Medical Library Association |
| OH—Hayes | The Manuscript Collections, Rutherford B. Hayes Presidential Center, Fremont |
| OH—Marietta Coll. | Dawes Memorial Library, Marietta College, Marietta |
| OH—Mount Pleasant Hist. Soc. | Mount Pleasant Historical Society, Mount Pleasant |
| OH—OH Hist. Soc. | Archives/Library Division, Ohio Historical Society, Columbus |

| | |
|---|---|
| OH—U. Cincinnati | Archives and Rare Books Department, University Libraries, University of Cincinnati |
| OH—U. Cincinnati Med. | Cincinnati Medical Heritage Center, Medical Center Libraries, University of Cincinnati Medical Center, Cincinnati |
| OH—Western Reserve Hist. Soc. | Western Reserve Historical Society, Cleveland |
| PA—APS | Manuscripts Department, American Philosophical Society, Philadelphia |
| PA—CPP | Historical Collections, The Library of the College of Physicians of Philadelphia |
| PA—Hahnemann | Hahnemann University Archives and Special Collections at Allegheny University of the Health Sciences, Philadelphia |
| PA—Hist. Soc. PA | Historical Society of Pennsylvania, Philadelphia |
| PA—U. PA Arch. | The University of Pennsylvania Archives, Philadelphia |
| PA—U. PA Lib. | Department of Special Collections, Van Pelt-Dietrich Library Center, University of Pennsylvania, Philadelphia |
| PA—Women in Med. Arch. | Archives and Special Collections on Women in Medicine of Allegheny University of the Health Sciences, Philadelphia |
| RI—Brown | Manuscripts Division, Brown University Library, Providence |
| SC—SC Hist. Soc. | The South Carolina Historical Society, Charleston |
| SC—U. SC | Manuscripts Division, South Caroliniana Library, The University of South Carolina, Columbia |
| SC—Waring | Waring Historical Library, Medical University of South Carolina, Charleston |
| TN—TN State Lib. | Tennessee State Library and Archives, Nashville |
| TN—Vanderbilt | Historical Collection, Eskind Biomedical Library, Vanderbilt University, Nashville |
| TX—U. TX | The Center for American History, The University of Texas at Austin |
| VA—U. VA | Special Collections Department, Alderman Library, University of Virginia Library, Charlottesville |
| VA—VA Hist. Soc. | Division of Archives and Manuscripts, Virginia Historical Society, Richmond |
| VT—VT Hist. Soc. | Vermont Historical Society, Montpelier |
| WI—WI Hist. Soc. | Archives Division, State Historical Society of Wisconsin, Madison |

REPOSITORIES OUTSIDE THE UNITED STATES

| | |
|---|---|
| Bedford—Bedfords. RO | Bedfordshire County Record Office, Bedford |
| Bristol—Bristol RO | Bristol Record Office, Bristol |
| Chichester—West Sussex RO | West Sussex Record Office, Chichester |
| Durham—Durham RO | Durham Record Office, Durham |
| Edinburgh—Nat. Lib. Scotland | National Library of Scotland, Edinburgh |
| Edinburgh—U. Edinburgh | Special Collections, Edinburgh University Library |
| Exeter—Devon RO | Devon Record Office, Exeter |
| Leeds—U. Leeds | Special Collections, Brotherton Library, University of Leeds |

| | |
|---|---|
| Leicester—Leicesters. RO | Leicestershire County Record Office, Leicester |
| Liverpool—Liverpool RO | Liverpool Record Office and Local History Department, Liverpool |
| Liverpool—U. Liverpool | University Archives, University Library, University of Liverpool |
| London—Guildhall | Guildhall Library, Corporation of London, London |
| London—Guy's | Wills Medical Library, Guy's Hospital, United Medical and Dental School Library Services, London |
| London—RCP | Library, Royal College of Physicians, London |
| London—RCS | Library, The Royal College of Surgeons of England, London |
| London—RSM | Royal Society of Medicine, London |
| London—St. Bartholomew's | Archives Department, St. Bartholomew's Hospital, London |
| Manchester—Chetham's Lib. | Chetham's Library, Manchester |
| Montreal—McGill | Osler Library of Medical History, McGill University |
| Northampton—Northamptons. RO | Northamptonshire Record Office, Northampton |
| Norwich—Norfolk RO | Norfolk Record Office, Norwich |
| Ottawa—Nat. Arch. Canada | National Archives of Canada, Ottawa |
| Oxford—Bodleian | Department of Western Manuscripts, Bodleian Library, University of Oxford, Oxford |
| Paris—AN | Centre parisien des Archives nationales, Paris |
| Toronto—U. Toronto | Academy of Medicine Collection, Thomas Fisher Rare Book Library, University of Toronto |

### JOURNALS

| | |
|---|---|
| *BMSJ* | *Boston Medical and Surgical Journal* |
| *CLO* | *Cincinnati Lancet and Observer* |
| *CMJR* | *Charleston Medical Journal and Review* |
| *LMG* | *London Medical Gazette* |
| *MT* | *Medical Times* |
| *NOMSJ* | *New Orleans Medical and Surgical Journal* |
| *SLMSJ* | *St. Louis Medical and Surgical Journal* |
| *WJMS* | *Western Journal of Medicine and Surgery* |
| *WL* | *Western Lancet* |

INTRODUCTION
STORYTELLING AND PROFESSIONAL
CULTURE: AMERICAN CONSTRUCTIONS OF
THE PARIS CLINICAL SCHOOL

1. John T. Morse, Jr., *Life and Letters of Oliver Wendell Holmes*, 2 vols. (Boston and New York: Houghton, Mifflin and Company, 1896), 1:108–109.

2. For example, Russell M. Jones, "American Doctors and the Parisian Medical World, 1830–1840," *Bulletin of the History of Medicine* 47 (1973): 40–65, 177–204, p. 40; and see Richard H. Shryock, *American Medical Research Past and Present* (New York: The Commonwealth Fund, 1947), pp. 21–36.

3. Erwin H. Ackerknecht, *Medicine at the Paris Hospital, 1794–1848* (Baltimore: Johns Hopkins University Press, 1967). For an excellent historiographic review of the literature on the Paris School, see Ann La Berge and Caroline Hannaway, "Constructing Paris Medicine," in Hannaway and La Berge, *Reinterpreting Paris Medicine, 1790–1850* (Amsterdam and Atlanta: Rodopi, in press).

4. Michel Foucault, *The Birth of the Clinic: An Archaeology of Medical Perception*, trans. A. M. Sheridan Smith (first French ed. 1963; New York: Pantheon Books, 1973), p. xiv.

5. N. D. Jewson, "The Disappearance of the Sick-Man from Medical Cosmology, 1770–1870," *Sociology* 10 (1976): 225–244; and, for the appraisal of an ethicist-historian, Stanley J. Reiser, *Medicine and the Reign of Technology* (Cambridge: Cambridge University Press, 1978), pp. 23–44.

6. [P.] L[ouis] to [H. I. Bowditch], Paris, 5 Feb. 1840, MA—Countway. For the author of the letter probably more than for its recipient, the phrase resonated with earlier battles Louis had fought against the Paris clinician François-J.-V. Broussais, arguably the last great medical system-builder.

7. Ackerknecht, *Medicine at the Paris Hospital*, p. xiii.

8. Helpful frameworks for analyzing travelers' reports include James Buzard, *The Beaten Track: European Tourism, Literature, and the Ways to Culture, 1800–1918* (Oxford: Clarendon Press of Oxford University Press, 1993); Ahmed M. Metwalli, "Americans Abroad: The Popular Art of Travel Writing in the Nineteenth Century," in *America: Exploration and Travel*, ed. Steven E. Kagle (Bowling Green, Ohio: Bowling Green State University Popular Press, 1979), pp. 68–82; and William W. Stowe, *Going Abroad: European Travel in Nineteenth-Century American Culture* (Princeton: Princeton University Press, 1994).

9. William Osler, "The Influence of Louis on American Medicine," in *An Alabama Student and Other Biographical Essays* (1897; London: Oxford University Press, 1908), pp. 189–201.

10. Ackerknecht, *Medicine at the Paris Hospital*, p. 123. Ackerknecht put the date of that event at 1848, adjusting the date from 1850 somewhere in the course of drafting his text to bring his medical story into line with a political narrative; see Erwin H. Ackerknecht to Henry E. Sigerist, Madison, Wisc., 13 Sept. 1956, and Madison, Wisc., 20 July 1956, Henry Ernest Sigerist Papers, CT—Yale.

11. Throughout, by English I mean *English*, not British, for despite the deep intercalation of English and Scottish medical worlds in the nineteenth century, medicine in Scotland retained its distinctiveness in intellectual character, professional organization, and, not least of all, relationships to French culture. Studies on the relationship between Scottish, Italian, Spanish, and particularly German physicians and French medicine would greatly enhance our comparative perspective. Helpful starting points include Ursula Geigenmüller, "Aussagen über die französische Medizin der Jahre 1820–1847 in Reiseberichten deutscher Ärzte" (Doctoral diss., Freien Universität Berlin, n.d.) (which includes a good bibliography of reports on Paris by German medical travelers); Stephen Jacyna, "*Au lit des malades*: A. F. Chomel's Clinic at the Charité, 1828–9," *Medical History* 33 (1989): 420–449; idem, *Philosophical Whigs: Medicine, Science and Citizenship in Edinburgh, 1789–1848* (London and New York: Routledge, 1994); and idem, "Robert Carswell and William Thomson at the Hôtel-Dieu of Lyons: Scottish Views of French

Medicine," in *British Medicine in an Age of Reform*, ed. Roger French and Andrew Wear (London and New York: Routledge, 1991), pp. 110–135.

12. See Marc Bloch, "Toward a Comparative History of European Societies," a translation of his 1925 paper in *Enterprise and Secular Change*, ed. Fredric C. Lane and Jelle C. Riemersma (Homewood, Ill.: Richard D. Irwin, 1953), pp. 494–521; and see William H. Sewell, Jr., "Marc Bloch and the Logic of Comparative History," *History and Theory* 6 (1967): 208–218. On the utility of a comparative perspective for understanding what was and was not singular about the Paris School itself, see Othmar Keel, *La généalogie de l'histopathologie. Une révision déchirante. Philippe Pinel, lecteur discret de James Carmichael Smyth (1741–1821)* (Paris: Vrin, 1979); idem, "The Politics of Health and the Institutionalization of Clinical Practice in Europe in the Second Half of the Eighteenth Century," in *William Hunter and the Eighteenth-Century Medical World*, ed. W. F. Bynum and R. Porter (Cambridge: Cambridge University Press, 1985), pp. 207–256; and Guenter B. Risse, *Hospital Life in Enlightenment Scotland: Care and Teaching at the Royal Infirmary of Edinburgh* (Cambridge: Cambridge University Press, 1986).

13. The growing and suggestive recent literature on storytelling in medical culture has tended to focus on illness narratives. See, for example, Howard Brodie, *Stories of Sickness* (New Haven: Yale University Press, 1988); Julia Epstein, *Altered Conditions: Disease, Medicine, and Storytelling* (New York: Routledge, 1995); Kathryn Montgomery Hunter, *Doctor's Stories: The Narrative Structure of Medical Knowledge* (Princeton: Princeton University Press, 1991); Arthur Kleinman, *The Illness Narratives: Suffering, Healing, and the Human Condition* (New York: Basic Books, 1988); and Steven M. Stowe, "Seeing Themselves at Work: Physicians and the Case Narrative in the Mid-Nineteenth-Century American South," *American Historical Review* 101 (1996): 41–79.

14. Richard H. Shryock, review of Thomas Neville Bonner, *American Doctors and German Universities* (1963), in *Journal of the History of Medicine and Allied Sciences* 19 (1964): 309–310, p. 310.

15. Walter Artelt, "Louis' amerikanische Schüler und der Krise der Therapie," *Sudhoffs*

*Archiv für Geschichte der Naturwissenschaft* 42 (1958): 291–301; Henry Blumenthal, *Americans and French Culture, 1800–1900: Interchanges in Art, Science, Literature, and Society* (Baton Rouge: Louisiana State University Press, 1975), pp. 402–467; Howard Mumford Jones, *Americans and French Culture, 1750–1848* (Chapel Hill: University of North Carolina Press, 1927); Russell M. Jones, "American Doctors and the Parisian Medical World"; idem, "American Doctors in Paris, 1820–1861: A Statistical Profile," *Journal of the History of Medicine and Allied Sciences* 25 (1970): 142–157; idem, "An American Medical Student in Paris, 1831–1833," *Harvard Library Bulletin* 15 (1967): 59–81; and idem, "Introduction," in *The Parisian Education of an American Surgeon: Letters of Jonathan Mason Warren (1832–1835)* (Philadelphia: American Philosophical Society, 1978), pp. 1–69; Ronald L. Numbers and John Harley Warner, "The Maturation of American Medical Science," in *Scientific Colonialism: A Cross-Cultural Comparison*, ed. Nathan Reingold and Marc Rothenberg (Washington, D.C.: Smithsonian Institution Press, 1987), pp. 191–214; Richard H. Shryock, "Empiricism versus Rationalism in American Medicine, 1650–1950," *Proceedings of the American Antiquarian Society*, n.s., 79 (1969): 99–150; idem, "The Influence of French Medicine in Europe and America," in *The Development of Modern Medicine: An Interpretation of the Social and Scientific Factors Involved* (1936; Madison: University of Wisconsin Press, 1979), pp. 170–191; idem, "The Advent of Modern Medicine in Philadelphia, 1800–1850," in *Medicine in America: Historical Essays* (Baltimore: Johns Hopkins University Press, 1966), pp. 203–232; Bruce Sinclair, "Americans Abroad: Science and Cultural Nationalism in the Early Nineteenth Century," in *The Sciences in the American Context: New Perspectives*, ed. Nathan Reingold (Washington, D.C.: Smithsonian Institution Press, 1979); John Harley Warner, "Science, Healing, and the Physician's Identity: A Problem of Professional Character in Nineteenth-Century America," *Clio Medica* 22 (1991): 65–88.

16. Charles E. Rosenberg, *The Care of Strangers: The Rise of America's Hospital System* (New York: Basic Books, 1988), pp. 82–90; James C. Mohr, *Doctors and the Law: Medical Jurisprudence in Nineteenth-Century America* (New York and Oxford: Oxford University Press, 1993); Barbara Gutmann Rosenkrantz,

*Public Health and the State: Changing Views in Massachusetts, 1842–1936* (Cambridge, Mass., and London: Harvard University Press, 1979); Dale Cary Smith, "The Emergence of Organized Clinical Instruction in the Nineteenth Century American Cities of Boston, New York, and Philadelphia" (Ph.D. diss., University of Minnesota, 1974); James H. Cassedy, *American Medicine and Statistical Thinking, 1800–1860* (Cambridge, Mass., and London: Harvard University Press, 1984); John Harley Warner, "The Selective Transport of Medical Knowledge: Antebellum American Physicians and Parisian Medical Therapeutics," *Bulletin of the History of Medicine* 59 (1985): 213–231; and idem, *The Therapeutic Perspective: Medical Practice, Knowledge, and Identity in America, 1820–1885* (Cambridge, Mass., and London: Harvard University Press, 1986), pp. 185–206.

17. Russell C. Maulitz, *Morbid Appearances: The Anatomy of Pathology in the Early Nineteenth Century* (Cambridge: Cambridge University Press, 1987); Adrian Desmond, *The Politics of Evolution: Morphology, Medicine, and Reform in Radical London* (Chicago: University of Chicago Press, 1989); Pierre Huard and M. D. Grmek, "Les élèves étrangers de Laennec," *Revue d'histoire des sciences* 26 (1973): 315–337; Ulrich Tröhler, "Quantification in British Medicine and Surgery, 1750–1830, with Special Reference to Its Introduction into Therapeutics" (Ph.D. diss, University of London, 1978); John Harley Warner, "The Idea of Science in English Medicine: The 'Decline of Science' and the Rhetoric of Reform, 1815–45," in French and Wear, *British Medicine in an Age of Reform,* pp. 136–164.

18. Among the most helpful studies on the background and formation of postrevolutionary French medicine are Lawrence W. B. Brockliss, "L'enseignement médical et la Révolution: essai de réévaluation," *Histoire de l'éducation* 42 (1989): 79–110; idem, "Medical Reform, the Enlightenment and Physician-Power in Late Eighteenth-Century France," in *Medicine and Enlightenment,* ed. Roy Porter (Amsterdam and Atlanta: Rodopi, 1995), pp. 64–112; Toby Gelfand, *Professionalizing Modern Medicine: Paris Surgeons and Medical Science and Institutions in the Eighteenth Century* (Westport, Conn.: Greenwood Press, 1980); Matthew Ramsey, *Professional and Popular Medicine in France, 1770–1830: The Social World of Medical Practice* (New York: Cambridge University Press, 1988);

Jean-Charles Sournia, *La médecine révolutionnaire, 1789–1799* (Paris: Payot, 1989); David M. Vess, *Medical Revolution in France, 1789–1796* (Gainesville: University Presses of Florida, 1975); and Dora B. Weiner, *The Citizen-Patient in Revolutionary and Imperial Paris* (Baltimore and London: Johns Hopkins University Press, 1993).

Of a large literature on early- and mid-nineteenth-century Paris medicine, important studies include William Coleman, *Death Is a Social Disease: Public Health and Political Economy in Early Industrial France* (Madison: University of Wisconsin Press, 1982); Paul Delaunay, *D'une révolution à l'autre, 1789–1848: l'évolution des théories et de la pratique médicales* (Paris: Editions Hippocrate, 1949); Jacalyn Duffin, *To See with a Better Eye: A Life of R.T.H. Laennec* (Princeton: Princeton University Press, in press); Jan Goldstein, *Console and Classify: The French Psychiatric Profession in the Nineteenth Century* (Cambridge: Cambridge University Press, 1987); Hannaway and La Berge, *Reinterpreting Paris Medicine, 1790–1850;* Pierre Huard and Marie-José Imbault-Huart, "L'enseignement libre de la médecine à Paris au XIXe siècle," *Revue d'histoire des sciences* 37 (1974): 45–62; Ann F. La Berge, *Mission and Method: The Early Nineteenth-Century French Public Health Movement* (New York: Cambridge University Press, 1992); Ann La Berge and Mordechai Feingold, eds., *French Medical Culture in the Nineteenth Century* (Amsterdam and Atlanta: Rodopi, 1994); Jacques Léonard, *La médecine entre les savoirs et les pouvoirs: histoire intellectuelle et politique de la médecine française au XIXe siècle* (Paris: Aubier Montaigne, 1981); John E. Lesch, *Science and Medicine in France: The Emergence of Experimental Physiology, 1790–1855* (Cambridge, Mass., and London: Harvard University Press, 1984); Russell C. Maulitz, "In the Clinic: Framing Disease at the Paris Hospital," *Annals of Science* 47 (1990): 127–137; Matthew Ramsey, "The Politics of Professional Monopoly in Nineteenth-Century Medicine: The French Model and Its Rivals," in *Professions and the French State, 1700–1900,* ed. Gerald L. Geison (Philadelphia: University of Pennsylvania Press, 1984); George Rosen, "The Philosophy of Ideology and the Emergence of Modern Medicine in France," *Bulletin of the History of Medicine* 20 (1946): 328–339; George Weisz, *The Medical Mandarins: The French Academy of Medicine in the Nineteenth* and *Early Twentieth Centuries* (New York and Oxford: Oxford University Press, 1995); and Mireille Wiriot, *L'enseignement clinique dans les hôpitaux de Paris entre 1794 et 1848 (d'après des documents de l'époque)* (Paris, 1970).

## CHAPTER 1
### PROFESSIONAL IMPROVEMENT AND THE ANTEBELLUM MEDICAL MARKETPLACE

1. The prevailing image of antebellum medical education is well depicted in, for example, William Frederick Norwood, *Medical Education in the United States before the Civil War* (Philadelphia: University of Pennsylvania Press, 1944); Ronald L. Numbers, ed., *The Education of American Physicians: Historical Essays* (Berkeley, Los Angeles, and London: University of California Press, 1980); William G. Rothstein, *American Physicians in the Nineteenth Century: From Sects to Science* (Boston and London: Johns Hopkins University Press, 1972); and Paul Starr, *The Social Transformation of American Medicine: The Rise of a Sovereign Profession and the Making of a Vast Industry* (New York: Basic Books, 1982).

2. Helpful overviews include Joseph F. Kett, *The Formation of the American Medical Profession: The Role of Institutions, 1780–1860* (New Haven and London: Yale University Press, 1968), and Rothstein, *American Physicians*, pp. 63–174.

3. E[lias] B[enson] Thompson to [Mary Eleanor (Benson) Thompson], [New Orleans], 13 Nov. 1866, Benson-Thompson Family Papers, NC—Duke.

4. Cincinnati College of Medicine and Surgery, Board of Trustees Minutes, 1851–1889, entry for 22 Jan. 1859, OH—U. Cincinnati.

5. Samuel Forwood to William Stump Forwood, Gosport, Alabama, 8 Oct. 1846, William Stump Forwood Papers, NC—SHC. A young man reading medicine in rural Louisiana could write to a friend in 1848 that he was "farming some and studying some," determined that poverty would not keep him from becoming a doctor; "I do not intend to let that discourage me for there has bin many men that has suceeded under advers fortune" (A. Addison to Jeptha McKinney, St. Helena Parish, Louisiana, 18 June 1848, Jeptha McKinney Papers, LA—LSU).

6. W. Abell to Anna Abell, Utica, 8 Mar. 1829, Abell Family Papers, NY—Cornell.

7. Geo. B. Wood to Franklin Bache, New Orleans, 17 May 1844, G. B. Wood Misc. Correspondence, PA—CPP; and, as an example from the West, see Sheldon Erwin Holmes to Henry M. Morfit, Chicago, 28 Mar. 1850, Chicago Letters from Physicians and Surgeons, IL—Chicago Hist. Soc.

8. Barton Randall to Alexander Randall, Williamsport, 26 Aug. 1828, Randall Family Papers (no. 9564), VA—U. VA.

9. A. Stillé to G. C. Shattuck, Philadelphia, 6 Aug. 1844, Shattuck Papers, vol. 18, MA—MA Hist. Soc.

10. See Geo. W. Holmes to Richard Smith, [Plymouth?], 8 Nov. 1831, and V. B. Webb to Richard Smith, London, 30 Apr. 1824, in Bristol Infirmary Biographical Memoirs, vols. 10 and 12, Bristol—Bristol RO.

11. James Norcom to D. D. Hosack, Edenton, North Carolina, 14 June 1819, Dr. James Norcom and Family Papers, NC—NC State Arch.

12. Penington Tucker to G. B. Wood, Livingston, Mississippi, 4 June 1847, Wood Misc. Correspondence.

13. Charles Harrod to [Simeon B. Evans], New Orleans, 1 Mar. 1845, Nathaniel Evans and Family Papers, LA—LSU. The kind of agonizing many antebellum Americans experienced as they sorted out how to acquire an adequate medical education is lucidly expressed in Horace A. Barrows, Diaries, vols. 1–5, 1829–1838, Horace Aurelius Barrows Papers, ME—ME Hist. Soc.

14. Benj. H. Pierson to C[hapman] J. Stuart, [St. Louis], 12 Feb. 1845, Stuart Family Papers, VA—VA Hist. Soc.

15. Samuel Brown to Orlando Brown, Lexington, 20 Jan. 1821, Orlando Brown Papers, KY—Filson Club.

16. J. C. Nott to James M. Gage, New Orleans, Mar. [1837], James McKibbin Gage Papers, NC—SHC. "But trust me," he continued, "you will find it a bitter pill to swallow . . . to see these triflers with human existence, alike ignorant of the common courtesies of life, as of the first principles of their profession, mounting with rapid strides, the ladder of worldly reputation, while you 'lie grovelling.'"

17. John P. Harrison to R. La Roche, Louisville, 3 Oct. 1825, R. La Roche Correspondence, PA—CPP.

18. Charles Johnson to Lou[die], Nashville, 1 Nov. 1860, Charles James Johnson Letters and Family Correspondence, LA—LSU. "When I think of the short time required of students to prepare for the profession (two years! how short for the enormity of the labor!) I am astonished at the Cupidity of Medical Professors," he continued. "In Georgia at some of the schools they have reduced the time to one year, and several students of Medicine who attended their first course here last winter graduated at the last spring. Oh! Money!"

19. J[efferson] Howard De Votie to [James H. De Votie], New Orleans, 15 Dec. 1861, and ibid., 26 Feb. 1862, James H. De Votie Papers, NC—Duke.

20. W. T. Holland, "Typhoid Fever" (M.D. thesis, Medical College of the State of South Carolina, 1856), SC—Waring; J. A. Long, "Eleven Years Practice" (M.D. thesis, University of Nashville, 1855), TN—Vanderbilt; Alfred Boyd, "Finale of Twenty Years Study and Practice of Medicine" (M.D. thesis, Medical College of the State of South Carolina, 1856), SC—Waring.

21. John M. Magnan, "The Principles of Medicine" (M.D. thesis, University of Pennsylvania, 1867), PA—U. PA Lib.

22. Edwin L. Mcall to Lemuel Kollock, Philadelphia, 19 Oct. 1805, Lemuel Kollock Papers, GA—GA Hist. Soc.

23. S. M. Van Wyck to My Own Darling, New York, 12 Dec. 1858, Maverick and Van Wyck Families Papers, SC—U. SC.

24. Printed form giving grades of "scale of preparation" for medicine; for chemistry and materia medica; and for physiology, anatomy and surgery, at the University of Virginia, 1 Dec. 1844, enclosed with letter from Philip C. Gooch to Mrs. M. R. Gooch, [Charlottesville], 9 Dec. 1844, Gooch Family Papers, VA—VA Hist. Soc.

25. "The lectures are fast approaching to a termination, & with it of course comes all the terrors of the Greene Box which ordeal I among others must soon undergo," one medical student reported from Philadelphia in 1843 (Matthew Gayle to W. B. Crawford, Philadelphia, 19 Feb. 1843, Sarah Ann and William B. Crawford Papers, AL—U. AL).

26. Proceedings of the Faculty of the Medical College of Louisiana, May 1835–Feb. 1847, entry for 15 Mar. 1845, LA—Tulane

Med.; Cincinnati College of Medicine and Surgery, Board of Trustees Minutes, 1851–1889, entry for 15 Feb. 1854, OH—U. Cincinnati. Instances of the rejection of M.D. degree candidates on the basis of their examinations are readily found in Cincinnati College of Medicine and Surgery, Faculty Minutes, 1851–1868, OH—U. Cincinnati; Homoeopathic Medical College of Pennsylvania, Faculty Minutes, 1850–1869, PA—Hahnemann; Miami Medical College, Faculty Minutes, 1852–1881, OH—U. Cincinnati; Medical College of Ohio, Faculty Minutes, 1831–1852, OH—U. Cincinnati; University of Pennsylvania, Minutes of the Medical School Faculty, 1829–1873, PA—U. PA Arch.; Rutgers Medical College, Minutes of the Board of Professors, Dec. 1826–Oct. 1827 BV Rutgers Medical College, NY—NY Hist. Soc.; and Transylvania University, Medical Department, Minute Book, 1819–1849, KY—Transylvania.

27. A. Dugas to Frederick E. Dugas, Philadelphia, 22 Aug. 1826, Dugas Papers, GA—GA Hist. Soc.

28. Notes appended to Abner Webb, Diary, 1821–1874, OH—Dittrick; Oliver H. Stout to James G. Taliaferro, Lexington, 11 Nov. 1820, Zachariah and James G. Taliaferro Papers, LA—LSU. And see Daniel Drake to Jared Mansfield, Cincinnati, 10 July 1813, Jared Mansfield Papers, OH—OH Hist. Soc.

29. W. C. Whetstone to My Dear Mother, Columbia, S.C., 10 Feb. 1854; ibid., Col[umbi]a 24 Feb. 1854, Whetstone Family Papers, SC—U. SC.

30. For a helpful overview, see John B. Blake, "Anatomy," in Numbers, *Education of American Physicians*, pp. 29–47.

31. Girard Dayers to Usher Parsons, Boston, 9 Jan. 1819, Parsons Family Papers, RI—Brown.

32. Ruel Smith to Smith Robertson, Rochester, 21 May 1841, Smith Robertson Papers, NY—Cornell. He went on to say that "the justice is satisfied by this time, that medical students are hard colts to break as they have the favor of the legal profession, and all the intelligent part of the community." And see Faculty Minutes, Medical Department, University of Louisville, 1857–1891, entry for 26 Dec. 1863, KY—U. Louisville.

33. Abiel Hall, Jr., to Usher Parsons, Alfred, 29 Aug. 1811, Parsons Family Papers.

34. Medical College of Ohio, Faculty Min-

utes, Feb. 1822–Feb. 1831, entry for 12 Dec. 1828, OH—U. Cincinnati.

35. Medical College of Ohio, Faculty Minutes, 1831–1852, entry for 21 Mar. 1843, OH—U. Cincinnati.

36. Ibid., entry for 27 Oct. 1849.

37. Medical College of Ohio, Faculty Minutes, 1852–1909, entry for 5 June 1878, OH—U. Cincinnati.

38. *Circular of the Medical College of Louisiana in the Ninth Session. 1842–3* (New-Orleans: Office of the Bee, 1842), p. 4.

39. Thomas G. Prioleau, Dean, Medical College of South Carolina, Circular to Legislature, Charleston, 19 June 1824, in Minute Book of the Medical Society of South Carolina, 2 July 1810–9 Dec. 1833, typescript, p. 240, SC—U. SC.

40. See Todd L. Savitt, "The Use of Blacks for Medical Experimentation and Demonstration in the Old South," *Journal of Southern History* 48 (1982): 331–348; and, for a revealing exploration of the British context, see Ruth Richardson, *Death, Dissection, and the Destitute* (London and New York: Routledge and Kegan Paul, 1987).

41. W. C. Whetstone to [Nathan Whetstone], Columbia, 23 Mar. 1855, Whetstone Family Papers.

42. Alexander Grieg to Dear Uncle [John Grieg], New York, 9 Dec. 1840, NY—NY Acad. Med.

43. Lunsford P. Yandell, Notes Taken on Lectures Given at Transylvania University, Prof. Richardson, Introductory in the Chapel, 9 Nov. 1825, Daniel Drake Papers, in Emmet Field Horine Collection, KY—U. KY.

44. George Bacon Wood, Introductory to the Course of Lectures on the Practice of Medicine in the University of Pennsylvania, 10 Oct. 1851 and 12 Oct. 1854, PA—U. PA Arch.

45. *Annual Circular of the Medical Department of the University of Louisiana, Session of 1859–60* (New Orleans: Picayune Print, 1858), p. 7.

46. Carter P. Johnson to Chapman J. Stuart, Richmond, 11 June 1845, Stuart Family Papers.

47. J. Milligan to Joseph A. S. Milligan, Augusta, 4 June 1846, Milligan Family Papers, NC—SHC.

48. Q. R. Calhoun to J.A.S. Milligan, Woodville P[ost] Off[ice], Greenwood, 4 June 1847, Milligan Family Papers.

49. Edwin L. Mcall to Lemuel Kollock, Philadelphia, 22 Feb. 1805, Kollock Papers.

50. "Private Med. School," *BMSJ* 3 (1830–1831): 344.

51. "Charleston and Columbia Preparatory Medical Schools," *CMJR* 14 (1859): 278–279, p. 278.

52. Joseph Parrish to [George B. Wood], Burlington, 19 Feb. 1852, Wood Misc. Correspondence.

53. C.G.W. Comegys to Scott Cook, Cincinnati, 30 Oct. 1848, Matthew Scott Cook Papers, OH—Western Reserve Hist. Soc.

54. Charles E. Rosenberg, *The Care of Strangers: The Rise of America's Hospital System* (New York: Basic Books, 1987), esp. pp. 58–68, 190–200.

55. Joseph T. Webb to [M. S. Cook], Cincinnati, 4 Feb. 1851, Cook Papers.

56. J. C. Nott to James M. Gage, Mobile, 5 Nov. 1836, Gage Papers.

57. Levin S. Joynes to Thomas R. Joynes, Baltimore, 19 Feb. 1845, Joynes Family Papers, VA—VA Hist. Soc.

58. Elisha Bartlett to Isaac Hays, Lowell, 27 Feb. 1838, Isaac Hays Papers, PA—APS. Bartlett went on to ask advice about opportunities for professional improvement in Philadelphia.

59. Elisha Bartlett to Elisabeth Bartlett, Philadelphia, 11 Sept. 1841; and see E. Bartlett to John O. Green, Philadelphia, 7 Sept. 1841, both in Bartlett (Elisha) Family Papers, NY—U. Rochester.

60. J. T. Updegraff, Day Book, Medical Practice, 15 Jan. 1846–31 Dec. 1853, entry for 31 Dec. 1847, OH—Mount Pleasant Hist. Soc.

## CHAPTER 2
## WHY PARIS?

1. Samuel Lewis, "List of the American Graduates in Medicine at the University of Edinburgh from 1705 to 1866, with Their Theses," *New England Historic Genealogical Register* 42 (1888): 159–165, cited in Russell M. Jones, "American Doctors in Paris, 1820–1861: A Statistical Profile," *Journal of the History of Medicine and Allied Sciences* 25 (1970): 143–157, p. 143. For a broad depiction of changing patterns of medical education in Europe and America, see Thomas Neville Bonner, *Becoming a Physician: Medical Education in Britain, France, Germany, and the United*

States, 1750–1945 (New York: Oxford University Press, 1995).

2. Whitfield J. Bell, Jr., *John Morgan: Continental Doctor* (Philadelphia: University of Pennsylvania Press, 1965), pp. 78–79.

3. James Jackson, Jr., to James Jackson, Sr., Paris, 26 June 1831, James Jackson Papers, MA—Countway.

4. Chandos Michael Brown, *Benjamin Silliman: A Life in the Young Republic* (Princeton: Princeton University Press, 1989), pp. 156–197.

5. George Watson to Joseph Shelton Watson, Edinburgh, 25 Sept. 1805, Watson Family Papers, VA—VA Hist. Soc. On John Collins Warren's surgical studies in Paris in 1802, see Edward Warren, ed., *The Life of John Collins Warren, M.D., Compiled Chiefly from His Autobiography and Journals*, 2 vols. (Boston: Ticknor and Fields, 1860), esp. 1:55–60.

6. George Watson to James Watson, Edinburgh, 31 Jan. 1806. For the Edinburgh context, see Guenter B. Risse, *Hospital Life in Enlightenment Scotland: Care and Teaching at the Royal Infirmary of Edinburgh* (Cambridge: Cambridge University Press, 1986), and Lisa Rosner, *Medical Education in the Age of Improvement: Edinburgh Students and Apprentices, 1760–1826* (Edinburgh: Edinburgh University Press, 1991).

7. George Watson to Joseph Shelton Watson, Edinburgh, 25 Sept. 1805.

8. George Watson to James Watson, Edinburgh, 31 Jan. 1806.

9. George Watson to David Watson, Edinburgh, 21 Dec. 1805.

10. George Watson to James Watson, Edinburgh, 31 Jan. 1806.

11. George Watson to David Watson, Edinburgh, 27 Mar. 1806.

12. George Watson to James Watson, Edinburgh, 29 Apr. 1806.

13. George Watson to David Watson, [Edinburgh], 27 Mar. 1806.

14. George Watson to James Watson, Edinburgh, 29 Apr. 1806. And see George Watson to David Watson, Edinburgh, 30 May 1806, and 16 July 1806.

15. George Watson to David Watson, London, 30 Sept. 1806.

16. George Watson to James Watson, Paris, 25 Nov. 1806.

17. George Watson to David Watson, Paris, 2 Apr. 1807 [misdated as 1806].

18. George Watson to James Watson, Paris, 3 Dec. 1806.

19. George Watson to David Watson, Paris, 8 May 1807.

20. Ibid.

21. Ibid., 2 Apr. 1807, and 23 Apr. 1807.

22. Ibid., 28 May 1807.

23. Ibid., Paris, 15 Feb. 1808. And see ibid., 2 Jan. 1808.

24. Ibid., 8 Apr. 1808.

25. Ibid., Edinburgh, 16 July 1806, and Philadelphia, 13 Jan. 1809.

26. Ibid., Philadelphia, 13 Jan. 1809. On family opposition to Philadelphia, see David Watson to George Watson, [Louisa Court House, Va.], 1 Jan. 1809.

27. Wyndham B. Blanton, *Medicine in Virginia in the Nineteenth Century* (Richmond: Garrett and Massie, 1933), pp. 320, 76, 238.

28. Samuel Low to John Barclay, New York, 25 Aug. 1815, John W. Francis Papers, NY—NY State Lib.

29. On his visits while abroad, see the collection of calling cards in Francis Papers; and see John B. Stevenson to John W. Francis, Paris, 8 Nov. 1818, John W. Francis Papers, NY—NY Pub. Lib.

30. Usher Parsons to Lyman Spalding, Paris, 29 Nov. 1819, Parsons Family Papers, RI—Brown; and see Williams Thayer Solomon Drowne, Paris, 16 Jan. and 4 Nov. 1818, Drowne Family Papers, RI—Brown. On Parsons's time abroad, see Seebert J. Goldowsky, *Yankee Surgeon: The Life and Times of Usher Parsons (1788–1868)* (Boston: Francis A. Countway Library of Medicine, 1988), pp. 120–145.

31. David S. Gittings to Richard Gittings, Edinburgh, 3 Oct. [1818], Richard and David S. Gittings Papers (MS 1667), MD—MD Hist. Soc. Reflecting on his American training, Gittings told his father that "though a Doctor by title I feel myself but ill qualified to enter the responsibilities attached to the practice of medicine."

32. Ibid., Oct. 1818.

33. Jones has not made available to me the list of names on which he based his statistical statements. For his figures, see Russell M. Jones, "American Doctors and the Parisian Medical World, 1830–1840," *Bulletin of the History of Medicine* 47 (1973): 40–65, 177–204, on pp. 46 and 48, and idem, ed., *The Parisian Education of an American Surgeon: The Let-*

ters of Jonathan Mason Warren 1832–1835 (Philadelphia: American Philosophical Society, 1979), p. 2. He gave slightly different figures—lower for the 1820s, 1830s, and 1850s but higher for the 1840s—in idem, "American Doctors in Paris, 1820–1861: A Statistical Profile," Journal of the History of Medicine and Allied Sciences 25 (1970): 143–157, p. 150.

34. Registres des Inscriptions, Faculté de Médecine, 1815–1839, (AJ$^{16}$ 6426–6451), Paris—AN. On Fisher, see 6432, N° 843, 4$^e$ trimestre, 1825, and on Jackson, 6438, N° 173, 4$^e$ trimestre, 1831. Of the Americans who inscribed for at least one term, 49 out of 108 gave Louisiana as their residence.

35. George H. Doane, "Comparative Advantages of Vienna and Paris, As Places for Medical Study, with Some Remarks on the Operation of Extraction for the Removal of Cataract," New Jersey Medical Reporter 7 (1854): 17–20, p. 18. Austin Flint estimated "not far from a hundred here during the winter" in "Foreign Correspondence" (Paris, 18 June 1854), WJMS 2 (1854): 89–99, p. 89.

36. R. Smith to Benjamin Travers, Philadelphia, 7 Apr. 1830; Roberts Vaux to William Allen, Philadelphia, 14 Apr. 1830; W. Gibson to Professor Bell, Philadelphia, 18 Apr. 1830; W. E. Horner to George Borthwick, Philadelphia, 16 Apr. 1830; Thomas Parke to Robert Barclay, Philadelphia, 20 Apr. 1830; Richard Harlan to J. J. Audubon, Philadelphia, 15 Apr. 1830; and Joseph G. Nancrede to Docteur Orfila, Philadelphia, 15 Apr. 1830, all in C. W. Pennock Papers, PA—APS.

37. Comments of Dr. J. B. Gaston at banquet honoring Dr. J. M. Sims, in Montgomery Daily Register, 22 Mar. 1877, p. 3, col. 3. "The empty distinction of having been to the schools in Paris," one physician suggested, "with many is the only substantial benefit they ever receive" (Will Geo. Wesley to [N. J. Pittman], Wilmington, N.C., 9 Oct. 1852, N. J. Pittman Papers, NC—Duke).

38. Charles Gideon Putnam to James Jackson, Jr., Salem, 27 Apr. 1833, MA—Countway.

39. Francis P. Porcher to Julian Henry Porcher, New York, June 1847, Porcher Papers, SC—SC Hist. Soc.

40. Charles T. Jackson to Lydia Jackson, Paris, 7 June 1832, Charles Thomas Jackson Papers, DC—LC; Edward E. Jenkins to [John Jenkins], Paris, 12 Aug. 1853, John Jenkins Papers, SC—U. SC.

41. F. P. P[orcher], "Editorial Correspondence of the Charleston Medical Journal and Review" (Paris, 6 Oct. 1852), CMJR 7 (1852): 859–864, p. 862.

42. F. Campbell Stewart, Eminent French Surgeons, with a Historical and Statistical Account of the Hospitals of Paris; together with Miscellaneous Information and Biographical Notices of the Most Eminent Living Parisian Surgeons (Buffalo: A. Burke, 1845), p. xvi.

43. Moses L. Linton, "Hospitals and Medical Schools of London, Paris, Dublin and Edinburgh," WJMS 1 (1840): 388–395, p. 388.

44. Augustus Kinsley Gardner, Old Wine in New Bottles; or, Spare Hours of a Student in Paris (New-York: C. S. Francis & Co.; Boston: J. H. Francis, 1848), pp. 160, 161, 163.

45. Wesley to [Pittman], 9 Oct. 1852. Knowledge, he continued, "particularly ensures that success in practice which, after all, is the safest and surest evidence of a man[']s qualifications for his business."

46. Thomas R. Joynes to Levin S. Joynes, Accomack, Va., 18 Mar. 1835, Joynes Family Papers, VA—VA Hist. Soc.

47. Ibid., 21 Oct. 1835.

48. Ibid., 29 Jan. 1836.

49. Ibid., 27 Jan. 1837; italics removed.

50. Ibid., Hot Springs, Battle County, 31 Aug. 1837.

51. Ibid., Accomack, 29 Jan. 1839.

52. Levin S. Joynes to Thomas R. Joynes, Philadelphia, 4 Nov. 1839.

53. Ibid.

54. Ibid., 10 Nov. 1839.

55. William Gibson, Rambles in Europe in 1839. With Sketches of Prominent Surgeons, Physicians, Medical Schools, Hospitals, Literary Personages, Scenery, Etc. (Philadelphia: Lea and Blanchard, 1841), p. 66.

56. Levin S. Joynes to [Thomas R. Joynes], Ship Columbus, Longitude 15 Degrees 36′, Latitude 50 Degrees 50′, 13 June 1840.

57. J. L. Cabell to Joseph C. Cabell, Baltimore, 29 Jan. 1834, James Lawrence Cabell Papers (no. 1640), VA—U. VA.

58. Ibid., 25 Feb. 1837.

59. Ibid., 13 Dec. 1834.

60. Ibid., 22 Feb. 1835.

61. Ibid.

62. Ibid., Richmond, 26 Oct. 1836.

63. Ibid.

64. Ibid., New York, 1 Dec. 1836.

65. Ibid., Paris, 26 Feb. 1837.

66. William P. Powell to Dr. Inman, Liverpool, 5 May 1852, letter inserted in Liverpool Royal Infirmary School of Medicine Minutes, 1845–1859 (S.3076), at entry for 29 May 1852, Liverpool—U. Liverpool.

67. Liverpool Royal Infirmary Minutes, entry for 29 May 1852.

68. See Herbert M. Morais, *The History of the Negro in Medicine* (New York: Publishers Company, 1967), pp. 31–32. Leslie Falk, who is writing a biography of Smith, says that while Smith proceeded from Glasgow to Paris for study, little is known of what he did in Paris beyond improving his French; personal communication, Falk to author, Shelburne, Vt., 1 June 1994.

69. M. O. Bousfield, "An Account of Physicians of Color in the United States," *Bulletin of the History of Medicine* 17 (1945): 61–84, p. 66; Leonard W. Johnson, "History of the Education of Negro Physicians,"*Journal of Medical Education* 42 (1967): 439–446, p. 440; Morais, *History of the Negro in Medicine*, p. 38.

70. Martin R. Delany, *The Condition, Elevation, Emigration, and Destiny of the Colored People of the United States, Politically Considered* (Philadelphia, 1852), 134–137, quoted in Morais, *History of the Negro in Medicine*, p. 216.

71. Particularly helpful studies include Thomas Neville Bonner, *To the Ends of the Earth: Women's Search for Education in Medicine* (Cambridge, Mass., and London: Harvard University Press, 1992); Virginia Drachman, *Hospital with a Heart: Women Doctors and the Paradox of Separatism at the New England Hospital, 1862–1969* (Ithaca: Cornell University Press, 1984); and Regina Markell Morantz-Sanchez, *Sympathy and Science: Women Physicians in American Medicine* (New York: Oxford University Press, 1985).

72. Frances Emily White, "The American Medical Woman," *Medical News* 67 (1895): 123–128, pp. 126–127.

73. Mary J. Reynolds, "The Duties and Responsibilities of the Physician" (M.D. thesis, Female Medical College of Pennsylvania, 1861), PA—Women in Med. Arch.

74. F. Nightingale to [Elizabeth Blackwell], General Hospital, Balaclava, 12 May 1856, Blackwell Family Papers (MC 411), MA—Schlesinger.

75. Elizabeth Blackwell, Journal, entry of 2 June 1847, excerpt in Elizabeth Blackwell, *Pioneer Work in Opening the Medical Profession to Women: Autobiographical Sketches by Dr. Elizabeth Blackwell* (1895; reprint, New York: Schocken Books, 1977), pp. 60–61, on p. 61. And see Nancy Sahli, "Elizabeth Blackwell, M.D. (1821–1910): A Biography" (Ph.D. diss., University of Pennsylvania, 1974).

76. [Elizabeth Blackwell] to [Emma Hart] Willard, Philadelphia, 24 May [1847], in Blackwell, *Pioneer Work*, pp. 62–64, on p. 63.

77. Blackwell, *Pioneer Work*, p. 61.

78. Ibid., pp. 61–62. She attributes this proposal to "Doctor Pankhurst," but it seems likely that his name, like many details in the autobiography she composed in her mid-seventies, was misremembered.

79. Blackwell to Willard, 24 May [1847], p. 64.

80. Ibid., p. 63.

81. Blackwell, Journal, entry for 2 June 1847, in Blackwell, *Pioneer Work*, pp. 60–61, on p. 60.

82. E. Blackwell] to Dear Milly [Emily Blackwell], Philadelphia, 27 Oct. 1847, Blackwell Family Papers.

83. On her admission and experiences, see Blackwell, *Pioneer Work*, pp. 76–81.

84. E. [Blackwell] to Emily [Blackwell], [Philadelphia], 16 Apr. 1848, Blackwell Family Papers.

85. Blackwell, *Pioneer Work*, pp. 80–81.

86. Blackwell to Blackwell, 16 Apr. 1848.

87. E. [Blackwell] to Emily Blackwell, Geneva, 15 Oct. 1848, Blackwell Family Papers.

88. Blackwell, Journal, entry for 10 Mar. 1849, excerpt in Blackwell, *Pioneer Work*, p. 92.

89. Blackwell, *Pioneer Work*, p. 94.

90. Blackwell to Blackwell, n.p., n.d. [archive dates as 1851, but at least 1852], Blackwell Family Papers. She described Clark as "the most promising of the female M.D., that I have yet seen—but she is young in all senses, knows nothing of practise, & is desirous of being [a] pupil for some time." On Clark, see Esther Pohl Lovejoy, *Women Doctors of the World* (New York: Macmillan Company, 1957), pp. 82–84. For a review of the literature on Fowler—who took advantage of her husband's lecture tour to Europe in 1860–1861 to study medicine in Paris before returning to teach midwifery at the hydropathic New York Hygeio-Therapeutic College—see

Naomi Rogers, "Women and Sectarian Medicine," in *Women, Health, and Medicine in America: A Historical Handbook*, ed. Rima D. Apple (New Brunswick, N.J.: Rutgers University Press, 1992), pp. 273–302, on pp. 288–289.

91. Elizabeth [Blackwell] to Emily [Blackwell], [New York], entry of 25 Apr. in letter of 20 Apr. 1854, Blackwell Family Papers.

92. Blackwell to Blackwell, n.d.

93. Emily Blackwell, Journal, 1850–1858, microfilm copy of transcript, Blackwell Family Papers (M-35), entry for 18 Sept. 1853.

94. Elizabeth [Blackwell] to Emily [Blackwell], [New York], 20 Apr. 1854, Blackwell Family Papers.

95. Emily Blackwell, Journal, entry for 16 July 1853.

96. Ibid., entry for 8 Oct. 1853.

97. Emily [Blackwell] to Dear People, Steamship Arabia, 26 Mar. 1854, Blackwell Family Papers; and see Emily Blackwell, Journal, entries for 28 and 29 Mar. 1854. Although the two had long known of each other, Blackwell first met Clark only five weeks earlier, when Clark showed up for the public reading of Blackwell's M.D. thesis (Blackwell, Journal, entry for 20 Feb. 1854).

98. She first visited Paget, who had fostered Elizabeth's studies, in London and reported that "he does not like France and says many difficulties are thrown in the way of students there" (Emily to Dear People, London, 15 Apr. 1854, Blackwell Family Papers). On her reception by Simpson, see Emily to Dear People, Maternity Hospital, [Edinburgh], 1 June [1854], and Emily to Dear Howard, Maternity House, [Edinburgh], 21 June 1854, Blackwell Family Papers, and Emily Blackwell, Journal, entries for 26 and 27 May, and 12 and 25 June.

99. Emily to Dear People, Maternity Hospital, Minto House, [Edinburgh], 7 July 1854, Blackwell Family Papers.

100. Ibid., Edinburgh, 28 Oct.–7 Nov. 1854, Blackwell Family Papers. "There are two physicians in France from whom I hope something," she continued; "one is M Jobert a skillful brute, who holds an important position in the Hotel Dieu, he is a detestable man, but quite celebrated, he was followed in his visits last year by a lady, so I rather hope to find him inclined to approve of me. The second is M Valleix who has taken up some of Simpsons ideas very enthusiastically, is an emi-

nent man, and a very decent one. . . . Still I am not excessively sanguine about the Parisian success." And see Emily to Dear People, Edinburgh, 1–29 Oct. 1854, Blackwell Family Papers.

101. For example, see Emily to Dear Friends, Edinburgh, 27–31 Nov. 1854; Emily to Dear People, London, 22 Jan.–2 Feb. 1855; Emily to Dear Friends, London, 22–25 May 1855; Emily to Dear Friends, Smethwick, June 1855, all in Blackwell Family Papers.

102. Emily to Dear People, Maternity Hospital, Minto House, [Edinburgh], 24 June 1854, Blackwell Family Papers.

103. Emily Blackwell, Journal, entry for 4 July 1854.

104. [Elizabeth Blackwell to Emily Blackwell, New York], 24 July [1854], in Blackwell, *Pioneer Work*, pp. 200–204, quotations on pp. 202, 201–202, 202, 203.

105. Emily to Dear Friends, [London], 8–15 June 1855, Blackwell Family Papers.

106. Their educational credentials, like those of their American-trained counterparts, are recorded in the Registre du Comité Médical de la Nouvelle Orléans, 29 Apr. 1816–14 Aug. 1854, LA—Tulane Med. The Registre lists some seventy physicians, at least half of them foreign born, who claimed to hold Paris medical diplomas. In addition, a number of the practitioners whose credentials were inscribed in the Registre held a medical diploma from Montpellier or French credentials as an *officier de santé*. Nearly half of the Americans who formally registered for medical instruction in Paris gave Louisiana as their residence (see Registres des Inscriptions, Faculté de Médecine, 1815–1839). Twenty-five M.D. theses, each identified as a "Thèse pour le Doctorat en Médecine, présentée et soutenue à la Faculté de Médecine de Paris," by students from New Orleans or its vicinity between 1832 and 1870 (but largely in the 1830s and 1840s) are deposited in Thèses de Médecine, 3 vols., LA—LA Coll. The medical culture these practitioners entered in Louisiana deserves close investigation; see, as one starting point, "Quelques mots au public," *L'Union médicale de la Louisiane* 1 (1852): 3–5.

107. See, for example, A. W. Cenas to W. W. Gerhard, New Orleans, 30 June 1830, W. W. Gerhard Papers, PA—CPP.

108. Benjamin J. Hicks to J. Y. Bassett,

Paris, 31 July 1837, John Young Bassett Papers, AL—AL State Arch.

109. D. D. Slade to George Lord, Cambridge, 21 Nov. 1845, George Lord Papers, NC—Duke.

110. Gabriel Manigault, typescript of Autobiography, 1834–1899, p. 100, SC—U. SC.

111. Gabriel Manigault to Louis Manigault, Paris, 1 Oct. 1854; and Gabriel Manigault to Charles Manigault, Paris, 15 Oct. 1854, Manigault Family Papers, SC—U. SC.

112. Manigault, Autobiography, pp. 308–309.

113. Charles T. Jackson to Charles Brown, Paris, 30 Mar. 1830, C. Jackson Papers; Edward E. Jenkins to [John Jenkins], Paris, 13 Jan. 1854, Jenkins Papers.

114. C.G.W. Comegys to Scott Cook, Cincinnati, 23 Nov. 1850, Matthew Scott Cook Papers, OH—Western Reserve Hist. Soc.

115. Ibid., 4 Nov. 1851.

116. Ibid., 25 Mar. 1852.

117. L. M. Lawson, "Foreign Correspondence" (Paris, Aug. 1845), WL 4 (1845–1846): 241–248, p. 247.

118. J. R. Atkins, "Monthly Report of the Proceedings of the Cincinnati Medical Society," WL 17 (1856): 90–106, p. 94.

119. Austin Flint, "Address at the Opening of the Session for 1854–55 in the Medical Department of the University of Louisville," WJMS, n.s., 2 (1854): 409–425, p. 423.

120. Courtney J. Clark, Notes Taken on Lectures Given by Chas. Caldwell, Medical Institute of Louisville, 1841–1842, entry for 1841, NC—Duke; Ja[me]s S. McLaury to A. J[ames] McCall, New York, 28 Nov. 1839, McCall Family Papers, NY—Cornell.

121. Henry Bryant to John Bryant, Paris, entry of 21 Dec. in letter of 11 Dec. 1843, William Sohier Bryant Papers (MS 45), MA—New England Hist. Gen. Soc.

122. George C. Shattuck, Journal, 1833, entry for 5 Mar. 1833, MA—Countway.

123. George C. Shattuck, Jr., Diary, 1834–1842, entry for 6 Apr. 1836, Shattuck Papers, MA—MA Hist. Soc.

124. Μελανιςκος to Editor (Paris, Jan. 1857), Nashville Journal of Medicine and Surgery 12 (1857): 304–308, p. 304. And see Austin Flint, "European Correspondence" (Paris, 18 May 1854), WJMS 2 (1854): 9–17, p. 17.

125. Elisha Bartlett to Robert Peter, Lowell, 15 May 1841, Bartlett (Elisha) Family Papers, NY—U. Rochester.

126. George B. Wood, Journal, 1817–1829, entry for 30 July 1818, George B. Wood Journals, PA—CPP.

127. C.G.W. Comegys to Diathea M. Tiffin, Cincinnati, 13 Jan. 1851, Cook Papers.

128. A consumptive man abroad for his health noted that "Dr Reese of N York told me previous to my leaving home that in Paris he had learned the Physicians cured tubercles of the Lungs but in this country we can not—adding that he had taken a partner for that purpose, so that he might have opportunity to go to Paris and make observations" (John Moffatt Howe, Diary of Trip to Europe, June–Sept. 1838, entry for London, 9 Sept. 1838, BV Howe, NY—NY Hist. Soc.).

129. Ashbel Smith to Father [Moses Smith], Paris, 26 Jan. 1832, Ashbel Smith Letters, TX—U. TX. And see Ashbel Smith to Dear Friends, Paris, 25 Feb. 1832.

130. Hardy Vickers Wooten, Diary, vol. 2, 1838–1845, entry for Lowndesboro, Alabama, 13 Oct. 1839, transcript in Hardy Vickers Wooten Papers, AL—AL State Arch.

131. G. F. Manning to John Y. Bassett, Philadelphia, 9 May 1835, Bassett Papers.

132. John Young Bassett, Autobiographical Notes, [1836].

133. Robert Battey to Mary Battey, Rome, Ga., 15 Oct. 1848, Robert Battey Family Papers, GA—Emory.

134. Robert Battey to Mary Battey Halsey, Rome, Ga., 29 Nov. 1857.

135. Robert Battey to Ma chère Belle [Martha (Smith) Battey], Paris, 14 Mar. 1860.

136. Robert Battey to My Dearest Love [Martha (Smith) Battey], Paris, 7 Feb. 1860. Obtaining an M.D. degree might also promise betterment to someone who had pursued another occupation. "I could have been content to have ploded on in that humble way—had I not been haunted by the ghosts of outraged duty, & neglected opportunities and urged on by the laudable Ambition to elevate *our* position and thus to secure to *our* children advantages which they could never have enjoyed had I remained in the Farming Business," a man attending medical lectures in New York wrote home to his wife in 1858. "It was a sense of the heavy responsibilities which devolved upon me to guide and govern *these best gifts of God Almighty* & to give them the posi-

tion in the world that they had a *right* to *claim* at my hand that has awakened me from my lethargy, spurred me on to action and imparted within me the fine determination to *excell*" (S. M. Van Wyck to My Own Darling, New York, 12 Dec. 1858, Maverick and Van Wyck Families Papers, SC—U. SC).

137. C.G.W. Comegys to Diathea M. Tiffin, Cincinnati, 13 Jan. 1851; and see C.G.W. Comegys to Scott Cook, Cincinnati, 30 Oct. 1848 and 30 Jan. 1851, Cook Papers.

138. Comegys to Tiffin, 13 Jan. 1851.

139. Audrey W. Davis, "Moses L. Linton," in *Dictionary of American Medical Biography*, ed. Howard A. Kelly and Walter L. Burrage (1928; Boston: Milford House, 1971), p. 748.

140. A. H. Cenas to W. W. Gerhard, New Orleans, 30 June 1830, Gerhard Papers.

141. R. Clark to R. La Roche, New Orleans, 5 May 1830, R. La Roche Correspondence, PA—CPP. On travel as a prescription for health, see Sheila M. Rothman, *Living in the Shadow of Death: Tuberculosis and the Social Experience of Illness in American History* (New York: Basic Books, 1994), esp. pp. 13–74.

142. M. W. Williams to Chandler B. Chapman, Syracuse, 25 Jan. 1851, Chandler B. Chapman Papers, WI—WI Hist. Soc.

143. See, for example, on William Valentine Keating, George B. Wood, Journal, 25 Mar. 1862–28 Aug. 1862, entry for Paris, 18 May 1862, Wood Journals; and on John W. Francis, Samuel Low to John Barclay, New York, 25 Aug. 1815, John W. Francis Papers, NY—NY State Lib.

144. Alden March, "For the Boston Medical and Surgical Journal," Albany, 11 Sept. 1856, Alden March Papers, NY—Albany Med.

145. Typescript biographical note in Colman (Anson) Papers, n.d., NY—U. Rochester.

146. A. Colman to Catherine K. Colman (Care of Nathaniel Rochester), Boston, 5 Dec. 1824, Colman Papers.

147. Ibid., Boston, 11 Jan. 1825.

148. Catherine Colman to Anson Colman, Rochester, 19 Jan. 1825.

149. A. Colman to Catherine Colman, Philadelphia, 15 and 19 Nov. 1831.

150. Ibid., Philadelphia, 19 Nov. 1831. Catherine, for her part, while Anson was in Paris, was dealing with the fear that she was consumptive.

151. Saml. Colman to Catherine Colman, East Richfield, 25 May 1833.

152. A. Colman to Catherine Colman, Paris, 6 Jan. 1833.

153. Catherine Colman to Anson Colman, Rochester, 25 Feb. 1833.

154. "To the Honorable the Trustees of the Med. Col. of Ohio," [ca. 1829], Manuscripts of the Medical College of Ohio, OH—U. Cincinnati. And see "Return of the Editor," *WL* 4 (1845–1846): 288.

155. Henry H. Smith to Geo. B. Wood, Philadelphia, 11 May 1855, Wood Misc. Correspondence, PA—CPP.

156. Henry H. Smith, *Professional Visit to London and Paris. Introductory Lecture to the Course on the Principles and Practice of Surgery. Delivered in the University of Pennsylvania, October. 9, 1855* (Philadelphia: T. K. and P. G. Collins, 1855), pp. 7, 6.

157. Oliver H. Stout to James S. Taliaferro, Lexington, 2 Mar. 1821, Zachariah and James G. Taliaferro Papers, LA—LSU.

158. Ibid., 16 Oct. 1821. And see *First Annual Announcement of the Medical Department of the University of Nashville* (Nashville: J.T.S. Fall, 1851), p. 6.

159. "Dr. E. D. Fenner," *New Orleans Medical News and Hospital Gazette* 6 (1859–1860): 307–310.

160. Chas. Wilkins Short to Wm. Short, [Lexington], 20 Mar. 1836, transcript in Daniel Drake Papers, Emmet Field Horine Collection, KY—U. KY. And see ibid., Louisville, 11 June 1839.

161. Robert Peter to Frances Peter, Paris, 22 June 1839, Evans Papers, KY—U. KY. On this collecting, see Roemol Henry, "Introduction," in *Catalogue of the Transylvania University Medical Library* (Lexington: Transylvania University Press, 1987), pp. v–x.

162. Robert Peter to Frances Peter, Philadelphia, 19 Apr. 1839.

163. Ibid., Paris, 7 July 1839, Evans Papers.

164. A fuller treatment of the issues explored in this section is John Harley Warner, "American Physicians in London during the Age of Paris Medicine," in *The History of Medical Education in Britain*, ed. Roy Porter and Vivian Nutton (London: Rodopi, 1995), pp. 341–365.

165. Richard H. Shryock, *The Development of Modern Medicine: An Interpretation of the So-*

*cial and Scientific Factors Involved* (1936; Madison: University of Wisconsin Press, 1979), pp. 193 and 171.

166. Smith, *Professional Visit to London and Paris*, p. 9.

167. E. Williams, "Foreign Correspondence" (Vienna, 20 Oct. 1854), *WJMS* 2 (1854): 441–458, p. 445.

168. Joshua B. Flint, *Address Delivered to the Students of the Louisville Medical Institute, in Presence of the Citizens of the Place, at the Commencement of the Second Session of the Institute, November 13th, 1838* (Louisville: Prentice and Weissenger, 1838), 24.

169. P. to the Editor, "Foreign Correspondence" (Paris, 10 July 1855), *Stethoscope and Virginia Medical Gazette*, 5 (1855): 624–633, p. 631.

170. Edward E. Jenkins to [John Jenkins], Paris, 25 June 1855, Jenkins Papers.

171. Robert Peter to Francis Peter, Paris, 14 July 1839, and London, entry of 21 Aug. in letter of 11 Aug. 1839, Evans Papers.

172. P., "Foreign Correspondence," p. 632.

173. Frank J. Lutz, ed., *The Autobiography and Reminiscences of S. Pollack, M.D.* (St. Louis: Reprinted from the St. Louis Medical Review, 1904). Pollack's observations were from a trip to London and Paris begun in 1859.

174. Levin S. Joynes to Thomas R. Joynes, Paris, 12 Dec. 1841, Joynes Family Papers.

175. Levin S. Joynes to William Joynes, Paris, 9 Jan. 1842.

176. Louis Alexandre Dugas to Dear Mama, Paris, 6 July 1829, typescript translation in GA—Med. Coll. GA. And see James Jackson, Jr., to James Jackson, Sr., Paris, 27 June 1833, J. Jackson Papers.

177. Philip Claiborne Gooch, Diary, 20 Feb. 1845–22 Dec. 1847, entry for Edinburgh, 4 Jan. 1847, VA—VA Hist. Soc.

178. T. Stewardson to W. W. Gerhard, London, 9 Sept. 1834, Gerhard Papers.

179. John B. Stevenson to John W. Francis, Paris, 8 Nov. 1818, John W. Francis Papers, NY—NY Pub. Lib.

180. A. Smith to James Jackson, Paris, 11 June 1832, Putnam, Jackson and Lowell Papers, MA—MA Hist. Soc.

181. E. Williams, "Foreign Correspondence" (Vienna, 20 Oct. 1854), *WJMS* 2 (1854): 441–458, p. 444.

182. John Ware, "Success in the Medical Profession. An Introductory Lecture, Delivered at the Massachusetts Med. College, Nov. 6, 1850," *BMSJ* 43 (1850): 496–505, 509–522, p. 510.

183. J. Y. Bassett to Wells A. Thompson, Paris, 10 Mar. 1836, Bassett Papers.

184. Gooch, Diary, 23 Feb. 1847–30 Dec. 1847, entries for London, 6–15 Oct. 1847.

185. James Jackson, Sr., to James Jackson, Jr., Waltham, 12 Aug. 1832, J. Jackson Papers.

186. Oliver Wendell Holmes to Dear Father and Mother, Paris, 22 Oct. 1833, in John T. Morse, Jr., *Life and Letters of Oliver Wendell Holmes*, 2 vols. (Boston and New York: Houghton, Mifflin and Company, 1896), 1:117.

187. Gibson, *Rambles in Europe*, p. 66.

188. Ibid., pp. 63–64, 64.

189. Charles T. Jackson to Lydia Jackson, Paris, 23 July 1832, C. Jackson Papers.

190. T. J. Cogley, "To the Editors of the Lancet" (Paris, 10 Oct. 1853), *WL* 15 (1854): 45–47, p. 45.

191. David W. Yandell, "Clinical Instruction in the London and Paris Hospitals," *WJMS*, ser. 3, 3 (1848): 392–400, p. 393.

192. James Jackson, Jr., to James Jackson, Sr., London, 12 Sept. 1832, J. Jackson Papers.

193. Yandell, "Clinical Instruction," p. 395.

194. Ibid., p. 393.

195. Jackson to Jackson, London, 12 Sept. 1832; first emphasis is added.

196. C. B. Chapman, "Medical Travels in Europe" (Edinburgh, July 1851), *BMSJ* 45 (1851–1852): 72–75, p. 73.

197. Charles T. Jackson to Lydia Jackson, Paris, 13 May 1831, C. Jackson Papers.

198. David W. Yandell, "Notes on Medical Matters and Medical Men in London and Paris," *Southern Medical and Surgical Journal*, n.s., 5 (1849): 211–225, pp. 223, 221. *Concours*, introduced with the Revolution, had a checkered career and at various times was abolished, reinstated, and circumvented.

199. Minutes of the Medical College, St Bartholomew's Hospital, Sept. 1834–Aug. 1843, meeting of 29 Sept. 1837, London—St. Bartholomew's.

200. "With the Physicians & Surgeons to whom I either had letters or to whom I have been introduced since I have been here I am

particularly well pleased," Colman wrote from London. "Every facility is afforded me of seeing, not only their sick and their operations, but of attending their Lectures, examining their museums, or whateverelse, connected with Medical Science, that I desire" (A. Colman to Catherine K. Colman, London, 24 Apr. 1833, Colman Papers).

201. Oliver Wendell Holmes to Dear Father and Mother, London, 21 June 1834, in Morse, *Holmes*, 1:134.

202. "The Hospitals of London," *BMSJ* 42 (1850): 461–466, pp. 462, 466.

203. Jackson to Jackson, London, 12 Sept. 1832.

204. James Jackson, Jr., to James Jackson, Sr., Bangor, Wales, 27 Aug. 1832, J. Jackson Papers. The case histories Robert Carswell recorded abroad, which include references to the corresponding drawings, are in his Notes of Medical Cases Made in France, 1822–1825, 2 vols. (Gen. 590–591), Edinburgh—U. Edinburgh.

205. "Defects of the London Hospital System," *London Medical and Surgical Journal*, n.s., 7 (1835): 316–317, p. 316.

206. James Jackson, Jr., to James Jackson Sr., Paris, 22 Feb. 1833, J. Jackson Papers.

207. Alfred Stillé to G. C. Shattuck, Philadelphia, 1 Sept. 1843, Shattuck Papers, vol. 18, MA—MA Hist. Soc.

## CHAPTER 3
### ERRAND TO PARIS

1. Ashbel Smith to John Beard, Jr., Paris, 23 Feb. 1832, Ashbel Smith Letters, TX—U. TX.

2. Henri Meding, *Paris médical: vade-mecum des médecins étrangers*, 2 vols. (Paris: J.-B. Ballière, 1852–1853). Meding wrote a number of German guides for the medical student in Paris; the Gallicized "Henri" appeared only in the French version of his guidebook.

3. Francis Peyre Porcher, Travel Journal, 1852–1853, entry for Versailles, 13 Oct. 1852, transcript in SC—Waring.

4. George C. Shattuck, Jr., Diary, 1834–1842, entry for 6 Apr. 1836, Shattuck Papers, MA—MA Hist. Soc.

5. Robert Peter to Frances Peter, Paris, 27 June 1839, Evans Papers, KY—U. KY.

6. Charlotte Henrietta Horlbeck, Travel Diary, 1857, 2 vols., vol. 1, entry for 11 Apr.

1857, SC—SC Hist. Soc. She was crossing from Charleston to Liverpool with her father (Dr. Horlbeck), Dr. Ogier, and a party of thirteen family members.

7. Gabriel Manigault, Autobiography, transcript, pp. 101–102, SC—U. SC. He crossed from Jersey City to Liverpool. George B. Wood, who kept a meticulously detailed account of his voyage, reported a crossing in only ten days and nineteen hours (entry for 27 Apr. in Journal, 15 Apr.–19 May 1853, PA—CPP).

8. Morton N. Waring, Travel Journal, 1856–1857, SC—SC Hist. Soc. This, he wrote, was "the first time that I was ever far remote from the approving smile of a kind & tender Mother, or a Fathers mild approbation or reproof. By Some I know this is counted as a gain but as to myself I feel it one of those gains where one loses all."

9. Horlbeck, Diary, vol. 1, entry for 11 Apr. 1857.

10. Waring, Travel Journal, 1856.

11. F. Peyre Porcher to Mother, U.S. Ship Baltic at Sea off New York, 4 Apr. 1854, Porcher Papers, SC—SC Hist. Soc. This was his return trip.

12. Emily [Blackwell] to Dear Friends, Steamer Arabia, 1–13 Apr. 1854, Blackwell Family Papers, MA—Schlesinger. "We have been passing icebergs all the morning, White islands and mountains of all shapes and sizes," she continued; "yesterday night we nearly ran into one."

13. John K. Kane to Dear People, [Southampton], 10 May 1857, Kane Family Papers, MI—Clements, U. MI.

14. Henry Bryant to John Bryant, London, 17 Nov. 1843, William Sohier Bryant Papers (MS 45), MA—New England Hist. Gen. Soc.

15. Philip Claiborne Gooch, Diary, 20 Feb. 1844–22 Feb. 1847, 23 Feb.–30 Dec. 1847, 1 Jan.–1 Sept. 1848, 1 Sept. 1848–31 Jan. 1855, entry for Atlantic Ocean, Lat 42′ Long 50′, 26 Sept. 1846, Philip Claiborne Gooch Diaries, VA—VA Hist. Soc. The collection contains both Gooch's manuscript diaries and a partial transcription (as well as translation of the entries that, starting in 1848, he kept entirely in French). I have retranscribed and retranslated some passages.

16. Edward E. Jenkins to [John Jenkins], Paris, 25 June 1855, John Jenkins Papers, SC—U. SC. Gooch (Diary, entry for 21 Nov.

1848) also worked as a surgeon for his return passage, noting that "many captains wanted me."

17. Charles T. Jackson to Lydia Jackson, On board Ship Charlemagne, off Havre, 20 Oct. 1829, Charles Thomas Jackson Papers, DC—LC.

18. Levin S. Joynes to Thomas R. Joynes, Paris, 11 July 1840, Joynes Family Papers, VA—VA Hist. Soc.

19. Typical examples include Elisha Bartlett to Caroline Bartlett, Paris, 24 July 1826, Bartlett (Elisha) Family Papers, NY—U. Rochester; Henry Bryant to John Bryant, Paris, 28 Nov. 1843, Bryant Papers; Levin S. Joynes to Thomas R. Joynes, Paris, 11 July 1840, Joynes Family Papers; and Robert Peter to Frances Peter, Paris, entry for 28 July in letter of 25 July 1839, Evans Papers.

20. L. A. Dugas to Ma chère Maman, Paris, 28 Aug. 1828, Dugas Papers, GA—GA Hist. Soc.

21. Levin S. Joynes to Thomas R. Joynes, Paris, 11 July 1840, Joynes Family Papers. The fare, eighteen francs, he judged to be modest.

22. W. Parker, Diary of a Trip to France, 1837, entry for Paris, 10 Apr. 1837, NY—NY Acad. Med.

23. James Jackson, Jr., to James Jackson, Sr., Paris, 30 May 1831, James Jackson Papers, MA—Countway.

24. L. A. Dugas to Frederick Dugas, Paris, 11 Sept. 1828, Dugas Papers.

25. Robert Peter to Frances Peter, Paris, 9 June 1839, Evans Papers.

26. J. Y. Bassett to Isaphoena Bassett, Paris, 7 Mar. 1836, John Young Bassett Papers, AL—AL State Arch.

27. Levin S. Joynes to Thomas R. Joynes, Paris, 11 July 1840, Joynes Family Papers.

28. Waring, Travel Journal, n.d., 1856.

29. Edward E. Jenkins to [John Jenkins], Paris, 12 Aug. 1853, Jenkins Papers.

30. Henry W. Williams to A[bigail] O[sood] Williams [but written to Sisters Three, that is, Lizzie, Margarette, and Abbie Williams], Cabin of Ship Baltimore at Sea, 9 Apr. 1846 (with subsequent entries on 22 and 28 Apr.), Henry Willard Williams Papers, MA—Countway. The instructions that they keep his letters are in Henry W. Williams to A. O. Williams, Paris, May 1846.

31. Entries of 4 and 5 May in ibid., Paris, 4 May 1846.

32. Henri [sic] W. Williams to A. O. Williams, Paris, 6 May 1846.

33. Entry of 7 May in ibid.

34. Entry of 8 May 1846 in ibid.

35. Entries for 11 and 15 May 1846 in ibid.

36. Entry of 3 June in ibid., 25 May 1846.

37. Ibid., 20 June 1846.

38. Entry of 23 June in ibid.

39. Ibid., 13 July 1846.

40. Ibid., entry of 10 Aug. in letter of 28 July 1846.

41. Ibid., 4 and 10 Oct. in letter of 10 Oct., and ibid., entry of 25 Nov. in letter of 20 Nov. 1846.

42. See, for example, ibid., Antwerp, 4 May 1847; Cologne, 5 Aug. 1847; Milano, 30 Sept. 1847; Firenze, 27 Oct. 1847; and Rome, Nov. 1847. He wrote from Paris on 15 Dec. 1847 to report his return.

43. Ibid., Paris, entry of 26 Feb. in letter of 23 Feb. 1848, and see also ibid., 16 Mar. 1848.

44. Ibid., 16 Mar. 1848; London, 5 June 1848; and n.d. June 1848.

45. Ibid., Paris, 1 July 1846. He would also study diseases of the eye in Vienna and London.

46. Entry of 4 Oct. in ibid., 25 Sept. 1846. His drawings are preserved at MA—Countway.

47. Henrie Williams to A. O. Williams, London, n.d. [but late spring / early summer 1848].

48. A. L. Peirson to Harriet Peirson, entry made On Ship, South of Newfoundland, 24 Sept. 1832, in Abel Lawrence Peirson, Letterbook (logbook kept in diary form of letters to Harriet Peirson, his wife), 1832–1833, MA—Countway. And see A. L. Peirson to Edward Brooks Peirson, Leghorn, 29 Jan. 1833, Peirson Papers, MA—Peabody Essex.

49. Entry for Paris, 21 Oct. 1832, in Peirson Letterbook.

50. Ibid. "I can make out to speak a little french, but I cannot catch the words as they are pronounced."

51. Entry for 22 Oct. in ibid.

52. Entry of 23 Oct.

53. Entries for 24–28 Oct.

54. Entries for 29 Oct. and 3 Nov.

55. Entry for Paris, 6 Mar. in entry begun Lyons, 1 Mar. 1833; and see entries for Rome, 18 Dec. 1832; Florence, 3 Feb. 1833; and Lyons, 1 Mar. 1833.

56. See entries of 11–18 Mar. 1833, in entry begun Lyons, 1 Mar. 1833.

57. Entry for Amiens, 21 Mar. 1833.

58. He quotes this in the entry of 11 May. On his Paris studies, see A. L. Peirson, untitled volume in the Peirson Papers, in which he recorded observations he made at the Hôpital St. Louis, La Pitié, and the Hôtel des Invalides.

59. Robert P. Harris, "Letter from Paris" (Paris, 19 Nov. 1855), *Medical Examiner*, n.s., 12 (1856): 10–13, p. 10. And see L. A. Dugas to Ma chère Maman, Baltimore, 21 Feb. [1826], and Paris, 27 Sept. 1828, Dugas Papers.

60. Manigault, Autobiography, p. 125.

61. Austin Flint, "European Correspondence" (Paris, 18 May 1854), *WJMS* 2 (1854): 9–17, p. 9. The formulaic quality assumed by "reports" on Paris suggests that in substantial measure they came to be not only conventionalized but cribbed, partly from guidebooks such as *Galignani's New Paris Guide for 1855* (Paris: A. and W. Galignani and Co., 1855) and *Chaix's Guide, Traveller's Library: New Guide to Paris with Maps, Plans, and Wood-Cuts* (Paris: Napoléon Chaix and Co., [1855]).

62. In the 1840s and 1850s such guides formalized what had been word-of-mouth advice. Meding noted that he had decided to publish his guide because, as president of the German Medical Society in Paris, "nous avons été presque quotidiennement consulté, par chaque confrère arrivant, sur la topographie médicale de cette capitale et généralement sur ce qu'elle offre d'intéressant en fait de médecine et d'hygiène" (Meding, *Paris médical*, 1:5).

63. F. H. Hamilton, "Notes of an European Tour" (Paris [1846]), *Buffalo Medical Journal and Monthly Review* 2 (1846): 396–409, p. 409.

64. William Gibson, *Rambles in Europe in 1839. With Sketches of Prominent Surgeons, Physicians, Medical Schools, Hospitals, Literary Personages, Scenery, Etc.* (Philadelphia: Lea and Blanchard, 1841), p. 65.

65. A variety of public conveyances—hackney carriages, omnibuses, and so on—provided alternatives to travel by foot (see *Chaix's Guide*, pp. 406–409, and *Galignani's New Paris Guide*, pp. 4–7); distance, however, remained a key ingredient in choices about plans of study.

66. Robert P. Harris, "Letter from Paris" (Paris, 25 Dec. 1855), *Medical Examiner*, n.s., 12 (1856): 70–75, p. 72.

67. One guidebook for American doctors recommended the Hôtel Meurice as a place where one could count on English's being spoken (F. Campbell Stewart, *Eminent French Surgeons, with a Historical and Statistical Account of the Hospitals of Paris; together with Miscellaneous Information and Biographical Notices of the Most Eminent Living Parisian Surgeons* [Buffalo: A. Burke, 1845], p. 170).

68. The young and disoriented Morton Waring took quite a while to figure this out. Distressed on arriving in Paris to discover that the friend he was counting on for advice, physician John S. Stoney, was away in Switzerland, he moved after a few days out of the Meurice into a residence on the Place Madeleine. It was only when his friend finally returned to Paris that Waring moved into the Latin Quarter, writing in his diary that when Stoney returned, "he informed me that I was too remote from my duties, and must move into the Latin quarter during the winter months at any rate" (Waring, Travel Journal, n.d., 1856).

69. A. Colman to Catherine K. Colman, Paris, 6 Jan. 1833, Colman (Anson) Papers, NY—U. Rochester.

70. Edward E. Jenkins to [John Jenkins], Paris, 7 Aug. 1854, Jenkins Papers.

71. Entries of 11 and 21 Dec. in Henry Bryant to John Bryant, Paris, 11 Dec. 1843, Bryant Papers.

72. Ibid., Paris, 25 Jan. 1844, and ibid., 21 Dec. 1843 in letter of 11 Dec. 1843. Williams also wanted to lodge with a family for the sake of his French.

73. Ibid., 25 Jan. 1844.

74. Ibid., 1 July 1844; and see entries of 22 and 23 May in letter of 17 May 1844.

75. Ibid., 17 Jan. and 23 Feb. 1845.

76. Elisha Bartlett to Caroline Bartlett, Paris, 29 Nov. 1826, Elisha Bartlett Papers, CT—Yale; J. L. Cabell to Joseph C. Cabell, Paris, 28 Jan. 1837, James Lawrence Cabell Papers (no. 1640), VA—U. VA.

77. Flint, "European Correspondence," pp. 16–17.

78. Ashbel Smith to John Beard, Jr., Paris, 23 Feb. 1832, Smith Letters.

79. Quoted in John T. Morse, Jr., ed., *Life and Letters of Oliver Wendell Holmes*, 2 vols.

(Boston and New York: Houghton, Mifflin and Company, 1896), 1:94.

80. Erwin H. Ackerknecht, *Medicine at the Paris Hospital, 1794–1848* (Baltimore: Johns Hopkins University Press, 1967), p. 44.

81. Henry W. Williams to A. O. Williams, Paris, entry of 2 Aug. in letter of Paris, 28 July 1846, Williams Papers.

82. Flint, "European Correspondence," p. 16.

83. Saml. G. Howe to Father, Paris, 26 Oct. 1830, in *Letters and Journals of Samuel Gridley Howe*, ed. Laura E. Richards, 2 vols. (Boston: Dana Estes and Company, 1906), 1:380.

84. James L. Kitchen, Notes Taken on Lectures Delivered by Chapman (1820–1821), Laennec (1823), and Broussais (1823), PA—Hahnemann.

85. Quoted in Morse, *Holmes*, 1:89.

86. Alexander Wilcox, "Miscellaneous" ([Philadelphia], 15 Nov. 1845), WL 4 (1846): 425–428, p. 426. And see Harris, "Letter from Paris" (Paris, 19 Nov. 1855), p. 11.

87. Augustus Kinsley Gardner, *Old Wine in New Bottles; or, Spare Hours of a Student in Paris* (New-York: C. S. Francis & Co.; Boston: J. H. Francis, 1848), p. 205. The complaint about the *duration* of courses at the École de Médecine was one Americans commonly voiced about other scientific lectures in Paris. Having heard Dumas lecture at the Jardin des Plantes for two hours on wine, alcohol, and vinegar, Robert Peter reported that "you can judge from this that they do not travel rapidly—I have indeed been told that a full course on chemistry occupies four years, and I believe it" (Robert Peter to Frances Peter, Paris, 22 June 1839, Evans Papers). And see Edward E. Jenkins to John Jenkins, Paris, 13 Jan. 1854, Jenkins Papers.

88. Elisha Bartlett to Caroline Bartlett, Paris, 29 Nov. 1826, Bartlett Papers. "These establishments are so numerous and employ so many lecturers and professors that a stranger at first sight would believe that attention of the whole city is directed toward them," Usher Parsons, having taken advantage of the medical institutions of Paris for several months in 1819, wrote home. "I have seen 2500 persons at Beclard's lectures and not more than three fourths of those who go to hear Thenard can gain admittance" (Usher Parsons to Lyman Spalding, Paris, 29 Nov. 1819, Parsons Family Papers, RI—Brown).

89. William B. Crawford, Journal, entry for 17 Nov. 1832, in Paris, 1832–1833, Sarah Ann (Gayle) Crawford Papers, NC—Duke.

90. M. M. Rodgers, "Letter from a Correspondent in Paris" (Paris, 6 Feb. 1851), *Buffalo Medical Journal* 6 (1850–1851): 644–646, p. 644.

91. Hamilton, "Notes of an European Tour," p. 398.

92. John K. Kane to Father and Mother, [Paris], 21 Oct. 1857, Kane Family Papers. He was dissecting at the École Pratique, noting in a letter of 14 Oct. 1857 that the Clamart was too far away.

93. Ibid., [Paris], 21 Oct. [1857].

94. Stewart, *Eminent French Surgeons*, p. 142. Helpful descriptions of the dissection facilities include ibid., pp. 142–145; Meding, *Paris médical*, 2:323–324; and David W. Yandell, "Clinical Instruction in the London and Paris Hospitals," *WJMS*, ser. 3, 5 (1848): 392–400, pp. 397–399.

95. Stewart, *Eminent French Surgeons*, p. 143. And, for example, see the description in George B. Wood, Journal, vol. 7, 25 Aug.–4 Oct. 1853, entry for Paris, 8 Sept. 1853, Wood Journals.

96. M. L. L[inton], "Hospitals and Medical Schools of London, Paris, Dublin and Edinburgh," *WJMS* 1 (1840): 388–395, p. 394.

97. See, for example, Edward E. Jenkins to John Jenkins, Paris, 12 Aug. 1853, Jenkins Papers; Austin Flint, "Foreign Correspondence" (Paris, 18 May 1854), *WJMS*, n.s., 2 (1854): 88–89, pp. 96–97; and John A. Murphy, [Letter to Editors] (Paris, Mar. 1854), WL 15 (1854): 529–540, p. 535.

98. J. Y. Bassett to Marguerite Bassett, Paris, 3 July 1836, Bassett Papers.

99. Charles T. Jackson to Charles Brown, Paris, 18 Feb. and 6 Mar. 1830, C. Jackson Papers. And see ibid., 8 Mar. 1830.

100. Henry Bryant to John Bryant, Paris, 23 Feb. 1845, Bryant Papers.

101. Stewart, *Eminent French Surgeons*, p. 126. And see Elisha Bartlett to Caroline Bartlett, Paris, 27 Sept. 1826, Bartlett Papers.

102. Oliver Wendell Holmes to Parents, Paris, 14 May 1835, in Morse, *Holmes*, 1:150–152, on pp. 151–152.

103. James Duncan, "Clinical and Miscellaneous Notes Taken at the Ecole de Medicine & Various Hospitals, Paris, Winter Semestre, 1846–1847," entry for 22 Nov. 1847, Lon-

don—St. Bartholomew's; "Comparative Merits of the French and English Schools," *LMG* 19 (1836–1837): 319–322, p. 319.

104. See Russell C. Maulitz, *Morbid Appearances: The Anatomy of Pathology in the Early Nineteenth Century* (Cambridge: Cambridge University Press, 1987), pp. 109–157.

105. Austin Flint, "Foreign Correspondence" (Paris, Apr. 1854), *WJMS* 2 (1854): 169–174, p. 172. Those who went to Paris before receiving an M.D. gained ready admission to the medical institutions. "I have found no difficulty whatsoever from not having my degree," reported Holmes, who earned his diploma only in 1836, after returning to Boston. "They are not taken the least notice of,—nobody uses the title of Doctor, and I would not give a copper for the advantages it would give me" (Oliver Wendell Holmes to John Holmes, Paris, 21 June 1833, in Morse, *Holmes*, 1:100–103, on pp. 101–102).

106. Cabell to Cabell, Paris, 28 Jan. 1837.

107. A. Colman to Catherine K. Colman, 6 Jan. 1833, Colman Papers.

108. Robert P. Harris, "Letter from Paris" (Paris, 19 Nov. 1855), *American Medical Gazette and Journal of Health* 7 (1856): 168–171, p. 171.

109. Ibid., p. 169.

110. J. Y. Bassett to Isaphoena Bassett, Paris, 16 Mar. 1836, Bassett Papers.

111. Jenkins to [Jenkins], Paris, 12 Aug. 1853.

112. A. L. Peirson, entry for 26 Oct. 1832, in Peirson Letterbook.

113. J. H. Richardson to John Rolph, Paris, 29 July 1846, John Rolph Papers (MG24 B24), Ottawa—Nat. Arch. Canada. I am grateful to Jacalyn Duffin for spotting this letter.

114. Wilcox, "Miscellaneous," pp. 425–426.

115. David W. Yandell, "Notes on Medical Matters in Paris" (Paris, Feb. 1847), *WJMS*, n.s., 7 (1847): 93–113, p. 99.

116. Yandell, "Clinical Instruction," p. 396.

117. I.H.D., "The Hospitals and Professors of Paris" (Paris, Oct. 1849), *BMSJ* 41 (1850): 341–343, p. 342. "There are some hospitals which are very little visited, on account of distance, that have very eminent physicians and surgeons, and whose instructions are perhaps, more valuable, as there is a much better opportunity of studying the cases, on account of

their being no crowd of visitors," wrote another American who particularly singled out the St. Louis (Harris, "Letter from Paris" [Paris, 25 Dec. 1855], p. 72). Stewart (*Eminent French Surgeons*, p. 41) also noted that the Hôpital de la Pitié, "very much out of the way," was frequented "particularly by English students."

118. Henry Bryant to John Bryant, entry of 21 Dec. in letter of Paris, 11 Dec. 1843, Bryant Papers.

119. Stewart, *Eminent French Surgeons*, pp. 325, 202.

120. Bryant, for example, attended the meeting at which Ricord gave his address as president; Henry Bryant to John Bryant, entry of 23 May in letter of Paris, 17 May 1844, Bryant Papers.

121. M. L. Linton, "Hospitals of Paris" (Paris, 24 Dec. 1840), *WJMS* 3 (1841): 65–74, p. 67.

122. Gardner, *Old Wine*, p. 163. George B. Wood, though, noted that "Dr. B. Velpeau is always pleasant, often jocose, and makes us laugh by his occasional attempts to speak English" (entry for 1–4 May 1862, Journal, 25 Mar. 1862–28 Aug. 1862, Wood Journals).

123. Stewart, *Eminent French Surgeons*, p. 42. On the limited opportunities for students to gain obstetric experience in America, see Judith Walzer Leavitt, *Brought to Bed: Childbearing in America, 1750–1950* (New York and Oxford: Oxford University Press, 1986), pp. 36–63.

124. Gooch, Diary, entry for 30 June 1848. The audience was unusually large, Gooch noted, because the weather outside was very bad. On 3 July he observed that "I found the poor woman who was operated for a delivery by caesarian section died." Gardner reported, "Whenever a female is in labor, a signal is placed at the door indicating the fact. All, who see the notice, enter. The first comer is the *accoucheur* under the direction of the resident *sage-femme*. Around the bed a railing keeps off the multitude, who often number fifty or more. I have seen the room crowded during the performance of such operations as are necessary. The patient is uncovered, as the labor advances, for the benefit of those around. How many of the very lowest classes in the United States would be thus willingly exposed?" (*Old Wine*, p. 203).

125. Waring, Travel Journal, n.d., 1856.

126. Austin Flint, "Address at the Opening of the Session for 1854–55 in the Medical Department of the University of Louisville," *WJMS*, n.s., 2 (1854): 409–425, p. 418.

127. Flint, "European Correspondence," p. 14.

128. Cabell to Cabell, Paris, 28 Jan. 1837.

129. Yandell, "Clinical Instruction," p. 399. And see Manigault, Autobiography, p. 130.

130. F. P. P[orcher], "Editorial Correspondence of the Charleston Medical Journal and Review" (Paris, 5 Mar. 1853), *CMJR* 8 (1853): 416–429, pp. 416–417.

131. Cabell to Cabell, Paris, 28 Jan. 1837.

132. C. B. Chapman, "Medical Study in Paris," *BMSJ* 47 (1853): 286–287, p. 287.

133. Henry Bryant to John Bryant, Paris, 6 Feb. 1844, Bryant Papers.

134. Ibid., 13 Aug.; 2 Oct.; and 22 Nov. 1844.

135. Yandell, "Clinical Instruction," p. 399.

136. Stewart, *Eminent French Surgeons*, p. 140.

137. C. T. Jackson to Charles Brown, Paris, 29 June 1830, C. Jackson Papers.

138. Ibid., Paris, 6 Dec. 1829.

139. "Editorial Correspondence of the Charleston Medical Journal and Review" ([Letter to the Editor], Paris, 5 Mar. 1853), *CMJR* 8 (1853): 416–429, pp. 423–424.

140. Waring, Travel Journal, entry for 22 Dec. 1856.

141. J. Y. Bassett to Marguerite Bassett, Paris, 29 Apr. 1836, Bassett Papers. The judgment on his midwifery course is in J. Y. Bassett to Isaphoena Bassett, Paris, 27 Mar. 1836. He added, "I have also entered another private class of six with Mons. *Robecchi* for anatomical instruction; these gentlemen are both aiming at Professorships & Mons. *Chassaignac* aspiring at present for the Chair of Anatomy, & consequently they spare no pains."

142. Wilcox, "Miscellaneous," pp. 426, 427.

143. [Lundsford P. Yandell], editorial note in Austin Flint, "Foreign Correspondence" (Paris, 18 June 1854), *WJMS*, ser. 4, 2 (1854): 89–99, p. 97.

144. P., "The Advantages and Disadvantages of Paris as a Place of Resort for Medical Students" (Paris, 10 July 1853), *SLMSJ* 12 (1854): 79–84, p. 80.

145. Jenkins to [Jenkins], 12 Aug. 1853.

146. Ibid. Paris, 13 Jan. 1854. "I live as economically as I can," Kane told his parents, "but private courses are expensive beyond all conception" (John K. Kane to Mother and Father, [Paris], 22 Aug. [1857], Kane Family Papers).

147. Elizabeth Blackwell, "Copy of a Letter from Elizabeth Blackwell, M.D., Late Graduate of Geneva College" (Paris, 28 Feb. 1850), *BMSJ* 42 (1850): 351–354, p. 353; emphasis added.

148. [Elizabeth Blackwell to Family], Paris, May 1849, in Elizabeth Blackwell, *Pioneer Work in Opening the Medical Profession to Women: Autobiographical Sketches by Dr. Elizabeth Blackwell* (1895; reprint, New York: Schocken Books, 1977), pp. 111–114, on pp. 113, 117.

149. [Elizabeth Blackwell to Emily Blackwell, New York], 24 July [1854], in Blackwell, *Pioneer Work*, pp. 201–204, quotation on p. 201. Trousseau's suggestion that Blackwell disguise herself as a man gained currency among the rumors passed around the wider community of American physicians in Paris. As one wrote back in 1851, another student had "remarked that a female, he believed from the United States, applied for permission to attend the lectures generally. The professor said he had no objection, provided she would put on a coat and pantaloons" ("Editorial Correspondence. Hospitals of Paris," *BMSJ* 43 [1851]: 22–24, p. 24).

150. Blackwell, *Pioneer Work*, p. 18; on her decision making, see pp. 114–123.

151. Blackwell, "Copy of a Letter," p. 353.

152. Ibid., and Elizabeth Blackwell to Dear Cousin [Kenyon Blackwell], [Paris], 15 June [1849], in Blackwell, *Pioneer Work*, pp. 120–121, quotation on p. 120.

153. On the Maternité, see Meding, *Paris médical*, 2: 92–96, and Stewart, *Eminent French Surgeons*, pp. 61–63. James Jackson, Jr., reported in 1831 from Paris that the Maternité once had been more open to male medical students, but that he had been told such access had ended "on account of the constant difficulties which arose from the assemblage of these same gentlemen and the young sage-femmes who attend there—the complaint is that 'il font plus d'enfans que d'accouchements'" (Jackson, Jr., to James Jackson, Sr., Paris, 7 Oct. 1831, J. Jackson Papers).

154. [Elizabeth Blackwell] to Dear Mother, [Paris], à la Maternité, 1 July 1849, in Blackwell, *Pioneer Work*, pp. 124–130, quotation on p. 124. On her time at the Maternité, see Blackwell, *Pioneer Work*, pp. 124–157.

155. Blackwell, *Pioneer Work*, p. 135. "Let me sketch a day for you. From 5 to 6 in the morning, I dressed and arranged my patients in the long galleries devoted to cases of natural labor; from 6 to 7, followed the visit of the sage-femme en chef through these same galleries; from 7 to 8, her lecture; 8 to 9, I followed the physician's visit through the infirmaries (breakfast whenever I could snatch it); 9 to 10, Dubois's lecture; 10 to 11, visited the nursery, or the salle for the femmes enceintes; 11 to 12, another lecture; 12 to 1, dinner and a breath of fresh air in the wood; 1 to 2, the interne's lecture; 2 to 3, wrote observations on interesting cases, composition, &c.; 3 to 4, tended my patients and followed Mad. Charrier's second visit; 4 to 5, attended the reception of patients, ascertaining the stage of pregnancy, &c.; 5 to 6, a second visit to the infirmaries; after that, tea, and study during the evening" (Blackwell, "Copy of a Letter," p. 354).

156. [Elizabeth Blackwell] to Dear Friends, [Paris], 22 Oct. 1849, in Blackwell, *Pioneer Work*, pp. 148–153, quotations on pp. 148, 149, 153. Students were permitted to leave the institution during the day a few times each year, and then only "with their mothers and fathers and husbands, or with persons expressly designated by them" (Meding, *Paris médical*, 2:96).

157. Bessie Parkes to Barbara Leigh Smith, Compton Terrace, [London?], 13 Nov. 1850, Elizabeth Blackwell Letters, NY—Columbia.

158. Elizabeth Blackwell, Journal, entry for 4 July [1849], excerpt in Blackwell, *Pioneer Work*, pp. 143–144, quotations on p. 143.

159. [Elizabeth Blackwell] to Dear Mother, entry of 3 July in letter of 1 July [1849], in Blackwell, *Pioneer Work*, pp. 124–130, on p. 129.

160. Meding, *Paris médical*, 2:94; the figures are for 1850.

161. Blackwell, Journal, entry for 12 Aug. [1849], excerpt in Blackwell, *Pioneer Work*, p. 144.

162. Blackwell, Journal, entry for 21 Sept. [1849], in Blackwell, *Pioneer Work*, pp. 146–147.

163. Blackwell, "Copy of a Letter"; idem, *Pioneer Work*, pp. 154–163; and Parkes to Smith, 13 Nov. 1850.

164. Blackwell, Journal, entry for 22 [Nov. 1849], excerpt in Blackwell, *Pioneer Work*, p. 156.

165. Elizabeth Blackwell to Dear Uncle, [Paris, n.d but around late Nov. 1849], in Blackwell, *Pioneer Work*, pp. 157–158, quotation on p. 158.

166. [Elizabeth Blackwell to Emily Blackwell, New York], 24 July [1854], in Blackwell, *Pioneer Work*, pp. 201–204, quotations on p. 202; and cf. Blackwell, *Pioneer Work*, p. 158.

167. On her London studies, see Blackwell, *Pioneer Work*, pp. 163–189. She wrote to her American preceptor, however, "I cannot wonder that students throng to Paris, instead of to the immense smoke-hidden London; here there is no excitement, all moves steadily onward, constantly but without enthusiasm" ([Elizabeth Blackwell] to [Samuel Henry] Dickson, 28 Thavies Inn [London], 1850, in ibid., pp. 173–175, quotation on p. 174).

168. James Paget, Entry Book of Students in the College of St. Bartholomew's Hospital, 1843–1859, entry no. 521, London—RCS, reproduced by kind permission of the President and Council of the Royal College of Surgeons of England.

169. Blackwell, *Pioneer Work*, p. 123.

170. Elizabeth [Blackwell] to Dear Emily, [New York, 1852?]; Elizabeth [Blackwell] to Dear Emily, [New York], entry of 25 Apr. in letter of 20 Apr. 1854, Blackwell Family Papers (MC 411), MA—Schlesinger. Clark, Elizabeth explained to Emily, "feels quite a tie to you from having graduated where she did & has great respect for your abilities—I think you might do her good."

171. Ibid.

172. R. A. Kinloch, "Medical News From Paris France" (Paris, 20 Nov. 1854), *CMJR* 10 (1855): 58–66, p. 65. Kinloch commented that Clark "looks rather more interesting I imagine, than most of the few of her sex, who have thus thrown aside the most prominent feature in the character of woman, and entered the domains of our science." He noted that "M. Dubois, and also his excellent 'Chef de Clinique,' Dr. Campbell, treat her with much attention, often troubling themselves to explain to her in English, as she understands at present but little French" (p. 65). And see

R. A. Kinloch, "Medical News from Paris" (Paris, 13 Jan. 1855), *CMJR* 10 (1855): 159–170, p. 159. Helpful treatments of Clark are in Esther Pohl Lovejoy, *Women Doctors of the World* (New York: Macmillan Company, 1957), pp. 82–84, and Frederick C. Waite, "Dr. Nancy E. (Talbot) Clark: The Second Woman Graduate in Medicine to Practice in Boston," *New England Journal of Medicine* 205 (1931): 1195–1198. Waite suggests that Clark spent a year at the Maternité.

173. Emily [Blackwell] to Dear Friends, [London], 8–15 June 1855, Blackwell Family Papers.

174. Elizabeth Blackwell had advised her sister to spend six months at the Maternité, but as her sister's visit to Paris approached, the elder Blackwell had second thoughts. Concerned for her sister's "freedom," she wrote, "I almost doubt the propriety of your entering the Maternité, or rather I hope that the necessity may be obviated by your finding other openings." At the least, she proposed, "I would not think of doing so until I had seen all the others and tried for better openings" ([Elizabeth Blackwell to Emily Blackwell], 13 Nov. 1854, in Blackwell, *Pioneer Work*, pp. 204–205, on p. 204; and cf. Elizabeth [Blackwell] to Dear Emily, [New York, 1852?], Blackwell Family Papers).

175. [Elizabeth Blackwell] to Dear M., [Paris], July 1849, in Blackwell, *Pioneer Work*, pp. 130–143, on p. 130. Framing her time at the Maternité this way in no way diminished its importance in her mind and, indeed, perhaps enhanced it through the implications of martyrdom for a cause; it was her time abroad that, along with her earlier studies in America, she saw as "Pioneer work," more so than her later efforts in New York and in England; see Elizabeth [Blackwell] to Emily [Blackwell], Rock House, [Hastings], 17 Feb. [1895], Blackwell Family Papers.

176. [Elizabeth Blackwell] to Dear Mother, entry of 3 July in letter begun [Paris] à la Maternité, 1 July 1849, in Blackwell, *Pioneer Work*, pp. 124–130, on p. 130.

177. Elisha Bartlett to George Bartlett, Paris, 24 Apr. 1846, Bartlett Family Papers.

178. Charles T. Jackson to Charles Brown, Paris, 28 Jan. 1830, and Charles T. Jackson to Lydia Jackson, Paris, 13 May 1831, C. Jackson Papers.

179. Samuel [Wigglesworth] to Thomas

Wigglesworth, Paris, 24 Apr. 1836, Wigglesworth Letters, NY—NY Acad. Med.; Porcher, Travel Journal, entry for 11 Oct. 1852.

180. F. H. Hamilton, "Notes of an European Tour.—No. 3," *Buffalo Medical Journal* 1 (1846): 21–30, p. 26.

181. Robert Peter to Frances Peter, Paris, 22 June 1839, Evans Papers.

182. Levin S. Joynes to Thomas R. Joynes, Paris, 20 May 1841, Joynes Family Papers.

183. Henry Bryant to John Bryant, Paris, 1 July 1844, Bryant Papers.

184. Manigault, Autobiography, pp. 128–129.

185. Gabriel Manigault to Charles Manigault, Paris, 15 Oct. 1854, Manigault Family Papers, SC—U. SC.

186. Manigault, Autobiography, p. 276. "The great dissecting place known as Clamart, where most of my acquaintances spent their days, was only visited by me once, the visit having been simply one of curiosity" (p. 131).

187. Jeffries Wyman to Morrill Wyman, Paris, 14 Jan. 1841, Wyman Papers, MA—Countway.

188. Jeffries Wyman to David Humphreys Storer, Paris, 31 Aug. 1841, in George E. Gifford, Jr., ed., "An American in Paris, 1841–1842: Four Letters from Jeffries Wyman," *Journal of the History of Medicine and Allied Sciences* 22 (1967): 274–285, pp. 275–279, on pp. 279, 277.

189. Jeffries Wyman to Morrill Wyman, Paris, 31 Oct. 1841, Wyman Papers.

190. Ibid., Paris, 14 Apr. 1842.

191. Samuel [Wigglesworth] to Thomas Wigglesworth, Paris, 9 Jan. 1836, Wigglesworth Letters.

192. Ashbel Smith to John Beard, Jr., Paris, 23 Feb. 1832, Smith Letters.

193. Ibid.

194. Waring, Travel Journal, n.d., 1856.

195. For example, William B. Crawford (Sarah [Gayle] Crawford, Journal, 1849, entry for Paris, 28 Sept. 1853, Sarah Ann and William B. Crawford Papers, AL—U. AL); Dr. Jarvis (Elisha Bartlett to Caroline Bartlett, Paris, 29 Nov. 1826, Bartlett Papers); and Austin Flint (Austin Flint, "Foreign Correspondence" [Paris, 26 June 1854], *WJMS*, ser. 4, 2 [1854]: 273–277, p. 273).

196. For example, J. Y. Bassett to Indiana Manning, Paris, 7 June 1836; and cf. letters to his sister: J. Y. Bassett to Marguerite Bassett,

Paris, 16 Oct. 1836; 29 Apr. 1836; 3 July 1836; 28 Aug. 1836, all in Bassett Papers.

197. J. Y. Bassett to Isaphoena Bassett, Paris, 1 Feb. 1836, Bassett Papers.

198. Ibid., 12 June 1836.

199. Ibid., 28 Aug. 1836.

200. Ibid., 11 Sept. and 16 Oct. 1836.

201. Oliver Wendell Holmes to Parents, Paris, 14 Feb. 1834, in Morse, *Holmes*, 1:127–130, on p. 130.

202. The phrase comes from John Moffatt Howe, Diary of Trip to Europe, June–Sept. 1838, BV Howe, NY—NY Hist. Soc. Although he would later study medicine, at this point Howe, having been chaplain to the New York Hospital, went to Paris for his own health.

203. See C. T. Jackson to Charles Brown, Paris, 26 Feb. 1831, C. Jackson Papers.

204. Blackwell, "Copy of a Letter," p. 351.

205. See Blackwell, *Pioneer Work*, pp. 154–163, and Parkes to Smith, 13 Nov. 1850.

206. Henry Bryant to John Bryant, Paris, 17 Jan. 1845, Bryant Papers.

207. Ibid., [Paris], July 1845.

208. Henry Williams to A. O. Williams, Paris, entry of 23 Jan. in letter of 20 Jan. 1847, Williams Papers.

209. George C. Shattuck, Jr., to Mrs. A. H. Shattuck, Paris, 29 Oct. 1837, Shattuck Papers, vol. 15. And see David P. Holton to Emeline R. Turner, Paris, 18 June 1856, in which the secretary of the American Medical Society in Paris recounted the last illness and death of a young American physician to his sister. "Laboring hard for breath," Holton wrote, the young man "attempted to utter some sentences, his words were indistinct and none could be recognized but that very precious word mother—mother— . . . " (David Parsons Holton Papers, NY—NY Gen. & Biogr. Soc.).

210. Flint, "Address," pp. 423–424.

211. E.L.D., "Foreign Correspondence" (Paris, May 1850), *Transylvania Medical Journal* 2 (1850–1852): 129–134, pp. 130–131.

212. Frances Peter to Robert Peter, [Lexington, Kentucky], 29 May 1839, Evans Papers.

213. Robert Battey to My dearest Love [Martha (Smith) Battey], Paris, 4 Mar. 1860, Robert Battey Family Papers, GA—Emory.

214. Porcher, Travel Journal, entry for Paris, 26 Sept. 1852. "Paris is a free City!" he commented. "Though there are more Police and they know more about you in a public and less in a private way than any where else

in the world. If you offend not politically you are really & truly *free* for society has culpably [*sic*] few restraints. Their habit being to indulge socially in vice, license & excess, no strict mentor frowns upon it in others. In America we are politically free & liberal—socially puritanical & exacting both in religion & morals."

215. Saml. G. Howe to William [Sampson], Paris, 14 Nov. 1831, in Richards, *Letters and Journals of Samuel Gridley Howe*, 1:391; Oliver Wendell Holmes to Mother and Father, Paris, 14 Feb. 1834, in Morse, *Holmes*, 1:127–130, on p. 129.

216. L. S. Joynes to Louisa A. S. Joynes, Paris, 14 Dec. 1840, Joynes Family Papers.

217. Levin S. Joynes to Anne B. Joynes, Paris, 18 July 1840. "This is Sunday, and the only thing that distinguishes it from any other day here, is that there is rather more dissipation & a greater display in the shop windows, which are all open," Bassett observed (J. Y. Bassett to Isaphoena Bassett, Paris, 13 Mar. 1836, Bassett Papers); and see Robert Peter to Frances Peter, Paris, 14 July 1839, Evans Papers; and A. Colman to Catherine Colman, Paris, 15 Apr. 1833, Colman Papers.

218. H. I. Bowditch to J. Jackson, Jr., [Paris], 11 June 1832, Putnam, Jackson and Lowell Papers, MA—MA Hist. Soc.

219. A. Smith to James Jackson, Paris, 11 June 1832, Putnam, Jackson and Lowell Papers.

220. Charles T. Jackson to Charles Brown, Paris, 4 Sept. 1830, and ibid., Paris, 30 Oct. 1830, C. Jackson Papers. See Guillaume de Bertier de Sauvigny, *La révolution de 1830 en France* (Paris: Armand Colin, 1970).

221. Edward E. Jenkins to [John Jenkins], Paris, 26 July 1854, Jenkins Papers.

222. William Joseph Holt, Journal of My Voyage in Europe, entry for Crakov, 9 Aug. 1854, William Joseph Holt Papers, SC—U. SC.

223. See William Holt, Journal, 19 July 1854–12 Sept. 1855; W. J. Holt, Medical Notes, 1856; and Joseph I. Waring, "The Journal of Dr. William Joseph Holt in the Crimean War," edited transcript, all in Holt Papers.

224. L. A. Dugas to Pauline Dugas, Paris, 27 Sept. 1828, Dugas Papers.

225. Henry Bryant to John Bryant, Paris, 11 Dec. 1843, Bryant Papers. "An Englishman never wears a moustache," another American

physician noted in Paris, "and he is easily known" (Iatros, "Medical Heads and Medical Life in Paris," *CMJR* 9 [1854]: 476–483, p. 477).

226. Manigault, Autobiography, esp. pp. 131–133.

227. Henry W. Williams to Sisters, entry of 6 Mar. in letter of Paris, 23 Feb. 1848, Williams Papers.

228. Oliver Wendell Holmes to Parents, Paris, 12 Feb. 1834, in Morse, *Holmes*, 1:127–130, on pp. 127–128. See, for example, J. L. Cabell to C. Cabell, Paris, 28 Jan. 1837, Cabell Papers; and Gardner, *Old Wine*, p. 58. And see G. de Bertier de Sauvigny, *La France et les Français vus par les voyageurs américains* (Paris: Flammarion, 1982), and Robert C. L. Scott, "American Travellers in France, 1830–1860: A Study of Some American Ideas against a European Background" (Ph.D. diss., Yale University, 1940).

229. [Wigglesworth] to Wigglesworth, Paris, 9 Jan. 1836.

230. Charles T. Jackson to Charles Brown, New York, 17 Nov. 1832, C. Jackson Papers. He noted that "I did not mention to you in my letter from Paris that I was engaged in such business, lest you should have some fears on my account as you knew our subjects were furnished by the dreaded cholera."

231. Gardner, *Old Wine*, p. 18. On American visits to Lafayette, see, for example, George Rosen, ed., "An American Doctor in Paris in 1828: Selections from the Diary of Peter Solomon Townsend, M.D.," *Journal of the History of Medicine and Allied Sciences* 6 (1951): 64–115, 209–252, p. 231.

232. Williams to Sisters, entry of 8 May in letter of 6 May 1846.

233. H. W. Williams to Sister, Paris, 11 Sept. 1846.

234. L. J. Frazee, *The Medical Student in Europe* (Maysville, Ky.: Richard U. Collins, 1849), p. 116.

235. See, for example, John Hamilton to G. C. Shattuck, Dublin, 20 Jan. 1840, Shattuck Papers, vol. 16.

236. Henry W. Williams to Sisters, London, [Apr. or May 1848], Williams Papers; Henry Bryant to John Bryant, Paris, entry of 21 May in letter of 17 May 1844, Bryant Papers. Louis was married to Zoé Duridal de Montferrier, the sister of Victor Hugo's brother's wife.

237. James Jackson, Jr., to James Jackson, Sr., Paris, 15 Jan. 1832, J. Jackson Papers.

238. [P.] Louis to [H. I. Bowditch], Paris, 23 Mar. 1846, MA—Countway. Attending dinner at Louis's house, Bryant was asked "if I should like to become a member of the Société medicale d'observation—I am affraid as yet to attempt it as it is necessary to write a paper on some thing or other and read it before the society and I imagine that my French would not be very good whatever my ideas were" (Henry Bryant to John Bryant, Paris, entry of 21 May in letter of 17 May 1844, Bryant Papers). Stewardson, who did join, reported, "I find the advantage very great and only wish I had become a member much sooner—not the least advantage is my being brought into more close connection with Louis, with whom by the by I expect to have the pleasure of dining this evening" (T. Stewardson to W. W. Gerhard, Paris, 22 Mar. 1834, W. W. Gerhard Papers, PA—CPP).

239. Henry Bryant to John Bryant, Paris, entry of 23 May in letter of 17 May 1844, Bryant Papers. On the society, see especially Meding, *Paris médical*, 2:398–399.

240. The best-represented states were South Carolina (16), Ohio (14), Pennsylvania (14), New York (12), Massachusetts (10), Kentucky (8), Louisiana (6), and Virginia (6); *Constitution of the American Medical Society in Paris. Instituted November 15, 1851* (Paris: S. Raçon, 1854). And see the manuscript draft "Constitution de la Société Médicale Americaine de Paris, 1854," PA—CPP; "The American Medical Society in Paris," *CMJR* 11 (1856): 280–281; "American Medical Society in Paris," *BMSJ* 49 (1854): 66; W. E. Johnston, David P. Holton, and Saml. Gourdin, [Letter to Editor], [Assembly] Hall of the "American Medical Society in Paris," Paris, 4 July 1855, *Medical Examiner*, n.s., 12 (1856): 246–247; and Meding, *Paris médical*, 2:401–402.

241. Gooch, Diary, entry for University of Virginia, 20 Feb. 1845.

242. Ibid., Edinburgh, 4 Nov. 1846.

243. Ibid., 13 Jan. 1847.

244. Ibid., 19 Jan. 1847.

245. Ibid., 21 Jan. 1847.

246. Gooch, having just passed through the customshouse in Le Havre, wrote in his diary, "Well, here I am in *France*,—no difficulte in talking, which I had anticipated."

Yet he soon learned that listening was more difficult, writing of a morning spent at the Hôtel Dieu that he "saw very many cases examined & some operation[s]—heard part of 2 cliniques, not understanding much" (ibid., entries of Havre, 19 Oct. 1847 and Paris, 10 Nov. 1847).

247. Ibid., Paris, 13 Dec. 1847.

248. Ibid., 19 Jan. 1848.

249. Ibid., 26 Jan. 1848.

250. Ibid., 27 Jan. 1848.

251. Ibid., 1 Feb. 1848.

252. Ibid., 5 Feb. 1848.

253. Ibid., 3 Feb. 1848.

254. Ibid., 21 Feb. 1848.

255. Ibid., 24 Feb. 1848.

256. Ibid., 25 Feb. 1848.

257. Ibid., 26 Feb. 1848.

258. Ibid., 6 Mar. 1848.

259. Ibid., 23 Mar. 1848.

260. Ibid., 5 May 1848.

261. Ibid., 26–27 May 1848.

262. Ibid., 9 June 1848.

263. Ibid., 23 June 1848.

264. Ibid., 24 June 1848.

265. Ibid., 25 June 1848.

266. Ibid., 6 Aug. 1848.

267. Ibid., 11 Aug. 1848.

268. Ibid., 21 Aug. 1848.

269. P. C. Gooch to Maria R. R. Gooch, [Paris, n.d., but summer of 1848], Gooch Family Papers, VA—VA Hist. Soc. He said that he planned to send the letter by way of Dr. Hume, who was still with him in Paris (Gooch, Diary, entry for Paris, 17 June 1848).

270. Gooch, Diary, entry for Paris, 1 Sept. 1848.

271. Ibid., 6 Sept. 1848.

272. Ibid., 7 Sept. 1848.

273. Ibid., 30 Sept. 1848.

274. Ibid., 6 Oct. 1848.

275. Ibid., 23 Oct. 1848.

276. Ibid., 24 Oct. 1848.

277. Ibid., 12 Nov. 1848.

278. Oliver Wendell Holmes to John Holmes, Paris, 21 June 1833, in Morse, *Holmes*, 1:100–103, on p. 102.

279. Oliver Wendell Holmes to Parents, Paris, 28 Sept. 1833, in Morse, *Holmes*, 1:112–114, on p. 113.

280. James Norcom to John Norcom, Edenton, N.C., 18 Feb. 1846, Dr. James Norcom and Family Papers, NC—NC State Arch.; and on discipleship, see G. F. Manning to John Y.

Bassett, Philadelphia, 9 May 1835, Bassett Papers, and Lundsford Pitt Yandell, Diary, 1824–1843, entry for Craggy Bluffs, 19 Apr. 1825, Yandell Family Papers, KY—Filson Club.

281. William Osler, "The Influence of Louis on American Medicine" (1896), in *An Alabama Student and Other Biographical Essays* (London: Oxford University Press, 1908), pp. 189–210.

282. Henry W. Williams to A. O. Williams, Paris, entry of 10 Aug. in letter of 28 July 1846, Williams Papers.

283. Oliver Wendell Holmes, *Medical Essays, 1842–1882* (1861; Boston and New York: Houghton, Mifflin and Company, 1895), p. 431.

284. Williams to Williams, entry of 10 Aug. in letter of 28 July 1846.

285. James Jackson, Jr., to James Jackson, Sr., Paris, 30 May 1831, J. Jackson Papers.

286. James Jackson, Jr., to Mother, [Paris], 9 July 1831; and see James Jackson, Jr., to James Jackson, Sr., Paris, 29 July 1831, and ibid., 7 July 1831.

287. Ibid., 27 July 1831.

288. Ibid., 5 Aug. 1831.

289. Ibid., 27 July 1831; and see ibid. 18 Oct. 1831 and 26 Jan. 1832.

290. Ibid., 7 Oct. 1831.

291. Ibid., 15 Nov. 1831.

292. Ibid., 11 Aug. 1831; and see ibid., 28 Oct. 1831.

293. Ibid., 6 Nov. 1831.

294. Ibid., 26 Jan. 1832.

295. Wigglesworth to Wigglesworth, Paris, 9 Jan. 1836.

296. James Jackson, Jr., to James Jackson, Sr., Paris, 15 Jan. 1832; and see ibid., 26 Jan. 1832, J. Jackson Papers.

297. Ibid., 14 Dec. 1831.

298. Ibid., 3 Feb. 1832.

299. Ibid., 27 Feb. 1832.

300. Ibid., 18 Mar. 1832.

301. Ibid., 20 Mar. 1832.

302. Ibid., Havre, 25 Apr. 1832.

303. Ibid., London, 3 May 1832; ibid., 5 Sept. 1832.

304. Ibid., Paris, 21 Oct. 1832.

305. Ibid., 1 Dec. 1832.

306. Ibid., 22 Mar. 1832.

307. Ibid., 29 Apr. 1833.

308. Ibid., 20 Apr. 1833; and see ibid., 27 June 1833.

309. Ibid., 13 July 1833.

310. See, for example, Alfred Stillé, *Elements of General Pathology: A Practical Treatise* (Philadelphia: Lindsay and Blakiston, 1848), pp. 46–48.

311. Charles T. Jackson to David Henshaw, Paris, 15 June 1832, C. Jackson Papers.

312. Charles T. Jackson to Charles Brown, New York, 17 Nov. 1832, C. Jackson Papers.

313. G. Roberts Smith to William Gerhard, Paris, 6 July 1834, Gerhard Papers.

314. J. Y. Mason to Count Walewski, Paris, 20 June 1856; M. Baroche to Mr. Mason, Paris, 4 July 1856; Mr. Mason to Count Walewski, Paris, 8 May 1856; and Count Walewski to Mr. Mason, Paris, 3 June 1856, all in James Mason Young, Letterbook, 5 Jan. 1856–28 Mar. 1857, VA—VA Hist. Soc.

315. Edward E. Jenkins to Dear Father, Paris, 16 June 1854, Jenkins Papers. And see Edward E. Jenkins to Dear Bunch, Paris, 21 June 1854, and Edward E. Jenkins to [John Jenkins], Paris, 7 Oct. 1853.

316. John K. Kane to Parents, [Paris], 15 Oct. 1857, Kane Family Papers.

317. L. A. Dugas to P[auline] Dugas, Paris, 27 Sept. 1829, Dugas Papers.

318. L. A. Dugas to Ma chère Maman, Havre, 29 Oct. 1829.

319. A. Colman to Catherine K. Colman, Paris, 15 Apr. 1833, Colman Papers.

CHAPTER 4
CONTEXTS OF TRANSMISSION:
DUTY AND DISTINCTION

1. Saml. Henry Dickson to John A. Dickson, New York, 3 Nov. 1848, Dickson Family Papers, NC—SHC.

2. Henry Bryant to John Bryant, entry of 17 Feb. in letter from Paris, 1 Feb. 1844, William Sohier Bryant Papers (MS 45), MA—New England Hist. Gen. Soc.

3. Joseph Winthrop to Gabriel E. Manigault, Charleston, 24 Feb. 1855, SC—Waring.

4. Thomas Lincoln to George C. Shattuck, Dennysville, 26 Sept. 1837, Shattuck Papers, vol. 15, MA—MA Hist. Soc.

5. G. Roberts Smith to W. W. Gerhard, Paris, 6 July 1834, W. W. Gerhard Papers, PA—CPP.

6. T. Stewardson to W. W. Gerhard, Paris, 22 Mar., 1834, Gerhard Papers. Stewardson noted of Louis that "Broussais has himself

placed him at the head of all living physicians by devoting double the space (nearly 200 pages) to the examination of his works."

7. For example, J. C. Nott, "Letter from Doctor Nott," Munich, 30 July 1859, *Mobile Daily Register*, 2 Sept. 1859.

8. Levin S. Joynes to Thomas R. Joynes, Paris, 20 May 1841, and L. S. Joynes to Louisa A. S. Joynes, Paris, 14 Dec. 1840, Joynes Family Papers, VA—VA Hist. Soc.

9. Austin Flint, "Foreign Correspondence," *WJMS*, n.s., 2 (1854): 331–339. The French text was Maria-Guillaume-Alphonse Devergie, *Traité pratique des maladies de la peau* (Paris: V. Masson, 1854).

10. B. Allen, "Foreign Correspondence" (Paris, 25 Jan. 1854), *SLMSJ* 12 (1854): 226–231, p. 226.

11. Alden March, "For the Boston Medical and Surgical Journal," Albany, 11 Sept. 1856, Alden March Papers, NY—Albany Med.

12. J. C. W[arren], "Foreign Correspondence.—Parisian Hospitals" (Paris, 30 Dec. 1837), *BMSJ* 18 (1838): 42–46, p. 44.

13. [Lundsford] Y[andell], prefatory note to M. L. L[inton], "Hospitals and Medical Schools of London, Paris, Dublin and Edinburgh," *WJMS* 1 (1840): 388–395, p. 388.

14. David W. Yandell, "Notes on Medical Matters and Medical Men in Paris," *WJMS*, n.s., 8 (1847): 19–42, p. 20.

15. David W. Yandell, *Notes on Medical Matters and Medical Men in London and Paris* (Louisville, Ky.: Prentice and Weissinger, 1848). L. P. Yandell, like other medical journal editors, clearly welcomed his son's letters from Paris as a steady source of all-too-scarce original copy. "In the midst of engrossing studies, which left me but little leisure," the son explained in prefacing the collected letters, "I was induced to continue the correspondence, not more by the evidence afforded me that my contributions were well received, than by the assurance of the working Editor, that they lightened his onerous labors" ("Preface").

16. Augustus Kinsley Gardner, *Old Wine in New Bottles; or, Spare Hours of a Student in Paris* (New York: C. S. Francis & Co.; Boston: J. H. Francis, 1848).

17. [James Jackson], *A Memoir of James Jackson, Jr., M.D., with Extracts from His Letters to His Father; and Medical Cases, Collected by Him* (Boston: I. R. Butts, 1835).

18. William Gibson, *Rambles in Europe in 1839. With Sketches of Prominent Surgeons, Physicians, Medical Schools, Hospitals, Literary Personages, Scenery, Etc.* (Philadelphia: Lea and Blanchard, 1841), p. iv.

19. F. Campbell Stewart, *Eminent French Surgeons, with a Historical and Statistical Account of the Hospitals of Paris; together with Miscellaneous Information and Biographical Notices of the Most Eminent Living Parisian Surgeons* (Buffalo: A. Burke, 1845), p. vii. Stewart first published his observations as *The Hospitals and Surgeons of Paris* (New York: J. and H. G. Langley; Philadelphia: Carey and Hart, 1843).

20. C.G.W. Comegys to Scott Cook, Cincinnati, 20 Apr. 1852, Matthew Scott Cook Papers, OH—Western Reserve Hist. Soc.

21. J. Bell to Usher Parsons, Paris, 14 May 1822, Parsons Family Papers, RI—Brown.

22. Josiah C. Nott to John W. Kirk, Columbia, South Carolina, 18 Aug. 1833, SC—Waring.

23. Samuel Brown, Diary, entry for Paris, 7 July 1824, KY—U. KY.

24. S[amuel] Brown to R. La Roche, Paris, 8 July 1824, R. La Roche Correspondence, PA—CPP.

25. Louis Alexander Dugas to Dear Mama, Paris, 6 July 1829, typescript translation in GA—Med. Coll. GA; and see Robert Peter to Frances Peter, Paris, 27 June 1839, Evans Papers, KY—U. KY; C. T. Jackson to Charles Brown, Paris, 18 Feb. 1830, Charles Thomas Jackson Papers, DC—LC; Henry Bryant to John Bryant, Paris, 1 July 1844, Bryant Papers; Civiale to Isaac Hays Paris, 1 Dec. 1834, and ibid., 16 Jan. 1848, Isaac Hays Papers, PA—APS.

26. George B. Wood, Journal, 15 Apr. 1853 to 19 May 1853, entry for Paris, 11 May 1853, George B. Wood Journals, PA—CPP.

27. Ibid., 25 Aug.–4 Oct. 1853, entries for Paris, 2 and 8 Sept. 1853, and ibid., 8 Oct.–21 Nov. 1860, entry for 4 Nov. 1860. And see Nott, "Letter from Doctor Nott"; Robert Peter to Frances Peter, Paris, 22 June 1839, Evans Papers; Isaac Taylor to Alden March, New York, 8 Sept. 1841, March Papers; and J. M. Warren to J. C. Warren, Paris, 27 Nov. 1832, 9 Jan. 1833, 14 Mar. 1833 and 28 Apr. 1834, in *The Parisian Education of an American Surgeon: Letters of Jonathan Mason Warren (1832–1835)*, ed. Russell M. Jones (Philadelphia:

American Philosophical Society, 1978), pp. 86–89, 95–99, 108–110, 197–202.

28. For example, Benjamin J. Hicks to J. Y. Bassett, Paris, 31 July 1837, John Young Bassett Papers, AL—AL State Arch.

29. Robert Peter to Frances Peter, Paris, 14 July 1839, Evans Papers.

30. Ibid., London, 11 Aug. 1839.

31. Levin S. Joynes to Tho. R. Joynes, Philadelphia, 4 Nov. 1839, Joynes Family Papers.

32. Saml. Hazard [to C. W. Pennock], Extract from the Minutes of a Meeting of the Board of Guardians of the Philadelphia Almshouse, 22 Mar. 1831, C. W. Pennock Papers, PA—APS.

33. The place of museums in nineteenth-century American medical culture deserves vastly more attention than it has received. Suggestive for interpreting the meanings of such collections is Susan Stewart, *On Longing: Narratives of the Miniature, the Gigantic, the Souvenir, the Collection* (Baltimore: Johns Hopkins University Press, 1984; Durham and London: Duke University Press, 1993).

34. Charles T. Jackson to James Jackson, Jr., Vienna, 23 Sept. 1831, Putnam, Jackson and Lowell Papers, MA—MA Hist. Soc.

35. Ibid.

36. James Jackson, Sr., to James Jackson, Jr., Boston, 25 Nov. 1831, James Jackson Papers, MA—Countway.

37. Erwin H. Ackerknecht, *Medicine at the Paris Hospital, 1794–1848* (Baltimore: Johns Hopkins University Press, 1967), p. 158. On the cholera epidemic in Paris, see François Delaporte, *Disease and Civilization: The Cholera in Paris, 1832*, trans. Arthur Goldhammer (Cambridge, Mass., and London: MIT Press, 1986), and Catherine J. Kudlick, *Cholera in Post-Revolutionary Paris: A Cultural History* (Berkeley, Los Angeles, and London: University of California Press, 1996).

38. James Jackson, Jr., to James Jackson Sr., Paris, 1 Apr. 1832, J. Jackson Papers.

39. Ibid., entry for Paris, 3 Apr. 1832, in cholera letter-log dated Paris, 5 Apr. 1832.

40. Ibid., entry for Paris, 5 Apr. 1832.

41. Ibid., entry for Paris, 3 Apr. 1832.

42. Jackson, Jr., to Jackson, Sr., Paris, 8 Apr. 1832.

43. Jackson, Jr., to Jackson, Sr., London, 3 May 1832; and see ibid., 10 May 1832.

44. Jackson, Sr., to Jackson, Jr., Boston, 16 June 1832.

45. Charles T. Jackson to Charles Brown, Missina, 14 Apr. 1832, C. Jackson Papers.

46. A. Smith to James Jackson, Paris, 11 June 1832, Putnam, Jackson and Lowell Papers; and see James Jackson, Jr., to James Jackson, Sr., London, 18 May 1832, J. Jackson Papers.

47. C. W. Pennock and W. W. Gerhard, "Observations on the Cholera of Paris" (Paris, 5 May 1832), *American Journal of the Medical Sciences* 10 (1832): 319–390, p. 319.

48. W. W. Gerhard to James Jackson, Jr., Paris, 26 Aug. 1832, Putnam, Jackson and Lowell Papers.

49. Ibid.

50. See J. L. Cabell to Joseph C. Cabell, Paris, 14 May 1837, James Lawrence Cabell Papers (no. 1640), VA—U. VA, and Edward E. Jenkins to [John Jenkins], Paris, 13 Jan. 1854, Jenkins Papers, SC—U. SC.

51. Levin S. Joynes to Thomas R. Joynes, Paris, 19 Aug. 1841, Joynes Family Papers.

52. Ibid., Dublin, 1 July 1842; and see ibid., Paris, 12 Dec. 1841.

53. Ibid., Paris, 12 Dec. 1841.

54. L. S. Joynes to Louisa A. S. Joynes, Paris, 14 Dec. 1840.

55. Smith to Gerhard, Paris, 6 July 1834.

56. L. A. Dugas to L. Charles Dugas, Paris, 28 July 1829, Dugas Papers, GA—GA Hist. Soc.

57. John Y. Bassett to Theodore Parker, Huntsville, 15 Dec. 1849, Theodore Parker Papers, vol. 8, MA—MA Hist. Soc.

58. G. C. Shattuck, Jr., to Thomas Hun, Boston, 11 Dec. 1839, Thomas Hun Letters, NY—NY State Lib.

59. T. Stewardson to W. W. Gerhard, London, 22 May [1834], Gerhard Papers.

60. Samuel Parkman to Thomas Hun, Boston, 4 June 1839, Hun Letters.

61. Park Benjamin to John O. Sargent, 13 Sept. 1833, quoted in Thomas Franklin Currier, *Bibliography of Oliver Wendell Holmes* (New York: New York University Press, 1953), p. 312.

62. "La Grisette," first published in 1836, began, "Ah Clemence! when I saw thee last / Trip down the Rue de Seine, / And turning, when thy form had past, / I said, 'We will meet again,'— /I dreamed not in that idle glance / Thy latest image came, / And only left to memory's trance / A shadow and a name" (reprinted in *The Poems of Oliver Wendell*

*Holmes* [Boston: Ticknor and Fields, 1864], pp. 38–39).

63. Eleanor Shattuck to George C. Shattuck, Boston, 26 Jan. 1838, vol. 15, Shattuck Papers.

64. Joynes to Joynes, Paris, 12 Dec. 1841.

65. Quoted (and unidentified) family correspondence in Gardner, *Old Wine*, p. 293.

66. John Bryant to Henry Bryant, Boston 1 June 1846, Bryant Papers.

67. J. O. Green to Elisha Bartlett, Lowell, 16 Feb. 1848, Bartlett (Elisha) Family Papers, NY—U. Rochester.

68. Edward E. Jenkins to Mother, Paris, 11 Nov. 1853, Jenkins Papers.

69. Smith to Gerhard, Paris, 6 July 1834.

70. Edward E. Jenkins to [John Jenkins], Paris, 12 Aug. 1853, Jenkins Papers.

71. Note from S. Parkman to Thomas Hun, in Shattuck to Hun, Boston, 11 Dec. 1839, and Samuel Parkman to Thomas Hun, Boston, 29 July 1839, Hun Letters.

72. J. Jackson to C. W. Pennock, Boston, 5 Dec. 1833, Pennock Papers. Jackson had written to his father from Paris, "I believe that in 'Fever' the Plaques de Peyer are as uniformly diseased as the lungs are in Pneumonia—(I believe it, because I have never seen *one* case in wh. they were not, I have never read *one* wh. they were not, I have seen & read *many* in wh. they were—I know of no other evidence than this" (Jackson, Jr., to Jackson, Sr., Paris, 5 Apr. 1833, J. Jackson Papers); and see ibid., Paris, 18 Dec. 1832.

73. William Wood Gerhard, Journal Medical, 11 Mar. 1833–17 Mar. 1839, entries for 10 Apr. 1834 and 17 June 1834, PA—CPP.

74. Alfred Stillé to George C. Shattuck, Philadelphia, 6 Aug. 1842, Shattuck Papers, vol. 17.

75. A. Stillé to George C. Shattuck, Philadelphia, 6 Aug. 1844, Shattuck Papers, vol. 18.

76. Comments of Dr. Bonner, Sr., in J. A. Thacher, "Proceedings of the Cincinnati Academy of Medicine, Regular Meeting, December 5th, 1859," *CLO* 21 (1860): 22–27, p. 25.

77. Elisha Bartlett to John O. Green, Lexington, 18 Mar. 1847, Bartlett Family Papers.

78. Gardner, *Old Wine*, p. 161.

79. Joshua B. Flint, *Address Delivered to the Students of the Louisville Medical Institute, in Presence of the Citizens of the Place, at the Commencement of the Second Session of the Institute,*

November 13th, 1838 (Louisville: Prentice and
Weissenger, 1838), pp. 22–23.

80. C. C[aldwell], "Medicine in Paris"
(London, 29 May 1841), WJMS 4 (1841):
237–240, p. 240.

81. Courtney J. Clark, Notes Taken on
Medical Lectures Given by Chas. Caldwell,
Medical Institute of Louisville, 1841–1842,
entry for 6 Nov. 1841, NC—Duke.

82. A. Stillé to G. C. Shattuck, Philadelphia, 7 May 1842, Shattuck Papers, vol. 17.

83. T. Stewardson to W. W. Gerhard, London, 9 Sept. 1834, Gerhard Papers.

84. Whitfield J. Bell, The College of Physicians of Philadelphia: A Bicentennial History
(Canton, Mass.: Science History Publications,
1987), pp. 61–69.

85. Peter Martin to James Jackson, Sr.,
Reigate, 20 Aug. 1837, J. Jackson Papers.

86. George B. Wood, Diary, 1836–1839,
entry for 1836, PA—APS.

87. Philip Claiborne Gooch, Diary, 20 Feb.
1845–1 Sept. 1848, entry for 10 July 1848,
VA—VA Hist. Soc.

88. J. Y. Bassett to Theodore Parker,
Huntsville, Alabama, 7 Oct. 1849, Parker Papers; and see C. F. Winslow to John Y. Bassett, Nantucket, 22 Nov. 1840, John Young
Bassett Papers, AL—AL State Arch.

89. Gabriel Manigault, Autobiography, transcript, pp. 308–527, SC—U. SC.

90. See Alejandro Bolaños-Geyer, William
Walker: The Gray-Eyed Man of Destiny (Lake
Saint Louis, Mo.: Privately published, 1988);
William O. Scroggs, Filibusteros y financieros:
la historia de William Walker y sus asociados
([Managua]: El Fondo de Promocion, 1974);
and, for an extensive bibliography of studies
on Walker, Rafael Obregón, Costa Rica y la
guerra contra los filibusteros (Alajuela, Costa
Rica: Museo Histórico Cultural Juan San-
tamaría, 1991).

91. John Christopher Faber to Christina
Faber Smith, Paris, 13 Dec. 1837, Elihu
Penquite Smith Papers, SC—U. SC.

92. Ibid., Charleston, 10 Apr. 1840 and 18
Mar. 1841.

93. Ibid., 11 Nov. 1841.

94. Ibid., 24 June 1842.

95. Ibid., 3 Aug. 1842.

96. Oliver W. Holmes to Theodore Parker,
Boston, 14 Sept. 1857, Parker Papers. See
R.-T.-H. Laennec, A Treatise on the Diseases of
the Chest, in Which They Are Described According to Their Anatomical Characteristics, and

Their Diagnosis Established on a New Principle
by Means of Acoustic Instruments, trans. with a
preface and notes by John Forbes (London: T.
and G. Underwood, 1821); the first American
edition was published Philadelphia: J. Webster, 1823.

97. The time he lavished on sorting out
what could be done with the new instrument
is evident in the physical examination of patients recorded in John Forbes, In-Patient
Case Book, 22 Nov. 1826–11 Aug. [1829],
and John Forbes, Out-Patient Prescription
Books, 3 Oct. 1823–2 Feb. 1825, Chichester—
West Sussex RO.

98. Russell C. Maulitz, Morbid Appearances:
The Anatomy of Pathology in the Early Nineteenth Century (Cambridge: Cambridge University Press, 1987), esp. pp. 168–169.

99. F.-J.-V. Broussais, On Irritation and In-
sanity. A Work, wherein the Relations of the
Physical with the Moral Conditions of Man, Are
Established on the Basis of Physiological Medi-
cine, trans. Thomas Cooper, To Which Are
Added Two Tracts on Materialism, and an Out-
line of the Association of Ideas. By Thomas Coo-
per (Columbia, S.C.: S. J. M'Morris, 1831).
And see Thomas Jefferson to Thomas Cooper,
Monticello, 29 Mar. 1824, SC—U. SC.

100. Charles Caldwell to Lemuel Kollock,
Philadelphia, 31 Jan. 1805, Lemuel Kollock Papers, GA—GA Hist. Soc.

101. Ibid., Philadelphia, 2 Oct. 1804.

102. J. Glen to Kollock, Philadelphia, 2
Mar. 1807, Kollock Papers.

103. Subscription list dated Boston, 26
May 1819, MA—Countway. The translation
was published three years later as Xavier Bichat, General Anatomy Applied to Physiology
and Medicine, trans. George Hayward (Boston:
Richardson and Lord, 1822).

104. A. Stillé to G. C. Shattuck, Philadelphia, 1 Sept. 1843, and ibid., 26 Mar. 1844,
Shattuck Papers, vol. 18. And see ibid., 8 Apr.
1841, 7 May 1842, and 21 July 1842, Shattuck
Papers, vol. 17.

105. Dugas to Dear Mama, Paris, 6 July
1829.

106. Parkman to Hun, Boston, 29 July
1839.

107. William Baly to Mother, [London], 15
Aug. [1836], William Baly Papers, London—
RCP.

108. William Baly to Father, [London], 22
Sept. [1836].

109. John H. Packard to G. B. Wood, Phila-

delphia, 6 Jan. 1861, G. B. Wood Misc. Correspondence, PA—CPP.

110. Elisha Bartlett to O. W. Holmes, Baltimore, 13 Jan. 1845; and see Elisha Bartlett to John O. Green, Lexington, 31 Mar. 1843, and Roby to Elisha Bartlett, Boston, 15 Mar. 1845, all in Bartlett Family Papers.

111. J. Bell to R. La Roche, Philadelphia, 2 July 1828, La Roche Correspondence.

112. J. D. Fisher to Isaac Hays, Boston, 17 Oct. 1838, Hays Papers.

113. See, for example, Inventory of the Estate of J.H.P. Shackelford, [1849], Augusta Co., Ala., John H. P. Shackelford Collection, AL—AL State Arch., and S. H. Dickson, Catalogue of Library, 1843, in his Memoranda, SC—Waring.

114. Civiale to R. La Roche, Paris, 8 Mar. 1830, La Roche Correspondence.

115. Paul F. Eve to Monsieur Le Professeur Dobleau, Nashville, Tennessee, n.d., TN—TN State Lib.

116. For example, see Medical College of Ohio, Register of Property in 1847, OH—U. Cincinnati; and Proceedings of the Faculty of the Medical College of Louisiana, May 1835–16 Feb. 1847, entry for 31 Mar. 1841, LA—Tulane Med.

117. Alden March to Dear Sir, 14 July 1830, March Papers.

118. T[heodric] Romeyn Beck to John W. Francis, [Albany, 1812], John W. Francis Papers, NY—NY State Lib.

119. Ibid., [Albany, 1820], 4 July, Francis Papers.

120. K.L.H. to R. La Roche, Philadelphia, 29 Aug. 1828, La Roche Correspondence.

121. A. Brigham to Isaac Hays, New York, 22 June 1838, Hays Papers.

122. Joseph M. Smith to Isaac Hays, New York, 3 Dec. 1834, Hays Papers.

123. Faculty Minutes, Medical Department, University of Louisville, 1857–1891, entry for 30 June 1857, KY—U. Louisville; and see Usher Parsons to Dear Sir, Providence, 12 Jan. 1834, Parsons Papers.

124. See Minute Book of Richmond, Virginia Board of Health, 1 June–11 Aug. 1849, entry of 1 June 1849 and passim, VA—VA Hist. Soc.; and Gooch, Diary, 1 Sept. 1848–16 May 1852, entries for 31 May and 1 June 1849.

125. Ibid., entry for Richmond, 7 June 1849.

126. For the autopsy and letter to Paris, see ibid., 20 May 1849 and 8 Mar. 1850.

127. Ibid., 6 Mar. 1850.

128. Ibid., 31 Mar. 1850.

129. Ibid., 9 Nov. 1850.

130. P. Claiborne Gooch, Richmond, 12 Nov. 1850 (printed circular soliciting subscriptions for the *Stethoscope*, Gooch Family Papers, VA—VA Hist. Soc.).

131. Gooch, Diary, 1 Sept. 1848–16 May 1852, entries for Richmond, 5 Dec. 1850, 26 Nov. 1850, and 1 Jan. 1851.

132. Ibid., 28 Apr. 1852.

133. "The Great Medical Center of the South," *Stethoscope* 2 (1852): 468–476; and see the accusation of "*sectional* rivalry" in "The Stethoscope, and Virginia Medical Gazette," *Western Lancet and Hospital Reporter* 18 (1851): 203.

134. See *Stethoscope* 1 (1851), title page.

135. Undated manuscript, Gooch Family Papers.

136. Quotations are from R[obert] W[illiam] Haxall, Richmond, 12 Sept. 1849; Ch. Bell Gibson to Sirs, 7 Sept. 1849; Edw. H. Carmichael to Doctor Crous, Richmond, 8 Sept. 1849; others include James Beale to P. C. Gooch, Richmond, 15 Sept. 1849; R[ichard] L[afou] Bohannon, Richmond, 15 Sept. 1849; Corbin Braxton, 24 Sept. 1849; J. L. Cabell to the Faculty of the Medical Department of the University of Missouri, University of Virginia, 20 Sept. 1849; and Carter P[age] Johnson to the Dean of the Medical Faculty of the University of Missouri, Richmond, 10 Sept. 1849; all are in Gooch Papers, VA—VA Hist. Soc.

137. This pattern was common in self-presentation as well; see, for example, Francis Peyre Porcher to the Trustees and Faculty of the Medical College of the State of South Carolina, Charleston South Bay, June 1866, Francis Peyre Porcher Letters, SC—U. SC; James L. Cabell to Chapman Johnson, Member of the Board of Visitors of the University of Virginia, Paris, 14 May 1837, Cabell Papers; and manuscript sheet announcing that "Dr W W Gerhard will return to this country by the 1st of October next," Sept. 1844, Gerhard Papers.

138. Russell M. Jones, "American Doctors in Paris, 1820–1861: A Statistical Profile," *Journal of the History of Medicine and Allied Sciences* 25 (1970): 143–157, on pp. 151–152. Jones's sample had an inbuilt bias favoring physicians who became prominent.

139. William G. Rothstein, *American Physicians in the Nineteenth Century: From Sects to*

*Science* (Baltimore and London: Johns Hopkins University Press, 1972), p. 92.

140. J. P. Kirtland to S. P. Hildreth, Cincinnati, 8 Nov. 1837, Samuel P. Hildreth Papers, OH—Marietta Coll.; John D. Fisher to Isaac Hays, Boston, 5 Dec. 1838, Hays Papers.

141. Oliver H. Stout to James S. Taliaferro, Lexington, 16 Mar. 1822, Zachariah and James G. Taliaferro Papers, LA-LSU.

142. University of Pennsylvania, Minutes of the Medical Faculty, vol. 4, 1846–1853, entry for meeting of 7 Feb. 1852, PA—U. PA Arch. The books were by Hermann Pidoux and Armand Trousseau.

143. J. Jackson to W. W. Gerhard, Waltham, Mass., 4 Sept. 1834, Gerhard Papers. On students buying texts, see for example J. L. Cabell to Joseph C. Cabell, Baltimore, 29 Jan. 1834, Cabell Papers.

144. For example, James W. Dunklin to N[athaniel] E. McLeeland, Lowndes Co., Alabama, 3 May 1830, McCleeland Family Papers, NC—SHC.

145. Samuel Brown to Orlando Brown, Lexington, 20 Jan. 1821, Orlando Brown Papers, KY—Filson Club.

146. "The following is a list of Books required to be read by the Medical Student in order to a by Law of the Massachusetts Medical Society," one New York medical student recorded in his class notebook (Thomas A. Brayton, Notes taken on Medical Lectures Given by Drs. Batchelor, Childs, and Dewey, New York, 1822, Thomas Brayton Papers, NY—NY Pub. Lib.).

147. "Massachusetts Medical Society," *BMSJ* 14 (1836): 113.

148. And see Baltimore Pathological Society Minutes, 2 vols., 1853–1858, vol. 1, entry for 4 June 1855, NC—Duke, and Robert Peter to Frances Peter, Paris, 27 June 1839, Evans Papers.

149. George Lord to Melvin Lord, Paris, 9 Oct. 1844, Evans Papers; Samuel A. Cartwright to Wm. N. Mercer, Paris, 2 Jan. 1837, William Newton Mercer Papers, LA—Tulane; John Moffatt Howe, Diary of a Trip to Europe, June–Sept. 1838, BV Howe, NY—NY Hist. Soc.; George B. Wood, Journal, 25 Mar.–28 Aug. 1862, entries for 9 Apr., 11 Apr., 16 Apr., and 3–4 May 1862; J. Howard to Usher Parsons, Genoa, 10 Apr. 1828, Parsons Papers. The travel of these American health-seekers to Europe deserves investigation.

150. Tho. Harris, Thuiry[?—illegible] Neill, and Ch. D. Meigs to R. La Roche, Philadelphia, 8 May 1827, La Roche Correspondence.

151. Franklin Bache to George B. Wood, Philadelphia, 31 Aug. 1842, Wood Misc. Correspondence.

152. For example, John Leonard Riddell, Notes Taken on Lectures Delivered at the Medical College of Ohio, 1834–1835, notes on practice by Eberle, John Leonard Riddell Volumes, vol. 26, LA—Tulane; Michael William Holt, Notes Taken on Lectures Given by Samuel Jackson, Philadelphia, 1836–1837, Michael William Holt Notes, NC—Duke; R. T. Dismukes, Notes Taken on Lectures Given by [B. W.] Dudley, Transylvania University, 1838–1839, NC—Duke; Benjm. S. Downing, Notes Taken on Lectures Given by Joseph Mather Smith on the Theory and Practice of Medicine, College of Physicians and Surgeons at the University of the State of New York, 1826, NY—Columbia Med.; Titus Munson Coan, Notes Taken on Lectures Given by Alonzo Clark, College of Physicians and Surgeons, New York, 1859–1860, BV Coan, NY—NY Hist. Soc.

153. The same pattern is also clear in the practice of young graduates whose professors had Parisian experience. Following a common course, one Albany graduate in practice only seventeen months wrote back to his professor, Paris-experienced Thomas Hun, asking advice about a difficult case. No doubt echoing his teacher's precepts, he reported that in cases of typhoid fever, "I have no routine method of treatment. I endeavor to adapt the treatment to the nature of the case. As a general rule, when there is no complication that I can discover, I follow Andral's expectant method, and thus far I have been successful" (Robert Morris, Jun. to Prof. Thos. Hun, Hammond, 30 Dec. 1847, Hun Letters).

CHAPTER 5
TELLING A HISTORICAL STORY

1. George H. Daniels, *American Science in the Age of Jackson* (London and New York: Columbia University Press, 1968), esp. pp. 63–85; Theodore Dwight Bozeman, *Protestants in an Age of Science: The Baconian Ideal and Antebellum American Religious Thought* (Chapel Hill: University of North Carolina Press, 1977).

2. See John Harley Warner, *The Therapeutic Perspective: Medical Practice, Knowledge, and Identity in America, 1820–1885* (Cambridge, Mass., and London: Harvard University Press, 1986), pp. 162–184.

3. J. Jackson to C. W. Pennock, Boston, 5 Dec. 1833, C. W. Pennock Papers, PA—APS.

4. For example, C. F. Winslow to John Y. Bassett, Nantucket, 22 Nov. 1840, John Young Bassett Papers, AL—AL State Arch.; Valliex to G. Shattuck, [Paris], 8 Sept. 1841, Shattuck Papers, vol. 17, MA—MA Hist. Soc.; E. Rufz to W. W. Gerhard, [Paris] 6 Nov. n.y., W. W. Gerhard Papers, PA—CPP; G. C. Shattuck to Thomas Hun, Boston, 11 Dec. 1839, Thomas Hun Letters, NY—NY State Lib.; T. Stewardson to W. W. Gerhard, London, 22 May [1834], Gerhard Papers; J. Jackson to W. W. Gerhard, Boston, 26 Oct. 1835, in ibid.

5. For example, James Hamilton to G. C. Shattuck, Dublin, 20 Jan. 1840, and Shattuck Papers, vol. 16, and Samuel Wigglesworth to Thomas Wigglesworth, Paris, 9 Jan. 1836, Wigglesworth Letters, NY—NY Acad. Med.

6. W. W. Gerhard to P. Louis, Philadelphia, 23 Apr. 1848, G. B. Wood Misc. Correspondence, PA—CPP; and see Louis to [Wood], 18 July [1848], in ibid.

7. For example, Alfred Stillé to R. La Roche, Philadelphia, 12 May 1860, R. La Roche Correspondence, PA—CPP; and see J. C. W[arren], "Foreign Correspondence.—Parisian Hospitals" (Paris, 30 Dec. 1837), *BMSJ* 18 (1838): 42–46, p. 44.

8. James Jackson, Jr., to James Jackson, Sr., Paris, 20 Apr. 1833, James Jackson Papers, MA—Countway.

9. W. W. Gerhard to J. Jackson, Paris, 13 Aug. 1833, Putnam, Jackson and Lowell Papers, MA—MA Hist. Soc.

10. John Hamilton to G. C. Shattuck, Dublin, 1 Mar. 1841, Shattuck Papers, vol. 17; and see "Dr. Shattuck's Translation of M. Louis," *BMSJ* 21 (1839): 294, and [P.] Louis to [H. I. Bowditch], Paris, 30 May 1836, MA—Countway. See P.-Ch.-A. Louis, *Anatomical, Pathological and Therapeutic Researches on the Yellow Fever of Gibraltar of 1828*, trans. G. C. Shattuck, Jr. (Boston: C. C. Little and J. Brown, 1839).

11. David W. Yandell, "Notes on Medical Matters and Medical Men in Paris" (Paris, July 1847), *WJMS*, n.s., 8 (1847): 369–395, p. 374.

12. Henry Bryant to John Bryant, Paris, 24 Mar. 1844, William Sohier Bryant Papers (MS 45), MA—New England Hist. Gen. Soc. For a seconding of this appraisal of Louis, see Yandell, "Notes on Medical Matters," p. 376.

13. Henry Bryant to John Bryant, Paris, 2 May 1844, Bryant Papers; ibid., entry for 21 May in letter of 17 May 1844. And see ibid., Paris, 9 June 1844.

14. Ibid., entry for 18 May in letter begun 17 May 1844.

15. A. Stillé to G. C. Shattuck, Philadelphia, 24 Oct. 1844, Shattuck Papers, vol. 17.

16. John P. Barratt, "An Address Delivered before the Medical Society, of Abbeville District, S. C. at Their Second Anniversary, in May, 1837," *Southern Medical and Surgical Journal* 2 (1838): 585–594, p. 588.

17. L. M. Whiting, "Investigation of Disease," *BMSJ* 14 (1836): 181–190, p. 181; emphasis removed.

18. C. D., Review of "*A Treatise on Pathological Anatomy. By G. Andral,*" *American Journal of the Medical Sciences* 9 (1831): 389–419, pp. 389, 389, 389, 389, 390, 391–392. The "French school," he went on, citing in particular Laennec, Louis, Andral, and Cruveilhier, were "giving to the healing art the stability of a science, and to the practitioner surer and more palpable principles of conduct at the bed-side of sickness" (p. 391).

19. Alfred Stillé, *Elements of General Pathology: A Practical Treatise* (Philadelphia: Lindsay and Blackiston, 1848), p. 27.

20. Ibid., p. 34.

21. Ibid., p. 35.

22. Ibid., pp. 31, 163.

23. Lundsford P. Yandell, Notes Taken on Lectures Given at Transylvania University, introductory lecture of Caldwell, 7 Nov. 1825, Daniel Drake Papers, Emmet Field Horine Collection, KY—U. KY.

24. John A. Lyle, "Exclusive Systems of Medicine" (M.D. thesis, Transylvania University, 1841), KY—Transylvania.

25. John Williams, "Systems of Medicine" (M.D. thesis, Transylvania University, 1842), KY—Transylvania.

26. Brett Randolph, "Violation of the Natural Laws" (M.D. thesis, Transylvania University, 1848), KY—Transylvania.

27. Henry J. Hawley, "Science vs. Empiricism" (M.D. thesis, Albany Medical College, 1850), NY—Albany Med.

28. D. Bryan Baker, "Medical Reform"

(M.D. thesis, Albany Medical College, 1843), NY—Albany Med.

29. S. C. Furman, "The Improvements to the Progress of Medical Science" (M.D. thesis, Medical College of the State of South Carolina, 1852), SC—Waring.

30. George K. G. Todd, "Young Physic" (M.D. thesis, Transylvania University, 1848), KY—Transylvania.

31. See Russell C. Maulitz, *Morbid Appearances: The Anatomy of Pathology in the Nineteenth Century* (Cambridge: Cambridge University Press, 1987), pp. 109–229.

32. "Medical Reform.—Minutes of the Proceedings of the Medico-Chirurgical Society of Cincinnati," *WL* 6 (1847): 220–226, p. 222.

33. G[eorge] Watson to Joseph Shelton Watson, Edinburgh, 25 Sept. 1805, Watson Family Papers, VA—VA Hist. Soc.

34. Robert Peter to Frances Peter, London, 11 Aug. 1839, Evans Papers, KY—U. KY.

35. B. B. Smith, "What of Theory!" (M.D. Thesis, University of Nashville, 1857), TN—Vanderbilt.

36. Austin Flint, "Foreign Correspondence" (Paris, 18 June 1854), *WJMS* 2 (1854): 89–99, p. 98.

37. Henry Gilson, "Medical Science" (M.D. thesis, Albany Medical College, 1840), NY—Albany Med.

38. Victor J. Fouregaud, "An Introductory Lecture on the History of Medicine, Delivered on the 23d December, 1845, before the Medico-Chirugical Society of St. Louis, Mo.," *SLMSJ* 4 (1847): 481–496, p. 482.

39. Review of "*The Writings of Hippocrates and Galen*. Epitomised from the Original Latin Translations. By John Redman Coxe," *WJMS*, ser. 2, 5 (1846): 485–515, p. 507.

40. Eugene Henderson, "Honorable Medicine" (M.D. thesis, University of Nashville, 1858), TN—Vanderbilt.

41. Marvin Meyes long ago made this suggestion in *The Jacksonian Persuasion: Politics and Belief* (Stanford: Stanford University Press, 1951). See also Lawrence Frederick Kohl, *The Politics of Individualism: Parties and the American Character in the Jacksonian Era* (New York and Oxford: Oxford University Press, 1989), and Lewis Perry, *Boats against the Current: American Culture between Revolution and Modernity, 1820–1860* (New York and Oxford: Oxford University Press, 1993).

42. Erwin H. Ackerknecht, "Elisha Bartlett and the Philosophy of the Paris Clinical School," *Bulletin of the History of Medicine* 24 (1950): 43–60, pp. 43, 60.

43. Elisha Bartlett, address that begins "Gentlemen of the Class," n.d. Bartlett (Elisha) Family Papers, NY—U. Rochester.

44. Elisha Bartlett, *An Essay on the Philosophy of Medical Science* (Philadelphia: Lea and Blanchard, 1844), p. 182. On the distribution of the text, including three copies sent to Louis, see Elisha Bartlett to Gentlemen [his publishers], Lowell, 3 Sept. 1844, Gratz Collection, PA—Hist. Soc. PA.

45. Bartlett, *Philosophy of Medical Science*, p. 218.

46. Ibid., pp. 201, 290.

47. Ibid., p. 205.

48. Ibid., p. 224; uppercasing not reproduced.

49. E. Leigh, "The Philosophy of Medical Science, Considered with Special Reference to Dr. Elisha Bartlett's 'Essay on the Philosophy of Medical Science,'" *BMSJ* 48 (1853): 69–74, 89–95, 115–121, p. 71; "Review of Elisha Bartlett, *An Essay on the Philosophy of Medical Science* (1844)," *WL* 3 (1844–1845): 386–388, p. 387.

50. J.C.N., Review of "An Essay on the Philosophy of Medical Science, by Elisha Bartlett," *New Orleans Medical Journal* 1 (1844): 490–494, pp. 491, 492.

51. Stillé to Shattuck, Philadelphia, 24 Oct. 1844.

52. Elisha Bartlett, *A Discourse on the Times, Character and Writings of Hippocrates. Read before the Trustees, Faculty and Medical Class of the College of Physicians and Surgeons, at the Opening of the Term of 1852–3* (New York: H. Baillière, 1852), pp. 23, 23, 24, 25, 25, 25–26.

53. Ibid., pp. 47, 35, 47.

54. F.-J.-V. Broussais, *History of Phlegmasiae or Chronic Inflammations, Founded on Clinical Experience and Pathological Anatomy, Exhibiting a View of the Different Varieties of and Complications of These Diseases, with Their Various Methods of Treatment*, trans. from the 4th French ed. by Isaac Hays and R. Eglesfeld Griffith, vol. 2 (Philadelphia: Carey and Lea, 1831), p. 10; and see p. xx.

55. Ibid., p. 10.

56. See Erwin H. Ackerknecht, *Medicine at the Paris Hospital, 1794–1848* (Baltimore: Johns Hopkins University Press, 1967), pp. 61–80; idem, "Broussais or a Forgotten Medical Revolution," *Bulletin of the History of Medi-*

*cine* 27 (1953): 320–343; Jean-François Braunstein, *Broussais et le matérialisme: médecine et philosophie au XIXe siècle* (Paris: Meridiens Klinksieck, 1986); Michel Foucault, *Birth of the Clinic: An Archaelology of Medical Perception*, trans. A. M. Sheridan Smith (first French ed. 1963; New York: Pantheon Books, 1973), pp. 184–192; Michel Valentin, *François Broussais, 1772–1838: empereur de la médecine* (Cesson-Sévigné: La Presse de Bretagne, 1988); and Elizabeth Williams, *The Physical and the Moral: Anthropology, Physiology, and Philosophical Medicine in France, 1750–1850* (Cambridge: Cambridge University Press, 1994), pp. 166–175.

57. E. D. Faust, Review of *"Exposition des Principles de la Nouvelle Doctrine Médicale, avec un précis des thèses soutenues sur ses différentes parties. Par. J. M. A. Goupil,"* *American Journal of the Medical Sciences* 8 (1831): 156–158, pp. 156, 156. For Hays's translations, see Broussais, *History of Phlegmasiae*, and idem, *Principles of Physiological Medicine, in the Form of Propositions*, trans. Isaac Hays and R. Eglesfeld Griffith (Philadelphia: Carey and Lea, 1832).

58. Reginald Horsman, *Josiah Nott of Mobile: Southerner, Physician, and Racial Theorist* (Baton Rouge and London: Louisiana State University Press, 1987), p. 4; on Josiah's later studies in Paris, see pp. 43–52. And see J.-M.-A. Goupil, *The Exposition of the Principles of the New Medical Doctrine, with an Analysis of the Thesis Sustained on Its Different Parts. To Which is Appended a Short Essay on Leeches*, trans. Josiah C. Nott (Columbia: Times and Gazette Office, 1831).

59. See, for example, Pierre-Frédéric Thomas (de Royan, Départment de la Charente-Inférieure) ... (Président de la Société médicale de la Nouvelle-Orléans), *Considérations sur la maladie connue sons le nom de fièvre jaune. Thèses pour le Doctorat en Médecine, présentée et soutenue à la Faculté de Médecine de Paris* (Paris: Pidot le Jeune, 1834), which Thomas dedicated to Broussais (LA—LA Coll.).

60. See Edward H. Barton, *The Application of Physiological Medicine to the Diseases of Louisiana* (Philadelphia: Skerrett, 1832), and L. J. Bégin, *Application of the Physiological Doctrine to Surgery*, trans. Wm. Sims Reynolds (Charleston: E. J. Van Brunt, 1835).

61. James Norcom to Benjamin Rush Norcom, Edenton, N.C., 1 Jan. 1832, Dr.

James Norcom and Family Papers, NC—NC State Arch.

62. W. S. Sobdell to William Abell, St. Francisville, [La.], 7 Sept. 1831, Abell Family Papers, NY—Cornell.

63. J[ohn] Bell to R. La Roche, Philadelphia, 2 July 1828, La Roche Correspondence; and see John D. Goodman to Isaac Hays, New York, 2 Jan. 1827, Isaac Hays Papers, PA—APS; F.-J.-V. Broussais, *On Irritation and Insanity*, trans. Thomas Cooper (Charleston: J. J. M'Morris, 1831); Broussais, *History of Phlegmasiae*; idem, *Principles of Physiological Medicine*; and idem, *Cholera. Two Clinical Lectures upon the Nature, Treatment, and Symptoms of spasmodic Cholera*, trans. John S. Bartlett (New York: W. Stodart, 1832).

64. For example, John Y. Bassett to Marguerite Bassett, Paris, 5 Sept. 1836, Bassett Papers.

65. For example, Benjamin J. Hicks to John Y. Bassett, Paris, 31 July 1837, Bassett Papers; John Leonard Riddell, Journal commenced Worthington, Ohio, 1832, John Leonard Riddell Manuscript Volumes, vol. 5, LA—Tulane; James W. Dunklin to N[athaniel] E. McClelland, Lowndes Co., Ala., 3 May 1830, McClelland Family Papers, NC—SHC; John P. Schermerhorn, Notes Taken on Dr. Stevens's Lectures on Surgery, 1829–1830, BV Schermerhorn, NY—NY Hist. Soc.; Benjm. S. Downing, Notes Taken on Lectures Given by Joseph Mather Smith on the Theory and Practice of Medicine, College of Physicians and Surgeons at the University of the State of New York, vol. 1, 1826, NY—Columbia Med.; D. Drake to Isaac Hays, New York, 12 Feb. 1831, Hays Papers.

66. H. I. Bowditch, Notes Taken on Lectures Given by [James] Jackson, Boston, 1831–1832, MA—Countway; John Leonard Riddell, Notes Taken on Lectures Given on Practice by Eberle, Medical College of Ohio, 1834–1835, Riddell Volumes, vol. 26; John Custis Darby, Medical Notebook, Lexington, Kentucky, 1839–1846, Notes Taken on Lectures on Surgery Given by Dudley, 1839, NC—Duke Med.

67. With Broussais, Barratt urged, "the light of philosophic truth bursts through the accumulated mists of ages, and sheds its general influence on our too long and too much benighted profession" ("Address," p. 590).

68. James Jackson, Jr., to James Jackson, Sr., Paris, 13 Nov. 1832, J. Jackson Papers.

69. T. Stewardson to W. W. Gerhard, Paris, 22 Mar. 1834, Gerhard Papers.

70. J. M. Warren to J. C. Warren, Paris, 23 Mar. 1834, in Russell M. Jones, ed., *The Parisian Education of an American Surgeon: Letters of Jonathan Mason Warren (1832–1835)* (Philadelphia: American Philosophical Society, 1978), pp. 185–188, on p. 187.

71. T. Stewardson to W. W. Gerhard, London, 9 Sept. 1834, Gerhard Papers.

72. Pierre Louis, *Examen de l'examen de M. Broussais relativement à la phthisie et à l'affection typhoïde* (Paris: J. B. Baillière, 1834).

73. Joshua B. Flint, *Address Delivered to the Students of the Louisville Medical Institute, in Presence of the Citizens of the Place, at the Commencement of the Second Session of the Institute, November 13th, 1838* (Louisville: Prentice and Weissenger, 1838), p. 20.

74. Elisha B. Stedman, "The Theory of Broussais" (M.D. thesis, Transylvania University, 1835), KY—Transylvania.

75. For example, John C. Cardwell, Notes Taken on Lectures Given by James Conquest Gross, Transylvania University Medical Department, Lexington, Kentucky, 1843–1844, Drake Papers; and John H. Claiborne, Notes Taken on Lectures on Physiology Given by James D. Cabell, [University of Virginia], 1849 (no. 337), VA—U. VA.

76. "From the Medical Examiner. Death of Broussais," *Southern Medical and Surgical Journal* 3 (1839): 318–320, pp. 319, 320; and see A. Stillé to G. C. Shattuck, Philadelphia, 24 May 1842, Shattuck Papers, vol. 17; and Jacob Bigelow, "Introductory Lecture, Delivered at the Medical College, Boston, November 6th," *BMSJ* 31 (1844–1845): 329–336, p. 332.

77. M. L. L[inton], "Medicine in Paris" (Paris, 25 July 1840), *WJMS* 2 (1840): 69–73, pp. 69, 70, 72, 72.

78. Review of "*The History, Diagnosis and Treatment of the Fevers of the United States*. By Elisha Bartlett," *CMJR* 3 (1848): 171–185, p. 171.

79. A[yres] P[hillips] Merrill to R. La Roche, Memphis, 15 Jan. 1857, and Memphis, 15 May 1857, La Roche Correspondence.

80. "Letter from Dr. Cartwright" (Saml. A. Cartwright to Rezin Thompson, New Orleans, 15 June 1856), *Nashville Journal of Medicine and Surgery* 1 (1851): 212–216, p. 213; and see S. P. Crawford, "Southern Medical Litera-

ture," *Nashville Medical and Surgical Journal* 18 (1860): 195–198.

81. Alexander Means, "An Address, Introductory to the Second Course of Lectures in the Atlanta Medical College," *Atlanta Medical and Surgical Journal* 1 (1855–1856): 707–723, p. 707. The development of this theme by southern physicians is explored in John Harley Warner, "The Idea of Southern Medical Distinctiveness: Medical Knowledge and Practice in the Old South," in *Science and Medicine in the Old South*, ed. Ronald L. Numbers and Todd L. Savitt (Baton Rouge and London: Louisiana State University Press, 1989), pp. 179–205.

82. W. Taylor, "Annual Oration," *Transactions of the Medical Association of the State of Alabama at Its Eighth Annual Session, Begun and Held in the City of Mobile, February 5,-6,-7, 1855* (Mobile: Middleton, Harris and Company, 1855), p. 120.

83. Means, "Address," p. 708.

84. Samuel A. Cartwright, "Malum Egyptiàcum, Cold Plague, Diphtheria, or Black Tongue," *NOMSJ* 16 (1859): 378–388, 797–821, p. 815.

85. Taylor, "Annual Oration," p. 120.

86. [Robley] Dunglison, *An Introductory Lecture to the Course of Institutes of Medicine, &c. in Jefferson Medical College, Delivered Nov. 4, 1844* (Philadelphia: B. E. Smith, 1844), p. 15.

87. Ibid., p. 16.

88. Ibid., p. 17.

89. Ibid., pp. 20–21.

90. Ibid., pp. 24, 20.

91. Flint, *Address*, p. 20.

92. Ibid.

93. Ibid., p. 21.

94. Ibid.

95. Ibid., pp. 21, 23, 22.

96. Ibid., pp. 26, 27.

97. Ibid., pp. 21, 28.

98. Dunglison, *Introductory Lecture*, p. 19.

99. L. M. Lawson, "Remarks on the Treatment of the Inflammation, with Special Reference to Pneumonia," *American Journal of the Medical Sciences* 77 (1860): 17–42, p. 17.

100. H.I.B., "Medical and Physiological Commentaries," *BMSJ* 23 (1840–1841): 73–84, 89–98, 106–110, p. 73.

101. "Dr. Paine's Reply to H.I.B.," *BMSJ* 23 (1840–1841): 185–193, 201–210, 217–221, 233–239, 269–278, 329–331, p. 235. And see

Martyn Paine, *Medical and Physiological Commentaries*, 2 vols. (New York: Collins, Keese and Co.; London: John Churchill, 1840), and a third volume bearing the same title (New York: Printed for the Author, 1841–1844).

102. Hamilton to Shattuck, Dublin, 1 Mar. 1841.

103. [P.] Louis to [H. I. Bowditch], Paris, 3 June 1841, MA—Countway. On Bowditch's defense, see Bowditch, "Medical and Physiological Commentaries"; M.C.R. to [Elisha Bartlett], Hanover, 6 Sept. 1847, Bartlett Family Papers; and A. Stillé to G. C. Shattuck, Philadelphia, 26 Mar. 1844, and ibid., Philadelphia, 24 Oct. 1844, Shattuck Papers, vol. 17.

104. Elisha Bartlett to L. M. Lawson, Lexington, 8 Jan. 1847, Bartlett Family Papers.

CHAPTER 6
"THEY MANAGE THESE THINGS BETTER IN
FRANCE": POLITY AND REFORM

1. On the migration of English students to Paris, see Pierre Huard and Mirko D. Grmek, "Les élèves étrangers de Laennec," *Revue d'histoire des sciences* 26 (1973): 315–337, and Russell C. Maulitz, *Morbid Appearances: The Anatomy of Pathology in the Early Nineteenth Century* (Cambridge: Cambridge University Press, 1987), esp. pp. 134–157. I draw heavily in this section on John Harley Warner, "The Idea of Science in English Medicine: The 'Decline of Science' and the Rhetoric of Reform, 1815–45," in *British Medicine in an Age of Reform*, ed. Roger French and Andrew Wear (London: Routledge, 1991), pp. 136–164.

2. William Baly to Mother, Paris, 2 Feb. [1835]; and see ibid., 7 Jan. 1835, in William Baly Papers, London—RCP.

3. John Dunlop, Journal, 1845–1846, entry for Paris, 24 Oct. 1845, Edinburgh—Nat. Lib. Scotland. The underlying message was a common one; as one class of English medical students were told in 1839, "More may be learnt of the true nature, progress, principles, and treatment of disease, by three months spent in the hospitals of Paris, than in three sessions devoted to many of the London institutions" (Rutherford Alcock, "Observations on Clinical Instruction. *The Substance of an Introductory Lecture to the Course of Surgery, at Sydenham College School of Medicine*," *Lancet* 1 [1839–1840]: 694–700, p. 700).

4. See, for example, certificates for John

Griffith Leete, 1830, in Leete Correspondence (Markham Papers 1941/4 and 22), Northampton—Northamptons. RO, and John Liddell Robinson, 1845, in Miscellaneous Papers (D/X 376/18), Durham—Durham RO.

5. Benjamin Phillips to Henry Daniel, Paris, 29 May 1830, Bristol Infirmary Biographical Memoirs, vol. 10 (1825–1830), Bristol—Bristol RO.

6. John Green Crosse, "Lettre 12ème," Paris, 26 Jan. 1815, in "Letters from Paris," 1814–1815, 2 vols., vol. 1, John Green Crosse Papers (MS 473, T132F, L8510), Norwich—Norfolk RO.

7. Crosse, "Lettre 6ème," Paris, [Jan. 1815], and "Lettre 10ème," Paris, 21 Jan. 1815, in ibid.

8. Crosse to Dear Shaw, "Lettre 8ème," Paris, [Jan.] 1815, in ibid.

9. Crosse, "Lettre 16ème," in ibid., vol. 2 (MS 474, T132F, L8511).

10. Crosse, "Lettre 12ème," Paris, 26 Jan. 1815, in ibid., vol. 1.

11. J. H. James, Diary, Paris, 1815, John Haddy James Papers (64/8/8/10), Exeter—Devon RO. His military service and studies in Paris are recounted in Richard Gough to the Governors of the Devon and Exeter Infirmary, London, 27 May 1816, James Papers (64/8/8/7).

12. J. H. James to Benjamin Fuller, [Paris], 18 Oct. 1815, James Papers (64/8/8/10).

13. For accounts written in Paris, see, for example, Anglais, "Paris Letter" (Paris, 12 Jan. 1831 and 9 Feb. 1831), *LMG* 7 (1830–1831): 534–536, 659–662; "Copy of a Letter to a Physician, on the Comparative Positions of the Medical Profession in France and England" (Mountaubon, France, 10 May 1828), *Lancet* 2 (1827–1828): 586–588; "The French Schools," *Lancet* 11 (1826–1827): 107–109, 258–259, 445–448, 569–571, 699–701; "Medical Letters from Paris," *Quarterly Journal of Foreign Medicine and Surgery* 2 (1819–1820): 256–266; and Viator, "Present State of Medicine in Paris" (Paris, 2 Jan. 1828), *LMG* 1 (1827–1828): 177–179.

14. T. Pridgin Teale, Notes on Paris Hospitals, commenced 26 Jan. 1856, entry for Paris, 26 Jan. 1856 (MS 563), Leeds—U. Leeds. Such complaints were voiced about the London hospitals as well. One British observer at Guy's Hospital in 1833 commented in his journal that "I know not how sufficiently to express my abhorrence of the manner in which

the students rushed through the wards and crowded round the wretched patients, thrusting, and elbowing and sometimes standing upon the truckle of the sufferer; what a mockery of misery!" (Thomas Laycock, Journal, 1833–[1857] [Gen. 1813], entry for London, 30 Sept. 1833, Edinburgh—U. Edinburgh).

15. See William Baly to Mother, Paris, 7 Dec. 1834 and 2 Feb. [1835], Baly Papers; "Medical Schools of Paris" (extract of letter from Paris), *LMG* 1 (1827–1828): 31–32; Teale, Notes on Paris Hospitals, entries for 1 and 8 Feb. 1857; and J[ohn] Thomson to Margaret Thomson, Paris, 13 Aug. 1814, Thomson Papers (Gen. 1813), Edinburgh—Nat. Lib. Scotland.

16. Broadside headed "Medical Education, in Paris" (and, on the verso, "Outline of the Advantages Enjoyed by Medical Students *In Paris*"); n.d., but the testimonial is dated 14 Dec. 1827, NY—NY Acad. Med.

17. Maulitz, *Morbid Appearances*, p. 227.

18. Adrian Desmond, *The Politics of Evolution: Morphology, Medicine, and Reform in Radical London* (Chicago: University of Chicago Press, 1989).

19. "Parallel between the English and French Hospitals," *Lancet* 1 (1837–1838): 314–317, on pp. 314, 315.

20. "Medical Reform—Education," *LMG* 11 (1832–1833): 89–92, on pp. 89, 90.

21. Of a large literature on professional structure and reform in English medicine during the first half of the nineteenth century, especially helpful are S.W.F. Holloway, "Medical Education in England, 1830–1858: A Sociological Analysis," *History* 49 (1964): 299–324; Ian Inkster, "Marginal Men: Aspects of the Social Role of the Medical Community in Sheffield 1790–1850," in *Health Care and Popular Medicine in Nineteenth Century England*, ed. John Woodward and David Richards (London: Croom Helm, 1977), pp. 128–163; Irvine Loudon, *Medical Care and the General Practitioner 1750–1850* (Oxford: Clarendon Press, 1986); M. Jeanne Peterson, *The Medical Profession in Mid-Victorian London* (Berkeley, Los Angeles, and London: University of California Press, 1978); Matthew Ramsey, "The Politics of Professional Monopoly in Nineteenth-Century Medicine: The French Model and Its Rivals," in *Professions and the French State, 1700–1900*, ed. Gerald L. Geison (Philadelphia: University of Pennsylvania Press, 1984),

pp. 225–305; Edwina Sherrington, "Thomas Wakley and Reform, 1823–62" (D. Phil. thesis, University of Oxford, 1973); and Ivan Waddington, *The Medical Profession in the Industrial Revolution* (Dublin: Gull & Macmillan, 1984).

22. "The Medical Practitioners Act," *Lancet* 2 (1858): 147–149, p. 148. See especially Loudon, *Medical Care and the General Practitioner*, pp. 297–301, and other sources cited in n. 21.

23. "Fundamental Government of the Profession," *MT* 5 (1841–1842): 6–7, p. 6; my italics.

24. "Medical Reform in France," *Lancet* 1 (1847): 681–683, p. 683.

25. On the use of the decline argument to further provincial interests, see, for example, [William Sands Cox], *Remarks on the Importance of Extending the Means for the Cultivation of Medical Science in Birmingham, by One of the Lecturers of the School of Medicine* (Birmingham: J. C. Barlow, 1831), and "*An Address Delivered to the Members of the Worcestershire Natural History Society, &c.*, By Charles Hastings, M.D.," *British Annals of Medicine* 1 (1837): 656–657.

26. Of a large literature on the decline-of-science controversy, particularly helpful is Susan Faye Cannon, *Science in Culture: The Early Victorian Period* (New York: Dawson and Science History Publications, 1978).

27. "State of Medical Science in England," *LMG* 7 (1830–1831): 274–278, pp. 275, 278.

28. "The French Hospitals and Medical Schools," *MT* 1 (1839–1840): 2–4, p. 4.

29. "The National Association of General Practitioners," *MT* 13 (1845–1846): 176–177, p. 176.

30. "Dinner of Medical Practitioners. British Medical Association," *Lancet* 1 (1836–1837): 224–230, p. 226. The connection between science and the corporate aspirations of general practitioners was made in some of the earliest clear demands to put general practitioners on an equal footing with physicians and surgeons; see, for example, Edward Barlow to [Samuel Whitbread], Bath, 30 Dec. 1813, in Samuel Whitbread Correspondence (W 1/4632), by the kind permission of Mr. S. C. Whitbread, Bedford—Bedfords. RO.

31. "Anatomical Report," *LMG* 2 (1828): 406–413, pp. 410; and see "Anatomy," *London Medical and Physical Journal* 59 (1828): 554–557.

32. This was true of not only normal but also pathological and surgical anatomy; as London surgeon John Abernethy told students at St. Bartholomew's Hospital, "The French who have great opportunities for practicing operations on the dead body are so expert that they will take off an arm in a minute" (J. F. South, Notes Taken on Lectures Given by John Abernethy on Natural and Morbid Anatomy and Physiology, Delivered in the Anatomical Theatre at St Bartholomew's Hospital in the years 1819 & 1820, 4 vols., vol. 4, entry for 14 Jan. 1820, London—RCS, reproduced by kind permission of the President and Council of the Royal College of Surgeons of England).

33. "The Anatomy Bill," *London Medical and Surgical Journal*, n.s., 1 (1832): 481–482, p. 482.

34. Comments of Dr. Traill in Literary and Philosophical Society of Liverpool, Minute Book (typescript excerpts), vol. 3, 1823–1836, meeting of 4 Feb. 1825, Liverpool—Liverpool RO.

35. "Anatomical Report," p. 411; and see "Anatomy," *London Medical and Physical Journal* 60 (1828): 373–383; "London Hospital Surgeons and Pupils," *Lancet* 2 (1831–1832): 55–60; and H. W. Rush, "Clinical Instruction in London and Paris," *Lancet* 2 (1833–1834): 321–322, p. 321.

36. Sir Sidney Smith to Sir Henry Halford, Paris, 20 Jan. 1832, Halford Manuscripts, Leicester—Leicesters. RO.

37. "The Supply of Subjects for Dissection," *LMG*, n.s., 1 (1837–1838): 177–183, p. 180; and see "The Anatomy Act," *Lancet* 1 (1844): 194–196, and "Supply of Subjects to the Schools—The Anatomy Act," *LMG*, n.s., 3 (1846): 882–883. And see Ruth Richardson, *Death, Dissection and the Destitute* (London and New York: Routledge and Kegan Paul, 1987).

38. "Meeting of the Medical Profession at the Freemason's Tavern," *London Medical and Surgical Journal*, n.s., 4 (1833–1834): 376–377, p. 377.

39. "Causes of the Slow Advancement of Medical Science," *Lancet* 2 (1837–1838): 778–782, p. 779.

40. "Poverty of English Medical Literature," *Lancet* 2 (1842–1843): 197–199, p. 198. "It is not the want of opportunity that renders our hospital physicians infinitely inferior to those of France as observers of disease," Wakley argued, "but the lack of *scientific enthusiasm*" (p. 197). "We blame, then, the system of medical legislation under which hospitals that should be national blessings, fraught with liberal aid for the poor, and boundless information for the profession,—are allowed to be used for perpetration of private jobs, while the medical functionaries connected with them, who ought to be the high-priests of medical science, slumber on in torpid neglect, amid the rich and interminable fields of observation that they occupy" (p. 198).

41. George Webster, "Address," in "Public Meeting Held at Exeter Hall, London, on Thursday Evening, January 19, 1837, of the British Medical Association," *Lancet* 2 (1835–1836): 593–608, p. 596. And see "Hospitals Should be National Institutions," *London Medical and Surgical Journal*, n.s., 7 (1835): 345; "Administration of the Parisian Hospitals, and Mode of Electing a Surgeon to the Bureau Central d'Admission," *Lancet* 2 (1828–1829): 5–7; and Spectator, "Reforms in the Hospitals" (letter to the editor, 14 Sept. 1837), *Lancet* 1 (1837–1838): 24–25.

42. William Baly to Dear Mother, London, 29 Mar. [1834], Baly Papers. Students also privately protested against the irregularity of clinical instruction in London, a contrast to praise for Parisian arrangements; see, for example, the complaints of a pupil from Sheffield in Medical Student Diary, London, 1820, entry for 6 Oct. 1820, Manchester—Chetham's Lib.

43. "Causes of the Slow Advancement of Medical Science," p. 779; and see "Monopolies in Medical Education," *Lancet* 1 (1837–1838): 873–877. As Wakley put it, "Instead of making the offices of dresser, of house-surgeon, of apothecary, of surgeon, and of physician, the rewards of merit, and temptations to exertion in the cause of science, the mercenary officers sell several of these places" ("Defects in Medical Education," *Lancet* 1 [1838–1839]: 125–128, p. 127).

44. "Contrast between Medical Receptions in London and Paris," *Lancet* 1 (1834–1835): 168–170, p. 168.

45. "Parallel between the English and French Hospitals," p. 316. As a Bloomsbury practitioner asserted, "In France the desideratum which the system espouses is talent—talent making the way to preferment; in England it is money and family patronage" (G. D. Dermott, "The National System of Medical Educa-

tion in France," *MT* 13 [1845–1846]: 37–39, p. 38). As he continued, "In the hospitals of France, the *externes*, or dressers, are chosen by *concours*; in England, where money is the test of respectability and professional talent, they *purchace* their appointments by the twelvemonth, the responsibility of dressing wounds, &c., often thus falling to the lot of the '*higher class*' of English pupils, i.e., often the most idle, dissolute, and monied." And see "Dupuytren's Lectures," *Lancet* 1 (1832–1833): 369.

46. "Defects in Medical Education," pp. 128, 127.

47. See "Clinical Lectures in London and Paris," *Lancet* 1 (1844): 227–228, p. 227. Some reformers also hoped that state support for the intertwined activities of patient care, teaching, and clinical investigation would obviate the suspicion medical officers at English hospitals perennially encountered from lay boards of governors that their pursuit of science in the wards threatened to undermine the charitable aim of caring for the deserving sick poor; see, for example, J. E. Stock to the Committee of the Bristol Infirmary, Clifton [Bristol], 28 Sept. 1816, Bristol—Bristol RO.

48. *Lancet* 1 (1832–1833): 2; and, for example, "Preface," *Lancet* 1 (1838–1839): 1–5, p. 2.

49. *MT* 14 (1846): 220.

50. *MT* 8 (1843): 90–93, p. 90.

51. See Report from the Committee of Examiners to the Chairman of the Bill Committee, 11 June 1811, Act of Parliament Committee, Minutes, 1814–1834 (MS 8211/1); Special Court of Assistants, 28 July 1821, and Court of Assistants, 1 Aug. 1828, Court of Assistants, Minute Book, 1817–1833 (MS 8200/1); and Report to the Court of Assistants, 21 July 1831, Court of Examiners, Minutes, vol. 4, 1828–1833 (MS 8239/4), all in Society of Apothecaries Records, London—Guildhall.

52. For a typical criticism of such proceedings, see "Neglect of the Interests of the Students at St. Bartholomew's Hospital," *Lancet* 2 (1831–1832): 24–26.

53. "Medical Organization," *British and Foreign Medical and Chirurgical Review* 3 (1849): 31–48, pp. 40, 31; "Depressed State of Medical Literature in England," *London Medical and Surgical Journal*, n.s., 6 (1835): 376–378, p. 377. And see "Corruption Totters," *Lancet* 2 (1830–1831): 243–248, and "The Incorpo-

rated General Practitioners," *Lancet* 2 (1844): 342–343. On the unification of surgery and physic in France, see especially Toby Gelfand, *Professionalizing Modern Medicine: Paris Surgeons and Medical Science and Institutions in the Eighteenth Century* (Westport, Conn.: Greenwood Press, 1980).

54. *MT* 8 (1843): 90–91, p. 90. And see "Dr. Ryan on State of the Medical Profession," *London Medical and Surgical Journal* 5 (1830): 223–240, and "Causes of the Depressed State of the Medical Profession in Great Britain," *Lancet* 2 (1831–1832): 88–92.

55. "Narrative of a Journey to London, in 1814, . . . By Philibert Joseph Roux," *Monthly Medico-Chirurgical Review and Chemico-Philosophical Magazine*, n.s., 1 (1824): 156–159, 202–208, p. 202.

56. J. B[illegible] to [John S. Soden], Bristol, 15 Dec. 1842, J. S. Soden, Medical Tracts and Letters, London—RSM.

57. "English and French Medical Students," *LMG* 7 (1830–1831): 474–477, pp. 476, 475. For the celebration by elite surgeons of an *English* tradition of science, however, see L. S. Jacyna, "Images of John Hunter in the Nineteenth Century," *History of Science* 21 (1983): 85–108.

58. Benjamin C. Brodie, *An Introductory Discourse, on the Studies Required for the Medical Profession. Addressed to the Students of the Medical School of St. George's Hospital, October 1, 1838* (London: T. Brettell, 1838), pp. 6–7; my emphasis.

59. "Medical Education in England," *LMG* 1 (1827–1828): 10–11, p. 11.

60. "The One Faculty—Instar Omnium," *LMG* 13 (1833–1834): 402–407, p. 406.

61. "Practice of Physic," *Anderson's Quarterly Journal of Medical Science*, n.s., 1 (1824): 139–147, p. 140; "Review of *Physiologie de l'Homme*, par N. P. Adelon," *Anderson's Quarterly Journal of Medical Science* 2 (1825): 89–93, p. 93.

62. "Reform—College of Physicians," *LMG* (1832–1833): 485–489, p. 485; and see "Medical Reform in Germany," *LMG* 13 (1833–1834): 723–727, pp. 723, 726, which proposed that Prussia offered better models for emulation than those of "the French levellers" who sought to bring to English soil "French reform—or rather revolution."

63. "French Mode of Medical Education," *LMG* 11 (1832–1833): 891–894, p. 893.

64. For example, see "The Concours," *LMG* 7 (1830–1831): 153–157; "The Concours in Paris," *LMG*, n.s., 2 (1841–1842): 438–441; and "Working of the Concours System," *LMG* 12 (1833): 153–165.

65. This unity amidst diversity is clear in the testimony presented in the *Report from the Select Committee on Medical Education: With the Minutes of Evidence, and Appendix*, 4 vols. (London: House of Commons, 1834), in which Henry Warburton, as chair, pressed questions on the neglect of science in England and comparison between medical science in that nation and in France.

66. "Preface," *Lancet* 1 (1842–1843): 1–4, p. 1.

67. T. K. Chambers to [Henry] Acland, [London], 16 Mar. 1841, Acland Manuscripts (MS Acland d62), Oxford—Bodleian.

68. While I have not focused on certain fields such as forensic medicine, psychiatry, and public health in which American attention to French polity was particularly robust, what remains striking is that American physicians overall gave much less attention to Parisian polity than did their English counterparts.

69. A. Stillé to G. C. Shattuck, Philadelphia, 6 Oct. 1844, Shattuck Papers, vol. 18, MA—MA Hist. Soc.

70. Samuel Henry Dickson to John A. Dickson, Chestnut Hill, 14 Sept. 1846, Dickson Family Papers, NC—SHC.

71. The phrase appears in his journal the *Telescope*, which was devoted to radical religious and political causes; quoted in Joseph F. Kett, *The Formation of the American Medical Profession: The Role of Institutions, 1780–1860* (New Haven and London: Yale University Press, 1968), p. 105.

72. "Medical Monopoly," *Botanico-Medical Recorder* 9 (1841): 309. And see "Memorial of the American Eclectic Medical Convention," *Eclectic Medical Journal* 2 (1849): 50–61; "The Monster Threatened," *Boston Thomsonian Manual and Lady's Companion* 5 (1838–1839): 153; "Address," *Western Medical Reformer* 4 (1844): 1–2; and "The Two Systems," *Water Cure Journal, and Herald of Reforms* 17 (1854): 98–99.

73. John King, "The Progress of Medical Reform," *Western Medical Reformer* 6 (1846): 79–82, pp. 80–81.

74. Helpful studies on botanic medical movements include Alex Berman, "The Impact of the Nineteenth Century Botanico-Medical Movement on American Pharmacy and Medicine" (Ph.D. diss., University of Wisconsin–Madison, 1954); John S. Haller, *Medical Protestants: The Eclectics in American Medicine, 1825–1939* (Carbondale: Southern Illinois University Press, 1994); Kett, *Formation of the American Medical Profession*, pp. 97–131; and William G. Rothstein, *American Physicians in the Nineteenth Century: From Sects to Science* (Baltimore and London: Johns Hopkins University Press, 1972), pp. 125–151. On hydropathy, see Susan E. Cayleff, *Wash and Be Healed: The Water-Cure and Women's Health* (Philadelphia: Temple University Press, 1987), and Jane B. Donegan, *"Hydropathic Highway to Health": Women and Water-Cure in Antebellum America* (New York and Westport, Conn.: Greenwood Press, 1986). On the broader health reform movement and its criticism of orthodox medicine, see Stephen Nissenbaum, *Sex, Diet, and Debility in Jacksonian America: Sylvester Graham and Health Reform* (Westport, Conn.: Greenwood Press, 1980), and Ronald L. Numbers, *Prophetess of Health: A Study of Ellen G. White* (New York: Harper and Row, 1976). Homeopaths shared in the assault upon orthodox monopoly, theory, and practice, and claimed empirical testing or proving of drugs as the core of homeopathic epistemology, but their movement was not marked by an animus against professionalism; see Harris L. Coulter, *Divided Legacy: A History of the Schism in Medical Thought*, 3 vols. (Washington, D.C.: McGrath, 1973), vol. 3, *Science and Ethics in American Medicine, 1800–1914*; Martin Kaufman, *Homeopathy in America: The Rise and Fall of a Medical Heresy* (Baltimore and London: Johns Hopkins University Press, 1971); and Kett, *Formation of the American Medical Profession*, pp. 132–164.

75. Ramsey, "The Politics of Professional Monopoly," p. 251.

76. On licensing and its decline, see Samuel Lee Baker, "Medical Licensing in America: An Early Liberal Reform" (Ph.D. diss., Harvard University, 1977); Kett, *Formation of the American Medical Profession*, pp. 1–96; Rothstein, *American Physicians*, pp. 63–100; and Richard Harrison Shryock, *Medical Licensing in America, 1650–1965* (Baltimore: Johns Hopkins University Press, 1967).

77. Samuel Thomson, *New Guide to Health*;

or, *Botanic Family Physician* (Boston: J. Q. Adams, 1835), p. 5.

78. B., "Medical Despotism," *Western Medical Reformer* 6 (1847): 265–270, p. 266.

79. C.G.W. Comegys to Scott Cook, Cincinnati, 23 Nov. 1850, Matthew Scott Cook Papers, OH—Western Reserve Hist. Soc.

80. Samuel Clark Oliver, "An Essay on the Causes Which Prevent the Progress and Usefulness of Medical Science in the United States" (M.D. thesis, University of Pennsylvania, 1820), PA—U. PA Lib.

81. Augustus Kinsley Gardner, *Old Wine in New Bottles: or, Spare Hours of a Student in Paris* (New-York: C. S. Francis & Co.; Boston: J. H. Francis, 1848), p. 160.

82. For example, "Legal Regulation of Medicine and Surgery," *WL* 2 (1843–1844): 435–438, and W. C. Smith, "Remarks on Empiricism" (M.D. thesis, Medical College of the State of South Carolina, 1850), SC—Waring.

83. "State Legislation Respecting Medical Practice," *Illinois Medical and Surgical Journal* 1 (1844): 97–105, p. 103.

84. "Medical Despotism," pp. 268, 268, 266, 265.

85. William Tully to Alden March, New Haven, 11 July 1846, Alden March Papers, NY—Albany Med.

86. Thomas Hun, Joel A. Wing, and Mason F. Cogswell, [Report of a Committee of the Albany Medical Society], in "State Legislation Respecting Medical Practice," pp. 99–105, pp. 104, 105.

87. Rob Peter to Elisha Bartlett, Lexington, 5 June 1847, Bartlett (Elisha) Family Papers, NY—U. Rochester.

88. For example, see Jacob Bigelow to Isaac Hays, Boston, 25 Apr. 1847, Isaac Hays Papers, PA—APS.

89. "Medical Reform," *Western Lancet and Medical Library* 5 (1846): 67–72, pp. 68, 67.

90. Joseph Pancoast, *Professional Glimpses Abroad. A Lecture Introductory to the Course on Anatomy, in the Jefferson Medical College of Philadelphia, Delivered October 17, 1856* (Philadelphia: Joseph M. Wilson, 1856), p. 10.

91. This is clear both in the intensifying emphasis on hands-on anatomical experience in the curricula of medical schools and in published guides to dissection and surgical practice on the dead body. See, for example, Thomas L. Ogier, *A Compendium of Operative Surgery Intended for the Use of Students, and*

*Containing Descriptions of All Surgical Operations* (Charleston: E. J. Van Brunt, 1834), which, citing French precedents, was intended "chiefly to assist the student in operating on the dead subject" (p. 5).

92. "Editorial Correspondence" (Paris), *BMSJ* 41 (1849–1850): 44–45, p. 44. And see Paul F. Eve, *An Introductory Lecture Delivered in the Medical College of Georgia, November 6th, 1849* (Augusta: Jas. McCafferty, 1849), p. 18, and Cornelius S. Younglove, "Medical Science" (M.D. thesis, Albany Medical College, 1849), NY—Albany Med.

93. J. Y. Bassett to Isaphoena Bassett, Paris, 11 Sept. 1836, John Young Bassett Papers, AL—AL State Arch. George Weisz has explored the prominence of "the rise from humble origins" theme within France, in the *éloges* of the Académie de Médecine, in *The Medical Mandarins: The French Academy of Medicine in the Nineteenth and Early Twentieth Centuries* (New York and Oxford: Oxford University Press, 1995), pp. 215–236, esp. on pp. 219–222.

94. L. S. Joynes, Journal, [Paris, 1840], Joynes Family Papers, VA—VA Hist. Soc. And see Gardner, *Old Wine*, pp. 77–81.

95. William Gibson, *Rambles in Europe in 1839. With Sketches of Prominent Surgeons, Physicians, Medical Schools, Hospitals, Literary Personages, Scenery, Etc.* (Philadelphia: Lea and Blanchard, 1841), pp. 74–75.

96. See Karen Halttunen, *Confidence Men and Painted Women: A Study of Middle-Class Culture in America, 1830–1870* (New Haven and London: Yale University Press, 1982), pp. 198–205.

97. M. L. Linton, "Hospitals of Paris" (Paris, 24 Dec. 1840), *WJMS* 3 (1841): 65–74, p. 68.

98. F. Campbell Stewart, *Eminent French Surgeons, with a Historical and Statistical Account of the Hospitals of Paris; Together with Miscellaneous Information and Biographical Notices of the Most Eminent Living Parisian Surgeons* (Buffalo: A. Burke, 1845), p. 214.

99. Valentine Mott, *Travels in Europe and the East* (New-York: Harper and Brothers, 1842), p. 38.

100. Stewart, *Eminent French Surgeons*, p. 128.

101. Gardner, *Old Wine*, p. 78.

102. "Letter from S. S. Satchwell, M.D." (Paris, 20 Feb. 1861), *Medical Journal of North Carolina* 3 (1861): 340–345, p. 342.

103. Gardner, *Old Wine*, pp. 77, 78. And see R[ené] La R[oche], "An Account of the Origin, Progress, and Present State of the Medical Schools of Paris," *American Journal of Medical Sciences* 9 (1831): 109–124, 351–388, 401–418, pp. 379–381, and John A. Murphy, "[Letter to the Editors]" (Paris, Mar. 1854), *WL* 15 (1854): 481–491, p. 483.

104. "Response to Memorial," [n.d., but ca. 1829–1832], in College Faculty Papers, 1829–1835, Ford-Ravenal Papers, SC—SC Hist. Soc.

105. George Sidney Doane to George C. Shattuck, New York, 29 Jan. [1839], Shattuck Papers, vol. 16.

106. C. B. Chapman, "Medical Institutions of Paris," *BMSJ* 45 (1851–1852): 279–281, pp. 280–281.

107. Austin Flint, "Address at the Opening of the Session for 1854–55 in the Medical Department of the University of Louisville," *WJMS*, n.s., 2 (1854): 409–425, p. 413; and see p. 414.

108. Montrose A. Pallen, "Letter from Our European Correspondent" (Paris, 29 May 1857), *SLMSJ* 15 (1857): 356–366, p. 359.

109. Ibid.

110. Gardner, *Old Wine*, p. 161.

111. [F. Peyre Porcher], "[Letter to the Editor]," *CMJR* 8 (1853): 416–429, p. 424.

112. Levin S. Joynes to Thomas R. Joynes, Paris, 12 Dec. 1841, Joynes Family Papers.

113. William B. Crawford to Margaret Crawford, Paris, 14 Feb. 1833, Sarah Ann (Gayle) Crawford Papers, NC—Duke.

114. Richard Cary Morse, "Journal of 8 Months in Europe," entry for Paris, 1838, Morse Family Papers, CT—Yale.

115. Alfred Stillé to [G. C.] Shattuck, Philadelphia, 5 Dec. 1857, MA—Countway.

116. Robert Peter to Frances Peter, London, 11 Aug. 1839, Evans Papers, KY—U. KY.

117. James Jackson, Jr., to James Jackson, Sr., Paris, 15 Jan. 1832, James Jackson Papers, MA—Countway.

118. See Russell M. Jones, "American Doctors and the Parisian Medical World, 1830–1840," *Bulletin of the History of Medicine* 47 (1973): 40–65, 177–204, pp. 202–203.

119. For example, see Baltimore Pathological Society Minutes, 2 vols., 1853–1858, 1867–1872, NC—Duke.

120. Alfred Stillé to G. C. Shattuck, 26 Mar. 1844, Shattuck Papers, vol. 18.

121. See Ohio State Medical Society, Min-

utes, entry for 4 June 1853, OH—Dittrick, and "Transactions of the South Carolina Medical Association" [address by J. P. Barratt], *Charleston Medical and Surgical Review* 11 (1856): 178–198.

122. Proceedings of the Faculty of the Medical College of Louisiana, May 1835–Feb. 1847, entry for 15 Oct. 1836, LA—Tulane Med.

123. Medical College of Ohio, Faculty Minutes, 1831–1852, entry for 4 Mar. 1842, OH—U. Cincinnati.

124. Charles E. Rosenberg, *The Care of Strangers: The Rise of America's Hospital System* (New York: Basic Books, 1987); Dale Cary Smith, "The Emergence of Organized Clinical Instruction in the Nineteenth Century American Cities of Boston, New York and Philadelphia" (Ph.D. diss., University of Minnesota, 1979).

125. Edwin L. Mcall to Lemuel Kollock, Philadelphia, 22 Feb. 1805, Lemuel Kollock Papers, GA—GA Hist. Soc.

126. John Manning to Charles Bolles, Waldoboro, Maine, 13 Aug. 1824, Manning Family Papers, MA—Peabody Essex.

127. Essex Southern District Medical Society, Minutes of the Society, vol. 1, 1805–1871, entry for 3 Mar. 1829, MA—Peabody Essex; James Jackson, Jr., to James Jackson, Sr., entry of 29 Oct. in letter of Paris, 21 Oct. 1832, J. Jackson Papers. And see Jackson, Jr., to Jackson, Sr., Havre, 25 Apr. 1832, and Jackson, Sr., to Jackson, Jr., Boston, 15 Nov. 1831.

128. Richard Maris, Notes of a Course of Lectures on the Materia Medica Given by Samuel Jackson, 1826–1828, to Which Are Added Three Lectures on the Stethoscope, by the Same, 1827, PA—CPP.

129. For example, William Wood Gerhard, "Journal Medical," 11 Mar. 1833–17 Mar. 1839, PA—CPP; "Lectures, 1850. Bart, Ricord, Bernard's Lectures," Paris, 1850–1851, and continued with clinical observations at the Roper Hospital, Charleston, 1852, SC—Waring.

130. John P. Caffry, "Calomel in Southern Fevers" (M.D. thesis, Medical College of the State of South Carolina, 1839), SC—Waring.

131. Philip Claiborne Gooch, Diary, 1 Sept. 1848–16 May 1852, entry for Richmond, 20 May 1849, Philip Claiborne Gooch Diaries, VA—VA Hist. Soc.; Lundsford Pitts Yandell, Diary, 1824–1843, entry for 1826, KY—Filson Club.

132. Wm M. Boling to E. Bartlett, Mont-

gomery, Ala., 27 Dec. 1847, Bartlett Family Papers.

133. M. H. Aikins to L. S. Aikins, Philadelphia, 5 Jan. 1857, Aikins Papers, Toronto—U. Toronto. Demands for increased access abounded; see, for example, Daniel Drake to Samuel P. Hildreth, Cincinnati, 14 Nov. 1838, Daniel Drake Papers, OH—OH Hist. Soc., and J. Harrison to John B. Sawson, New Orleans, 10 Nov., 1843, Butler (Thomas and Family) Papers, LA—LSU.

134. Smith, "The Emergence of Organized Clinical Instruction."

135. J. C. Nott to James M. Gage, New Orleans, Mar. [1837], James McKibbin Gage Papers, NC—SHC.

136. M. H. Aikins to L. S. Aikins, Philadelphia, 20 Nov. 1856, Aikins Papers.

137. Quoted in Edward C. Atwater, "Internal Medicine," in *The Education of American Physicians: Historical Essays*, ed. Ronald L. Numbers (Berkeley, Los Angeles, and London: University of California Press, 1980), pp. 143–174, on p. 155.

138. Robt Peter to Elisha Bartlett, Lexington, 2 Feb. 1846, Elisha Bartlett Papers, CT—Yale.

139. Ibid., 28 July 1848.

140. For examples of college *cliniques*, see Minute Book of the Faculty of the Female Medical College of Pennsylvania, 1850–1864, meeting of 9 Oct. 1850, PA—Women in Med. Arch.; Minutes of the Faculty of the Savannah Medical College, entries for 28 July and 7 Aug. 1854, GA—GA Hist. Soc.; Medical College of Ohio, Faculty Minutes, 1852–1909, entry for 15 Oct. 1852, OH—U. Cincinnati; William Pepper to George B. Wood, [Philadelphia], 11 Feb. 1856, G. B. Wood Miscellaneous Correspondence, PA—CPP; F. P. Porcher to Louis Peyre Porcher, New York, June 1847, Porcher Papers, SC—SC Hist. Soc.

141. "*Cliniques*," *Buffalo Medical Journal and Monthly Review* 2 (1847): 623–626, pp. 623–625.

142. C., "What Medical School Shall I Attend?" *Southern Journal of the Medical and Physical Sciences* 3 (1855): 361–365, pp. 363, 364. And see Henry Ingersoll Bowditch, "Lectures. 1858. Mass. Gen. Hospital. Introductory &c to the Clinical Course No 1," MA—Countway.

143. Cincinnati General Hospital, Medical Staff Minute book, 1861–1891, entries for 27 June 1872 and 13 June 1874, OH—U. Cincinnati.

144. A. A. Marrett, Notes Taken on Lectures on Clinical Medicine Delivered at the Louisville City Hospital and the Medical University of Louisville by Prof. L. P. Yandell Jr., Session 1873–4, entries for 16 Sept. and 6 Nov. 1873, KY—U. Louisville.

145. Samuel Bard, *Two Discourses Dealing with Medical Education in Early New York* (New York: Columbia University Press, 1921), quoted in Rosenberg, *Care of Strangers*, pp. 194–195.

146. "Medical Department of the University of Louisiana," *NOMSJ* 6 (1849): 816–819, p. 816.

147. John Barber, "Medicine Clinique" (M.D. thesis, University of Pennsylvania, 1862), PA—U. PA Lib.

148. Medical College of Ohio, Faculty Minutes, 1831–1852, entry for 18 Aug. 1831, OH—U. Cincinnati.

149. Almshouse Medical Reports, 1833–1837, [Baltimore, Case Notes of Dr. James H. Miller], entry for 1 Feb. 1834, Almshouse Medical Records (MS 2474), MD—MD Hist. Soc.

150. W. M. Carpenter, "Introductory Lecture Delivered before the Medical Class of the Louisiana Medical College on the 20th Nov. 1844," *New Orleans Medical Journal* 1 (1844–1845): 364–369, p. 367. On regional separatism in medical education, see Ronald L. Numbers and John Harley Warner, "The Maturation of American Medical Science," in *Scientific Colonialism, 1800–1930: A Cross-Cultural Comparison*, ed. Nathan Reingold and Marc Rothenberg (Washington, D.C.: Smithsonian Institution Press, 1987), pp. 191–214, and John Harley Warner, "A Southern Medical Reform: The Meaning of the Antebellum Argument for Southern Medical Education," *Bulletin of the History of Medicine* 57 (1983): 364–381.

151. Jas. C. Billingslea, "An Appeal on Behalf of Southern Medical Colleges and Southern Medical Literature," *Southern Medical and Surgical Journal*, n.s., 12 (1856): 398–402, p. 401.

152. E. D. Fenner, "Remarks on Clinical Medicine," *New Orleans Medical News and Hospital Gazette* 4 (1857–1858): 458–472, p. 468.

153. "The Lecture Season," *New Orleans Medical News and Hospital Gazette* 4 (1857–1858): 551–553, p. 552.

154. E. D. Fenner, "Introductory Lecture, Delivered at the Opening of the New Orleans School of Medicine, on the 17th Nov., '56," *New Orleans Medical News and Hospital Gazette* 3 (1856–1857): 577–600, p. 579.

CHAPTER 7
"AGAINST THE SPIRIT OF SYSTEM":
EPISTEMOLOGY AND REFORM

1. "The One Faculty—Instar Omnium," *LMG* 13 (1833–1834): 402–407, p. 406; "Medical Reform in Germany," *LMG* 13 (1833–1834): 723–727, p. 726.

2. "Medical Reform," *Lancet* 1 (1836–1837): 489–492, p. 491.

3. J. G. Crosse, "Lettre 13ᵉᵐᵉ," Paris, 28 Jan. 1815, John Green Crosse, Letters from Paris, 2 vols., vol. 2, 1815, John Green Crosse Papers (MS474, T132F, L8511), Norwich—Norfolk RO.

4. J.S.F., "Descartes," *Weekly Medico-Chirurgical and Philosophical Magazine* 1 (1823): 2–4, pp. 3, 4, 3.

5. Notes Taken on Introductory Lecture on the Practice of Physic by Charles Fergusson Forbes M.D. Delivered January 20th 1819, London—RCP.

6. "Present State of the Practice of Medicine," *Lancet* 1 (1844): 163–165, p. 164.

7. J. F. South, Notes Taken on Lectures Given by John Abernethy on Natural and Morbid Anatomy and Physiology Delivered by John Abernethy Esq FRS. in the Anatomical Theatre at St Bartholomew's Hospital in the Years 1819 & 1820, 4 vols., vol. 1, entry for 2 Oct. 1819, London—RCS. On the long-standing emphasis on practical medical instruction in London, see Susan C. Lawrence, *Charitable Knowledge: Hospital Pupils and Practitioners in Eighteenth-Century London* (Cambridge and New York: Cambridge University Press, 1996).

8. Thomas Wakley, "Address to Those Students in Medicine Who Are About to Commence or Resume Their Studies in the Medical Schools of the British Empire" (London, 27 Sept. 1834), *Lancet* 2 (1833–1834): 1–6, p. 5; Medical Student Diary, London, 1820–1821, entry on John Bostock's lecture on

chemistry, 16 Oct. 1820, and see entries 2, 9, and 14 Oct. 1820, Manchester—Chetham's Lib.

9. W. H. Walshe, "Lectures on Clinical Medicine, Delivered at University College Hospital," *Lancet* 1 (1849): 1–5, p. 3. See P.-Ch.-A. Louis, *Researches on Phthisis, Anatomical, Pathological, and Therapeutical,* 2d ed., trans. Walter Hayle Walshe (London: Sydenham Society, 1844).

10. "Pathological Society of London" (remarks of C.J.B. Williams at meeting of 20 Oct. 1846), *Lancet* 2 (1846): 481–483, pp. 481, 482. Williams described himself as a "*conservative* reformer" (Charles J. B. Williams, "On the State of the Medical Profession and on the Best Means of Improvement," *LMG* 1 [1841–1842]: 22–26, p. 22). The objective of the society was to cultivate pathology, not to promote professional reform, and its meetings were to center on "the exhibition and examination of specimens . . . with accompanying written or oral descriptions illustrative of Pathological Science" (The Pathological Society of London, Minute Book, 1846, minutes for meeting of 8 May 1846, London—RSM).

11. Edward Henry Sieveking, Notebook, 1846–1857, London—RCP.

12. T. Hodgkin, "First Report of the Committee," 8 Oct. 1836, in General Reports of the [Guy's Hospital] Clinical Society from Oct. 1836 to Oct. 1845, London—Guy's.

13. [Richard] Bright, "Ninth Report of the Committee," Oct. 1840, in General Reports of the Clinical Society.

14. Samuel Ashwell, "Seventh Report of the Committee," 12 Oct. 1839, in General Reports of the Clinical Society.

15. Bright, "Second Report of the Committee," Apr. 1837, and B. G. Babington, "Sixth Report of the Committee," 27 Apr. 1839, both in General Reports of the Clinical Society.

16. C. Aster Key, "Third Annual Report of the Committee," 11 Oct. 1837, in General Reports of the Clinical Society. For the French influence on Bright and Hodgkin, see Pamela Bright, *Dr. Richard Bright (1789–1858)* (London: The Bodley Head, 1983), and Amalie M. Kass and Edward H. Kass, *Perfecting the World: The Life and Times of Dr. Thomas Hodgkin, 1798–1866* (Boston: Harcourt Brace Jovanovich, 1988). And see J.M.H. Campbell, "The History of the Physical Society," *Guy's*

*Hospital Gazette* (1925): 107–119; and J. R. Wall, "The Guy's Hospital Physical Society (1771–1852)," *Guy's Hospital Reports* 123 (1974): 159–170.

17. "Medical Statistics," *LMG* 1 (1842–1843): 336–340, p. 338.

18. Review of "*Mémoires de la Société Médicale d'Observation, de Paris.* Tome premier— Paris, 1836," *British and Foreign Medical and Surgical Review* 5 (1839): 154–162, pp. 154, 160.

19. "The Lancet's Anti-Quackery Era," *Lancet* 2 (1846): 487; and see "Duty of the Profession to Exterminate Quackery," *Lancet* 2 (1846): 537–538, p. 537.

20. J. C. Prichard, "An Address Delivered at the Third Anniversary Meeting of the Provincial Medical and Surgical Association, July 23rd 1835," *Transactions of the Provincial Medical and Surgical Association* 4 (1836): 1–54, pp. 5, 33.

21. Quoted in "Preface," *Lancet* 1 (1837–1838): 1–3, p. 3.

22. Review of "*An Essay on Clinical Instruction,* by P. Ch. A. Louis," *British and Foreign Medical Review* 1 (1836): 397–424, p. 404.

23. John Taylor, "Introductory Lecture, on the Opening of the Medical Session of 1841–42, in University College," *Lancet* 1 (1841–1842): 41–48, pp. 111–112; and see Review of "*Recherches sur les Effets de la Saignée dans quelques Maladies Inflammatoires,*" *Lancet* 1 (1834–1835): 828–835, p. 828.

24. Review of "*Pathological Researches on Phthisis. By E.* [sic] *Ch. Louis . . . ,*" *British and Foreign Medical Review* 1 (1836): 165–172, p. 165.

25. "Practitioners at Home and Abroad," *LMG* 2 (1838–1839): 393–396, p. 394.

26. See, for example, "Reform—College of Physicians," *LMG* 11 (1832–1833): 485–489, p. 486.

27. A typical summary is "Causes of the Depressed State of the Medical Profession in Great Britain," *Lancet* 2 (1832–1833): 88–92. The closest to being an exception was the argument that adherents of nonorthodox medical movements such as homeopathy were followers of systems and that the pursuit of sound medical knowledge would put an end to quackery. Reformers, however, looked chiefly to legislative, legal solutions to the problem of heterodoxy.

28. A. Colman to Catherine K. Colman, Paris, 6 Jan. 1833, Colman (Anson) Papers, NY—U. Rochester.

29. Alden March, Diary of a Tour of Europe, entry for Paris, 1841, Alden March Papers, NY—Albany Med.

30. R. A. Kinloch, "Medical News in Paris" (Paris, 2 July 1854), *CMJR* 9 (1854): 587–596, p. 587.

31. Henry H. Smith, *A Professional Visit to London and Paris: Introductory Lecture to the Course on the Principles and Practice of Surgery Delivered in the University of Pennsylvania, October 9, 1855* (Philadelphia: T. K. & P. G. Collins, 1855), p. 7.

32. David W. Yandell, "Clinical Instruction in the London and Paris Hospitals," *WJMS*, ser. 3, 3 (1848): 392–400, pp. 396–397.

33. M. L. L[inton], "Medicine in Paris" (Paris, 25 July 1840), *WJMS* 2 (1840): 69–73, p. 70.

34. T. Stewardson to W. W. Gerhard, London, 9 Sept. 1834, W. W. Gerhard Papers, PA—CPP.

35. [Linton], "Medicine in Paris," p. 72.

36. James Jackson, Jr., to James Jackson, Sr., Paris, 21 Oct. 1832, James Jackson Papers, MA—Countway; and see ibid., Paris, 22 Feb. 1833.

37. Elisha Bartlett, "Letter from Paris" (Paris, 20 Apr. 1846), *WL* 5 (1846–1847): 107–111, pp. 107–108.

38. Augustus Kinsley Gardner, *Old Wine in New Bottles: or, Spare Hours of a Student in Paris* (New-York: C. S. Francis & Co.; Boston: J. H. Francis, 1848), title page and p. 20.

39. Committee (William Taft, James Boykin, and Jns. Patterssbroff[?: illegible]) to Prof. Bartlett, Medical Department, [Transylvania University, Lexington Kentucky], 16 Nov. 1841, with reply from Bartlett attached, Elisha Bartlett Papers, CT—Yale.

40. George R. C. Todd, "Young Physic" (M.D. thesis, Transylvania University, 1848), KY—Transylvania.

41. S. C. Furman, "The Impediments to the Progress of Medical Science" (M.D. thesis, Medical College of the State of South Carolina, 1852), SC—Waring.

42. Daniel H. Whitney, *The Family Physician, or Every Man His Own Doctor* (New York: N. and J. White, 1834), p. iv.

43. Samuel North, *The Family Physician and Guide to Health* (Waterloo, N.Y.: William Child, 1830), p. iii.

44. *Boston Thomsonian Manual and Lady's Companion* 5 (1838–1839): 137.

45. "Address of the American Hydropathic Convention to the People of the United States," *Water Cure Journal, and Herald of Reforms* 10 (1850): 79–81, p. 81.

46. Ellen M. Snow, "Duties of Physicians," *Water Cure Journal, and Herald of Reforms* 21 (1856): 55–56, as quoted in Regina Markell Morantz, "Nineteenth Century Health Reform and Women: A Program of Self-Help," in *Medicine without Doctors: Home Health Care in American History*, ed. Guenter B. Risse, Ronald L. Numbers, and Judith Walzer Leavitt (New York: Science History Publications, 1977), pp. 73–93, on p. 76; and see G. H. Taylor, "Medical Credulity," *Water Cure Journal, and Herald of Reforms* 16 (1853): 75, and "Physic and Prevention," *Water Cure Journal, and Herald of Reforms* 11 (1851): 90–91.

47. Samuel Thomson, *New Guide to Health: or Botanic Family Physician* (Boston: J. Q. Adams, 1835), p. 5.

48. George Washington Bowen, Notes Taken on Lectures Given by Chas. D. Williams on the Institutes and Practice of Homoeopathy, Cleveland Institute of Homoeopathy, 1851–2, OH—Western Reserve Hist. Soc.; John Wesley Lykes, "The Decline of Allopathy" (M.D. thesis, Homoeopathic Medical College of Pennsylvania, 1849), PA—Hahnemann.

49. John Harley Warner, "Medical Sectarianism, Therapeutic Conflict, and the Shaping of Orthodox Professional Identity in Antebellum American Medicine," in *Medical Fringe and Medical Orthodoxy 1750–1850*, ed. W. F. Bynum and Roy Porter (London: Croom Helm, 1987), pp. 234–260, and John Harley Warner, "Power, Conflict, and Identity in Mid-Nineteenth-Century American Medicine: Therapeutic Change at the Commercial Hospital of Cincinnati," *Journal of American History* 73 (1987): 934–956.

50. Paul F. Eve, *An Introductory Lecture, Delivered in the Medical College of Georgia, November 6th, 1849* (Augusta: Jas. McCafferty, 1849), p. 22.

51. "Code of Medical Ethics," *Transactions of the New York State Medical Association* 1 (1884): 570–584, p. 577. This was taken from the Code of Ethics of the American Medical Association, drafted after it was founded in 1847 and adopted by many local and state medical societies.

52. Samantha S. Nivison, "Priest of Nature and Her Interpreter" (M.D. thesis, Female Medical College of Pennsylvania, 1855), PA—Women in Med. Arch.

53. W.A.A., "Thomsonism," *BMSJ* 19 (1839): 379–383, p. 382.

54. Review of "*The Principles of Medicine, founded on the Structure and Functions of the Animal Organism.* By Samuel Jackson," *American Journal of the Medical Sciences* 10 (1832): 157–196, p. 157.

55. Alfred Stillé, *Elements of General Pathology: A Practical Treatise* (Philadelphia: Lindsay and Blackiston, 1848), pp. 23, 46, 27.

56. Elisha Bartlett, *An Essay on the Philosophy of Medical Science* (Philadelphia: Lea and Blanchard, 1844), p. 291.

57. J. Jackson to E. Bartlett, Boston, 25 Jan. 1844, Bartlett Papers.

58. E. D. Faust, "[Review of] *Exposition des Principes de la Nouvelle Doctrine Medicale,*" *American Journal of the Medical Sciences* 8 (1831): 156–158, p. 156.

59. Alfred T. Hamilton to Father, Franklin Water Cure (near Winchester, Tennessee), 2 Sept. 1858, Alfred T. Hamilton Papers, TN—TN State Lib.

60. Wm. M. M'Pheeters, "Heroic Medicine," *SLMSJ* 4 (1847): 385–388, pp. 385–386.

61. See, for example, William G. Rothstein, *American Physicians in the Nineteenth Century: From Sects to Science* (Baltimore and London: Johns Hopkins University Press, 1972). On therapeutic change, see Charles E. Rosenberg, "The Therapeutic Revolution: Medicine, Meaning, and Social Change in Nineteenth-Century America," in *The Therapeutic Revolution: Essays in the Social History of American Medicine*, ed. Morris J. Vogel and Charles E. Rosenberg (Philadelphia: University of Pennsylvania Press, 1979), pp. 3–25, and John Harley Warner, *The Therapeutic Perspective: Medical Practice, Knowledge, and Identity in America, 1820–1885* (Cambridge, Mass., and London: Harvard University Press, 1986).

62. B. S. Woodworth, "The Best Way to Oppose Homoeopathy and Its Kindred Delusions," *CLO*, n.s., 1 (1858): 400–404, p. 403.

63. John A. Lyle, "Exclusive Systems of Medicine" (M.D. thesis, Transylvania University, 1841), KY—Transylvania; and see D. Bryan Baker, "Medical Reform" (M.D. thesis, Albany Medical College, 1843), NY—Albany Med.

64. J.S.J. Guerard, "Defence of Medicine" (M.D. thesis, Medical College of the State of South Carolina, 1845), SC—Waring; M. B. Wooldridge, "The Medical Student" (M.D. thesis, University of Nashville, 1857), TN—Vanderbilt.

65. Bowen, Notes on Lectures by Williams, introductory lecture, 1851.

66. John W. Kennedy, "The Maladministration of Cathartics, and Especially Mercurials" (M.D. thesis, Transylvania University, 1846), KY—Transylvania; and see Samuel L. McKeehan, "Nosology" (M.D. thesis, Washington Medical College of Baltimore, 1820), Joseph M. Toner Papers, DC—LC.

67. H. M. Bullitt, "The Art of Observing, or the Proper Method of Examining Patients, with a View to Correct Diagnosis," WL 3 (1844–1845): 397–409, p. 409.

68. Furman, "Impediments to the Progress of Medical Science."

69. Lyle, "Exclusive Systems of Medicine."

70. James Jackson, Jr., to James Jackson, Sr., Paris, 22 Feb. 1833, J. Jackson Papers.

71. "The True Value of Medical Experience," BMSJ 19 (1839): 351–354, p. 353.

72. Elisha Bartlett, "[Address] to Gentleman of the Medical Class," n.d. [but 1840s], Bartlett (Elisha) Family Papers, NY—U. Rochester.

73. W. C. Smith, "Remarks on Empiricism" (M.D. thesis, Medical College of the State of South Carolina, 1850), SC—Waring; Thos. S. Weston, "Homeopathy" (M.D. thesis, University of Nashville, 1856), TN—Vanderbilt.

74. W. Taylor, "Changeability of Disease," in Proceedings of the Medical Association of the State of Alabama, at Its Sixth Annual Meeting, Begun and Held in the City of Selma, Dec. 13–15, 1852, with an Appendix and List of Members (Mobile: Dade, Thompson, & C., 1853), pp. 68–81, on p. 79.

75. James C. Heicklin, "The Necessary Connexion between Theory and Practice in Medicine" (M.D. thesis, Medical University of the State of South Carolina, 1845), SC—Waring.

76. George B. Barrns, "Superstition & Credulity" (M.D. thesis, Albany Medical College, 1854), NY—Albany Med.

77. Danl. U. Foles, "The Progress of Medical Science" (M.D. thesis, Albany Medical College, 1840), NY—Albany Med.

78. Cornelius S. Younglove, "Medical Science" (M.D. thesis, Albany Medical College, 1849), NY—Albany Med.

79. E. D. F[enner], Review of "Homoeopathy, Allopathy, and 'Young Physic'," By John Forbes," NOMSJ 2 (1845–1846): 745–761, p. 760.

80. Samuel Clark Oliver, "The Causes which Prevent the Progress and Usefulness of Medical Science in the United States" (M.D. thesis, University of Pennsylvania, 1820), PA—U. PA Lib.; and see Alfred Patten Monson, "Empiricism" (M.D. thesis, Medical Institution of Yale College, 1847), CT—Yale Med.

81. Peter S. Stanley, "The Physician" (M.D. thesis, Albany Medical College, 1853), NY—Albany Med.

82. Henry Gilson, "Medical Science" (M.D. thesis, Albany Medical College, 1840), NY—Albany Med.

83. Elisha B. Stedman, "Theory of Broussais" (M.D. thesis, Transylvania University, 1835), KY—Transylvania.

84. M. B. Wooldridge, "The Medical Student" (M.D. thesis, University of Nashville, 1857), TN—Vanderbilt.

85. Karen Halttunen, Confidence Men and Painted Women: A Study of Middle-Class Culture in America, 1830–1870 (New Haven and London: Yale University Press, 1982); Neil Harris, Humbug: The Art of P. T. Barnum (Boston: Little, Brown and Co, 1973); Lawrence Frederick Kohl, The Politics of Individualism: Parties and the American Character in the Jacksonian Era (New York and Oxford: Oxford University Press, 1989); Lewis Perry, Boats against the Current: American Culture between Revolution and Modernity, 1820–1860 (New York: Oxford University Press, 1993).

86. Benjamin G. Bruce, "Medical Science, Its Improvements: and the Spirit of Progress" (M.D. thesis, Transylvania University, 1850), KY—Transylvania.

87. A. Stillé to G. C. Shattuck, Philadelphia, 8 July 1848, Shattuck Papers, vol. 21; and see A. Stillé to Shattuck, Philadelphia, 5 Oct. 1857, MA—Countway.

88. A. Stillé to Geo. C. Shattuck, Philadelphia, 3 June 1840, Shattuck Papers, vol. 16.

89. Alfred Stillé, An Introductory Lecture Delivered at the Pennsylvania College,—Medical Department, Philadelphia, October 13th, 1854 (Philadelphia: Kind & Baird, 1854), p. 13.

90. James R. R. Horne, "Specifics in Medi-

cine" (M.D. thesis, University of Nashville, 1857), TN—Vanderbilt.

91. Stillé, *Elements of General Pathology*, pp. 165, 166.

92. Ibid., p. viii. The intercalation of medical with theological opposition to *superstition* in antebellum thinking deserves exploration; it is particularly clear in, for example, physician Frederick W. Adams's "Journal and Theological Essays," Montpelier, Vermont, 1840–1846 (MS 17, no. 4), VT—VT Hist. Soc.

93. Stillé, *Elements of General Pathology*, p. 46.

94. Saml. Clark, "Medical Science in the United States" (M.D. thesis, University of Pennsylvania, 1820), PA—U. PA Lib.

95. A. Stillé to G. C. Shattuck, Philadelphia, 24 Oct. 1844, Shattuck Papers, vol. 18, MA—MA Hist. Soc.

96. Smith, "Remarks on Empiricism."

97. Gardner, *Old Wine*, p. 160.

98. R. F. McGuire, Diary, 1818–1852, Ouachita Parish, Monroe, Louisiana, entry for July 1837, LA—LSU; and see S. W. Brown to Hannah [Brown], Sacramento City, 25 Jan. 1850, Samuel W. Brown Papers (MS 236/1), CA—CA Hist. Soc.

99. Charles A. Lee, *Homeopathy. An Introductory Address to the Students of Starling Medical College, November 2, 1853* (Columbus: Osgood, Blake and Knapp, 1853), pp. 30, 31.

100. *The Anatomy of a Humbug, of the Genus Germanicus, Species Homeopathia* (New York: Printed for the author, 1837), pp. 8, 7, 15, 16. The best-known denunciation of homeopathy as delusion was Oliver Wendell Holmes, *Homeopathy and Its Kindred Delusions: Two Lectures Delivered before the Boston Society for the Diffusion of Useful Knowledge* (Boston: William D. Ticknor, 1842).

101. H. V. Wooten, *Character: A Valedictory Address to the Graduating Class of the Memphis Medical College Delivered by H. V. Wooten, M.D. Professor of the Principles and Practice of Medicine, at the Annual Commencement February 26th, 1853* (Memphis: Eagle and Enquirer Steam Printing House, 1853), p. 6. Wooten, like some other regular physicians who believed their character to be sound, also engaged in periodic assessments of their own behavior in the privacy of their diaries; see, for example, H. V. Wooten, Diary, transcript, vol. 2, entry for 30 May 1839, and vol. 3,

entry for Dec. 1847, Hardy Vickers Wooten Papers, AL—AL State Arch.

102. Joseph P. Logan, "Medicine As It Is," *Atlanta Medical and Surgical Journal* 1 (1855): 1–11, pp. 1–2, 3, 6, 10.

103. Richard M. Jones, "The Moral Responsibilities and the Proper Qualifications of the Physician" (M.D. thesis, Transylvania University, 1844), KY—Transylvania.

104. James Jackson, Jr., to James Jackson, Sr., Paris, 18 Mar. 1832, J. Jackson Papers.

105. Elisha Bartlett, "Letter from Paris" (Paris, 4 May 1846), WL 5 (1846–1847): 172–176, p. 174.

106. James Jackson, Jr., to James Jackson, Sr., Paris, 21 Oct. 1832, J. Jackson Papers.

107. Ibid., 13 Nov. 1832.

108. Ibid., London, 19 May 1832; ibid., entry for 26 Dec. in letter of Paris, 21 Dec. 1832.

109. Ibid., Paris, 24 Nov. 1832; ibid., 22 Feb. 1833. "In the notes of the introductory part of my course of Lectures," Stillé told Shattuck, "I had developed the idea of Rousseau used by Louis as an epigraph, to this effect, that 'truth resides in the subject not in us,' consult Nature honestly & she will reply truly:—an idea which is the *Resumé* of Bartlett's treatise" (A. Stillé to G. C. Shattuck, Philadelphia, 24 Oct. 1844, Shattuck Papers, vol. 18).

110. M.C.R. to [Bartlett], Hanover, 6 Sept. 1847, Bartlett Family Papers.

111. Jamie V. Ingham, "An Essay on Empiricism" (M.D. thesis, University of Pennsylvania, 1866), PA—U. PA Lib.

112. For a fuller discussion of the use of the terms *rational, empirical*, and *rational empiricism* in antebellum medical rhetoric, see Warner, *The Therapeutic Perspective*, pp. 41–46. "Rational empiricism" was not an exclusively American compromise; see, as one example, "Principles of Medical Education," *British and Foreign Medical Review* 10 (1840): 175–203, p. 183.

113. Stillé, *Elements of General Pathology*, pp. 163, 165.

114. James H. Jerome, Notebook, address copied under entry for Peach Orchard, Hector, Tompkins County, 8 Aug. 1834, NY—NY State Lib. Suggestive studies of much earlier deployments of different versions of empiricism are Harold J. Cook, *The Decline of the*

*Old Medical Regime in Stuart London* (Ithaca and London: Cornell University Press, 1986), and idem, "The New Philosophy and Medicine in Seventeenth-Century England," in *Reappraisals of the Scientific Revolution*, ed. David C. Lindberg and Robert S. Westman (Cambridge: Cambridge University Press, 1990), pp. 397–436.

115. Smith, "Remarks on Empiricism."

116. James Jackson, Jr., to James Jackson, Sr., Paris, entry for 26 Nov. in letter of 24 Nov. 1832, J. Jackson Papers.

117. Younglove, "Medical Science."

118. B. K. Mynatt, "Malarial Dropsy" (M.D. thesis, University of Nashville, 1853), TN—Vanderbilt.

119. Elisha Bartlett, *An Enquiry into the Degree of Certainty in Medicine* (Philadelphia: Lea and Blanchard, 1848).

120. G[ilman] Kimball to Elisha Bartlett, Lowell, 19 Nov. 1844; and see Elisha Bartlett to Caroline Bartlett, Lowell, 4 Sept. 1837, both in Bartlett Family Papers.

121. P.-J.-G. Cabanis, *Du degré de certitude de médecine* (Paris: Firmin Pidot, 1798), which became more accessible to American physicians as *An Essay on the Certainty of Medicine*, trans. R. La Roche (Philadelphia: Robert Desilver, 1823). See Martin Staum, *Cabanis: Enlightenment and Medical Philosophy in the French Republic* (Princeton: Princeton University Press, 1980).

122. C.G.W. Comegys to Scott Cook, Cincinnati, 7 Jan. 1851, Matthew Scott Cook Papers, OH—Western Reserve Hist. Soc.

123. Thos. T. Beall, "An Essay on the Physician's Calling" (M.D. thesis, University of Pennsylvania, 1858), PA—U. PA Lib.

124. Bartlett, "[Address] to Gentlemen of the Medical Class."

125. James Jackson, Jr., to William Henry Channing, Paris, 16 Feb. 1832, MA—Countway.

126. Jackson, Jr., to Jackson, Sr., entry of 26 Nov. in letter of Paris, 24 Nov. 1832. And see W. W. Gerhard to James Jackson, Jr., Paris, 13 Aug. 1833, Putnam, Jackson & Lowell Papers, MA—MA Hist. Soc.

127. Jackson, Jr., to Jackson, Sr., entry for 28 Nov. in letter of Paris, 24 Nov., J. Jackson Papers.

128. Ashbel Smith to James Jackson, Jr., Salisbury, North Carolina, 21 Feb. 1834, MA—Countway.

129. John Y. Bassett, "Report on the Topography, Climate, and Diseases of Madison County, Ala.," *Southern Medical Reports* 1 (1849): 256–282; and idem, "On the Climate and Diseases of Huntsville, Ala., and Its Vicinity, for the Year 1850," ibid. 2 (1850): 315–323. And see E. D. Fenner to John Y. Bassett, New Orleans, 24 Oct. 1849, Bassett Papers, NC—SHC.

130. W. W. Gerhard to James Jackson, Sr., Philadelphia, 19 Apr. 1834, J. Jackson Papers.

131. For example, A. H. Cenas to W. W. Gerhard, New Orleans, 24 Sept. 1834; J. Jackson to W. W. Gerhard, Waltham, 16 July 1834; ibid., Boston, 26 Oct. 1834; Stewardson to Gerhard, London, 9 Sept. 1834, all in Gerhard Papers; and J. Jackson to W. W. Gerhard, Waltham, 4 Sept. 1834, J. Jackson Papers.

132. W. W. Gerhard to James Jackson, Sr., Philadelphia, 1 Feb. 1835, J. Jackson Papers.

133. "[Review of Three Books on Auscultation and Diagnosis of Diseases of the Chest]," *NOMSJ* 3 (1846–1847): 84–85, p. 85.

134. Stillé, *Elements of General Pathology*, p. 166.

135. W. W. Gerhard to James Jackson, Sr., Philadelphia, 11 July 1834, J. Jackson Papers.

CHAPTER 8
SCIENCE, HEALING, AND THE
MORAL ORDER OF MEDICINE

1. John Asplin, Journals, 1819–1824, 3 vols., vol. 3, entry for Paris, 17 July 1824, Montreal—McGill.

2. "Poverty of English Medical Literature," *Lancet* 2 (1842–1843): 197–199, p. 197. And see "Medical Education in England," *LMG* 1 (1827–1828): 10–11, p. 11, and "Practice of Physic," *Anderson's Quarterly Journal of Medical Sciences*, n.s., 1 (1824): 139–147, pp. 139–140.

3. Review of "*Darstellungen und Ansichten zur Vergleichung der Medicin in Frankreich, England, und Deutschland, nach einer Reise in diesen Ländern im Jahre 1835*. Von Dr. Adolph Mühry," *British and Foreign Medical Review* 3 (1837): 447–452, p. 449; and see "Medical Reform. Meeting of the North of England Medical Association," *Lancet* 1 (1839–1840): 737–739, p. 737.

4. Voyageur, "Parisian News" (Paris, 1 May 1828), *LMG* 2 (1828): 695–697, p. 695.

5. J. L. Cabell to Joseph C. Cabell, Paris, 28

Jan. 1837, James Lawrence Cabell Papers (no. 1640), VA—U. VA.

6. For example, Samuel Grant, "Topical Bleeding" (M.D. thesis, Medical University of the State of South Carolina, 1827), SC—Waring.

7. Robert P. Harris, "Letter from Paris," (Paris, 19 Nov. 1855), *American Medical Gazette and Journal of Health* 7, no. 3 (1856): 168–171, p. 171.

8. On the broader belief that therapeutics had to be individuated according to variables such as ethnicity, class, and region, see John Harley Warner, *The Therapeutic Perspective: Medical Practice, Knowledge, and Identity in America, 1820–1885* (Cambridge, Mass., and London: Harvard University Press, 1986), pp. 58–80.

9. James Rackliffe, Notes on the Lectures of Benjamin S. Barton, Philadelphia, 1 Nov. 1815, NC—Duke Med. On the larger context of this thinking, see Antonello Gerbi, *The Dispute of the New World: The History of a Polemic, 1750–1900*, trans. Jeremy Moyle (1955; [Pittsburgh]: Pittsburgh University Press, 1973).

10. [Lawrence] Jefferson Trotti, Notes on Lectures by [Benjamin] Dudley, in Notebook, bound with Catalogue for Transylvania University, 1828, KY—Transylvania.

11. See Anonymous, Notes Taken on Lectures Given by Benjamin Dudley, 1830, LA—Tulane Med.; R. T. Dismukes, Notes Taken on Lectures Given by B. W. Dudley, Prof. of Anatomy & Surgery, Medical Department of Transylvania University, 1838–1839, NC—Duke; Daniel D. Slauson, Notes Taken on Introductory Lecture, Geneva College, 1846, By Prof. Webster, in Medical Daybook, 1846–1877, Daniel D. Slauson Papers, LA—LSU; and John George Metcalf, Medical Lectures, Boston, 1825–1826, 2 vols., vol. 2, [James Jackson], Cases at the Massachusetts General Hospital, 21 Nov. 1825, MA—Countway.

12. Courtney J. Clark, Notes Taken on Lectures Given by Chas Caldwell, Medical Institute of Louisville, 1841–1842, entry of 6 Nov. 1841, Courtney J. Clark Papers, NC—Duke.

13. Samuel A. Cartwright, "Alcohol and the Ethiopian; or, the Moral and Physical Effects of Ardent Spirits on the Negro Race, and Some Account of the Peculiarity of That People," *NOMSJ* 10 (1853–1854): 150–165, p. 161.

14. Henry Bryant to John Bryant, Paris, entry of 21 Dec. in letter of 11 Dec. 1843, William Sohier Bryant Papers (MS 45), MA—New England Hist. Gen. Soc. And see Edward Keller, Diary as a Student at S[outh] C[arolina] College and Lecture Notes, 1849–1859; the quotation is from "Remarks and Lectures of Dr. Laborde for the Sopho[mo]re Class of 1854 Concerning Physiology," SC—U. SC.

15. F.P.P., "Editorial Correspondence of Charleston Medical Journal and Review" (Paris, 6 Oct. 1852), *CMJR* 7 (1852): 859–864, p. 861; Geo. Suckley, "On Matters of Novelty or General Interest, As at Present Exhibited in the Practice of the Hospitals of Paris" (Paris, 27 Mar. 1858), *New York Journal of Medicine* 5 (1853): 21–32, p. 24.

16. C. C[aldwell], "Medicine in Paris" (London, 29 May 1841), *WJMS* 4 (1841): 237–240, pp. 239, 240.

17. Joshua B. Flint, *Address Delivered to the Students of the Louisville Medical Institute, in Presence of the Citizens of the Place, at the Commencement of the Second Session of the Institute, November 13th, 1838* (Louisville: Prentice and Weissenger, 1838), pp. 19, 19–20, 20.

18. James Jackson, Jr., to James Jackson, Sr., Paris, 26 June 1831, James Jackson Papers, MA—Countway. And see ibid., Paris, entry of 8 June in letter of 7 June 1831; Paris, 18 Feb. 1832; and London, 12 Sept. 1832.

19. F. Campbell Stewart, *Eminent French Surgeons, with a Historical and Statistical Account of the Hospitals of Paris; together with Miscellaneous Information and Biographical Notes of the Most Eminent of the Living Paris Surgeons* (Buffalo: A. Burke, 1845), p. 122.

20. Levin S. Joynes to Thomas R. Joynes, Paris, 12 Dec. 1841, Joynes Family Papers, VA—VA Hist. Soc.

21. Flint, *Address*, p. 25.

22. C[aldwell], "Medicine in Paris," p. 239.

23. Robert Peter to Frances Peter, Paris, 27 June 1839, Evans Papers, KY—U. KY.

24. William Williams Keen to Parents, undated typescript [Paris, 1864 or 1865], William Williams Keen Papers, RI—Brown.

25. A. Colman to Catherine K. Colman, Paris, 28 Jan. 1833, Colman (Anson) Papers, NY—U. Rochester.

26. C[aldwell], "Medicine in Paris," pp. 237, 237–238.

27. Ibid., p. 238.

28. For a compelling analysis of this cost-

benefit trade-off and its place in professionalism, see Martin S. Pernick, *A Calculus of Suffering: Pain, Professionalism, and Anesthesia in Nineteenth-Century America* (New York: Columbia University Press, 1985).

29. George Suckley, "Notes on the Practice in the Hospitals of Paris. The 'Ecraseur,' 'Electric Cautery,' Maisonneuve's Method of Dividing Strictures, Etc., Etc.," *New York Journal of Medicine*, ser. 3, 4 (1858): 341–355, p. 344.

30. Valentine Mott, *Travels in Europe and the East* (New-York: Harper and Brothers, 1842), p. 45.

31. Edward Warren, *A Doctor's Experiences in Three Continents* (Baltimore: Cushings and Bailey, 1885), p. 170.

32. Cf. James Jackson, Jr., to James Jackson, Sr., Paris, 6 Nov. 1831, J. Jackson Papers, and the published version of the same letter in James Jackson, *A Memoir of James Jackson, Jr., M.D., with Extracts from His Letters to His Father: and Medical Cases, Collected by Him* (Boston: I. R. Butts, 1835), pp. 86–88.

33. [Robley Dunglison], *An Introductory Lecture to the Course of Institutes of Medicine, &c. in Jefferson Medical College, Delivered Nov. 4, 1844, by Professor Dunglison* (Philadelphia: B. E. Smith, 1844), p. 26.

34. Henry H. Smith, *A Professional Visit to London and Paris: Introductory Lecture to the Course on the Principles and Practice of Surgery. Delivered in the University of Pennsylvania, October 9, 1855* (Philadelphia: T. K. and P. G. Collins, 1855), pp. 18–19.

35. Robert Peter to Frances Peter, Paris, 22 June 1839, Evans Papers. And see Benjamin J. Hicks to J. Y. Bassett, Paris, 31 July 1837, John Young Bassett Papers, AL—AL State Arch.

36. Flint, *Address*, p. 19.

37. M. M. Rodgers, "Letter from a Correspondent at Paris" (Paris, 6 Feb. 1851), *Buffalo Medical Journal* 6 (1850–1851): 644–646, p. 646.

38. Eugène Sue, *The Mysteries of Paris*, 3 vols. (Paris, 1843; London, 1846, 3:291–307. I discuss this scene more fully in *The Therapeutic Perspective*, pp. 193–195. On Sue (who came from a medical family) and the animus of his social reformism, see Nora Atkinson, *Eugène Sue et le roman-feuilleton* (Nemours: André Lesot, 1929); Charles Arlo Isetts, "Eugène Sue: A Writer for the People" (Ph.D. diss., Miami University, 1974); and John

Moody, *Les idées sociales d'Eugène Sue* (Paris: Presses Universitaires de France, 1938).

39. Henry Bryant to John Bryant, Paris, 11 Dec. 1843, Bryant Papers. And see, for example, Augustus Kinsley Gardner, *Old Wine in New Bottles; or, Spare Hours of a Student in Paris* (New-York: C. S. Francis & Co.; Boston: J. H. Francis, 1848), pp. 51, 109.

40. O. W. Holmes, "Experiments in Medicine," *BMSJ* 30 (1844): 201–203, pp. 203, 202.

41. Rodgers, "Letter from a Correspondent," p. 646.

42. Benjamin G. Bruse, "Medical Science, Its Improvements, and the Spirit of Progress" (M.D. thesis, Transylvania University, 1850), KY—Transylvania.

43. H. V. Wooten, "Address before the Alabama State Medical Association at Its First Regular Session in Selma, on the 9th Day of March 1848," Hardy Vickers Wooten Papers, AL—AL State Arch.

44. Daniel Drake, "A Discourse on the Necessity and Value of Professional Morality," Transylvania University, 1823, Drake Manuscripts, OH—U. Cincinnati Med.

45. John Ware, "Success in the Medical Profession. An Introductory Lecture, Delivered at the Massachusetts Med. College, Nov. 6, 1850," *BMSJ* 43 (1850–1851): 496–505, 509–522, on pp. 497–498.

46. George G. Todd, "Young Physic" (M.D. thesis, Transylvania University, 1848), KY—Transylvania. On the shifting place of character in depictions of the proper physician, see Rebecca J. Tannenbaum, "Earnestness, Temperance, Industry: The Definition and Uses of Professional Character among Nineteenth-Century American Physicians," *Journal of the History of Medicine and Allied Sciences* 49 (1994): 251–283.

47. Thos. T. Beall, "An Essay on the Physician's Calling" (M.D. thesis, University of Pennsylvania, 1858), PA—U. PA Lib.; and see John Adams Betts, "The Character and Duties of the Physician" (M.D. thesis, Medical Institution of Yale College, 1848), CT—Yale Med.

48. Elisha Bartlett to Otis Bartlett, Lowell, Mass., 17 Jan. 1828, Elisha Bartlett Family Papers, NY—U. Rochester.

49. H. V. Wooten, *Character: A Valedictory Address to the Graduating Class of the Memphis Medical College Delivered by H. V. Wooten, M.D. Professor of the Principles and Practice of*

*Medicine, at the Annual Commencement February 26th, 1853* (Memphis: Eagle and Enquirer Steam Printing House, 1853), pp. 21, 22, 22.

50. Joseph Jones to C. C. Jones, Philadelphia, 13 Dec. 1853, Joseph Jones Collection, LA—Tulane. And see Thomas J. Griffith, Diary, Ann Arbor, Mich., 1865, entry for 4 Nov. 1865, IN—IN U., and E. L. Mcall to Lemuel Kollock, Philadelphia, 2 Jan. 1805, Lemuel Kollock Papers, GA—GA Hist. Soc.

51. H.V.M. Miller, "Valedictory Address, to the First Graduating Class of the Medical College of Memphis, Delivered on the 5th Day of March, 1847," *South-Western Medical Advocate* 1 (1847): 49–67, p. 63.

52. Ware, "Success in the Medical Profession," p. 518.

53. Dandridge A. Bibb, "The Effects of the Study and Practice of Medicine on the Mind and Character" (M.D. thesis, Medical College of the State of South Carolina, 1846), SC—Waring.

54. Ware, "Success in the Medical Profession," p. 500.

55. Regina Markell Morantz-Sanchez, *Sympathy and Science: Women Physicians in American Medicine* (New York and Oxford: Oxford University Press, 1985), and idem, "Feminist Theory and Historical Practice: Rereading Elizabeth Blackwell," *History and Theory*, Beiheft 31 (1992): 51–69. And see Ellen Singer More and Maureen A. Milligan, eds., *The Empathic Practitioner: Empathy, Gender, and the Therapeutic Relationship* (New Brunswick, N.J.: Rutgers University Press, 1994).

56. Ware, "Success in the Medical Profession," pp. 518, 519.

57. Mark Twain and Charles Dudley Warner, *The Gilded Age*, 2 vols. (1873; New York and Boston: Harper and Brothers, 1901), 1:177; Elizabeth Stuart Phelps, *Doctor Zay* (1882; New York: Feminist Press, 1987), p. 78; and William D. Howells, *Dr. Breen's Practice* (1881; Boston and New York: Houghton, Mifflin and Company, 1891), p. 12.

58. Max Adeler [Charles Heber Clark], *Out of the Hurly-Burly; or, Life in an Odd Corner* (Philadelphia: George Maclean and Co., 1874), chap. 5, pp. 68–83, on pp. 71–72.

59. Ibid., pp. 72–73.

60. Ibid., p. 74.

61. Ibid., pp. 79, 73, 81.

62. Nathaniel Hawthorne, "The Birthmark" (1843), in *Mosses from an Old Manse* (Columbus: Ohio State University Press, 1974), 10:36–56.

63. The images appear in Adeler, *Out of the Hurly-Burly*, pp. 68 and 83. Sonya S. Erickson notes the masculinization of these depictions in "The Image of Women Physicians in Ten Victorian American Novels, 1871–1886" (M.D. thesis, Yale University, 1991), p. 100.

64. See ibid., esp. pp. xiii–xx, 1–19, 185–193.

65. Sophia Jex-Blake, "Medical Women in Fiction," *The Nineteenth Century* 33 (1893): 261–272, p. 261. "The public have a right to require," she insisted, "that such portraits should be in some sense taken from life" (pp. 261–262).

66. Ibid., p. 268.

67. Graham Travers, *Mona Maclean, Medical Student*, 2d ed. (1892; 1893), quoted in ibid., p. 270.

68. E. H. Cleveland, *Introductory Lecture on Behalf of the Faculty to the Class of the Female Medical College of Pennsylvania, for the Session of 1858–59* (Philadelphia: Merrihew and Thompson, 1858), pp. 10–11, 6.

69. Emeline H. Cleveland, *Valedictory Address to the Graduating Class of the Woman's Medical College of Pennsylvania, at the Sixteenth Annual Commencement, March 14, 1868* (Philadelphia: Jas. B. Rodgers, 1868), p. 5–6. "The natural tendency of medical studies upon a pure and healthful mind is to refine, and elevate, and cause it to realize that we live amid holy things," Ann Preston, professor of physiology and hygiene at the same college, similarly urged, encouraging students to believe that focusing on what was spiritually "enriching and ennobling" in their calling would develop their "womanly character" (*Introductory Lecture to the Class of the Female Medical College, of Pennsylvania. Delivered at the Opening of the Tenth Annual Session, Oct. 19, 1859* [Philadelphia: A. Ketterlinus, 1859], pp. 14, 13).

70. "New York Medical College for Women," *Frank Leslie's Illustrated Newspaper*, vol. 30 (16 Apr. 1870), p. 71. Of the four plates illustrating instruction at the college, three depicted student dissection; and see illustrations on pp. 65, 72, and 73. And, in the same issue, note A. K. Gardner's supportive article titled "Women Doctors," pp. 66–67, which comments on the sketches.

71. Flint, *Address*, p. 9.

72. Henry Edwin Morril, "The Formation of Medical Character" (M.D. thesis, University of Pennsylvania, 1840), PA—U. PA Lib.

73. Gardner, *Old Wine*, p. 69.

74. Henry W. Williams to A. O. Williams, Paris, 20 June 1846, Henry Williard Williams Papers, MA—Countway.

75. Ibid., Paris, 20 Nov. 1846.

76. Auguste Shurtleff, [Journal of a Trip to Europe], 1850–1852, 2 vols., vol. 1, entry for 20 Jan. 1851, MA—Countway.

77. Gardner, *Old Wine*, pp. 72, 73.

78. Warren, *A Doctor's Experiences*, p. 175. For denunciations of Lisfranc's treatment of women, see, for example, "Notice of Lisfranc's Clinics," *Southern Medical and Surgical Journal* 1 (1837): 370–374, p. 372.

79. Warren, *A Doctor's Experiences*, pp. 176, 175.

80. J.B.G., "Foreign Correspondence" (Paris, 1 Feb. 1857), *New Hampshire Journal of Medicine* 7 (1857): 138–143, p. 140.

81. Stephen H. Bronson to Henry Bronson, Paris, 18 Dec. 1867, Stephen Henry Bronson Papers, CT—Yale Med.

82. M. L. Linton, "Hospitals of Paris" (Paris, 24 Dec. 1840), *WJMS* 3 (1841): 65–74, pp. 66, 67. Reactions to vivisectional work at Alfort, the veterinary school near Paris, were particularly powerful and deserve closer exploration.

83. J. Y. Bassett to Wells A. Thompson, Paris, 10 Mar. 1836; and see J. Y. Bassett to Isaphoena Bassett, Paris, 11 Mar. 1836, both in Bassett Papers.

84. L. H. Malchen to E. S. Cooper, Clinton, 19 Jan. 1855, Elias Samuel Cooper Papers (MS 458), CA—CA Hist. Soc.

85. Stephen Henry Bronson, Diary, Paris, vol. 1, 5 Oct. 1867–28 Feb. 1870, entry for 29 Nov. 1867, Stephen Henry Bronson Papers, CT—Yale.

86. Gardner, *Old Wine*, 203. And see A. Dugas to Ma chère Maman, Paris, 7 May 1829, Dugas Papers, GA—GA Hist. Soc.

87. S. S. Satchwell, "Letter from S. S. Satchwell, M.D." (Paris, 2 Jan. 1861), *Medical Journal of North Carolina* 3 (1861): 245–252, p. 249.

88. Elisha Bartlett to Caroline Bartlett, Paris, 25 Oct. 1826, Elisha Bartlett Papers, CT—Yale.

89. "Biscaccianti—Paris Generally," *Daily Crescent*, 14 Jan. 1850, p. 2, quoted in Alejandro Bolaños-Geyer, *William Walker: The Gray-Eyed Man of Destiny* (Lake Saint Louis, Mo.: Privately published, 1988), p. 32.

90. William Henry Channing to James Jackson, Jr., Cambridge, 26 Apr. 1832, and James Jackson, Jr., to William Henry Channing, Paris, 1 July 1832, J. Jackson Papers.

91. Austin Flint, "European Correspondence" (Paris, 18 May 1854), *WJMS* 2 (1854): 9–17, p. 17; and see Austin Flint, "Address at the Opening of the Session for 1854–55 in the Medical Department of the University of Louisville," *WJMS* 2 (1854): 409–425, pp. 423–424.

92. P., "The Advantages and Disadvantages of Paris As a Place of Resort for Medical Students," *SLMSJ* 14 (1856): 79–85, p. 84.

93. James Jackson, Jr., to James Jackson, Sr., Paris, 27 June 1833, J. Jackson Papers.

94. Henry Ingersoll Bowditch, Introductory to the Course on Clinical Medicine Nov 1861 Course of 1861–2, MA—Countway. Bowditch pointed to the Viennese clinician Skoda as the best representative of the pure Naturalist; "a frightful exhibition of human nature is presented by such a man."

95. Ibid.

96. M. L. L[inton], "Medicine in Paris" (Paris, 25 July 1840), *WJMS* 2 (1840): 69–73, p. 72.

97. Henry Bryant to John Bryant, Paris, entry of 21 Dec. 1829 in letter of 11 Dec. 1843, Bryant Papers; A. Dugas to L. Charles Dugas, Paris, 28 July 1829, Dugas Papers.

98. Gabriel Manigault, Autobiography, transcript, p. 130, SC—U. SC.

99. Gardner, *Old Wine*, p. 206.

100. Henry W. Williams to A. O. Williams, Paris, 10 Oct. 1846, Williams Papers.

101. "Here in Paris," a St. Louis physician reported the commonplace American perception of hospital arrangements, "for the benefit of the student all are infinitely superior to those of the United States, but for the patients far otherwise" (Montrose A. Pallen, "Letter from Our European Correspondent" [Paris, 29 May 1857], *SLMSJ* 15 [1857]: 356–366, p. 359).

102. James Jackson, Jr., to James Jackson, Sr., Paris, 7 Oct. 1831, J. Jackson Papers.

103. J. Y. Bassett to Isaphoena Bassett, Paris, 27 Mar. 1836, Bassett Papers.

104. J. Y. Bassett to Indiana Manning, Paris, 7 June 1836, Bassett Papers.

105. John Young Bassett, Autobiographical Notes, [1836], Bassett Papers.

106. J.B.G., "Foreign Correspondence," p. 140.

107. Gardner, *Old Wine*, p. 203.

108. Suckley, "Notes on the Practice in the Hospitals of Paris," pp. 344, 345.

109. T. Stewardson to W. W. Gerhard, London, 9 Sept. 1834, W. W. Gerhard Papers, PA—CPP.

110. Charles T. Jackson to Charles Brown, Paris, 8 Aug. 1832, Charles Thomas Jackson Papers, DC—LC.

111. James Jackson, Jr., to William H. Channing, London, [May or June] 1832, J. Jackson Papers. Jackson added: "I shd. burn this letter if my fire had not gone out while writing it and I have not time to write another."

112. William Henry Channing to James Jackson, Jr., Cambridge, 10 Mar. 1832, J. Jackson Papers.

113. James Jackson, Jr., to James Jackson, Sr., Paris, 17 Feb. 1832, J. Jackson Papers.

114. Ibid., Paris, 18 Feb. 1832.

115. James Jackson, Sr., to James Jackson, Jr., Waltham, 24 June 1832.

116. James Jackson, Jr., to James Jackson, Sr., Paris, entry of 8 Nov. in letter of 1 Nov. 1832. For the proposed plan, see Pierre Louis to James Jackson, Sr., Paris, 28 Oct. 1832, in [James Jackson], ed., *Memoir of James Jackson, Jr. M.D. Written by His Father, with Extracts from His Letters, and Reminiscences of Him, by a Fellow Student. For the Warren Street Chapel* (Boston: Hilliard, Gray & Co., 1836), pp. 27–30.

117. James Jackson, Jr., to James Jackson, Sr., Paris, 16 Jan. 1833; and see ibid., Paris, 25 Jan. 1833, J. Jackson Papers.

118. Ibid., 22 Feb. 1833.

119. Pierre Louis to James Jackson, Sr., Paris, 22 Mar. 1833, in [Jackson], *Memoir of James Jackson, Jr.*, pp. 31–33, pp. 31, 32; emphasis added.

120. James Jackson, Jr., to James Jackson, Sr., Paris, 22 Mar. 1833, J. Jackson Papers.

121. James Jackson, Sr., to James Jackson, Jr., Boston, 12 Apr. 1833.

122. Ibid., Waltham, 12 June 1833.

123. Ibid., 20 June 1833. The younger Jackson remained unwavering in his ardor to pursue Louis's plan; see James Jackson, Jr., to James Jackson, Sr., Paris, 27 June 1833, written only a fortnight before his departure for Boston.

124. [Jackson], *Memoir of James Jackson, Jr.*, p. 80; emphasis added.

125. Ibid.

126. Z., "Medical Improvement.—No. VII," *BMSJ* 9 (1834): 192–194, pp. 192, 194.

127. "Southern Medical Schools—Southern Toadyism," *Georgia Blister and Critic* 1 (1854): 34–35, p. 34; and see "P. H. Lewis, "Reply to Doctor W. M. Boling's Review of Doctor Lewis' Medical History of Alabama, with Some New Facts and Remarks, in Relation to the Diagnosis and Identity of the Fevers of the State," *NOMSJ* 4 (1847–1848): 601–640, p. 639; Review of "*Pneumonia: Its Supposed Connexion, Pathological and Aetiological with Autumnal Fevers . . . By R. La Roche*," *NOMSJ* 11 (1855): 103–108, p. 103.

128. Linton, "Hospitals of Paris," p. 70.

129. Dunglison, *An Introductory Lecture*, p. 24.

130. J. C. Warren to [Isaac] Hays, Boston, 7 Jan. 1850, Isaac Hays Papers, PA—APS.

131. Alfred Stillé, *Valedictory Address to the Graduates of the Medical Department of Pennsylvania College, Delivered at the Public Commencement, March 6, 1857* (Philadelphia: T. K. and P. G. Collins, 1857), p. 10. On the subsequent trajectory of this theme, see Susan E. Lederer, *Subjected to Science: Human Experimentation in America before the Second World War* (Baltimore and London: Johns Hopkins University Press, 1995).

132. Williams to Williams, entry of 26 June in letter of 20 June 1846.

133. James Jackson, Jr., to William H. Channing, Paris, 16 Feb. 1832, J. Jackson Papers.

134. W. W. Gerhard to James Jackson, Sr., Philadelphia, 11 July 1834, J. Jackson Papers.

135. W. W. Gerhard to J. Jackson, Paris, 13 Aug. 1833, Putnam, Jackson and Lowell Papers, MA—MA Hist. Soc. See also J. Jackson to W. W. Gerhard, Waltham, 4 Sept. 1834, Gerhard Papers.

136. See John Harley Warner, "The Selective Transport of Medical Knowledge: Antebellum American Physicians and Parisian Medical Therapeutics," *Bulletin of the History of Medicine* 59 (1985): 213–231.

137. [P.] Louis to James Jackson, Paris, 12 May 1834, MA—Countway.

138. H. I. Bowditch, Introductory to the

Clinical Course of Harvards Course of 1861, MA—Countway.

139. Warner, *The Therapeutic Perspective*, esp. pp. 21–31.

140. See ibid., pp. 219–220. For the development of Bowditch's appraisal in the 1860s and 1870s, see, for example, Henry I. Bowditch, Introductory to the Course on Clinical Medicine, Nov. 1861, Course of 1861–1862, MA—Countway, and idem, *Venesection, Its Abuse—Formerly—Its Neglect at the Present Day* (Boston: D. Clapp and Son, 1872). The letters of support the latter publication elicited make it clear that his stance was far from singular: for example, see Willard Parker to H. I. Bowditch, N.Y., 20 Mar. 1872; James A. Stetson to H. I. Bowditch, Quincy, Mass., 22 Apr. 1872; and Wm. G. White, Chelsea, Mass., 7 Mar. 1872, all in H. I. Bowditch, Collection of Autograph Letters and Portraits, MA—Countway. And see his treatment of skepticism in Henry I. Bowditch, *Public Hygiene in America: Being a Centennial Discourse Delivered before the International Medical Congress, Philadelphia, September, 1876* (Boston: Little, Brown, and Company, 1877), which he dedicated to Pierre Louis. And see Warner, *The Therapeutic Perspective*, pp. 28–35.

141. For example, Prof. Mitchell, "Typhoid Fever, an Objectionable Term," *NOMSJ* 2 (1845–1846): 391–393, p. 391.

142. "The Hospitals of London," *BMSJ* 42 (1850): 461–466, p. 464. The correspondent, though writing from England, was reflecting on American practice. See, however, Robert Southgate, "An Essay on Bloodletting, Read Before the Medical Association of the State of Georgia, at Their Annual Meeting, Held at Rome, April 11th, 1860," *Southern Medical and Surgical Journal* 16 (1860): 484–505, 577–581, pp. 496, 497.

143. John A. Lyle, "Exclusive Systems of Medicine" (M.D. thesis, Transylvania University, 1841), KY—Transylvania.

144. Quoted in John Spare, "Dr. Spare's Dissertation," in *Dissertations on the Part Performed by Nature and Time in the Cure of Disease; for Which Prizes Were Awarded by the Massachusetts Medical Society* (Boston: D. Clapp and Son, 1868), pp. 97–155, on p. 137.

145. A. L. Peirson, Notes Taken by Lectures on the Theory and Practice of Physic by James Jackson, Boston, 1814–1816, 4 vols., vol. 1, 1814–1815, entry for 18 Nov. 1815, MA—Countway.

146. Elisha Bartlett, Notes Taken by Lectures Given by James Jackson on the Theory and Practice of Physick, 1824–1825, lecture of 11 Dec. 1824, Bartlett Papers.

147. H. I. Bowditch, Notes Taken on Lectures Given by James Jackson, Boston, 1831–1832, MA—Countway. And see J[ohn] C[all] D[alton], Notes Taken on Lectures Given by James Jackson, 1816–1817, 2 vols., vol. 2, entry of 20 Dec. 1816, MA—Countway; Jonathan Greely Stevenson, Notes Taken on Lectures Given by James Jackson on the Theory and Practice of Physic, 1817–1819, 2 vols., vol. 2, MA—Countway; Aaron Cornish, Notes Taken by Lectures Given by James Jackson, Boston, 1818–1819, MD—NLM; and James Jackson, Jr., Notes Taken on Lectures Given by James Jackson, Sr., [1830–1831], MA—Countway. Similarly, a student attending Joseph Mather Smith's lectures in New York in 1826 recorded that in therapeutics there were two plans, "Active & Expectant." Active treatment, which he identified with the English, involved "interrupting the morbid action, by the application of artificial means," whereas in the expectant, the plan principally pursued by the French, "the Physician[']s only duty is to watch the action of the vis medicatrix & promote its operation" (Benjm. S. Downing, Notes Taken by Lectures Given by Joseph M. Smith on the Theory and Practice of Medicine, College of Physicians and Surgeons at the University of the State of New York, 1826, NY—Columbia Med.).

148. See John Harley Warner, "'The Nature-Trusting Heresy': American Physicians and the Concept of the Healing Power of Nature in the 1850's and 1860's," *Perspectives in American History* 11 (1977–1978): 291–324. During the 1840s and 1850s typhoid fever, which pathological researches by Paris clinicians and their disciples had shown to exemplify a self-limited disease, was the central pivot upon which debate over the expectant method turned. See Dale C. Smith, "Gerhard's Distinction between Typhoid and Typhus and Its Reception in America, 1833–1860," *Bulletin of the History of Medicine* 54 (1980): 368–385, and Lloyd G. Stevenson, "Exemplary Disease: The Typhoid Pattern," *Journal of the History of Medicine and Allied Sciences* 37 (1982):

159–181. This debate deserves attention in the context of regional support for the expectant plan (in the Northeast) and animosity against it (particularly in the South and West).

149. C. Grant, "The Fallacy of a Supposed Vis Medicatrix Naturae," *WL* 11 (1850): 348–357, p. 351; Review of *"An Address on the Bonds of Professional Union, Delivered before the Medical Association of Adams, Brown and Clermont Counties, Ohio, at Batavia, October 30th, 1847,"* *WL* 7 (1847): 287–290, p. 289; "Typhoid and Typhus Fever, Thirty-Two Years Ago," *WL* 1 (1842–1843): 420–421, p. 420.

150. Massachusetts General Hospital, Medical Case Records, vols. 48 and 50 (1832), MA—Countway. Nor did those who urged the expectant method on their students portray it as passive; see, for example, Walter Gilman Curtis, Notes Taken on Lectures Given by [John] Ware and [Jacob] Bigelow, Massachusetts Medical College, [n.d., between 1847 and 1853], notes on Bigelow, NC—SHC. As Ruben D. Mussey told his students in 1819, "If a fever has once got established we cant do much to shorten it for the fever must have its course. The Physician should not be an idle spectator but be ready to take hold & lend any assistance in his power. He should not be too officious in cramming his patient with Medicine, unless to allay the apprehensions of the friends or patient and in such cases the Medicine should be inert (a placebo)" (John Wheeler, Jr., Notes Taken on Lectures Given by Ruben D. Mussey on the Theory and Practice of Physic, Medical Institution of Dartmouth College, Oct. 1819, NH—NH Hist. Soc.).

151. George Eliot, *Middlemarch: A Study in Provincial Life* (1871–1872; Harmondsworth: Penguin Books, 1965), pp. 193, 118.

152. Ibid., pp. 186, 481, 486.

153. This discussion draws heavily on John Harley Warner, "Medical Sectarianism, Therapeutic Conflict, and the Shaping of Orthodox Professional Identity in Antebellum American Medicine," in *Medical Fringe and Medical Orthodoxy, 1750–1850,* ed. W. F. Bynum and Roy Porter (London: Croom Helm, 1987), pp. 234–260. The celebration of these therapies in principle at the moment of their near demise in practice is developed in Warner, *The Thera-*

*peutic Perspective,* esp. pp. 4–7, 162–184, 207–232. When the sectarian challenge to orthodoxy became especially severe, precipitating an awareness of professional crisis, regular physicians may have returned to traditional heroic remedies in practice, not just principle; see John Harley Warner, "Power, Conflict, and Identity in Mid-Nineteenth-Century American Medicine: Therapeutic Change at the Commercial Hospital of Cincinnati," *Journal of American History* 73 (1987): 934–956.

154. Oliver Wendell Holmes, *Currents and Counter Currents in Medical Science, an Address Delivered before the Massachusetts Medical Society, at the Annual Meeting, May 30, 1860* (Boston: Ticknor and Fields, 1860), p. 16. One critic tellingly denounced Holmes for his "free thinking" in therapeutics ("Dr. Holmes vs. the Medical Profession," *Medical Journal of North Carolina* 3 [1860]: 619–624, p. 619). On the charge of heresy, see, for example, review of *"Science and Success: A Valedictory Address Delivered to the Medical Graduates of Harvard University, at the College in Boston. Wednesday, March 9, 1859. By Henry Jacob Bigelow,"* *Nashville Journal of Medicine and Surgery* 17 (1859): 252–253, p. 252, and "The Water Cure or Hydropathy," *WL* 5 (1846–1847): 392–394, p. 393.

155. Alex. McBride, "A Chemico-Pathological Classification of Fevers, and Hints at Treatment Based Thereon," *CLO* 25 (1864): 9–26, p. 23.

156. See, for example, [Charles] Neidhard, "Preface," *Miscellanies on Homoeopathy* 1 (1839): 1–2; "Progress of Homoeopathy and the Abandonment of Allopathy," *American Journal of Homoeopathy* 7 (1852): 108–110, p. 110; and the articles in *Indian Arcana; Devoted to Illustrations of Indian Life, Indian Medicine, Science, Art, Literature, and General Intelligence* 5, no. 7 (1860).

157. "Review of John Forbes, *Homoeopathy, Allopathy, and Young Physic* (1846)," *WL* 5 (1847): 181–213, p. 198.

158. Jas. W. Hughes, "A Few Thoughts Suggested by the Present Phase of Medical Skepticism," *CLO,* n.s., 1 (1858): 654–656, p. 655.

159. Remarks of John P. Harrison at meeting of 1 Mar. 1849, Hamilton County [Ohio] Medical Club, Minutes of Meetings, 21 May 1842–4 Apr. 1850, MD—NLM.

160. Dr. Gans, paper on puerperal fever in

"Proceedings of the Cincinnati Academy of Medicine," *CLO*, n.s., 5 (1862): 23–34, p. 24.

161. Review of "William Stokes (Dublin), *Lectures on the Theory and Practice of Physic*," *WL* 1 (1842–1843): 354–357, p. 354.

162. Flint, "Address," p. 414.

163. Southgate, "An Essay on Bloodletting," p. 496.

164. "Nature and the Physician in the Cure of Disease" [extracts from Samuel Jackson's Annual Report on the Theory and Practice of Medicine to the College of Physicians of Philadelphia], *BMSJ* 33 (1845–1846): 461–463, pp. 461, 463.

165. [Lorenzo N. Henderson], Notes Taken on Lectures Given by Daniel Drake, 1830–1831, 2 vols., vol. 1, MD—NLM.

166. Notes Taken by Thomas J. Griffith on Lectures at the University of Michigan Department of Medicine and Surgery, 1 Oct. 1865–15 Mar. 1866, entry for lecture of Dr. Palmer on 1 Dec. 1865, Griffith Manuscripts, IN—IN U.; [A. W. Palmer], Notes Taken by Lectures Given by Geddings, Dickson, and Shepard, Charleston, South Carolina, 1851–1852, A. W. Palmer Collection, NC—SHC.

167. "Review of John Forbes, *Homoeopathy*," p. 191; emphasis added.

168. Samuel Murphy, Notes Taken on Lectures Given by Samuel Chapman, 1830, 2 vols., vol. 1., PA—U. PA Arch.

169. Samuel D. Gross to Benjamin P. Aydelott, Philadelphia, 25 Jan. 1862, Benjamin Parham Aydelott Papers, OH—Cincinnati Museum. "Opposed, as a general rule, to large doses & to heroic practice, I can, nevertheless, I think, see cases where prompt & decisive measures are absolutely necessary to save life," Gross continued. He felt that "the poet-doctor" deserved "the just indignation of an offended profession."

170. Warren Stone, "On Inflammation," *NOMSJ* 16 (1859): 761–777, p. 765.

171. A. M. Fauntleroy, "Annual Address of the President, on the Vis Medicatrix Naturae," *Transactions of the Medical Society of Virginia* 3 (1872): 29–34, p. 29.

172. Bowditch, Introductory to the Course on Clinical Medicine.

173. Augustus A. Gould, "Search Out the Secrets of Nature," *Medical Communications of the Massachusetts Medical Society* 9 (1855–1860): 1–45, p. 18. Asserting that "medicines can not, per se, cure disease; that their efficacy is limited to aiding Nature in her efforts to throw off her own maladies," a medical student urged that the physician's "administrations, to be available, must have the cooperation of Nature's consent. His object should be, to try to find out what she wants, what she would have done, for after all, she only looks to him to supply her with some support to her failing forces; and afterwards, if the conflict which is to be waged with the powers of disease is sustained at all, it is to be done thro' her *alone*" (Beall, "An Essay on the Physician's Calling").

174. Austin Flint, "Conservative Medicine as Applied to Therapeutics," *American Journal of the Medical Sciences*, n.s., 45 (1863): 22–43, p. 25.

175. J.T.W. Taylor, "Typhoid Fever" (M.D. thesis, University of Nashville, 1859), TN—Vanderbilt. On conservative medicine, see Pernick, *A Calculus of Suffering*, esp. pp. 21–22, 93–124.

176. Elisha Bartlett, *An Essay on the Philosophy of Medical Science* (Philadelphia: Lea and Blanchard, 1844), pp. 290, 286.

177. Samuel Clark Oliver, "On the Causes which Prevent the Progress and Usefulness of Medical Science in the United States" (M.D. thesis, University of Pennsylvania, 1820), PA—U. PA Lib.; and see John W. Williams, "Systems of Medicine" (M.D. thesis, Transylvania University, 1841), KY—Transylvania.

178. This statement is based on a study of the male medical wards case history books of the Massachusetts General Hospital in Boston (384 vols., 1823–1885, MA—Countway), and of the Commercial Hospital of Cincinnati (51 vols., 1837–1881, OH—U. Cincinnati Med.); see Warner, *The Therapeutic Perspective*, pp. 133–135, and idem, "Medical Sectarianism," pp. 245–246.

179. John Y. Bassett, "On the Climate and Diseases of Huntsville, Ala., and Its Vicinity, for the Year 1850," *Southern Medical Reports* 2 (1850): 315–323, p. 321.

180. It was with clear satisfaction, for example, that George B. Wood noted of a fellow diner at a party in Paris, who admitted that his son was a (regularly trained) homeopathic physician, that his dinner partner "agreed with me in the belief that homeopathy, practiced in accordance with its three recognized principles, was in fact simply leaving the patient to nature" (entry for Paris, 6 Nov. 1860,

425

in Journal, vol. 9, 8 Oct.–21 Nov. 1860, George B. Wood Journals, PA—CPP).

181. J.D.B. Stillman to Dear Brother, San Antonio, 1 June 1855, Jacob Davis Babcock Stillman Correspondence, CA—CA Hist. Soc.

182. I take the term from a later statement of "conservative medicine" by a Philadelphia medical student who asserted, "He only is the true physician who knows *when* to assist, and knowing when *not* to do anything, has the moral courage to let nature take her course, instead of giving sugar-powders, bread pills and making the patient believe he is working wonders with them" (John H. Fairfield, "Conservative Medicine" [M.D. thesis, University of Pennsylvania, 1880], PA—U. PA Lib.). And see the discussion of conservative medicine as a middle course in Pernick, *A Calculus of Suffering,* esp. pp. 21–22, 93–124.

CHAPTER 9
AMERICANS AND PARIS IN AN AGE OF
GERMAN ASCENDANCY

1. Erwin H. Ackerknecht, *Medicine at the Paris Hospital, 1794–1848* (Baltimore: Johns Hopkins University Press, 1967), pp. 123, xiii, dust jacket, and 123. On the migration to Germany, see Thomas Neville Bonner, *American Doctors and German Universities: A Chapter in International Intellectual Relations, 1870–1914* (Lincoln: University of Nebraska Press, 1963).

2. See Ann La Berge and Moti Feingold, eds., *French Medical Culture in the Nineteenth Century* (Amsterdam and Atlanta: Rodopi, 1994), and Caroline Hannaway and Ann La Berge, eds., *Reinterpreting Paris Medicine, 1790–1850* (Amsterdam and Atlanta: Rodopi, in press).

3. Richard H. Shryock, *The Development of Modern Medicine: An Interpretation of the Social and Scientific Factors Involved* (1936; Madison: University of Wisconsin Press, 1979), p. 193; and see p. 171.

4. Kenneth M. Ludmerer, *Learning to Heal: The Development of American Medical Education* (New York: Basic Books, 1985), p. 32.

5. David W. Yandell, "Notes on Medical Matters and Medical Men in Paris" (Paris, Apr. 1848), *WJMS,* ser. 3, 3 (1848): 1–27, p. 16; Henry W. Williams to Dearest Sister, Paris, 26 Feb. in letter of 23 Feb. 1848, William W. Williams Papers, MA—Countway.

6. Yandell, "Notes on Medical Matters,"

pp. 14–20; Henry W. Williams to Dearest Sisters, London, 5 June 1848, Williams Papers. For wider American perceptions, see Guillaume de Bertier de Sauvigny, *La révolution parisienne de 1848 vue par les Américains* (Paris: Ville de Paris Commission des Travaux Historiques, 1984).

7. Russell M. Jones, whose sample is eclectic and figures low, counted 123 medical Americans who traveled to Paris in the 1840s and 293 in the 1850s ("American Doctors in Paris, 1820–1861: A Statistical Profile," *Journal of the History of Medicine and Allied Sciences* 25 [1970]: 143–157, p. 150); by 1973 he had increased his tally for the 1840s to 128 and reduced the figure for the period 1850 to 1861 to 279 (idem, "American Doctors and the Parisian Medical World, 1830–1840," *Bulletin of the History of Medicine* 47 [1973]: 40–65, 177–204, p. 48).

8. "Correspondence" (Paris, 7 Dec. 1853), *New Jersey Medical Reporter* 7 (1854): 66–70, p. 66.

9. "American Physicians in Paris," *BMSJ* 45 (1851–1852): 456; and see "American Medical Society in Paris," *BMSJ* 47 (1853): 470, and Henri Meding, *Paris médical: vade-mecum des médecins étrangers,* 2 vols. (Paris: J.-B. Ballière, 1852–1853), 2:401–402.

10. For an overview of specialization in American medicine during this period, see Rosemary Stevens, *American Medicine and the Public Interest* (New Haven and London: Yale University Press, 1971), pp. 43–54; and on the French context, see George Weisz, "The Development of Medical Specialization in Nineteenth-Century Paris," in La Berge and Feingold, *French Medical Culture,* pp. 149–187.

11. Henry Bryant to John Bryant, Paris, 1 July 1844, William Sohier Bryant Papers (MS 45), MA—New England Hist. Gen. Soc.

12. Joseph Pancoast, *Professional Glimpses Abroad. A Lecture Introductory to the Course on Anatomy, in the Jefferson Medical College of Philadelphia, Delivered October 17, 1856* (Philadelphia: Joseph M. Wilson, 1856), p. 12; and see "Editorial Correspondence. Hospitals of Paris," *BMSJ* 43 (1851): 22–24.

13. Augustus Kinsley Gardner, *Old Wine in New Bottles: or, Spare Hours of a Student in Paris* (New-York: C. S. Francis & Co.; Boston: J. H. Francis, 1848), pp. 203, 159, 159, 159, 158, 158; and see Robert P. Harris, "Letter

from Paris" (25 Dec. 1855), *Medical Examiner,* n.s., 12 (1856): 70–75, p. 70.

14. Henry W. Williams to My Dearest Sister, Paris, 10 Oct. 1846, Williams Papers.

15. W. F. Westmoreland, "Foreign Correspondence" (Paris, 10 Jan. 1857), *Atlanta Medical and Surgical Journal* 2 (1857): 449–459, p. 459. And see A.B.H., "Foreign Correspondence—Letters from Paris," *BMSJ* 50 (1854): 154–160, 182–183, 220–221, 248–253, 320–323, 362–363, 377–380, 399–402, p. 220; Pancoast, *Professional Glimpses Abroad,* pp. 23–24; S. S. Satchwell, "Letter from S. S. Satchwell, M.D." (Paris, 2 Jan. 1861), *Medical Journal of North Carolina* 3 (1861): 245–252, p. 251.

16. Ackerknecht, *Medicine at the Paris Hospital,* pp. 42–43; Weisz, "The Development of Medical Specialization."

17. See Ann La Berge, "Dichotomy or Integration? Medical Microscopy and the Paris Clinical Tradition," in Hannaway and La Berge, *Reinterpreting Paris Medicine, 1790–1850;* idem, "Medical Microscopy in Paris, 1830–1855," in La Berge and Feingold, *French Medical Culture,* pp. 296–326; and John E. Lesch, *Science and Medicine in France: The Emergence of Experimental Physiology, 1790–1855* (Cambridge, Mass., and London: Harvard University Press, 1984). So too Paris-returned Americans were often more receptive to the laboratory than a model of polarization would suggest; see, for example, Thomas S. Huddle, "Competition and Reform at the Medical Department of the University of Pennsylvania, 1847–1877," *Journal of the History of Medicine and Allied Sciences* 51 (1996): 251–292.

18. George H. Doane, "Comparative Advantages of Vienna and Paris, as Places for Medical Study, with Some Remarks on the Operation of Extraction for the Removal of Cataract" (Burlington, 17 Nov. 1853), *New Jersey Medical Reporter* 7 (1854): 17–20, p. 18; and see the discussion of John Call Dalton in W. Bruce Fye, *The Development of American Physiology: Scientific Medicine in the Nineteenth Century* (Baltimore and London: Johns Hopkins University Press, 1987). And see A. C., "Parisian Correspondence" (Paris, 15 Mar. 1855), *American Medical Gazette and Journal of Health* 6 (1855): 203–205, p. 204; A. Peniston Notebook, Lectures by Claude Bernard, [Paris], 1854, LA—LSU; and Auguste Shurt-

leff, Journey of a Trip to Europe, 1850–1852, 2 vols., vol. 1, entry for 9 May 1851, MA—Countway.

19. Austin Flint, [Letter from Paris] (Paris, 28 June 1854), *WJMS,* n.s., 2 (1854): 277–286, p. 277. While Flint mentioned among others the letters of John Call Dalton of New York, not all of those who sent home full reports on Bernard's teachings were Northerners; see, for example, Julius T. Porcher, "The Influence Exerted by the Nervous System upon the Secretory Organs" (Paris, Feb. 1853), *CMJR* 8 (1853): 353–362.

20. John A. Murphy, [Letter to the Editor] (Paris, Mar. 1854), *WL* 15 (1854): 529–540, pp. 537, 538.

21. B., "Letter from Paris" (Paris, 13 Feb. 1854), *North-Western Medical and Surgical Journal* 3 (1854): 145–149, p. 146.

22. D. D. Slade to George Lord, Cambridge, Mass., 21 Nov. 1845, George Lord Papers, NC—Duke.

23. "Correspondence" (Paris, 7 Dec. 1853), p. 66.

24. [Letter to the Editor] (Paris, 14 Oct. 1868), *CLO,* n.s., 12 (1869): 32–38, p. 32.

25. Robert P. Harris, "Letter from Paris" (Paris, 19 Nov. 1855), *American Medical Gazette and Journal of Health* 7 (1856): 168–171, p. 168.

26. Edward E. Jenkins to John Jenkins, Paris, 12 Aug. 1853, John Jenkins Papers, SC—U. SC.

27. T. J. Cogley, "To the Editors of the Lancet" (Paris, 10 Aug. 1853), *WL* 15 (1854): 45–47, p. 45.

28. Harris, "Letter from Paris" (19 Nov. 1855), p. 169.

29. Iatros, "Medical Heads and Medical Life in Paris," *CMJR* 9 (1854): 476–483, p. 477.

30. John K. Kane, Jr., to Dear Father, Paris, 14 Oct. 1857, Kane Family Papers, MI—Clements, U. MI.

31. William Tully to Alden March, New Haven, 11 July 1846, Alden March Papers, NY—Albany Med.

32. "American Physicians in Paris," p. 456.

33. C. T. Jackson to David Henshaw, Paris, 15 June 1832, Charles Thomas Jackson Papers, DC—LC. The assessments by these American travelers of Italian medical figures, institutions, and practices deserves serious study.

34. Elisha Bartlett to [John Orne Green], Paris, 26 Apr. 1846, Bartlett (Elisha) Family Papers, NY—U. Rochester. And see Charles A. Pope, [Letter to the Editor] (Geneva, 4 Aug. 1846), *SLMSJ* 2 (1846): 214–219, p. 215.

35. A. Stillé to G. C. Shattuck, Vienna, 15 Jan. 1851, Shattuck Papers, vol. 22, MA—MA Hist. Soc.; and see Geo. B. Wood to Dear Doctor, Paris, 2 Sept. 1853, G. B. Wood Misc. Correspondence, PA—CPP.

36. James Jackson, Jr., to James Jackson, Sr., Paris, 17 Feb. 1832; ibid., 18 Feb. 1832. And see letters of Paris, 23 Jan. 1832; Paris, 26 Feb. 1832; Edinburgh, 15 July 1832; and Paris, 1 Dec. 1832. For the father's skepticism, see James Jackson, Sr., to James Jackson, Jr., Boston, 3 Apr. 1830, and ibid., 3 Apr. 1832; all in James Jackson Papers, MA—Countway.

37. In granting permission for the young man to go to Germany, the father's letters hint at his growing desire for his son to get away from Paris and the spell of Louis; see James Jackson, Sr., to James Jackson, Jr., Waltham, 8 Sept. 1832; Boston, 23 Oct. 1832; Boston, 14 Nov. 1832; and Boston, 12 Dec. 1832.

38. James Jackson, Jr., to James Jackson, Sr., Paris, 7 Jan. 1833; ibid., 25 Jan. 1833. And see ibid., entry of 29 Dec. in letter of Paris, 21 Dec. 1832; ibid., 25 Jan. 1833; and ibid., 22 Feb. 1833.

39. William E. Horner to G. B. Wood, Vienna, 4 Aug. 1848, Wood Correspondence. On the Viennese medical world, see Erna Lesky, *The Vienna Medical School of the Nineteenth Century*, trans. L. Williams and I. S. Levij (Baltimore and London: Johns Hopkins University Press, 1976).

40. Valentine Mott, *Travels in Europe and the East* (New-York: Harper and Brothers, 1842), p. 44; Harris, "Letter from Paris" (25 Dec. 1855), p. 74.

41. E. Williams, "Foreign Correspondence" (Vienna, 29 Oct. 1854), *WJMS*, n.s., 2 (1854): 441–458, p. 453.

42. Henry W. Williams to Sisters Three, entry of 8 June in letter of Paris, 26 May 1846, Williams Papers.

43. Levin S. Joynes to Thomas R. Joynes, Paris, 12 Dec. 1841, Joynes Family Papers, VA—VA Hist. Soc.

44. A. Stillé to G. C. Shattuck, Vienna, 15 Jan. 1851, Shattuck Papers, vol. 22.

45. Doane, "Comparative Advantages of Vienna and Paris," p. 18. The asterisk led to a note on the preponderance of Americans in Bernard's classes.

46. Austin Flint, "Address at the Opening of the Session for 1854–55 in the Medical Department of the University of Louisville," *WJMS*, n.s., 2 (1854): 409–425, pp. 412, 412–413, 413.

47. David W. Yandell, "Notes on Medical Matters and Medical Men in Paris" (Paris, July 1847), *WL*, n.s., 7 (1847): 369–395, p. 374.

48. Stillé to Shattuck, Vienna, 15 Jan. 1851. After his return Stillé reflected that in Paris, "politics are undermining & belittling science as they have done here" (ibid., Philadelphia, 28 Sept. 1851, Shattuck Papers, vol. 22).

49. B., "Letter from Paris," pp. 145, 146.

50. R. A. Kinloch, "Medical News from Paris" (Paris, 13 Jan. 1855), *CMJR* 10 (1855): 159–170, p. 159.

51. Ibid.; and see R. A. Kinloch, "Medical News from Paris, France," *CMJR* 10 (1855): 58–66, p. 65.

52. Henry H. Smith, *Professional Visit to London and Paris. Introductory Lecture to the Course on the Principles and Practice of Surgery. Delivered in the University of Pennsylvania, October 9, 1855* (Philadelphia: T. K. and P. G. Collins, 1855), p. 12.

53. Ibid., pp. 11, 12, 17, 18, 19. On the reorganization of private teaching from the 1860s onward, see George Weisz, "Reform and Conflict in French Medical Education, 1870–1914," in *The Organization of Science and Technology in France, 1808–1914*, ed. Robert Fox and George Weisz (Cambridge: Cambridge University Press, 1980), pp. 61–94.

54. Alexander Wilcox, "Miscellaneous" (13 Nov. 1845), *WL* 4 (1846): 425–428, p. 427.

55. Ibid., p. 427.

56. David W. Yandell, "Clinical Instruction in the London and Paris Hospitals," *WJMS*, ser. 3, 3 (1848): 392–400, p. 398. "A physician, who was *interne* during the existence of the law permitting it, told me, that so great was the love of money or the love of teaching, he could not say which, a short time before the law was repealed, the *internes* spent almost the entire day in the wards, examining and reexamining the patients, very often rousing them from sleep before it was fairly light to begin the work of investigating their diseases, and, not satisfied with prosecuting it

through the day, pursued it often by candle-light far into the night. Patients, at length, grew impatient and refused to submit to such torture."

57. Theodor Billroth, *The Medical Sciences in German Universities: A Study in the History of Civilization* (first German ed., 1876; New York: Macmillan, 1924). I am grateful to Thomas N. Bonner for this reference.

58. Edward E. Jenkins to Dear Sister, Paris, 27 Aug. 1854, Jenkins Papers. Jenkins was thinking about setting up practice in St. Louis and in another letter explained, "One of the best steps preliminary to settling in St Louis would be to spend sufficient time either at Berlin or Vienna to acquire the German language" (Edward Jenkins to [John Jenkins], Paris, 13 Jan. 1854). And see Clarence John Blake to Dear Pater and Mater, [Vienna], 8 Feb. 1866, Clarence John Blake Papers, MA—Countway, and William Williams Keen to Samuel C. and Mary Eastman, Vienna, 25 May 1865, William Williams Keen Papers, RI—Brown.

59. "The Vienna Hospitals—Letter from Henry K. Oliver, Jr., M.D., of Boston" (Vienna, 1 July 1857), *BMSJ* 57 (1857–1858): 49–58, 71–77, p. 50; Warren comments on p. 49.

60. H. Z. Gill, "Visiting Europe for the Purpose of Observation and Study of Medicine," *CLO*, n.s., 11 (1868): 546–554, pp. 551, 551–552, 548, 551, 552, 553.

61. Joseph T. Webb to Dear Mother, Vienna, 23 June 1868, Joseph Webb Letters in Rutherford B. Hayes Papers, OH—Hayes.

62. D. F. Lincoln, "Vienna Medical Education," *BMSJ*, n.s., 7 (1871): 273–278, p. 276.

63. Montrose A. Pallen, "European Correspondence" (Paris, 30 Sept. 1857), *SLMSJ* 15 (1857): 506–523, pp. 519–521.

64. "Medical Advantages of Vienna for American Students," *BMSJ* 63 (1860–1861): 51–53, p. 51; and see Frank J. Lutz, ed., *The Autobiography and Reminiscences of S. Pollak, M.D., St. Louis, Mo.* (Reprinted from the St. Louis Medical Review, 1904), pp. 213–214.

65. D. F. Lincoln, "A Letter from Vienna" (Vienna, 7 June 1871), *BMSJ* 85 (1871): 4–7, p. 6; and see Harris, "Letter from Paris" (25 Dec. 1855), pp. 71 and 74.

66. Patrick A. O'Connell, "A Letter from Vienna," *BMSJ* 86 (1872): 214–217, p. 216.

67. Lincoln, "A Letter from Vienna," p. 6;

and see Fred[eric]k Shattuck to George Cheyne Shattuck, Vienna, 14 Mar. 1874, Shattuck Papers, vol. 24.

68. Joseph T. Webb to Dear Mother, Berlin, 1 Aug. 1866, transcripts in Hayes Papers; and Wm. P. Thornton, "Letter to the Editors of the Lancet and Observer" (Vienna, 25 Feb. 1859), *CLO*, n.s., 2 (1859): 236–238, p. 238.

69. On Viennese therapeutic nihilism, see H. Buess, "Zur Frage des therapeutischen Nihilismus in 19. Jahrhundert," *Schweizerische Medizinische Wochenschrift* 87 (1957): 444–447; Erna Lesky, "Von den Ursprungen des therapeutischen Nihilismus," *Sudhoffs Archiv für Geschichte der Medizin und der Naturwissenschaften* 44 (1960): 1–20; and Lloyd G. Stevenson, "Joseph Dietl, William Osler and the Definition of Therapeutic Nihilism," in *Festschrift für Erna Lesky zum 70. Geburtstag*, ed. Kurt Ganzinger, Manfred Skopec, and Helmut Wyklicky (Vienna: Hollinck, 1981), pp. 149–152.

70. J. R. Black, "Remarks on the Semiology and Therapeutics of Chronic Diseases," *Cincinnati Lancet and Clinic*, n.s., 7 (1881): 109–115, pp. 110–111.

71. John Dole to [David] Lin[coln], Vienna, 15 Nov. 1865, MA—Countway; Lincoln, "Vienna Medical Education," p. 276.

72. Clare [Blake] to Dear Pater, Vienna, 9 Nov. [1865], Blake Papers.

73. In earlier instances in which the term denoted patients and not just cadavers, it seems most often to have referred to the entire complex of facilities for medical study that encompassed the hospitals and dissecting rooms themselves, the policies that governed their use, and both living and dead bodies; see, for example, L. M. Lawson, "Foreign Correspondence" (London, June 1845), *WL* 4 (1845): 145–153, p. 153.

74. William Williams Keen to Samuel C. and Mary Eastman, Vienna, 25 May 1865, Keen Papers.

75. Joseph T. Webb to Lu[cy Webb Hayes], Paris, 2 Apr. 1867, and Joseph T. Webb to James D. Webb, Paris, 21 Mar. 1867, Hayes Papers.

76. Bonner's fine *American Doctors and German Universities*, written over three decades ago, though he described it as "only suggestive" (p. vii), remains the fullest study we have of Americans and German medicine, and much of the further work he hoped his vol-

ume would stimulate remains to be done. The most insightful recent exploration, which focuses solely on the Americans who set out to study experimental physiology in Germany, is Robert G. Frank, "American Physiologists in German Laboratories, 1865–1914," in *Physiology in the American Context, 1850–1914*, ed. Gerald L. Geison (Bethesda: American Physiological Society, 1987), pp. 11–46; and see Fye, *Development of American Physiology*.

77. For example, see Ludmerer, *Learning to Heal*, p. 32. The best study of Bowditch and his European studies is W. Bruce Fye, "Why a Physiologist?—The Case of Henry P. Bowditch," *Bulletin of the History of Medicine* 56 (1982): 19–29; and see Frank, "American Physiologists."

78. Henry P. Bowditch to Henry I. Bowditch, Paris, 7 Feb. in letter of 26 Jan. 1869, Henry I. Bowditch Papers, MA—Countway.

79. Henry P. Bowditch to Henry I. Bowditch, Paris, 1 Nov. 1868. He reported on his routine in ibid., Paris, 29 Sept.; 4, 9, 15, and 25 Oct.; and 1 Nov. 1868, Bowditch Papers.

80. Ibid., Paris, 26 Jan. 1869.

81. H. P. Bowditch to Jeffries Wyman, Paris, 14 Jan. 1869, MA—Countway.

82. Ibid., Bonn, 23 May 1869, MA—Countway; Bowditch gave an almost identical report to his uncle just after he had received Professor Kühne's advice (H. P. Bowditch to H. I. Bowditch, Paris, 12 Apr. 1869, Bowditch Papers).

83. See Henry P. Bowditch to Editor [of *BMSJ*], Leipzig, 8 Mar. 1870, enclosed in Henry P. Bowditch to Henry I. Bowditch, Leipzig, 11 Mar. 1870, Bowditch Papers. He went on to explain that "Leipzig is a city very little visited by American medical men, for whom the larger cities such as Berlin & Vienna offer in general greater attractions in their superior opportunities for clinical observation. The student of Physiology & Chemistry however finds here facilities for prosecuting his studies which are not surpassed in any city in Germany." And see ibid., Leipzig, 5 Dec. 1869.

84. Ibid., Bonn, 30 May 1869; and see Henry P. Bowditch to Parents, Leipzig, 27 Feb. 1870.

85. Ibid., Leipzig, 2 Jan. 1870.

86. See, for example, William D. Somers to Henry Scott, Barnesville, Ga., 27 July 1864, William D. Somers Papers, NC—Duke; James

Howard De Votie to Father, Danville, Va., 15 June 1862, James H. De Votie Papers, NC—Duke; Robert Battey to Mary Battey, Rome, Ga., 19 July 1865, Robert Battey Family Papers, GA—Emory; Cornelius Kollock to Henrietta Kollock, Culpepper, Va., 20 July 1861, Cornelius Kollock Papers, SC—SC Hist. Soc.; and John K. Kane to Bess Kane, Cairo, Ill., 29 Nov. 1861, Kane Family Papers. Medical veterans often cited their war and European experiences in strikingly similar ways when applying for hospital or teaching posts; see, for example, Francis Peyre Porcher to The Trustees and Faculty of the Medical College of the State of South Carolina, Charleston, June 1866, Porcher Papers, SC—SC Hist. Soc.

87. Ethelred Philips to J. J. Philips, Marianna, Fla., 5 Oct. 1868, James Jones Philips Papers, NC—SHC. So too a St. Louis woman regarded her son's departure for hospital study in Vienna as a natural step in the struggle to build a medical career, an "ordeal" underscored by the experience of her other son in trying to establish his practice at a time when "doctors are crowding around us like flies" (Sarah L. Glasgow to William C. Glasgow, St. Louis, 11 Feb. 1871, William Carr Lane Papers, MO—MO Hist. Soc.).

88. Thus a young New Yorker in Strassburg who had already studied in Vienna and Berlin and judged Virchow "the greatest apostle of pathology" found himself enthralled by the microscopical work he was pursuing in Maldeyer's laboratory. "I sometimes feel as if I should never go back," he wrote to a compatriot studying in Germany. "I might discover something one day, who knows?" He recognized, however, that the microscope would not be his future work, and reflected that "I almost wish at times that I had been contented with knowing nothing at all about the thing as so many of my countrymen do who are all the happier for it" (W. T. Alexander to A. N. Blodgett, Strassburg, 11 June 1873; and see ibid., 30 Apr. 1873, in Albert Novatus Blodgett Letters, MA—Countway).

89. Charles E. Rosenberg gives a brief but very suggestive account of Blake's career-making choices in *The Care of Strangers: The Rise of America's Hospital System* (New York: Basic Books, 1987), pp. 166–168.

90. Clare [Blake] to Dear Pater, Mater, and Agnes, Vienna, 10 Oct. 1865, Blake Papers.

91. Ibid.

92. Blake to Pater, Vienna, 9 Nov. [1865].

93. Ibid., Vienna, 24 Oct. 1865.

94. Ibid. "The Syphilis wards illustrate this particularly. In the centre of those devoted to female patients are two high stands, like beds with long legs, so that the oil cloth mattress which covers them is on a level with the head of a person standing near. When the clinique opens the women who have been selected as illustrations ascend the stand in turn, stripped or with only a hospital wrapper, an assistant stands by with light and a speculum and Professor lectures and shows the class the points of interest in each succeeding case."

95. Ibid., Vienna, 9 Nov. 1865; and see ibid., 21 Jan. 1866.

96. Ibid.; ibid., 8 Feb. 1866.

97. Ibid., 18 Feb. [1865]; ibid., 7 Mar. 1866; ibid., 19 Mar. 1866. And see ibid., 22 Feb. 1866, and ibid., 19 Apr. 1866.

98. Blake to Poppet, Vienna, 25 Apr. 1866; Blake to Pater, Vienna, 29 Apr. 1866.

99. [Blake] to Pater and Mater, [Vienna], 8 Feb. 1866; and ibid., Vienna, 6 Feb. 1866. For a revealing example of the shaping of an early specialty practice, see Bonnie Ellen Blustein, *Preserve Your Love for Science: Life of William A. Hammond, American Neurologist* (Cambridge and New York: Cambridge University Press, 1991).

100. [Blake] to Pater and Mater, Vienna, 6 Feb. 1866; and ibid., [Vienna], 8 Feb. 1866.

101. Ibid.; and see Blake to Pater, Vienna, 21 Jan. 1866. On a group of Americans who did study chemistry in Liebig's laboratory, see Margaret W. Rossiter, *The Emergence of Agricultural Science: Justus Liebig and the Americans, 1840–1880* (New Haven and London: Yale University Press, 1975).

102. Blake to Pater and Mater, [Vienna], 8 Feb. 1866. He went on to note that "if a Dr has chemical work to be done he sends it to a Chemist, and however closely the two sciences may be related in mutual advancement they stand widely apart in practice." He was not quick to dismiss his father's recommendations, though, and proposed to pay attention to chemistry while in Vienna and then "spend a little time in Liebig's Laboratory as a finish" (and see Blake to Pater, [Vienna], 18 Feb. 1866, and Blake to Pater and Mater, Vienna, 7 Mar. 1866). Yet he would conclude, "I cannot see any opportunity to uniting chemistry with medicine and am every day less inclined to

practice any other than the medical profession" (Blake to Pater, [Vienna], 2 Apr. 1866).

103. Ibid., 19 Mar. 1866.

104. Ibid., 29 Apr. 1866.

105. Ibid., 5 June 1866; and see ibid., 18 June 1866.

106. Ibid., 3 July 1866. On his summer, see Blake to Pater, Mater and Ag, Munich, 27 July 1866, and Blake to Pater and Mater, Stuttgart, 14 Aug. 1866.

107. Blake to Pater, Vienna, 13 Dec. 1865.

108. Ibid., Vienna, 19 Apr. 1866; and see Blake to Mater, Vienna, 13 May 1866.

109. Blake to Pater, Vienna, 29 Apr. 1866.

110. Ibid., Vienna, 5 June 1866; and see ibid., 3 July 1866.

111. Blake to Mater, Pater and the Agni, Vienna, 21 Feb. 1869.

112. Note to Pater in Blake to Pater and Mater, Vienna, 11 Apr. 1869. "It should be made to rank with Ophthalmology."

113. Blake to Mater, [Vienna, n.d. but late Apr. or early May 1869].

114. Among others, see Blake's letters to Mater, Pater, and Agni, Vienna, 21 Feb. 1869; Mater, Vienna, 15 Mar. 1869; Mater, [Vienna], 4 Apr. 1869; Poppet [sister Agnes], [Vienna], n.d. [but probably Apr. 1869]; Pater, [Vienna], 26 Apr. 1869; Pater and Mater, Vienna, 4 May 1869; Pater and Mater, [Vienna], 9 May 1869; and Pater, Mater, and Agnes, Vienna, 28 May 1869.

115. Blake to Mater, Vienna, 24 May 1869.

116. Blake to Mater, Vienna, 24 May 1869. As Blake put it, "The education in the Hospital is principally in diagnosis, treatment seems to be a secondary consideration." And see Blake to Pater, Munich, 8 June 1869.

117. "A Hospital Picture," n.d. [but 1865–1866], Blake Papers.

118. Blake to Pater, Munich, 13 June 1869; Blake to Pater and Mater, Vienna, 4 May 1869.

119. Blake to Mater, Munich, 8 June 1869; and see [Blake] to Blessed Mater, Vienna, 8 Feb. 1869, and Blake to Poppet, [Vienna, Apr. 1869].

120. Blake to Blessed Mater, Vienna, 8 Feb. 1869; Blake to Pater, Vienna, 19 May 1869.

121. Ibid.

122. Blake to Pater, Munich, 8 June 1869; and see ibid., 13 June 1869.

123. Bonner, *American Doctors and German Universities*, p. 23.

124. Henry Hun, *A Guide to American Medi-*

*cal Students in Europe* (New York: William Wood and Co., 1883), p. 97, quoted in ibid., p. 18.

125. J. W. Humrichouse to C. W. Humrichouse, Strassburg, 26 June 1877, Ridgley Papers (MS 1908), MD—MD Hist. Soc.

126. John Burnham, "The Transit of Medical Ideas: Changes in Citation of European Publications in USA Biomedical Journals," in *Actas del XXXIII Congresso International de Historia de la Medicina*, ed. Juan L. Carrillo and Guillermo Olagüe de Ros (Seville, 1994), pp. 101–112.

127. Satchwell, "Letter," pp. 245, 246.

128. Even Blake looked forward to his departure from Vienna as an escape from "a nation of bloodsuckers" where he felt constantly cheated (Blake to Pater, Vienna, 19 Apr. 1866). On Paris, see Gill, "Visiting Europe," p. 548, and [Frank] Metcalfe to A. N. Blodgett, Paris, 14 Jan. 1873, Blodgett Letters.

129. [William Williams Keen] to Dear Parents, [typescript, Paris, 1864–1865], Keen Papers. And see Thomas Dwight to Dear Maman, Paris, 6 June [1867], MA—Countway.

130. J. T. Webb to Dear Lu, New York, 5 Feb. 1866, and Joseph Webb to Dear Jim, Paris, 21 Mar. 1868, Joseph Webb Letters, in Hayes Papers.

131. Bowditch to Wyman, 14 Jan. 1869.

132. Bowditch to Bowditch, 7 Feb. 1869. On the perception of decline, see Joseph Ben-David, "The Rise and Decline of France as a Scientific Center," *Minerva* 8 (1970): 160–179; Fox and Weisz, *The Organization of Science and Technology in France*; and Harry Paul, "The Issue of Decline in Nineteenth Century French Science," *French Historical Studies* 7 (1972): 416–450.

133. After telling his uncle of Lorain's pamphlet he went on to say that "M. Ranvier is giving a capital course of lectures on histology," which he described (Bowditch to Bowditch, 7 Feb. 1869); and, just before his oft-quoted indictment of Bernard's laboratory, the young Bowditch told Wyman that "there is a good deal that is interesting going on here," and cited in evidence Bernard's lectures on experimental physiology; Boste's lectures on embryogeny; Marey's lectures on the mechanism of flight; and his work on physiology with Ranvier (Bowditch to Wyman, Paris, 14 Jan. 1869).

134. See, for example, Henry Bronson, Diary, 20 Nov. 1839–26 May 1840, entry of Paris, 9 Mar. 1840, Stephen Henry Bronson Papers, CT—Yale.

135. [Stephen] Henry Bronson to Jeffries Wyman, New Haven, 16 Sept. 1867, MA—Countway.

136. Ibid., Paris, 26 Jan. 1868.

137. Stephen Henry Bronson, Diary, vol. 1, 5 Oct. 1867–28 Feb. 1870, entry for Paris, 16 Dec. 1867, Bronson Papers; and see, for example, entries for 28 Oct., 4 Nov., and 16 Nov. 1867; and Diary, vol. 2, 2 Mar.–12 June 1870, and 13 May–15 June 1871, entry for Paris, 4 May 1870, Bronson Papers.

138. Bronson, Diary, vol. 1, entry for Paris, 16 Nov. 1867. Later in the week he reported the unsettling incident to his parents: "While moving about from bed to bed, I noticed a young female, who with book and pencil seemed to be engaged in the same occupation as myself. Well! I thought to myself. Nothing is too strange for Paris" ([Stephen] Henry [Bronson] to Dr. and Mrs. Henry Bronson, Paris, 21 Nov. 1867, Bronson Papers). Gail Hamilton was the pen name of Mary Abigail Dodge.

139. [Stephen] Henry Bronson to Jeffries Wyman, Paris, 3 Nov. 1867, MA—Countway.

140. [Bronson] to Dr. and Mrs. Henry Bronson, Paris, 23 Oct. 1867; 31 Oct. 1867; 6 Nov. 1867; and 21 Nov. 1867.

141. Ibid., Paris, 15 Feb. 1869, and 7 Apr. 1868; Bronson, Diary, vol. 1, entry for Paris, 18 Jan. 1867.

142. On his encounter with Bowditch, see [Bronson] to Dr. and Mrs. Henry Bronson, Paris, 21 Jan. 1869; and see ibid., 6 Nov. 1867, 25 Dec. 1867, 5 May 1868, 25 Dec. 1868, 8 Jan. 1869, 15 Feb. 1869, and entries in Bronson, Diary, vol. 1, for 12 Nov. 1867, 21 Dec. 1867, 6 May 1868, 20 Jan. 1869, 6 July 1869.

143. See, for example, [Bronson] to Dr. and Mrs. Henry Bronson, Paris, 1 Dec. 1867, 18 Dec. 1867, 18 June 1868; and Bronson, Diary, vol. 1, entries of 18 Jan. 1867, 8 Apr. 1868, and 12 Oct. 1868.

144. [Bronson] to Dr. and Mrs. Henry Bronson, Paris, 1 Dec. 1867.

145. [Bronson] to My Dear Lottie, Paris, 16 Aug. 1868; and see [Bronson] to Dr. and Mrs. Henry Bronson, Paris, 18 Dec. 1867, and ibid., 25 Jan. 1868.

146. [Bronson] to Dr. and Mrs. Henry Bronson, Paris, 26 Nov. 1868.

147. Ibid., 21 Mar. 1869.

148. Bronson, Diary, vol. 1, entries starting "1 September, Mardi, 1868."

149. [Bronson] to Dr. and Mrs Henry Bronson, Paris, 21 Mar. 1869.

150. Bronson, Diary, vol. 1, entry of 9 June 1869.

151. See, for example, ibid., Berlin, 10 Mar. 1870; Berlin, 20 Mar. 1870; Dresden, 10 Apr. 1870; and Heidelberg, 28 Apr. 1870.

152. Ibid., London, 19 Mar. 1870.

153. Thomas Neville Bonner, "Medical Women Abroad: A New Dimension of Women's Push for Opportunity in Medicine, 1850–1914," Bulletin of the History of Medicine 62 (1988): 58–73, p. 65.

154. Elizabeth Blackwell, quoted in Virginia Perry, The Employments of Women: A Cyclopedia of Women's Work (Boston: Walker and Wise, Co., 1863), p. 29, quoted in Regina Markell Morantz-Sanchez, Sympathy and Science: Women Physicians in American Medicine (New York and Oxford: Oxford University Press, 1985), p. 64.

155. The experience of Americans is lucidly explored within a wider context that encompasses the education of Europeans in Thomas Neville Bonner, To the Ends of the Earth: Women's Search for Education in Medicine (Cambridge, Mass., and London: Harvard University Press, 1992).

156. Samuel Gregory, "Report," in Twentieth and Twenty-First Annual Catalogue and Report of the New-England Female Medical College (Cambridge: John Wilson and Son, 1869), pp. 11–16, on pp. 11, 12. On Parker, see Dorothy B. Porter, "Sarah Reymond Parker," in Notable American Women, ed. Edward T. James (Cambridge: Belknap Press of Harvard University Press, 1971), 3:136–137.

157. E. H. Cleveland, "Announcement," in Seventeenth Annual Announcement of the Female Medical College of Pennsylvania, North College Avenue and 22nd St., Philadelphia, for the Session of 1866–67 (Philadelphia: Jas. B. Rodgers, 1866), pp. 5–14, on p. 7.

158. See Bonner, To the Ends of the Earth; Virginia Drachman, Hospital with a Heart: Women Doctors and the Paradox of Separatism at the New England Hospital, 1862–1969 (Ithaca and London: Cornell University Press, 1984); Morantz-Sanchez, Sympathy and Science; Mary Roth Walsh, "Doctors Wanted: No Women Need Apply": Sexual Barriers in the Medical Profession, 1835–1975 (New Haven and London: Yale University Press, 1977).

159. Ann Preston, Introductory Lecture to the Class of the Female Medical College, of Pennsylvania. Delivered at the Opening of the Tenth Annual Session, Oct. 19, 1859 (Philadelphia: A. Ketterlinus, 1859), p. 9.

160. Samuel Gregory, "Report," in Seventeenth Annual Catalogue and Report of the New-England Female Medical College (Boston: The Trustees, 1865), pp. 11–22, on p. 20. And see idem, "Report," in Fourteenth Annual Catalogue and Report of the New-England Female Medical College (Boston: The Trustees, 1862), pp. 11–15, on p. 14.

161. See, for example, the survey of clinical instruction available to women students in Twenty-First Annual Announcement of the Woman's Medical College of Pennsylvania, North College Avenue and 22d Street, Philadelphia. Session of 1870–71 (Philadelphia: Loag, 1870), pp. 3–7.

162. Seventeenth Annual Catalogue and Report of the New-England Female Medical College (Boston: The Trustees, 1865), p. 12.

163. Nineteenth Annual Catalogue and Report of the New England Female Medical College (Boston: The Trustees, 1867), n.p.

164. Morantz-Sanchez, Sympathy and Science, p. 65; Agnes C. Vietor, ed., A Woman's Quest: The Life of Marie E. Zakrzewska, M.D. (New York and London: D. Appleton and Company, 1924), p. 279. On Cleveland's departure and reinstatement, see entries of 23 Sept. 1860, 17 Oct. 1860, and 13 Sept. 1862 in Minute Book of the Faculty of the Female Medical College of Pennsylvania, 1850–1864, and entry for 9 June 1862, in Female Medical College of Pennsylvania, Minutes of the Board of Corporators, vol. 2, 1857–1874, PA—Women in Med. Arch.

165. Elizabeth Blackwell to Emily Blackwell, [Paris], entry of 28 Sept. in letter of 21 Sept. 1866, Blackwell Family Papers (MC 411), MA—Schlesinger. And see entry of 16 Apr. 1851 in Female Medical College of Pennsylvania, Minutes of the Board of Corporators, vol. 1, 1850–1856.

166. Marie Zakrzewska to Lucy Sewall, Roxbury, 25 Jan. 1863, in Vietor, A Woman's Quest, pp. 306–308, on p. 308.

167. Cleveland, "Announcement," p. 7.

168. Morton's initial reaction to Paris is recounted in Marie Zakrzewska to Lucy Sewall, [Boston?], 21 Oct. [1862], in Vietor, *A Woman's Quest*, pp. 300–301; and see pp. 253, 490.

169. Emeline H. Cleveland, *Valedictory Address to the Graduating Class of the Female Medical College of Pennsylvania, at the Eleventh Annual Commencement, March 14, 1863* (Philadelphia: Crissy and Markley, 1863), p. 6. Cleveland's remarks were widely disseminated, for the Board of Corporators of the College authorized the printing of four thousand copies of her valedictory address (Minutes of the Board of Corporators, Female Medical College of Pennsylvania, vol. 2, 1857–1874, entry for 22 Apr. 1863).

170. Blackwell to Blackwell, [Paris], 28 Sept. 1866.

171. Mary Putnam to My Dear Little Mother [Victorine H. Putnam], Divonne, 3 Dec. 1866, in *Life and Letters of Mary Putnam Jacobi*, ed. Ruth Putnam (New York and London: G. P. Putnam's Sons, 1925), pp. 103–105, on p. 104. An insightful account of Putnam's Paris studies is Joy Harvey, "La Visite: Mary Putnam Jacobi and the Paris Medical Clinics," in La Berge and Feingold, *French Medical Culture*, pp. 350–371.

172. The petition created a furor. See the protest of Edwin Fussell to Dean, [Philadelphia] 10 Mar. 1864, in Female Medical College of Pennsylvania, Faculty Minute Book, 1850–1864, entry for 10 Mar. 1864; and see minutes of 26 Feb. 1864 and 12 Mar. 1864. Part of the minutes of the meeting of 12 Mar., at which the vote was taken, is missing—neatly cut out and removed from the Minute Book.

173. Putnam to Dear Mother and Father, [Steamer off the coast of Falmouth, England], 12 Sept. 1866, and Putnam to Father [George P. Putnam], Paris, 18 Sept. 1866, in Putnam, *Life and Letters*, pp. 86–89, 90–96; quotations on pp. 87, 93.

174. Putnam to Father, Paris, 18 Sept. 1866, and Putnam to Edith [G. Putnam], Paris, 30 Sept. 1866, in Putnam, *Life and Letters*, pp. 90–96, 96–98, quotation on p. 97.

175. Putnam to Mother, Paris, 15 Mar. 1867, in Putnam, *Life and Letters*, pp. 114–116.

176. Putnam to Mother, Paris, 21 Oct. 1866, in Putnam, *Life and Letters*, pp. 98–99,

quotation on p. 99. And see Blackwell to Blackwell, [Paris], 28 Sept. 1866.

177. Putnam to Mother, Paris, 13 Nov. 1866, in Putnam, *Life and Letters*, 100–103, quotations on p. 101.

178. Putnam to Mother, Divonne, 3 Dec. 1866, in Putnam, *Life and Letters*, pp. 103–105, quotations on p. 104.

179. Lucy E. Sewall to Caroline H. Dall, London, 1 Feb. 1863, Caroline H. Dall Papers, MA—MA Hist. Soc. "A few of them have urged me to stay in England and have said that if I could found a college here for women they would help me," Sewall added. "Miss Blackwell seems not to have left a pleasant impression on the Medical men here and not to have had as many friends in London as I supposed." And see S. E. Sewall to [Caroline] Dall, Melrose, 25 Dec. 1862, Dall Papers.

180. Putnam to Mother, Paris, 13 Nov. 1866, in Putnam, *Life and Letters*, pp. 100–103; and, on Sewall's arrival in Paris, Lucy E. Sewall to Caroline H. Dall, Paris, 17 Apr. [1863], Dall Papers.

181. Putnam to Mother, Divonne, 3 Dec. 1866, in Putnam, *Life and Letters*, pp. 103–105, quotation on p. 104.

182. Putnam to Mother, Paris, 9 Dec. 1866, in Putnam, *Life and Letters*, pp. 105–107, quotation on p. 107.

183. Putnam to Mother, Divonne, 13 Nov. 1866, in Putnam, *Life and Letters*, pp. 100–103, quotations on pp. 101, 102.

184. Putnam to Edith, Paris, 21 Feb. 1867, in Putnam, *Life and Letters*, pp. 112–114, quotation on p. 113.

185. Mary Putnam Jacobi, "Women in Medicine," in *Woman's Work in America*, ed. Annie Nathan Meyer (New York: Henry Holt, 1891), pp. 139–205, on p. 190.

186. Putnam to Mother, Paris, 16 Apr. 1867, in Putnam, *Life and Letters*, pp. 120–124, quotations on p. 121.

187. Putnam to Mother, Paris, 22 Dec. 1867, in Putnam, *Life and Letters*, pp. 157–161, quotation on p. 160.

188. The letters, which appeared in the *Medical Record* between 1867 and 1871, were later collected in *Mary Putnam Jacobi, M.D.: A Pathfinder in Medicine, with Selections from Her Writings and a Complete Bibliography*, ed. The Women's Medical Association of New York City (New York and London: G. P. Putnam's Sons, 1925), pp. 1–170; see especially letters

of 9 Sept. 1867, pp. 34–49, and 21 Aug. 1868, pp. 114–124 (quotation on p. 114). Undated clippings of some of the articles she was commissioned to write for American newspapers are included in the Mary (Putnam) Jacobi Papers (A-26), MA—Schlesinger; see, for example, "Gossip from Paris" (Paris, 2 Jan. 1867), *Evening Post*, and Mary Israel, "Our Paris Correspondent" (Paris, 7 Jan. 1867), *New Orleans Times*.

189. Minnie to Dear Father, Paris, 11 Mar. 1871, typescript in (Putnam) Jacobi Papers.

190. Putnam to Father, Paris, 1 Feb. 1867, in Putnam, *Life and Letters*, pp. 110–111, quotation on p. 111; and see Putnam to Mother, Divonne, 3 Dec. 1866, in Putnam, *Life and Letters*, pp. 110–111. On the constraints and possibilities of a woman's life in science in America, see Margaret W. Rossiter, *Women Scientists in America: Struggles and Strategies to 1940* (Baltimore and London: Johns Hopkins University Press, 1982), esp. pp. 1–99.

191. Putnam to Mother, Paris, 14 Feb. 1867, in Putnam, *Life and Letters*, pp. 111–112, quotations on pp. 111–112.

192. Putnam to Mother, Paris, 29 May 1867, in Putnam, *Life and Letters*, pp. 138–141, quotation on p. 139; and see ibid., 16 Apr. 1867, pp. 120–124, and Putnam to Father, Paris, 12 May 1867, pp. 133–137. Putnam too, however, one memorialist suggested, had to overcome the expectations of her anatomy teacher who initially took for granted that she would attend dissections wearing men's clothing (Richard Watson Gilder, "Introductory Remarks," in *In Memory of Mary Putnam Jacobi* [New York: Academy of Medicine, 1907], pp. 43–56, on pp. 52–53).

193. Putnam to Edith, Paris, 5 May 1867; Putnam to Father, Paris, 12 May 1867; and Putnam to Mother, 29 May 1867, in Putnam, *Life and Letters*, pp. 129–133, 133–137, and 138–141.

194. Putnam to Edith, Paris, 5 May 1867, quotation on p. 129.

195. Putnam to Father, Paris, 12 Nov. 1867, in Putnam, *Life and Letters*, pp. 151–154, quotations on pp. 152, 153, 153.

196. Putnam to Mother, Paris, 15 Dec. 1867, in Putnam, *Life and Letters*, pp. 155–157.

197. Putnam to Mother, Paris, 25 Jan. 1868, in Putnam, *Life and Letters*, pp. 167–171, quotation on p. 167. She had arrived in

Paris with a letter of introduction from Flint to Robin (Putnam to Mother, Divonne, 3 Dec. 1866, pp. 103–105, on p. 105).

198. Putnam to Edith, Paris, 24 Mar. 1868, in Putnam, *Life and Letters*, pp. 171–173, quotation on p. 172.

199. Putnam to Mother, Paris, 24 Oct. 1867, in Putnam, *Life and Letters*, pp. 150–151.

200. Elizabeth Blackwell to Emily Blackwell, n.p., n.d. [but early Sept. 1867], Blackwell Family Papers. The other two prospects Blackwell cited were Anita Tyng and Annette Buckel.

201. See Putnam to Mother, Paris, 22 Dec. 1867, in Putnam, *Life and Letters*, pp. 157–161; Paris, 12 June 1868, in Putnam, *Life and Letters*, pp. 176–178. Putnam, *Life and Letters*, provides the best chronicle of this process; an overview is Rhoda Truax, *The Doctors Jacobi* (Boston: Little Brown and Company, 1952), pp. 62–123. Putnam made a brief visit home in the summer of 1869; see Putnam, *Life and Letters*, pp. 215–216. Harvey, "La Visite," gives a fine sense of the critical role personal interactions played in Putnam's Parisian success.

202. Putnam to Mother, Paris, 7 Jan. 1868, pp. 167–171, on p. 170, and Putnam to Edith, Paris, 24 Mar. 1868, pp. 171–173, on p. 171, in Putnam, *Life and Letters*. For a wonderfully telling analysis of this relationship and its enduring place in Putnam's life, see Joy Harvey, "Medicine and Politics: Dr. Mary Putnam Jacobi and the Paris Commune," *Dialectical Anthropology* 15 (1990): 107–117; and see idem, "Clanging Eagles: The Marriage and Collaboration between Two Nineteenth-Century Physicians, Mary Putnam Jacobi and Abraham Jacobi," in *Creative Couples in the Sciences*, ed. Helena M. Pycior, Nancy G. Slack, and Pnina G. Abir-Am (New Brunswick, N.J.: Rutgers University Press, 1996), pp. 185–195.

203. Putnam to Father, Paris, 12 Nov. 1868, in Putnam, *Life and Letters*, pp. 200–202, on p. 201.

204. Putnam to Mother, Paris, 18 Oct. 1869, in Putnam, *Life and Letters*, pp. 218–221.

205. Putnam to Father, Paris, 4 Sept. 1870, pp. 256–269, and Putnam to Mother, Paris, 15 Sept. 1870, pp. 269–271, in Putnam, *Life and Letters*, quotation on p. 271.

206. Putnam to Father, Paris, 26 Dec.

1870, pp. 271–273; Putnam to Father, Paris, 2 Feb. 1871, pp. 273–277; Putnam to Brother [George Haven Putnam], Paris, 7 May 1871, pp. 277–279, in Putnam, *Life and Letters*, quotations on pp. 277 and 275.

207. See Putnam, *Life and Letters*, pp. 281–283, 292–293.

208. Putnam to Mother, [London, n.d. but summer 1871], in Putnam, *Life and Letters*, pp. 283–284.

209. Putnam to Mother, London, 29 July 1871, in Putnam, *Life and Letters*, pp. 286–288, on p. 286.

210. Putnam to Mother, London, 27 Dec. 1869, and ibid., 13 Jan. 1870, in Putnam, *Life and Letters*, pp. 226–229, 232–236. It was also in Paris that Putnam first met Susan Dimock, bound for medical study in Zurich (Mary Putnam-Jacobi, "Dr. Susan Dimock," in *Memoir of Susan Dimock, Resident Physician of the New England Hospital for Women and Children* [Boston, n.p., 1875], pp. 87–90, on p. 89).

211. *Twenty-Second Annual Catalogue and Report of the New-England Female Medical College* (Boston: John Wilson and Son, 1870), p. 17.

212. Sarah E. Palmer, "A Brief Account of the Doctors Emily and Augusta Pope," typescript in American Medical Women's Association Historic Collection, Biographical Files, Pope, PA—Women in Med. Arch.

213. Putnam to Mother, Paris, 27 Dec. 1869, in Putnam, *Life and Letters*, pp. 226–229; M. C. Putnam to [Elizabeth] Blackwell, [Paris], 4 Nov. [1869]; and, partly written onto blank spaces of the letter from Putnam to Blackwell, Elizabeth Blackwell to Emily Blackwell, [London], 9 Nov. [1869], Blackwell Family Papers.

214. Elizabeth Blackwell to Emily Blackwell, London, 14 May 1871; and see ibid., [London], 9 Nov. [1869], and ibid., New York, 18 Oct. [1869 or 1870].

215. Putnam to Mother, Paris, 15 Apr. 1870, in Putnam, *Life and Letters*, pp. 245–247, on p. 246; Putnam to Mother, Paris, 13 Jan. 1870, in Putnam, *Life and Letters*, pp. 232–235, on p. 233. The views of Blackwell and Putnam Jacobi are contrasted in Regina Morantz-Sanchez, "Feminist Theory and Historical Practice: Rereading Elizabeth Blackwell," *History and Theory*, Beiheft 31 (1992): 51–69, and idem, *Sympathy and Science*, pp. 184–202. Elizabeth Blackwell's judgment mel-

lowed when Putnam visited London deeply distraught over the course of political and personal affairs in France. "I do not think that you will have trouble with Miss Putnam, now that you are on your guard," Elizabeth told Emily after seeing Putnam in England. "She is awfully cut up by her disappointment, and I think, if she retain her health, that she will be very anxious to help you and the school. I shall hope for the best—and she may be of much service in encouraging the other young women physicians, for I think she is very unworldly, and has nothing of the medical shop keeper about her" (Elizabeth Blackwell to Emily Blackwell, [London], 23 July [1871], Blackwell Family Papers. See also ibid., Rome, 8 Dec. 1873).

216. "Dr. Mary Putnam Jacobi Dead. Well Known Women Physician Ends Four Years of Suffering," *New York Tribune*, 12 June 1906. A large number of obituaries featuring the same contribution are in (Putnam) Jacobi Papers.

217. The relative appeal of these elements was somewhat different in Britain, which still lacked the separate medical schools that gave American women access to an M.D. degree in their own country. In some respects, that enhanced the attraction of Paris for aspiring British women physicians. "By going to Paris, female students can get, without further difficulty or contention, at a very small cost, a first-class medical education, a choice of all the best hospital teachers of the place, a succession of stimulating and searching examinations, and a diploma of recognized value," Sophia Jex-Blake wrote to the London *Times* on 5 Aug. 1873, recognizing that English women were "seeking abroad that which is at present denied to them in their own country" (quoted in Shirley Roberts, *Sophia Jex-Blake: Woman Pioneer in Nineteenth-Century Medical Reform* [London and New York: Routledge, 1993], p. 138).

218. Harriet Beecher Stowe, *My Wife and I: or, Harry Henderson's History* (Boston: Houghton, Mifflin and Company, 1871), esp. pp. 272–273 and 403; quotation on p. 273.

219. William D. Howells, *Dr. Breen's Practice: A Novel* (Boston and New York: Houghton, Mifflin and Company, 1891), p. 97. It turned out, to his horror, that she had graduated from a New York homeopathic school.

220. Bonner, "Medical Women Abroad,"

p. 63. On the European training of the women doctors represented in late-nineteenth-century American fiction, see Sonya S. Erickson, "The Image of Women Physicians in Ten Victorian American Novels, 1871–1886" (M.D. thesis, Yale University, 1991).

221. J. E., "Foreign Correspondence" (Paris, 14 Dec. 1880), *Cincinnati Lancet and Clinic* 6 (1881): 82–85, p. 83. Having observed American women studying in the Paris hospitals, he argued that "woman is not here in her proper sphere," and that "one cannot entirely repress a feeling of revulsion when seeing one of these lady students in the midst of a crowd of the other sex at a female venereal hospital" (p. 83). For a representative counterargument that turned such concerns about modesty on their head, see Elizabeth C. Keller, "Clinical Instruction" (M.D. thesis, Woman's Medical College of Pennsylvania, 1871), PA—Women in Med. Arch.

222. Putnam to Mother, Paris, 22 Dec. 1867, in Putnam, *Life and Letters*, pp. 157–161, on pp. 157–158.

223. P.C.M. letter to the editor of the *Medical Record*, Paris, 18 June 1867, in Woman's Medical Association, *Mary Putnam Jacobi*, pp. 1–9, on p. 3.

224. J. E., "Foreign Correspondence" (Vienna, 26 May 1880), *Cincinnati Lancet and Clinic* 5 (1880): 13–14, p. 13. Another American in Vienna, echoing this point two years later, noted that "to me it seems as if Vienna has reached the height of its glory and popularity and is already slowly but unmistakably taking a down road," suggesting that "it is but a question of time to my mind when Vienna will lose its grip" and give way to other centers as "the shrines of medical worship" (Eric E. Sattler to Editors [Vienna, 29 Dec. 1882], *Cincinnati Lancet and Clinic* 10 [1883]: 83–85, p. 83).

225. J. W. Humrichouse to C. W. Humrichouse, Lucerne, 7 Sept. 1877, Ridgley Papers.

## CHAPTER 10
## REMEMBERING PARIS

1. "American Medical Periodicals," *BMSJ* 82 (1870): 83–84, p. 84.

2. [James Clark White], "The Past and Present of the School of Paris," *BMSJ* 72 (1866–1867): 389–390, p. 389.

3. Ibid., pp. 389–390.

4. On White's studies abroad, see James Clarke White, *Sketches from My Life, 1833–1913* (Cambridge: Riverside Press, 1914), pp. 74–109. White went to Vienna in the first place at the advice of Calvin Ellis, just returned from Europe where he had "spent a few week in Vienna and was greatly impressed by the advantages it offered" (p. 75). "In Paris," White later explained, "I remained only long enough to see the city and some of the distinguished teachers of medicine, and to visit the famous old hospitals, but did not really resume my studies there," a course he also followed in London (p. 109). Writing shortly after his return, he boasted that "I am happy to say that I was able to carry out an honorable and home virtue through dissolute Vienna and enticing Paris unsullied" (James C. White to H. I. Bowditch, Belfast, Maine, 27 Aug. 1857, in Henry I. Bowditch, Collection of Autograph Letters and Portraits, MA—Countway).

5. Clare Blake] to Dear Mater, n.p., n.d. [but Vienna, summer 1869], Clarence John Blake Papers, MA—Countway.

6. "Memorabilia des Wiener Clubs, Gegründet 1865," MA—Countway. The other founding members were Hasket Derby, Gustavus Hay, Benjamin J. Jeffries, Henry K. Oliver, and Francis P. Sprague.

7. Henry Ingersoll Bowditch, [Introductory Lecture on the Profession], 1864 & 5. College, MA—Countway.

8. B. to Editors (Boston, Mass., 11 Nov. 1870), *CLO*, n.s., 13 (1870): 751–755, p. 751. The address by White that prompted this comment was "An Introductory Lecture Delivered before the Medical Class of Harvard University, Nov., 2, 1870," *BMSJ* 83 (1870): 277–289; and see his earlier editorials, "Censorial Duties in Medical Education," *BMSJ* 75 (1866–1867): 105–107; "Election at Harvard University," *BMSJ* 74 (1866): 508–509; and "Medical Education—New Professorships in the Medical Department of Harvard University," *BMSJ* 74 (1866): 63–65. On the curriculum changes at Harvard, see Thomas S. Huddle, "Looking Backward: The 1871 Reforms at Harvard Medical School Reconsidered," *Bulletin of the History of Medicine* 65 (1991): 340–365, and Kenneth M. Ludmerer, *Learning to Heal: The Development of American Medical Education* (New York: Basic Books, 1985), esp. pp. 47–53.

9. See Henry P. Bowditch to Parents, Paris, 12 Feb. 1869, and ibid., Paris, 21 Mar. 1869, Bowditch Papers, MA—Countway. John V. Pickstone offers a suggestive framework for exploring the distinction in "Museological Science? The Place of the Analytical/Comparative in Nineteenth-Century Science, Technology and Medicine," *History of Science* 32 (1994): 111–138.

10. Henry P. Bowditch to Dear Father, Bonn, 19 July 1869, Bowditch Papers.

11. Henry P. Bowditch to Henry I. Bowditch, Leipzig, 5 Dec. 1869. He proceeded to write to Editor [*BMSJ*], Leipzig, 8 Mar. 1870, enclosed in Henry P. Bowditch to Henry I. Bowditch, Leipzig, 11 Mar. 1870.

12. Henry P. Bowditch to Dear Father, Leipzig, 2 Jan. 1870.

13. Bowditch to Editor, 8 Mar. 1870; emphasis added.

14. Blake to Mater, Vienna, 8 Feb. 1869, Blake Papers.

15. Blake to Pater and Mater, Vienna, 11 Apr. 1869.

16. Blake to Pater, Vienna, 19 May 1869.

17. [Blake] to Blessed Mater, Vienna, 8 Feb. 1869; Blake to Poppet, [Vienna, Apr. 1869].

18. I develop this point in "Narrative at the Bedside: The Transformation of the Patient Record in Nineteenth-Century America," paper for a conference titled "Narrative Medicine," Wellcome Institute for the History of Medicine, London, 2 June 1995. On the wider context for these shifts, see Lorraine Daston and Peter Galison, "The Image of Objectivity," *Representations* 40 (1992): 81–127, and David E. Shi, *Facing Facts: Realism in American Thought and Culture, 1850–1920* (New York and Oxford: Oxford University Press, 1995).

19. Claude Bernard, *Introduction to the Study of Experimental Medicine*, trans. Henry Copley Greene (Paris, 1865; New York: Macmillan, 1927), p. 139.

20. [Charles-Édward Brown-Séquard], "Introductory Lecture to the Winter Course at Harvard Medical School," *BMSJ* 75 (1866–1867): 307–308, p. 307; S. E. Chaille, Lectures on Physiology, Medical College, New Orleans, 1867, 5 vols., vol. 1, LA—Tulane Med.

21. Edward H. Dixon, *Back-Bone; Photographed from "The Scalpel"* (New York: Robert M. De Witt, 1866), pp. 180–181. The New York physician was Dr. Francis. Dixon, a physician turned professional satirist, edited the *Scalpel* between 1849 and 1864.

22. Edward H. Clarke, "Recent Progress in Materia Medica," *BMSJ* 71 (1864–1865): 309–323, p. 321.

23. "How to Study Medicine," *BMSJ* 79 (1868–1869): 74–76, p. 74. Just as historians have recently argued that in America during the final third of the nineteenth century the new scientific medicine of the experimental laboratory was gendered as masculine, so one can see in this same process evidence of a re-gendering of the older, empiricist program of the French tradition as feminine, a discursive regendering that functioned to contest both its epistemological authority and its power as a controlling science that directed intervention at the bedside. See Ellen Singer More, "'Empathy' Enters the Medical Profession," Regina Morantz-Sanchez, "The Gendering of Empathic Expertise: How Women Physicians Became More Empathic Than Men," and Susan E. Lederer, "Moral Sensibility and Medical Science: Gender, Animal Experimentation, and the Doctor-Patient Relationship," in *The Empathic Practitioner: Empathy, Gender, and Medicine*, ed. Ellen Singer More and Maureen A. Milligan (New Brunswick, N.J.: Rutgers University Press, 1994), pp. 19–39, 40–58, 59–73; and Regina Morantz-Sanchez, "Feminist Theory and Historical Practice: Rereading Elizabeth Blackwell," *History and Theory*, Beiheft 31 (1992): 51–69.

24. H. C. Wood, "The Principles of Modern Therapeusis," *Philadelphia Medical Times* 14 (1883–1884): 633–635, p. 633. See also Wood, "Preface to the First Edition," *A Treatise on Therapeutics, Comprising Materia Medica and Toxicology, with Especial Reference to the Application of the Physiological Action of Drugs to Clinical Medicine*, 3d ed. (Philadelphia: J. B. Lippincott, 1880), pp. 5–10, on pp. 5–6.

25. Wood, "Principles of Modern Therapeusis," p. 634.

26. Roberts Bartholow, "The Degree of Certainty in Therapeutics," *Transactions of the Medical and Chirurgical Faculty of the State of Maryland*, 1876, pp. 33–50, on pp. 33, 48. And see Jas. T. Whittaker, "The Relation of Physiology to Practice," *Transactions of the Ohio Medical Society* 27 (1872): 241–251, on p. 241.

27. C. D. Palmer, "The Unity of Medicine,"

extract in "College Commencements. Medical College of Ohio," *Cincinnati Lancet and Clinic*, n.s., 2 (1879): 187–194, p. 191.

28. E[lias] B. Thompson to Mother, New Orleans, 30 Dec. 1866, Benson-Thompson Family Papers, NC—Duke.

29. See A., Review of "*A Treatise on Therapeutics, Comprising Materia Medica and Toxicology.* By H. C. Wood, Jr. . . .," *BMSJ* 88 (1873): 577–579, p. 577.

30. "Poole's Physiological Therapeutics," *BMSJ* 101 (1879): 276; and see, for example, T. L. Wright, "Transcendental Medicine.—An Enquiry Concerning the Manner of Morbific and Remedial Agents Independently of Empiricism," *CLO* 20 (1877): 1015–1034, p. 1017, on the aim of creating a "rational therapeutics" by escaping empiricism.

31. "A System of Rational Therapeutics," *BMSJ* 87 (1872): 13–14, p. 13.

32. Burton J. Bledstein, *The Culture of Professionalism: The Middle Class and the Development of Higher Education in America* (New York: Norton, 1976), p. 80.

33. Samuel Haber, *The Quest for Authority and Honor in the American Professions, 1750–1900* (Chicago and London: University of Chicago Press, 1991), p. 191. On changing American attitudes in the Gilded Age and Progressive Era, see George M. Fredrickson, *The Inner Civil War: Northern Intellectuals and the Crisis of Union* (New York: Harper and Row, 1965), esp. pp. 183 ff.; Richard Hofstadter, *Anti-Intellectualism in American Life* (New York: Knopf, 1963); Morton Keller, *Affairs of State: Public Life in Late Nineteenth Century America* (Cambridge, Mass.: Belknap Press of Harvard University Press, 1977); Alexandra Oleson and John Voss, eds., *The Organization of Knowledge in Modern America, 1860–1920* (Baltimore: Johns Hopkins University Press, 1979); Charles E. Rosenberg, *No Other Gods: On Science and American Social Thought* (Baltimore: Johns Hopkins University Press, 1976), esp. pp. 135–172; and Robert H. Wiebe, *The Search for Order, 1877–1920* (New York: Hill and Wang, 1967).

34. W. F. Bynum, *Science and the Practice of Medicine in the Nineteenth Century* (Cambridge: Cambridge University Press, 1994); Gerald L. Geison, "'Divided We Stand': Physiologists and Clinicians in the American Context," in *The Therapeutic Revolution: Essays in the Social History of American Medicine*, ed.

Morris J. Vogel and Charles E. Rosenberg (Philadelphia: University of Pennsylvania Press, 1979), pp. 67–90; S.E.D. Shortt, "Physicians, Science, and Status: Issues in the Professionalization of Anglo-American Medicine in the Nineteenth-Century," *Medical History* 27 (1983): 51–68; John Harley Warner, "Science in Medicine," *Osiris*, n.s., 1 (1985): 37–58.

35. See Barbara Gutmann Rosenkrantz, "The Search for Professional Order in Nineteenth-Century American Medicine," in *Sickness and Health in America: Readings in the History of Medicine and Public Health*, ed. Ronald L. Numbers and Judith Walzer Leavitt (Madison: University of Wisconsin Press, 1985), pp. 219–232; John Harley Warner, "Ideals of Science and Their Discontents in Late Nineteenth-Century American Medicine," *Isis* 82 (1991): 454–478; and idem, *The Therapeutic Perspective: Medical Practice, Knowledge, and Identity in America, 1820–1885* (Cambridge, Mass., and London: Harvard University Press, 1986), pp. 258–283.

36. *Code of Ethics of the American Medical Association, Adopted May 1847* (Philadelphia: T. K. & P. G. Collins, 1848), pp. 18–19.

37. On the controversy over the code, see Toby A. Appel, "Biological and Medical Societies and the Founding of the American Physiological Society," in *Physiology in the American Context, 1850–1940*, ed. Gerald L. Geison (Bethesda: American Physiological Society, 1987), pp. 155–175; Kenneth Warren Hamstra, "The American Medical Association Code of Medical Ethics of 1847" (Ph.D. diss., University of Texas at Austin, 1987), pp. 60–85; Martin Kaufman, *Homeopathy in America: The Rise and Fall of a Medical Heresy* (Baltimore and London: Johns Hopkins University Press, 1971), pp. 125–140; Lester S. King, *American Medicine Comes of Age, 1840–1920* ([Chicago]: American Medical Association, 1984), pp. 37–45; and Warner, "Ideals of Science."

38. William S. Ely, "The Questionable Features of Our Medical Codes," in *An Ethical Symposium: Being a Series of Papers Concerning Medical Ethics and Etiquette from the Liberal Standpoint*, ed. Alfred C. Post et al. (New York: G. P. Putnam's Sons, 1883), pp. 8–25, on pp. 20, 21.

39. Abraham Jacobi, "The Anniversary Discourse: New York Academy of Medicine," *Medical Record* 30 (1886): 608–609, p. 608.

40. Wood, "Principles of Modern Thera-

peusis," p. 634. Wood stated clearly in his textbook that "the plan of the present work has been to make the physiological action of remedies the principal point of discussion" (*A Treatise on Therapeutics*, p. x); while Bartholow insisted that "the real and permanent advances in therapeutical art must be effected chiefly by the physiological method" (Roberts Bartholow, "Preface to the Fourth Edition," *A Practical Treatise on Materia Medica and Therapeutics*, 5th ed. [New York: D. Appleton, 1884], pp. vi–viii, on p. vii).

41. Roberts Bartholow, "Experimental Therapeutics," introductory address quoted in "Medical College of Ohio," *CLO*, n.s., 15 (1872): 635–636, p. 636. See also Horatio C. Wood, "General Therapeutic Considerations," in *A System of Practical Therapeutics*, ed. Hobart Amory Hare, 4 vols. (Philadelphia: Lea Brothers, 1891–1892), 1:17–52, on p. 19, and idem, "Principles of Modern Therapeusis," pp. 633–634.

42. Horatio R. Bigelow to C. R. Agnew, Washington, D.C., 9 May 1882, Cornelius Rea Agnew Papers, MD—NLM. And see Cornelius R. Agnew, "On Dr. Squibb's Resolutions to Abolish the Code of Ethics of the Medical Society of the State of New York," *New York Medical Journal* (1883): 345–347, p. 347, and C. R. Agnew to A. R. [illegible], 20 July 1882, Agnew Papers.

43. David Hunt to C. R. Agnew, Boston, 22 Nov. 1882, Agnew Papers.

44. John C. Minor to C. R. Agnew, n.d. [but 1882 or 1883], Agnew Papers. And see John Harley Warner, "Orthodoxy and Otherness: Homeopathy and Regular Medicine in Nineteenth-Century America," in *Culture, Knowledge, and Healing: Historical Perspectives of Homeopathic Medicine in Europe and North America*, ed. Robert Jütte, Guenter B. Risse, and John Woodward (European Association for the History of Medicine, in press).

45. Abraham Jacobi, "Requiescat in Pace," in Post et al., *An Ethical Symposium*, 156–175, p. 174. For Mary Putnam Jacobi's opposition to the code, see "Opponents of the Old Code," *New York Medical Journal* 37 (1883): 474–475, p. 474.

46. Thos. D. Parker to Geo. F. Shrady, Birmingham, Ala., 9 Dec. 1884, Agnew Papers; see also F. N. Smith to C. R. Agnew, Belmont, N.Y., 22 June 1882, Agnew Papers.

47. Joseph Davis Craig, "Modern Clinical

Research" (M.D. thesis, Albany Medical College, 1884), NY—Albany Med.

48. Ibid.

49. On shifting conceptions of what counted as *scientific medicine*, see John Harley Warner, "The History of Science and the Sciences of Medicine," *Osiris*, n.s., 10 (1995): 164–193.

50. A. Stillé to [G. C.] Shattuck, Philadelphia, 12 Jan. 1857, MA—Countway.

51. John A. Murphy, [Letter to the Editor] (Paris, Mar. 1854), *WL* 15 (1854): 529–540, p. 537.

52. "Parisian Correspondence," *American Medical Gazette and Journal of Health* 6 (1855): 209–213, p. 210. On the Parisian controversy, see Ann La Berge, "Medical Microscopy in Paris, 1830–1855," in *French Medical Culture in the Nineteenth Century*, ed. Ann La Berge and Mordechai Feingold (Amsterdam and Atlanta: Rodopi, 1994), pp. 296–326.

53. An Old Fogy, "OLD FOGYISM!—Cogitations and Vaticinations," *American Medical Gazette and Journal of Health* 7 (1856): 23–28, p. 26.

54. Ibid., p. 23.

55. Ibid., pp. 25, 26.

56. On early medical microscopy in the American context, see James H. Cassedy, "The Microscope in American Medical Science, 1840–1860," *Isis* 67 (1976): 76–97.

57. Henry Ingersoll Bowditch, Outline of Course for Winter 1860–1, MA—Countway.

58. Henry I. Bowditch, *Brief Memories of Louis and Some of His Contemporaries in the Parisian School of Medicine of Forty Years Ago* (Boston: John Wilson and Son, 1872), p. 30.

59. Quoted in John T. Morse, Jr., ed., *Life and Letters of Oliver Wendell Holmes*, 2 vols. (Boston and New York: Houghton, Mifflin and Company, 1896), 1:91; Oliver Wendell Holmes, *Our Hundred Days in Europe* (1887; Boston and New York: Houghton, Mifflin and Company, 1892), p. 164.

60. Elisha Bartlett, "Letter from Paris" (Paris, 20 Apr. 1846), *WL* 5 (1846–1847): 107–111, and ibid., (Paris, 4 May 1846) *WL* 5 (1846–1847): 172–176, p. 174.

61. Henry H. Smith, *Professional Visit to London and Paris: Introductory Lecture to the Course on the Principles and Practice of Surgery. Delivered in the University of Pennsylvania, October 9, 1855* (Philadelphia: T. K. and P. G. Collins, 1855), p. 11. And see B., "Letter

from Paris" (Paris, 13 Feb. 1854), *North-Western Medical and Surgical Journal* 3 (1854): 145–149, and Paul F. Eve, "Professional Letters from Paris," *NOMSJ* 9 (1852–1853): 409–413.

62. A. Stillé to G. C. Shattuck, Philadelphia, 28 Sept. 1851, Shattuck Papers, vol. 22, MA—MA Hist. Soc.

63. Ibid., Vienna, 15 Jan. 1851.

64. H. I. Bowditch, Introductory Lecture to the Clinical Course of Harvard's Course of 1861, MA—Countway.

65. Henry I. Bowditch to Henry P. Bowditch, [Boston], 18 Aug. 1868, Bowditch Papers.

66. Henry P. Bowditch to Henry I. Bowditch, Paris, 20 Sept. 1868.

67. Henry I. Bowditch to Henry P. Bowditch, Boston, 20 Oct. 1868.

68. Henry P. Bowditch to Henry I. Bowditch, entries of 9 Oct. and 2 Nov. in letter of Paris, 4 Oct. 1868.

69. Ibid., entry of 2 Nov. in letter of Paris, 15 Oct. 1868.

70. Henry I. Bowditch to Henry P. Bowditch, Boston, 30 Nov. 1868.

71. Henry P. Bowditch to Henry I. Bowditch, entry of 22 Nov. in letter of Paris, 15 Nov. 1868.

72. Henry P. Bowditch to Parents, Paris, 22 Nov. 1868.

73. Henry I. Bowditch to Henry P. Bowditch, [Boston], 21 Feb. 1869.

74. Ibid., Boston, 3 Mar. 1869.

75. Ibid., 30 Nov. 1868.

76. Henry P. Bowditch to Henry I. Bowditch, Paris, 13 Dec. 1868.

77. Ibid., entry of 7 Feb. in letter of 26 Jan. 1869.

78. Quoted in Mother [Lucy Orne Bowditch] to Henry P. Bowditch, Moss Hill, 7 Mar. 1869.

79. Henry I. Bowditch to Henry P. Bowditch, Boston, 3 Mar. 1869.

80. Ibid., 17 July 1871. The uncle acknowledged, though, that "of course, there is great doubt about the majority of the Profession being up to the mark of believing in a pure Physiologist being *able even* to help the *practicing* physician." And see Lucy Orne Bowditch to Henry P. Bowditch, [Moss Hill], 9 July 1871. The nephew gently dismissed the proposal; see Henry P. Bowditch to Parents, Leipzig, 6 Aug. 1871.

81. John LeConte, "'The Philosophy of Medicine'; An address, Delivered before the Graduates of the Medical College of Georgia, on the 20th of March, 1849," *Southern Medical and Surgical Journal*, n.s., 5 (1849): 257–277, pp. 264, 266.

82. For example, see S. C. Furman, "The Impediments to the Progress of Medical Science" (M.D. thesis, Medical College of the State of South Carolina, 1852), SC—Waring; Jamie V. Ingham, "An Essay on Empiricism" (M.D. thesis, University of Pennsylvania, 1866), PA—U. PA Lib.; and Elijah Evan Winn, "Theories of Idiopathic Fevers" (M.D. thesis, University of Nashville, 1858–1859), TN—Vanderbilt.

83. See, for example, Henry Alfred Hawley, "The Progress of Medicine" (M.D. thesis, Medical Department, University of Michigan, 1865–1866), MI—Bentley, U. MI.

84. Alfred Stillé, *Elements of General Pathology: A Practical Treatise* (Philadelphia: Lindsay and Blackiston, 1848), p. 27.

85. J. Jackson to H. I. Bowditch, [Boston], 15 Aug. 1857, H. I. Bowditch, Collection of Autograph Letters and Portraits.

86. Review of "*Therapeutics and Materia Medica* . . . by Alfred Stillé," *CLO*, 17 (1874): 764; Samuel Nickels, "Modern Therapeutics," *CLO* 7 (1881): 323–330, p. 330.

87. "Wood's Therapeutics," *BMSJ* 93 (1875): 645–646, p. 646.

88. T. C. M[inor], Review of "Materia Medica and Therapeutics. By Roberts Bartholow," *CLO* 37 (1876): 838–854, p. 842.

89. Ibid., p. 852.

90. Alfred Stillé, "An Address Delivered to the Medical Classes of the University of Pennsylvania, on Withdrawing from His Chair, April 10, 1884," *Medical News* 44 (1884): 433–438, p. 436.

91. Samuel S. Wallian, "The Therapeutics of the Future," *New York Medical Journal* 39 (1884): 265–270, p. 266.

92. Stillé, "Address Delivered to the Medical Classes," p. 435.

93. Chas. G. Stockton, "The Proper Attitude of Therapeutics," *Transactions of the New York State Medical Association* 3 (1886): 309–316, pp. 309, 310.

94. John Ashburton Cutter, "Clinical Morphology versus Bacteriology, with Some Therapeutic Deductions," *Medical Bulletin* 11 (1889): 307–317, p. 315. And see Austin

Flint, "Address on Medicine—Medicinal and Non-Medicinal Therapeutics," *Transactions of the New York State Medical Association* 1 (1884): 376–397, p. 382; John V. Lansing, *Therapeutic Skepticism: An Address, Introductory to the Course of 1869* (Albany: Joel Munsell, 1869), p. 11; and Alfred Stillé, *Therapeutics and Materia Medica: A Systematic Treatise on the Action and Uses of Medicinal Agents, Including Their Description and History*, 4th ed., 2 vols. (Philadelphia: Henry C. Lea, 1874), 1:vii.

95. Henry J. Bigelow, *Medical Education in America: Being the Annual Address Read before the Massachusetts Medical Society. June 7, 1871* (Cambridge: Welch, Bigelow, and Company, 1871), pp. 42, 43. And see Susan E. Lederer, *Subjected to Science: Human Experimentation in America before the Second World War* (Baltimore and London: Johns Hopkins University Press, 1995).

96. Alfred George Tebault, Notes on Medical Lectures Taken at the University of Virginia, Lecture Notebook, No. 4, n.d. [but ca. 1885–1895], Alfred George Tebault Papers (no. 9926), VA—U. VA.

97. See, for example, Henry I. Bowditch to A. N. Blodgett, Boston, 17 July 1887, Albert Novatus Blodgett Papers, MA—Countway. Positions on the code controversy were informed in part by the individual's posture toward liberalism; see Samuel Lee Baker, "Medical Licensing in America: An Early Liberal Reform" (Ph.D. diss., Harvard University, 1977).

98. Austin Flint, *Medical Ethics and Etiquette: The Code of Ethics Adopted by the American Medical Association, with Commentaries* (New York: D. Appleton, 1883), pp. 1–2. See, for example, Austin Flint, *The Clinical Study of the Heart Sounds in Health and Disease* (Philadelphia: Collins, 1859), and idem, *Compendium of Percussion and Auscultation*, 2d ed. (New York: William Wood and Company, 1865).

99. "Clarke County Medical Society—February Meeting," *CLO*, n.s., 18 (1875): 159–165, p. 161.

100. Austin Flint, in his textbook *Clinical Medicine*, spoke of "reasoning" from knowledge about the physiological action of drugs only as a source of error in therapeutic practice: *Clinical Medicine: A Systematic Treatise on the Diagnosis and Treatment of Diseases, Designed for the Use of Students and Practitioners*

*of Medicine* (Philadelphia: Henry C. Lea, 1879), p. 54; he virtually ignored it in the discussions on the sources of therapeutic knowledge in his *Treatise on the Principles and Practice of Medicine Designed for the Use of Practitioners and Students of Medicine*, 5th ed. (Philadelphia: Henry C. Lea's Sons, 1884), esp. pp. 111–112. See also Stillé, *Therapeutics and Materia Medica*, 1:viii.

101. Stillé, "Address Delivered to the Medical Classes," pp. 435, 436.

102. Ely Van de Warker, comments in *Minutes of a Convention Held in the City of Albany, February 4th and 6th, at Which the New York State Medical Association Was Organized on a Permanent Basis* [n.p., 1884], p. 21; and "Proceedings: First Annual Meeting of the New York State Medical Association, Held at the Murray Hill Hotel, in New York City, November 18, 19, and 20, 1884," *Transactions of the New York State Medical Association* 1 (1884): 585–609, p. 597.

103. "Truth" to the Editor, "Misstatements about the New York Code," *New York Medical Journal* 37 (1883): 54.

104. West Philadelphia Medical Society, Minutes, 1881–1890, resolution presented by Dr. John H. Mussen at meeting of 7 May 1883, PA—CPP. On Stillé's support, see minutes of 25 Apr. 1881.

105. H. W. Nichols to C. R. Agnew, Canandaigua, N.Y., 14 July 1882, H. W. Nichols Letter, NY—NY State Lib.

106. Henry D. Didama, "The President's Annual Address: Conservative Progress," *Transactions of the New York State Medical Association* 1 (1884): 19–32, p. 22. On the schism between this association and the established state medical society, see "Proceedings of the Medical Society of the State of New York, at Its Seventy-Eighth Annual Meeting, Held in Geological Hall, Albany, February 5, 6, and 7, 1884," *Transactions of the Medical Society of the State of New York* (1884): 37–65.

107. Austin Flint, *Medicine of the Future: An Address Prepared for the Annual Meeting of the British Medical Association in 1886* (New York: D. Appleton, 1886), pp. 16, 36.

108. A. Flint to C. R. Agnew, New York, 23 Oct. 1883, Agnew Papers.

109. Alfred Stillé, "Truth in Medicine and Truth in Life Inseparable," 1885, PA—CPP.

110. Augustus Kinsley Gardner, *Old Wine in New Bottles; or, Spare Hours of a Student in*

*Paris* (New-York: C. S. Francis & Co.; Boston: J. H. Francis, 1848), pp. 330–331. Suggestive of the wider context for understanding the place of memory in American culture is Michael G. Kammen, *Mystic Chords of Memory: The Transformation of Tradition in American Culture* (New York: Knopf, 1991).

111. H. I. Bowditch to William Henry Thayer, Boston, 5 Dec. 1857, in *Life and Correspondence of Henry Ingersoll Bowditch*, ed. Vincent Y. Bowditch, 2 vols. (Boston and New York: Houghton, Mifflin and Company, 1902), 1:260–262, on p. 261.

112. H. I. Bowditch, journal entry for [Paris], 26 Sept. [1867], in V. Y. Bowditch, *Life and Correspondence*, 2:142–145, on p. 144; and, on the lithograph, see journal entry for [Boston], 15 Sept. 1872, ibid., pp. 270–275, on p. 275.

113. Ibid., journal entry for Paris, 17 Sept. 1867, pp. 126–137, on p. 135.

114. Ibid., p. 126; ibid., journal entry for [Paris], 24 Sept. [1867], pp. 137–141, on p. 137; and ibid. (17 Sept.), p. 126.

115. Ibid., p. 126.

116. Holmes, *Our Hundred Days in Europe*, pp. 1, 164.

117. Edward Warren, *A Doctor's Experience in Three Continents* (Baltimore: Cushings and Bailey, 1885), p. 167.

118. A. Stillé to G. C. Shattuck, Philadelphia, 28 Sept. 1851, Shattuck Papers, vol. 22.

119. H. I. B[owditch] to Mary Hudson, [Boston], 31 Dec. 1863, in V. Y. Bowditch, *Life and Correspondence*, 2:20–22, on p. 21. "Now I feel bewildered and, almost without definite plan, I wend my way," he wrote to his nephew Henry, still in the army (H. I. Bowditch to H. P. Bowditch, [Boston, n.d. but spring or summer 1863]; and see idem, Boston, 6 Sept. 1863, both in Bowditch Papers).

120. Henry Ingersoll Bowditch, journal entry for 17 Mar. 1864, in V. Y. Bowditch, *Life and Correspondence*, 2:22.

121. A. Stillé to [G. C.] Shattuck, Philadelphia, 12 Jan. 1857, MA—Countway. This letter, clipped along one edge, is only partly legible.

122. A. Stillé to [G. C.] Shattuck, Philadelphia, 13 June 1871, Shattuck Papers, vol. 24; Jonathan Quinan to William Stump Forward, Logon County, 19 June 1884, William Stump Forward Papers, NC—SHC.

123. Kate Campbell Hurd-Mead, "Reminis-

cences of Medical Study in Europe (1880–1890)," in *Daughters of Aesculapius: Stories Written by Alumnae and Students of the Woman's Medical College of Pennsylvania, and Edited by a Committee Appointed by the Students Association of the College* (Philadelphia: George W. Jacobs, 1897), pp. 108–122, on p. 111. Helpful here is Jerome Bruner, *Actual Minds, Possible Worlds* (Cambridge, Mass., and London: Harvard University Press, 1986).

124. Henry Ingersoll Bowditch to Olivia Bowditch, [Philadelphia], 6 Sept. [1876], in V. Y. Bowditch, *Life and Correspondence*, 2:240; Henry Ingersoll Bowditch, quoted in V. Y. Bowditch, *Life and Correspondence*, 2:262–263; and Hurd-Mead, "Reminiscences," p. 121.

125. For example, A. A. Marrett, Lectures on Clinical Medicine Delivered at the Louisville City Hospital and the Medical University of Louisville by Prof. L. P. Yandell, Jr., Session 1873–1874, KY—U. Louisville.

126. H. I. Bowditch, Introductory Lecture to the Clinical Course of Harvard's Course of 1861.

127. O.W.H., "The Late Dr. Elisha Bartlett," *BMSJ* 53 (1855): 49–52, p. 51.

128. R. F. Michel, "Eulogy on Dr. James Berney, at Meeting of the Medical and Surgical Society of Montgomery, 20 July 1880," [Montgomery Alabama] *Advertiser and Mail*, 25 July 1880.

129. Henry Ingersoll Bowditch, extract from journal entry for [Boston], 15 Sept. 1872, in V. Y. Bowditch, *Life and Correspondence*, 2:270–275, on pp. 270, 275.

130. H. I. Bowditch, *Brief Memories of Louis*, pp. 1, 7, 16, 17, 18, 19. Louis's full inscription read, "Il y a quelque chose de plus rare que l'esprit de discernement, c'est le besoin de la vérité, cet état de l'âme qui ne nous permet pas de nous arrêter dans les travaux scientifiques à ce qui n'est que vraisemblable mais nous oblige à continuer nos recherches jusqu'à ce que nous soyons arrivés à l'évidence" (p. 19).

131. Z[oé Duridal Montferrier] Louis to Eleanor Shattuck, [Paris], 23 Oct. 1873; and see letter of 29 Oct. 1872, in Shattuck Papers, vol. 24. I am grateful to Virginia H. Smith at the Massachusetts Historical Society for clarifying the identities of the two Eleanor Shattucks, the sister and daughter of George Cheyne Shattuck, Jr.

132. A. Stillé to H. I. Bowditch, Philadelphia, 4 Jan. 1873, Bowditch, Collection of Autograph Letters and Portraits.

133. Henry I. Bowditch to Mrs. Pennock, Boston, 8 Sept. 1873, C. W. Pennock Papers, PA—APS.

134. Robert N. Butler and Myrna I. Lewis, *Aging and Mental Health* (New York: Mosby Medical Library, 1983), p. 53.

135. [Oliver Wendell Holmes], "Farewell Address of Dr. Oliver Wendell Holmes to the Medical School of Harvard University, Tuesday, November 28, 1882," *BMSJ* 107 (1882): 529–533, pp. 530, 531, 532, 533, 532.

136. Oliver Wendell Holmes to Samuel May, n.p., 20 June 1888, in Morse, *Holmes,* 2:71–72, on p. 72. For Holmes, as for others of his cohort, aging, dissolution, and remembrance became preoccupying themes, as in stanzas from his poem "The Last Leaf" (reprinted in Lewis W. Townsend, *Centenary Biography: Oliver Wendell Holmes* [London: Headley Brothers, 1909], pp. 94–95), which ends: "And if I should live to be / The last leaf upon the tree / In the spring, /Let them smile as I do now / At the old forsaken bough / Where I cling."

137. A. Stillé to Henry I. Bowditch, Philadelphia, 25 Feb. 1882, Bowditch, Collection of Autograph Letters and Portraits.

138. Stillé, "Address Delivered to the Medical Classes," p. 433.

139. Ibid., pp. 433, 435, 437, 438.

140. Stillé, "Truth in Medicine."

141. Alfred Stillé to William Osler, n.p., 27 June 1900, quoted in William Osler, "Alfred Stillé," *University of Pennsylvania Medical Bulletin* 15 (1902): 126–132, p. 131.

142. Stillé to Osler, 7 Feb. 1900, quoted in "Stillé," p. 131.

143. Osler, "Stillé," p. 126.

144. William Osler, *An Alabama Student and Other Biographical Essays* (New York: Oxford University Press, 1908), pp. 18, 189, 198, 190. Osler first presented the paper on Holmes in 1894, Bassett in 1895, and Bartlett in 1899; he first published the paper on the American students of Louis in 1897.

145. William Osler to Laura Bassett, Oxford, 25 Aug. 1906, John Young Bassett Papers, AL—AL State Arch. She was still living in Huntsville.

146. William Williams Keen to Samuel C. and Mary Eastman, Vienna, 25 May 1865, William Williams Keen Papers, RI—Brown.

147. A. C. Klebs, "Osler at the Tomb of Louis," *Journal of the American Medical Association* 46 (1906): 1716–1717. Klebs proceeded to claim the lineage of Louis for Osler and his American students. Osler, Klebs noted, had told them, "It was my privilege on several occasions to hear Henry I. Bowditch speak of Louis and of his extraordinary kindness to the young men from America who frequented his clinic, and Dr. Alfred Stillé, whose death a few years ago removed the last of this notable band, has often told me of the lifelong affection which he and all of the American pupils had for their great French master." Klebs asserted a similar role for Osler as mentor in the clinic, "surrounded by his boys, helping them as a friend in their struggles," guiding the student at the bedside "his arm around his shoulder." Drawing the link between present and past, Klebs proposed that "thus we imagine those *maitres* of the old French school, a school no longer limited by national boundaries, one of those men who have trodden the paths through the wards of the Salpetrière, the Charité and Lariboisière, the Necker, the Hotel Dieu, making apostles and missionaries in the great cause of scientific medicine" (pp. 1716–1717). See also Harvey Cushing, *The Life of Sir William Osler,* 2 vols. (Oxford: Clarendon Press, 1926), 2:21.

N.B.: Numbers in italics refer to figures.

rationalism: American assault on, 231–245, 347; Bartlett on, 175–177; clinical instruction as a counterforce to, 220; English assault on, 224–227; and experimental therapeutics, 337, 339, 348–349; heroic therapy blamed on, 232–233, 282, 288–289; Paris School identified by Americans with opposition to, 229–230; and specialized knowledge, 337–338

Réclus family, 325–326

religion, 68, 415n.92; in Paris, 271, 390n.217

Remond, Sarah Parker, 318

Revolution of 1830, 115

Revolution of 1848, 84, 116, 121–122, 291, 292, 299

Richmond Board of Health, 37, 125, 160

Ricord, Philippe, 82, 99, 260, 386n.120

Robin, Charles, 294, *295*, 316, 325, 354, 434n.197

Rodgers, M. M., 94, 260, 263

Roger, Henri-Louis, 82

Rokitansky, Carl von, 297, 298, 303

Rosenberg, Charles, 13, 29, 214

Rosenkrantz, Barbara Gutmann, 13–14

Rostan, Léon, 82

Roux, Philibert-Joseph, 107, 269, 343

Rufz, E., 118, 145, 168

Rush, Benjamin, 126, 179, 203, 255, 282; system of, 176, 180, 235, 347

St. Bartholomew's Hospital, 67, 70, 73, 107, 197, 225, 317

St. George's Hospital, 70, 200

St. John Roosa, Daniel B., 340, 352

St. Thomas's Hospital, 67, 70

Salpêtrière, La, 99, 323

San Francisco Hospital for Women and Children, 319

Satchwell, S. S., 271

science: as career in America, 53–55, 110–111, 151, 280–281, 306–307, 310, 323, 324, 346–347; devotion to, as threat to physician's character, 253–254, 256, 258–267, 272–273, 275–278; identified with empiricism, 175–176, 234, 342; identified with experimentalism, 306, 333, 334–336, 340–341, 346; identified with specialism, 311, 312, 333–334, 336–338, 339; and professional reform in England, 195–201, 405n.40; and shift in American migration to Germany, 291–292

Serres, Étienne-R.-A., 110, 316

Sewall, Lucy, 320, 322, 323, 324, 433n.179

Shattuck, Eleanor (sister of G. Shattuck, Jr.), 146

Shattuck, Eleanor (daughter of G. Shattuck, Jr.), 358

Shattuck, George Cheyne, Jr., 75, 76, 114, 135, 242, 342, 355: on dullness of Boston, 145; and Louis, 168, 185, 210, 358; on moral dangers of Paris, 57

Shrady, George F., 340

Shryock, Richard, 13, 67, 291

Sichel, Julius, 84, 102, 120, 123, 293

Sieveking, Edward Henry, 226

Simpson, James Y., 52–53, 119

skepticism, therapeutic: and conservative medicine, 288, 425n.182; critics of, 281, 283, 284–287, 343; and the healing power of nature, 281–289; and homeopathy, 284; and nihilism in Vienna, 303; proponents of, 281–282, 283, 287–290; as threat to physician's identity, 272–273, 281, 283–287. *See also* expectant method

skin diseases, 64, 136, 332; studied in Paris, 85, 86, 103, 316; studied in Vienna, 308

Skoda, Joseph, 297, 298, 303, 420n.94

Slade, Daniel, 294

Smith, Ashbel, 58, 76, 92, 111, 115, 143, 244, 249, 356

Smith, Barbara Leigh, 106

Smith, Dale, 14, 214

Smith, G. Roberts, 135, 145

Smith, Henry H., 65, 67, 260, 300, 343

Smith, James McCune, 48

Smith, Joseph Mather, 159, 422n.147

Société Médicale d'Observation, 86, 129, 213, 227, 391n.238

Society of Apothecaries (London), 193–194, 195, 198

southern medical separatism, 161, 180–182; and clinical instruction, 221

Spalding, Lyman, 37

specialism: and America, 292–294, 309–313, 332, 336–338, 339–340, 351–352; and experimental science, 346–347; and German medicine, 333–334; instruments and, 334, 336–337, 352; and Paris, 92, 292–294; as threatening, 351–352; and Vienna, 309–312

speculum, 103, 120, 121, 128, 138, 337

state, medicine and the: in America, 204–207, 210–212, 238, 251; in England, 71, 72, 251, 406n.47; in France, 35, 42, 71, 72, 93–94, 188, 189, 198, 205–207, 299, 315, 317

Sterne, Nicholas, 191, 194

## About the Author

JOHN HARLEY WARNER is Professor of the History of Medicine and Science and of American Studies at Yale University. He is the author of *The Therapeutic Perspective: Medical Practice, Knowledge, and Identity in America*, newly available in paperback through Princeton University Press.